THE JOURNAL OF

Pathology

A Journal of the Pathological Society of Great Britain and Ireland

1984 Volume 143

A WILEY MEDICAL PUBLICATION
JPTLAS 143(1–4) 1–331^A (1984)
ISSN 0022–3417

THE JOURNAL OF

Pathology

Published in association with the
Pathological Society of Great Britain and Ireland

Editor-in-Chief

Professor D. H. Wright
Department of Pathology, University of Southampton, South Laboratory/Pathology Block, Southampton General Hospital, Tremona Road, Southampton SO9 4XY, UK

Editors

Dr A. G. MacIver
Department of Pathology, University of Southampton, South Laboratory/Pathology Block, Southampton General Hospital, Tremona Road, Southampton SO9 4XY, UK

Professor F. Walker
Department of Pathology, University Medical Buildings, Foresterhill, Aberdeen AB9 2ZD, UK

Aims and Scope

The Journal of Pathology is a journal of the Pathological Society of Great Britain and Ireland. From January 1984, it will incorporate the other affiliated journal, *Diagnostic Histopathology*. The new group of Editors intend that the journal shall reflect the interests of the members of the Society. This will be no easy task since they cover the whole range of experimental and diagnostic histopathology.

High quality papers, written in English and dealing with descriptive histopathology will be welcome. Papers dealing with new techniques and those that elucidate the mechanisms underlying disease processes and histopathological appearance will be particularly encouraged. Single case reports will be accepted only when they are of exceptional interest with important new information and which contain a full, but concise, review of the literature. Good photo-micrographs are of particular value and interest to histopathologists and emphasis will be placed on the quality of the illustrations.

Original articles in the field of experimental pathology, relevant to human disease, will be welcome. Review articles dealing with general and experimental pathology, as well as diagnostic histopathology, will be solicited. Unsolicited reviews will also be accepted if they are clearly written and topical. Editorials, a letter column and reviews of recently published books will form regular features of the Journal. Meetings abstracts of the Pathological Society of Great Britain and Ireland will be published as they become available and the annual CL Oakley Lecture will continue to be included. Symposia proceedings may be published if the Editors consider them appropriate and relevant. The Editors wish to maintain the minimum delay between manuscript submission, decision and publication, and authors are therefore requested to follow the instructions for manuscript preparation as set out in the Notes for Contributors which are printed on the inside back cover.

JOURNAL OF PATHOLOGY, VOL. **143**: iv–vi (1984)

CONTENTS

Volume 143, Issue Nos 1–4, 1984

JOURNAL OF PATHOLOGY

Issue No. 1 MAY 1984

Editorial Policy i

Review Article
Oncogenes, J. PAUL 1

Original Articles
Post-mortem Prevalence of Lymphocytic Infiltration of the Lacrymal Gland: A Comparative Study in Autoimmune and Non-autoimmune Diseases, N. NASU, O. MATSUBARA AND H. YAMAMOTO 11

Cytoskeletal Control of Nuclear Arrangement in Langhans Multinucleate Giant Cells, P. J. RIGBY AND J. M. PAPADIMITRIOU 17

Histometrical Investigation of the Pulmonary Artery in Severe Hepatic Disease, O. MATSUBARA, T. NAKAMURA, T. UEHARA and T. KASUGA 31

The Histochemistry of Glycosidases in Human Benign and Malignant Breast Tissue, R. A. WALKER 39

On the Possible Origin of Extra-epithelial Enterochromaffin Cells by Budding from the Crypts of Lieberkuhn, P. D. MILLIKIN 51

Ultrastructural Localization of Anionic and Cationic Ferritin in the Rat Glomerular Basement Membrane in Protein-overload Proteinuria, D. J. BLISS AND D. B. BREWER 57

Synopses of Papers
Presented at the Joint Meeting of the Pathological Society of Great Britain and Ireland, the Dutch Pathological Society and the Norwegian Pathological Society A1

Issue No. 2 JUNE 1984

Review Article
Morphometric and Related Quantitative Techniques in the Study of Lymphoid Neoplasms. A Review, J. CROCKER 69

Original Articles
Pathological Aspects of Diffuse Nodular Hyperplasia of the Liver, K. WEINBREN AND S. S. MUTUM 81

Damage and Healing in the Conducting Tissue of the Heart (An Experimental Study in Dogs Infected with *Trypanosoma cruzi*), Z. A. ANDRADE, S. G. ANDRADE AND M. SADIGURSKY 93

The Subcellular Basis of Damage to the Human Urinary Bladder Induced by Irradiation, G. N. ANTONAKOPOULOS, R. M. HICKS and R. J. BERRY . . 103

Pathways of Cellular Efflux and Particulate Clearance After Carbon Instillation to the Lung, D. H. BOWDEN AND I. Y. R. ADAMSON 117

Sequential and Dose-dependent Alterations in Rat Bronchiolar Epithelium During *O,O,S*-Trimethyl Phosphorothioate Induced Delayed Toxicity, J. GANDY, T. R. FUKUTO AND T. IMAMURA 127

Book Reviews 139

Announcement 143

Issue No. 3 JULY 1984

Editorial
The Diagnosis of Malignant Mesothelioma, A. HERBERT 145

Review Article
Diagnosis of Pleural Malignant Mesothelioma in Life – A Practical Approach, D. WHITAKER AND K. B. SHILKIN 147

Original Articles
Hypertension, Cerebral Vascular Changes and Stroke in Ghana. 1 – Microaneurysm Formation and Stroke, J. T. ANIM AND A. D. KOFI 177

Age Related Detection of Tissue Amyloid P in the Skin, A. M. KHAN AND F. WALKER 183

The Routine Histopathological Investigation of Axillary Lymph Nodes for Metastatic Breast Cancer, F. HARTVEIT 187

Degradation of Basement Membrane Collagens by Metalloproteases Released by Human, Murine and Amphibian Tumours, S. E. SHIELDS, D. J. OGILVIE, R. G. MCKINNELL AND D. TARIN 193

Immunolocalization of Prealbumin as a Marker for Carcinoid Tumours, I. D. MILLER, W. A. REID, C. N. LIDDLE AND C. H. W. HORNE 199

Usefulness of Enzyme- and Immunohistochemistry in the Diagnosis of Juvenile Xanthogranuloma, C. DE WOLF-PEETERS, F. FACCHETTI, H. DEGREEF, J. J. VAN DEN OORD, A. VANNESTE AND V. J. DESMET 205

The Effects of Long-term Administration of Methyltestosterone on the Development of Liver Lesions in BALB/c Mice, W. TAYLOR, S. SNOWBALL AND M. LESNA 211

Book Reviews 219

Announcement 221

Issue No. 4 AUGUST 1984

Review Article

AIDS: Histopathological Aspects, P. R. MILLARD 223

Original Articles

The Immunocytochemical Detection of *Herpes simplex* Virus in Cervical Smears – A Valuable Technique for Routine Use, R. L. ADAMS, D. R. SPRINGALL, M. M. LEVENE AND T. E. C. BUSHELL 241

Yorkshire Regional Lymphoma Histopathology Panel: Analysis of Five Years' Experience, C. C. BIRD, I. LAUDER, H. S. KELLETT, I. CHORLTON, N. BARNES, C. DARWIN, R. A. CARTWRIGHT AND R. BOYKO 249

Immunostaining of Neuron-specific Enolase is a Valuable Aid to the Cytological Diagnosis of Neuroendocrine Tumours of the Lung, D. R. SPRINGALL, P. LACKIE, M. M. LEVENE, P. J. MARANGOS AND J. M. POLAK 259

Gastric Epithelial Cell Proliferation in Monkeys Fed 3,4,3′,4′-Tetrachlorobiphenyl, G. M. BECKER AND W. P. MCNULTY 267

The Monocyte/Macrophage Population of the Normal Human Kidney, R. J. MARSHALL AND A. G. MACIVER 275

Book Reviews 281

Announcements 287

Society Symposium Report

Regulatory Peptides 289

Synopses of Papers

Additional Synopses of Papers Presented at the Joint Meeting of the Pathological Society of Great Britain and Ireland, the Dutch Pathological Society and the Norwegian Pathological Society . . . . 291^A

Synopses of Papers Presented at the 149th Meeting of the Pathological Society of Great Britain and Ireland . . . . 293^A

JOURNAL OF PATHOLOGY, VOL. 143: 1–10 (1984)

ONCOGENES

JOHN PAUL

Beatson Institute for Cancer Research, Garscube Estate, Switchback Road, Bearsden, Glasgow G61 1BD, U.K.

Received 16 January 1984
Accepted 17 January 1984

KEY WORDS—Cancer, onogenesis, oncogenetic retroviruses.

INTRODUCTION

The idea of oncogenes was proposed by Huebner and Todaro[1] in 1969 in the context of tumorigenesis by tumour viruses. They proposed that viral genes could be integrated into the cellular genome where they might remain dormant or become 'activated', thus causing cancer. Although not absolutely correct in detail, this has proved to be a prophetic hypothesis.

The present model (Fig. 1), the evidence for which will be discussed, is as follows.[2–4] Eukaryotic cells contain certain genes (proto-oncogenes) concerned with the control (possibly cell-type specific) of growth and differentiation. Quantitative or qualitative anomalies of expression of these genes can give rise to malignant transformation. Anomalies may arise from the action of mutagens (carcinogens, radiations), viruses or random events on the genes themselves. Moreover, the gene sequences may be picked up by certain viruses (in which they occur as viral oncogenes) and transduced to other cells. Viruses which have acquired cellular sequences of this kind are recognized as oncogenic retroviruses.

ONCOGENIC RETROVIRUSES[5]

The background discoveries that led to this model arose mainly from the study of oncornaviruses, now usually called oncogenic retroviruses. In these viruses (Fig. 2) the genome is composed of RNA. It is present as two identical copies enclosed within a capsid which is itself enclosed within a glycoprotein envelope. On entry to a cell, the envelope and capsid are first removed (uncoating). The RNA is copied by the enzyme reverse transcriptase, also carried by the virus, into a DNA molecule, called a provirus, which becomes integrated into the cellular genome. The provirus is then treated as a cellular gene and transcribed by RNA polymerase into new RNA molecules identical with the original viral genome. These can have two different fates. Some act as messenger RNA molecules for the synthesis of new capsid and envelope proteins and viral reverse transcriptase. Others form the genomes for new viruses which assemble spontaneously from the different components. Finally the new virus particles bud off from the surface of the infected cells.

Two different classes of oncogenic retroviruses have been recognized. They are distinguished by their ability to induce tumours slowly or rapidly. The archetypic slow retrovirus contains only three genes, called Gag, Pol and Env. Gag (group specific antigen) genes carry the information for synthesis of capsid proteins; Pol (polymerase) genes carry information for reverse transcriptase (RNA dependent DNA polymerase); and Env (envelope) genes carry information for specific glycoproteins which form a component of the viral envelope, the rest of which is derived from cell membrane. Viruses which contain these three genes have all the components needed to proceed through the complete replicative cycle as described above. Typical examples are Avian Leukosis Virus (ALV), Murine Leukaemia Virus (MuLV) and Feline Leukaemia Virus (FeLV). They occur as natural wild-type viruses infecting populations of fowls, mice or cats in which they typically produce lymphomas or leukaemias. It is characteristic of these viruses that the incubation time of the disease is long, some months following inoculation.

0022–3417/84/050001–10$01.00

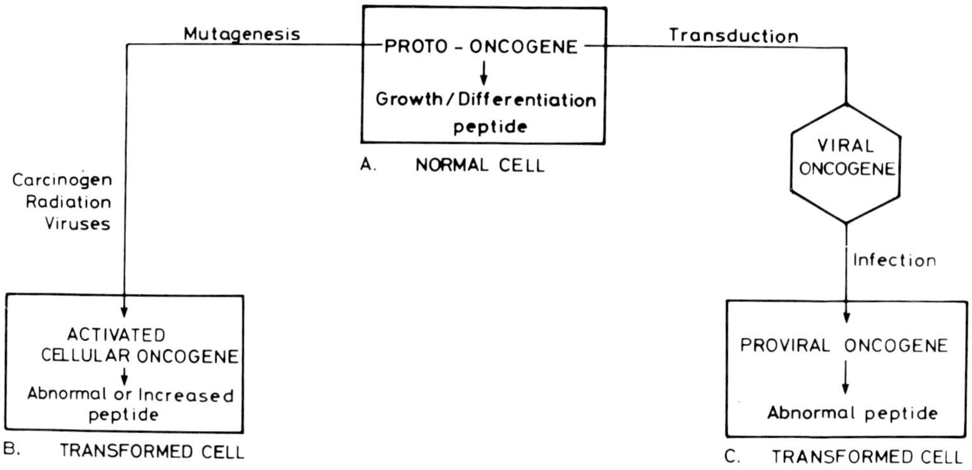

Fig. 1—A model to explain the possible role of oncogenes in carcinogenesis. See text for explanation

The second group, the rapidly transforming retroviruses, are closely related to the first but differ in important respects. They do not occur widely in wild populations but have nearly always been isolated from individual tumours. They do not readily infect animals by natural routes and have usually to be inoculated by injection. They produce tumours very rapidly, in days or weeks.

Only one rapidly transforming virus, the Rous Sarcoma Virus (RSV) is 'complete' (non-defective), all others being replication defective as described below. The Rous Sarcoma Virus contains four instead of three genes. Three of these are similar to the genes of ALV, the Gag, Pol and Env genes (Fig. 3). The fourth, called v-src, is particularly interesting because it can be shown that this gene is necessary and sufficient for the production of cellular transformation. The evidence for this statement is as follows (Fig. 4). RSV causes cellular transformation in cultured chick fibroblasts. The normal cells usually grow as sheets of fusiform cells orientated in parallel arrays. On infection with RSV this orderly appearance is lost. The cells round up and pile up on each other to form foci or colonies where individual infectious particles have entered cells. Fibroblastic transformation gives rise to cells which cause tumours when they are reinoculated into a chicken. Variants of RSV in which the v-src gene has been inactivated by deletion or mutation do not cause fibroblastic transformation. Moreover, temperature-sensitive mutants of the v-src gene have been produced and cells infected with the corresponding RSV show a transformed morphology at low (permissive) temperature but a normal morphology at a higher (non-permissive) temperature. Finally, by genetic engineering methods, it has proved possible to isolate the DNA corresponding to the v-src gene, to insert it into a bacterial plasmid and by this means to obtain quite large amounts of the pure gene as DNA. This by itself can be shown to transform fibroblasts (Fig. 4).

The v-src gene is now known to be one of the small family (about 20) of tranforming genes known together as viral oncogenes (v-oncs) each of which is typical of a particular acute transforming retrovirus. However, whereas v-src exists in RSV as an extra gene added to Gag, Pol and Env, all the other viral oncogenes are components of defective viruses in which part of the Gag, Pol and Env genes are deleted and replaced by the v-onc. Commonly, the Pol gene is completely absent from these viruses and also part of either the Gag gene or the Env gene. Typical genetic configurations of viruses of this kind are shown in Fig. 3. These viruses are 'defective'; they do not have the capacity to go through a replicative cycle by themselves but if cells are co-infected with them and a 'helper' virus such as ALV which provides the missing functions then they can be propagated and will produce tumours in infected animals. Individual viruses give rise to specific neoplasms, for example MuSV (Murine Sarcoma Virus) causes mainly sarcomas, AEV (Avian Erythroblastosis Virus) causes mainly erythroblastosis and so on. They are not completely specific for although the tumour most commonly produced is characteristic of each virus

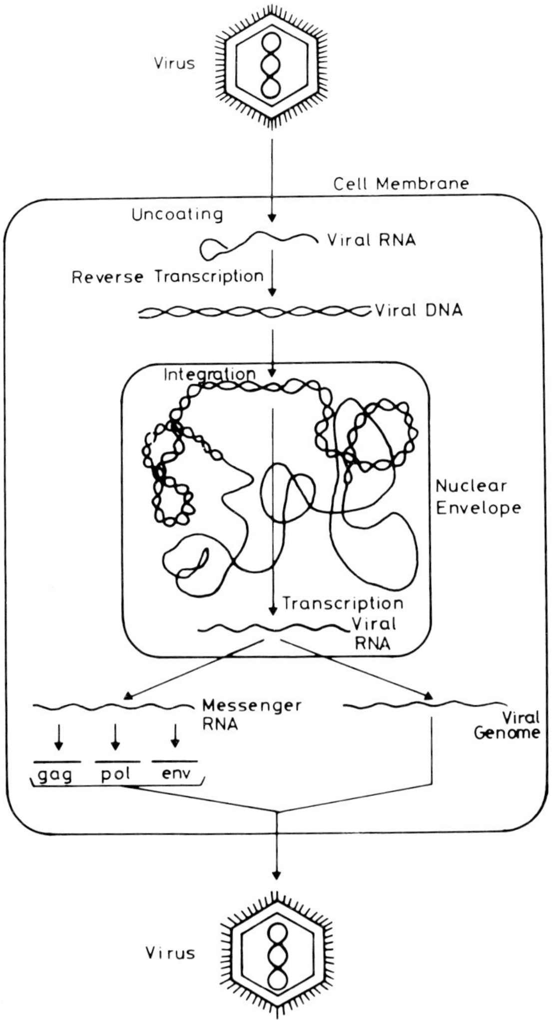

Fig. 2—A scheme summarizing the life cycle of a typical non-defective retrovirus. See text for explanation

and is directly correlated with the v-onc it contains, most will also give a low incidence of different tumours. Table I lists some known acute transforming retroviruses and their oncogenes.

A good deal has been learned about the protein products of v-oncs. Many of them, related to v-src, possess a particular enzymic activity, the ability to phosphorylate tyrosine in certain proteins. This tyrosine kinase is usually associated with the cell membrane and there are parallels with normal cellular functions. One of the most interesting of these relates to the receptor for epidermal growth factor which is apparently linked to a tyrosine kinase activity.

Among the oncogenes which code for tyrosine kinase activities are v-src, v-fps, v-fes, v-yes, v-abl and v-ros but not all oncogenes carry this kind of information and several quite different kinds of oncogene-related activities have so far been described.

PROTO-ONCOGENES

Current interest in cellular oncogenes (c-oncs) arose when it was found that DNA from normal tissues of all multicellular eukaryotes examined contains genes similar to v-oncs. This discovery[6] arose from the application of the technique of DNA hybridization and particularly a method known as Southern blotting.

DNA hybridization depends on the base-pairing relationship in double-stranded DNA. Adenine (A) in one DNA strand, always pairs with thymine (T) in the other strand and cytosine (C) in one strand with guanine (G) in the other. Consequently, the sequence of bases (such as CAGTACGCT) in one strand dictates the sequence of bases in the other strand (in this instance it would be GTCATGCGA according to the rules just stated). This relationship is very highly specific, almost exactly as specific as the relationship between a xerox copy of a page of a book and the original. Moreover, if DNA is heated the two strands separate and, if cooled, the complementary strands reassociate—but only if they are perfectly or nearly perfectly matched. It follows that a radioactively-labelled purified strand of DNA can be used as a tracer to recognize complementary sequences. If such a probe is added to a very complex mixture of DNA molecules and then put through the annealing procedure, radioactive double-stranded DNA will form only if a complementary (matching) strand is present in the mixture and there are techniques for identifying this.

Using DNA copied from v-onc RNA by reverse transcriptase as a probe, it became possible to determine whether DNA from normal animals contains matching sequences. This turns out to be the case and proves the existence of normal cellular sequences closely related to v-oncs which are referred to as proto-oncogenes.

The specially sensitive hybridization technique used to demonstrate these is known as the Southern blot. This exploits special endonucleases called restriction endonucleases which have the

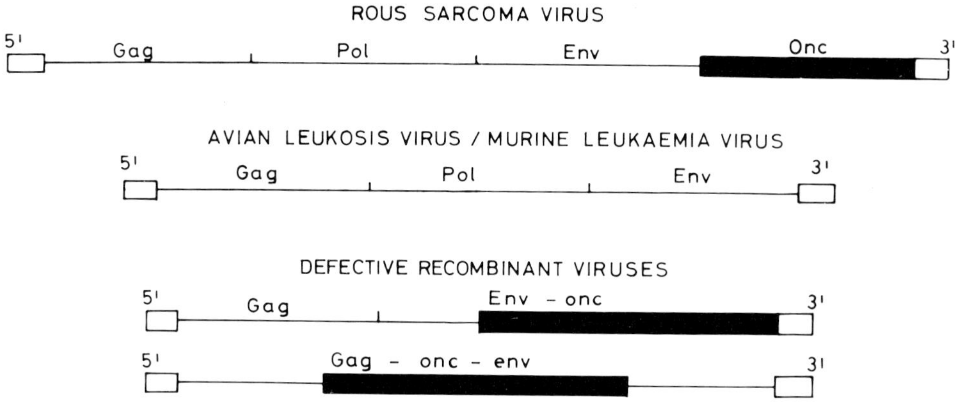

Fig. 3—Diagrams illustrating the arrangements of the genes in some retroviruses. The horizontal lines represent the RNA molecules which form the viral chromosomes. Filled in blocks represent viral oncogenes. Open blocks are special 5′ and 3′ sequences carrying transcriptional signals. The RNA is transcribed from the provirus (see text) from 5′ end to 3′ end

property of cleaving DNA molecules at unique sites defined by a sequence of bases (usually 4 or 6) which the enzyme can distinguish from other sequences. There are a large number of these restriction endonucleases and each one cleaves at a different site. A typical restriction enzyme, called EcoR1, cuts DNA wherever the sequence GAATTC occurs. This sequence occurs randomly in DNA but, on the average, roughly every 4000 base pairs. Consequently, if a piece of DNA is completely digested with the enzyme, it gives rise to many fragments varying from a few base pairs to many thousands of base pairs in length but averaging this size. A simple piece of DNA such as DNA from a bacteriophage 40 000–50 000 base pairs long may be cut into a small number of discrete pieces, roughly about 10. These can be separated into discrete fragments of specific size by electrophoresing them in an agarose gel. A more complex DNA preparation, such as that from human cells, also gives rise to fragments of unique size but with such complex material there may be more than 100 000 of them. Nevertheless, these can also be separated on a gel. The problem is that there are so many that they cannot readily be discriminated and if one simply looks at the distribution of all the DNA fragment they appear as a smear. The Southern technique solves this problem in an ingenious way. First, the DNA is transferred from the agarose to a sheet of cellulose acetate filter paper (this is the blotting component of the Southern blot technique). Unique fragments of DNA can then be identified by hybridizing a specific probe to this cellulose acetate sheet. For example, a probe for an oncogene may hybridize with only one of the 100 000 or so bands present on the paper. By the application of this method it has been shown that every single v-onc is related to sequences which occur in specific restriction fragments in every animal DNA tested, even in species as disparate as the human and Drosophila. These normal genes, related to v-oncs are called proto-oncogenes.

VIRAL ONCOGENES ARE DERIVED FROM NORMAL CELLULAR GENES

These are remarkable findings and their implications have had a profound impact on recent thinking about cancer. The first implication is that, since they are detected in DNA from a wide range of species the genes with which the v-onc DNAs hybridize must have been very rigorously conserved during evolution because the ability to hybridize depends on rather close similarity between the two DNAs used. The second implication is that either proto-oncogenes are derived from v-oncs or v-oncs are derived from proto-oncogenes. In view of the universal prevalence of these sequences in vertebrate DNAs it would seem much more likely that the v-oncs are derived from proto-oncogenes than the other way round. There is convincing independent evidence of this. By genetic engineering methods it is possible to clone individual genes from the genome

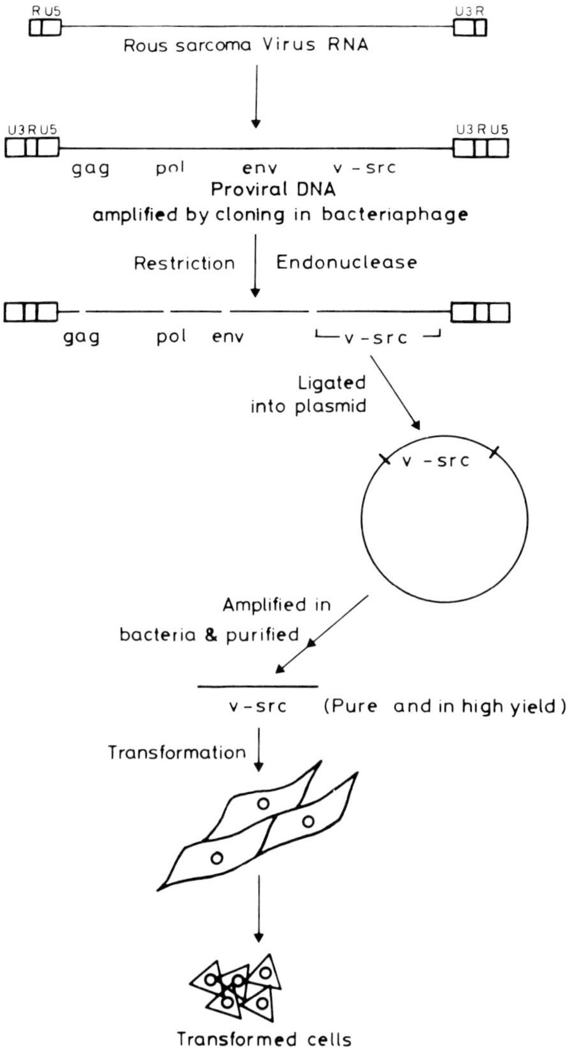

Fig. 4—Diagram of an experiment to test the function of v-src. The gene is isolated by genetic engineering methods which enable it to be purified in amounts which can be used to transform cells

of a vertebrate and in this way some of the proto-oncogenes from mice, humans and other species have been isolated, purified and analysed. It is these analyses which have provided revealing information about the nature of proto-oncogenes for not only are there striking resemblances between v-oncs and proto-oncogenes but there are also striking differences. In particular, in v-oncs the nucleotide sequences which code for a protein usually occur in one continuous block, a situation fairly typical of viruses. However, in proto-oncogene the information is split up, pieces of protein-coding sequences (exons) alternating with intervening sequences (IVS or introns). It is known that this is the typical structure of vertebrate genes.

The alternating exon-intron structure of a normal cellular gene is transcribed into a high molecular weight RNA molecule which is then 'processed' to remove the RNA corresponding to the introns to yield a cellular messenger RNA which is very similar indeed to the viral messenger RNA. These studies reveal, therefore, that proto-oncogenes have the structure of typical cellular genes and strongly suggest that the viral oncogenes arose by reverse transcription of a messenger RNA which was originally derived by processing of the transcript from a proto-oncogene.

Information about the kinds of proteins produced by v-oncs and their similarity to proto-oncogenes stimulated the speculation that the proteins coded by proto-oncogenes are in some way concerned with growth regulation. This idea has been very much strengthened by the recent finding that the v-sis gene codes for a protein very similar to a well-known growth factor, the Platelet Derived Growth Factor (PDGF).[7,8]

'ACTIVATED' CELLULAR ONCOGENES[9]

Since viral oncogenes have the ability to transform cells very rapidly, the question naturally arises—can cancer arise by inappropriate expression of the related proto-oncogenes? Much information has accumulated recently to show that inappropriate expression of these genes is, indeed, frequently associated with cancer and this will now be discussed.

The first evidence[10] arose from study of bursal lymphomatosis in chickens, a condition produced by infection with the Avian Leukosis Virus (ALV). It will be recollected that ALV does not contain an oncogene but that it can give rise to lymphomatosis after a long incubation period. When DNA from the lymphomas was analysed by the Southern blotting technique, it was discovered that restriction fragments in the avian genome which contained the ALV provirus also contained sequences which hybridized with a viral oncogene, v-myc. The startling implication was that in these particular tumours the ALV provirus must have integrated very near the proto-oncogene, c-myc, in

Table I—Viral oncogenes. Some are related, e.g. v-fps and v-fes appear to be the same oncogene from different species

Virus	Species of origin	v-onc	Type of tumour	Proto-oncogene
Rous sarcoma	Fowl	v-src	Sarcoma	Yes
Fujinama sarcoma	Fowl	v-fps	Sarcoma	Yes
Yamaguchi sarcoma	Fowl	v-yes	Sarcoma	Yes
Rochester-2 sarcoma	Fowl	v-ros	Sarcoma	Yes
Myelocytomatosis MC29	Fowl	v-myc	Carcinoma, sarcoma, leukaemia	Yes
Avian erythroblastosis	Fowl	v-erbB	Leukaemia, sarcoma	Yes
Myeloblastosis	Fowl	v-myb	Leukaemia	Yes
Avian SKV770	Fowl	v-ski		Yes
Reticulo-endotheliosis	Turkey	v-rel	Leukaemia	Yes
Moloney murine sarcoma	Mouse	v-mos	Sarcoma	Yes
Harvey murine sarcoma	Rat	v-H-ras	Sarcoma	Yes
Kirsten murine sarcoma	Rat	v-Ki-ras	Sarcoma	Yes
3611 murine sarcoma	Mouse	v-rab	Sarcoma	Yes
Abelson murine leukaemia	Mouse	v-abl	Leukaemia	Yes
FBJ murine osteosarcoma	Mouse	v-fos	Sarcoma	Yes
Feline sarcoma	Cat	v-fes	Sarcoma	Yes
Gardner–Pasheed feline sarcoma	Cat	v-fgr	Sarcoma	Yes
McDonough feline sarcoma	Cat	v-fms	Sarcoma	Yes
Simian sarcoma	Monkey	v-sis	Sarcoma	Yes

the cellular genome and this had somehow led to an alteration of the behaviour of the cell such that it became neoplastic. It was soon shown that at least part of this story was correct in that, in most lymphomas examined, ALV sequences were indeed integrated adjacent to the proto-oncogene, c-myc. Moreover, there was evidence that, in the infected cells, c-myc was expressed at a high level. This mechanism for the 'activation' of c-myc was further studied in the light of the structure of ALV.

The RNA genome of ALV, like all related retroviruses, has a short sequence (R) which is repeated at both end (see Fig. 4). At the 5′ end of the RNA the short repeat sequence is followed by a special unique sequence, U5, and at the 3′ end the short repeat is preceded by a unique sequence, called U3. When the RNA is transcribed into DNA and integrated into the host genome, the end sequences are duplicated in such a way that the proviral DNA sequences become flanked by identical sequences called long terminal repeats (LTR) at either end, consisting of the U3 sequence linked to an R sequence and followed by the U5 sequence. This long terminal repeat sequence with the U3RU5 structure has been found to have some extremely interesting properties. For one thing, it contains the promoter sequences from which transcription of RNA starts. (In the orientation shown in Fig. 4 the genes are usually transcribed from left—'upstream'—to right—'downstream'). It also contains a termination sequence where the RNA transcript stops. Besides these, it contains another kind of sequence called an enhancer which has the remarkable property of increasing the rate of expression of most DNA sequences within a few thousand base pairs in either direction.

In the first studies on bursal lymphomas, evidence was found that ALV sequences were inserted in front of the c-myc gene and this gave rise to the 'promoter insertion' model of carcinogenesis (Fig. 5). It was postulated that transcription could start not only at the 'upstream' LTR, giving rise to transcription of the viral genome, but also from the 'downstream' LTR, giving rise to a transcript which ran into the host genome and could account for transcription of the adjacent c-myc. This mechanism may indeed operate in certain cases but it soon turned out that it could not account for all because the LTR was active even when it was inserted downstream of the c-myc gene! It is now thought, therefore, that viral activation of a c-onc may only require proximity of an enhancer sequence such as that contained in the viral LTR.

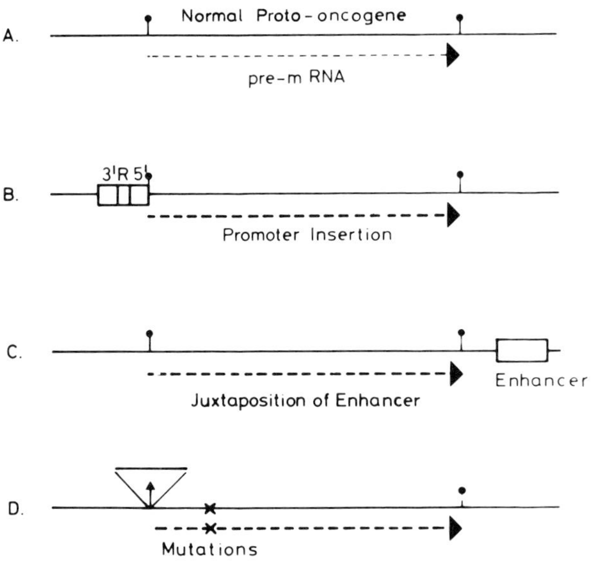

Fig. 5—Modes of activation of proto-oncogenes. (A) Represents a normal proto-oncogene with start and stop signals. The dotted line represents the transcript from it. (B) Represents a similar gene in which an LTR, usually associated with a proviral sequence, has been inserted in front of the gene causing an increased rate of transcription. (C) Illustrates another example of insertional mutagenesis in which an enhancer, usually associated with a retrovirus has been inserted near the gene. (D) Illustrates two possible mutations, one a deletion and the other a point mutation

TRANSFORMATION BY CELLULAR DNA

The next important observation was based on an assay for cell transformation using a special cell line called NIH 3T3. This cell line had been used for some years to study transformation by retroviruses and in the course of this work experiments were designed to investigate whether proviruses, i.e. integrated retrovirus sequences, could transform. These experiments involved taking DNA from transformed cells, and comparing the efficiency of this in transforming NIH 3T3 cells with DNA from untransformed cells. It was found that normal DNA cut into small fragments would not transform NIH 3T3 cells very effectively but DNA from transformed cells would do so.[11] The discovery was then made that DNA from many cell lines derived from tumours could also transform NIH 3T3 cells although they had not been treated with a virus. Some of the tumours which had this property included not only well-known experimental tumours in animals but also human spontaneous tumours.

These findings stimulated studies aimed at identifying the nature of the DNA which produced the transformation. By the application of genetic engineering methods the responsible genes were isolated and analysed. It was first discovered by Southern blotting that the transforming sequences in many cases were related to v-oncs, particularly to the v-oncs, Ki-ras and Ha-ras. These are closely related, the Ki-v-ras and Ha-v-ras being the oncogenes of viruses which produce sarcomas in rodents. When some of the transforming genes were isolated and the DNA sequences established, it became clear that they were not genes which had originated as v-oncs but were 'activated' c-oncs. The NIH 3T3 cell seems to be particularly sensitive to transformation by activated c-ras genes although it does also reveal the presence of some other transforming genes.

CHANGES ASSOCIATED WITH ACTIVATION OF c-oncs

The nature of the gene alteration which produces activation has obviously become a matter of intense study, particularly from two points of view. The first of these is: what is the normal function of the proto-oncogene? The second is: what alteration of the gene and of the gene product accounts for the cellular transformation?

Several different mechanisms have been uncovered which are associated with activation of proto-oncogenes (Fig. 5). Activation by an LTR has already been discussed and some very interesting experiments have been done in which a viral LTR has been chemically linked to Ha-c-ras. Whereas Ha-c-ras by itself will not normally transform NIH 3T3 cells, this complex will. However, it has to be mentioned that the efficiency of transformation with this combination is still considerably less than that of DNA containing Ha-v-ras and, moreover, most similar combinations between LTRs and other proto-oncogenes do not lead to cellular transformation. So this is not the whole story.

In some instances, amplification of proto-oncogenes, that is, an increase in the number of copies in the genome, has been correlated with transformation and in yet others point mutations would seem to be necessary and sufficient for oncogene activation. A particularly interesting case of the latter is a point mutation affecting the twelfth amino acid of the ras gene product, which results in activation of the Ha-c-ras gene. The same amino acid is altered in the product of Ha-v-ras and Ki-v-ras, although the rest of this peptide is very rigorously conserved.

CHROMOSOME TRANSLOCATION[12–14]

Perhaps the most interesting correlation has been found to be with certain chromosomal translocations. In Burkitt's lymphoma, chromosome 8 is very commonly involved in a reciprocal translocation with chromosome 2, chromosome 14 or chromosome 22 of which the 8 : 14 translocation is by far the commonest (Fig. 6). The myc proto-oncogene has been located on chromosome 8 near the point of translocation and chromosomes 2, 14 and 22 each are known to code for immunoglobulin chains, again in the region of the translocation. It has now been found that in many cases of Burkitt's lymphoma, this translocation involves the reorganization of the myc gene and indeed it has been found that frequently the immunoglobulin gene is fused (usually back-to-back) with the myc gene. Very recently immunoglobulin genes have been demonstrated to contain an enhancer element which acts over a considerable distance and it has, therefore, been postulated that this accounts for the activation of the myc gene

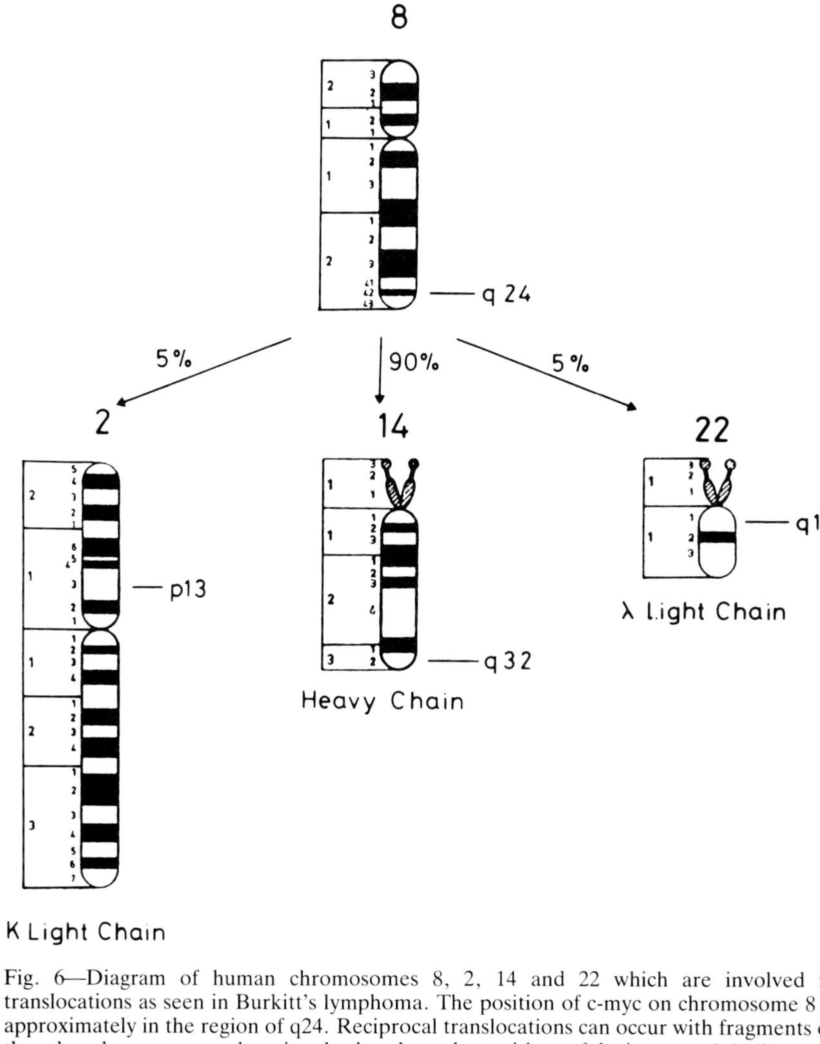

Fig. 6—Diagram of human chromosomes 8, 2, 14 and 22 which are involved in translocations as seen in Burkitt's lymphoma. The position of c-myc on chromosome 8 is approximately in the region of q24. Reciprocal translocations can occur with fragments of the other chromosomes: these involve breaks at the positions of the immunoglobulin genes shown

in this condition. However, it has to be mentioned that there are recent observations which conflict with this otherwise attractive hypothesis. Other chromosomal translocations have been shown to be regularly correlated with certain tumours and in many instances the translocation in one chromosome occurs in the region of a proto-oncogene.

HOW MANY EVENTS ARE NEEDED FOR TRANSFORMATION?

These and other observations have, therefore, led to the rather strong speculation that proto-oncogenes are genes concerned with cellular growth and that their activation by one of the means outlined gives rise to a partial relaxation of the control of growth of the cells in which the change has occurred. Many of the experimental findings still require to be pursued further to harden up the speculations and certain important questions remain outstanding. One of these relates to the number of events necessary to cause transformation of a normal cell to a malignant cell. In the natural evolution of human cancers there is evidence for a requirement for at least two and possibly several events. How then can this be reconciled with the observations on transformation of NIH 3T3 cells by a single event. Some experiments which have been done recently suggested that NIH 3T3 cells are unusual and that, indeed, more than one event is involved in transformation of normal cells. For example, although in the bursal lymphoma of chickens there is evidence for activation of the c-myc gene, this is not the gene which is identified when DNA from these cells is used to transform NIH 3T3 cells. Instead, a different transforming sequence, B-lym, has been isolated and purified. Moreover, in other instances involving malignancies arising from normal cells it has been claimed that a single activated oncogene may not be sufficient for transformation. Since the NIH 3T3 cell seems to be particularly sensitive to transformation by c-ras, the possibility has to be considered that it is already partly transformed.

The current feeling is that to transform normal cells at least two events are needed.[9] One is an alteration which 'immortalizes' cells, i.e. makes them capable of indefinite survival in culture although they are not capable of forming tumours in susceptible animals. If this is combined with a second transformation event which results in activation of a cellular oncogene then a transplantable tumour results. It is too early to say whether this is a scenario which applies to a significant number of 'spontaneous' naturally-occurring tumours and there are some experiments from this Institute which suggest it is an oversimplification but it provides a strong hypothesis for further investigations.

Not all questions about the molecular abnormalities in malignancy have therefore been answered by any means. Indeed we have a long way to go before we have anything like a complete understanding of the molecular nature of cancer but these findings have influenced our thinking dramatically and have provided both a theoretical framework and a wide range of experimental possibilities for further investigation. The field of cancer research has been altered for all time and there can be little doubt that within the next few years we will have a detailed understanding of at least some of the mechanisms concerned with the transformation of a normal cell to a malignant one.

ACKNOWLEDGEMENT

The Beatson Institute is supported by the Cancer Research Campaign.

REFERENCES

1. Huebner RJ, Todaro GJ. Oncogenes of RNA tumor viruses as determinants of cancer. *Proc Natl Acad Sci USA* 1969; **64:** 1087–1094.
2. Bishop JM. Cellular oncogenes and retroviruses. *Ann Rev Biochem* 1983; **52:** 301–354.
3. Bishop JM. Oncogenes. *Scientific American* 1982; **246:** 68–78.
4. Duesberg PH. Retroviral transforming genes in normal cells? *Nature* 1983; **304:** 219–226.
5. Weiss R, Teich N, Varmus HE, Coffin J. (Eds) RNA Tumor Viruses. Cold Spring Harbor, NY: Cold Spring Harbor, 1982.
6. Stehelin D, Varmus HE, Bishop JM, Vogt PK. DNA related to the transforming gene(s) of avian sarcoma viruses is present in normal avian DNA. *Nature* 1976; **260:** 170–173.
7. Doolittle RF, Hunkapiller MW, Hood Le, Devare SG, Robbins KC, Aaronson SA, Antoniades HN. Simian sarcoma virus onc gene, v-sis, is derived from the gene (or genes) encoding a platelet-derived growth factor. *Science* 1893; **221:** 275–277.

8. Waterfield MD, Scrace GT, Whittle N, Stroobant P, Johnsson A, Wasteson A, Westermark B, Heldin C-H, Huang JS, Deuel TF. Platelet-derived growth factor is structurally related to the putative transforming protein p28^{sis} of simian sarcoma virus. *Nature* 1983; **304:** 35–39.
9. Land H, Parada LF, Weinberg R.A. Cellular oncogenes and multistep carcinogenesis. *Science* 1983; **222:** 771–778.
10. Neel BG, Hayward WS, Robinson HL, Fang J, Astrin SM. Avian leukosis virus-induced tumors have common proviral integration sites and synthesize discrete new RNAs: oncogenesis by promoter insertion. *Cell* 1981; **23:** 323–324.
11. Shih C, Shilo B-Z, Goldfarb MP, Dannenberg A, Weinberg RA. Passage of phenotypes of chemically transformed cells via transfection of DNA and chromatin. *Proc Natl Acad Sci USA* 1979; **76:** 5714–1718.
12. Kirsch IR, Morton CC, Nakahara K, Leder P. Human immunoglobulin heavy chain genes map to a region of translocations in malignant B lymphocytes. *Science* 1982; **216:** 301–302.
13. Klein G. The role of gene dosage and genetic transpositions in carcinogenesis. *Nature* 1981; **294:** 313–318.
14. Lenoir GM, Preud'homme JL, Bernheim A, Berger R. Correlation between immunoglobulin light chain expression and variant translocation in Burkitt's lymphoma. *Nature* 1982; **298:** 474–476.

JOURNAL OF PATHOLOGY, VOL. **143:** 11–15 (1984)

POST-MORTEM PREVALENCE OF LYMPHOCYTIC INFILTRATION OF THE LACRYMAL GLAND: A COMPARATIVE STUDY IN AUTOIMMUNE AND NON-AUTOIMMUNE DISEASES

M. NASU, O. MATSUBARA AND H. YAMAMOTO

Department of Pathology, Tokyo Medical and Dental University, Tokyo, Japan

Received 4 October 1983
Accepted 21 October 1983

SUMMARY

The prevalence of focal lymphocytic infiltration of the lacrymal gland was investigated in 131 autopsy cases, 115 without and 16 with autoimmune diseases (nine cases of systemic lupus erythematosus, three of rheumatoid arthritis and four of Sjögren's syndrome). Focal lymphocytic infiltration was observed in 63·5 per cent of patients without autoimmune diseases and in all of those with autoimmune diseases. In those without autoimmune diseases, the frequency of lymphocytic infiltration was higher among those older than 40 years, and there was no sex difference in prevalence. The incidence of moderate or severe infiltration (grade III or IV) was 7·8 per cent in patients without autoimmune diseases; 55·6 per cent in systemic lupus erythematosus; 66·7 per cent in rheumatoid arthritis; and 100 per cent in Sjögren's syndrome. The present observation suggests that focal lymphocytic infiltration is indicative of an immunological disorder of the lacrymal gland in systemic lupus erythematosus and rheumatoid arthritis. Epimyoepithelial island formation was observed in only one patient with Sjögren's syndrome.

KEY WORDS—Lacrymal gland, lymphocytic infiltration, Sjögren's syndrome, autoimmune disease.

INTRODUCTION

Sjögren's syndrome is defined as consisting of keratoconjunctiva sicca, xerostomia and/or one of the connective tissue diseases. The pathohistology of the salivary gland in Sjögren's syndrome, connective tissue diseases and other diseases has been studied by many authors either using autopsy or biopsy materials.[1–6] However, there have been very few microscopic studies performed on the lacrymal gland.[7,8] This study is intended to report the prevalence of focal lymphocytic infiltration in the lacrymal glands taken from 131 autopsied patients, to examine the relationship between the grade of lymphocytic infiltration, sex, age and various coexisting diseases, and to study the significance of lymphocytic infiltration in the lacrymal gland.

0022–3417/84/050011–05$01.00

MATERIALS AND METHODS

Lacrymal glands (131), either left or right were taken at autopsy at Tokyo Medical and Dental University from 1978 to 1980. Of these, 115 patients had not been affected with autoimmune diseases, leukaemia, malignant lymphoma, or local tumour or infectious diseases of the orbit. There were 12 cases of autoimmune diseases: nine with systemic lupus erythematosus (SLE) and three with rheumatoid arthritis (RA). The diagnosis of these diseases was confirmed by clinical findings and autopsy examinations, but the diagnosis of Sjögren's syndrome was not made clinically. In addition, four patients with classical features of Sjögren's syndrome were examined. They consisted of two patients who had SLE coexisting, one patient with hepatic cirrhosis and one patient with meningoencephalitis. All the patients with autoimmune diseases had undergone long-term corticosteroid therapy. The lacrymal glands were fixed in 10 per cent neutral formalin and cut into pieces of about 10 × 10 × 3 mm in size. The sections were embedded in paraffin, serially cut in six micron-thick slices, and stained with haematoxylin and eosin. We examined 100 sections per case microscopically. We adopted a new grading standard for lymphocytic infiltration in the lacrymal glands (shown in Table I), based on Chisholm's[4] and Tarpley's[5] standards for the grading of the minor salivary glands.

The chi-square test was used to evaluate the relations among the degree of lymphocytic infiltration, sex, age and various diseases.

RESULTS

Histopathology of lacrymal glands

There was no basic difference in the lacrymal gland except the degree of lymphocytic infiltration. Mononuclear cells usually infiltrated in the periductal and/or perivascular regions of interlobular tissue (Figs 1 and 2) and then invaded the surrounding areas with acinar atrophy or destruction (Figs 3 and 4). The cellular population was mainly composed of small lymphocytes and a few plasma cells. Lymphocytes usually accumulated to make focal and folliculoid arrangements (Figs 1–3), and did not form germinal centres. Ductal cells showed moderate hyperplasia in several cases of SLE and Sjögren's syndrome (Fig. 5) and an epimyoepithelial island was recognized in one case of Sjögren's syndrome (Fig. 6).

Table I—Histological grading of lymphocytic infiltration in the lacrymal gland

Grade 0	No cellular infiltration
Grade I 'very slight'	One or two foci*
Grade II 'slight'	More than three foci (multiple) in all the sections
Grade III 'moderate'	Multiple foci or diffuse lymphocytic infiltration in all the sections with mildly destroyed tissue
Grade IV 'severe'	Multiple foci or diffuse lymphocytic infiltration in all sections with moderately or severely destroyed acinar tissue

* Each focus consists of an aggregate of 50 or more lymphocytes or plasma cells.

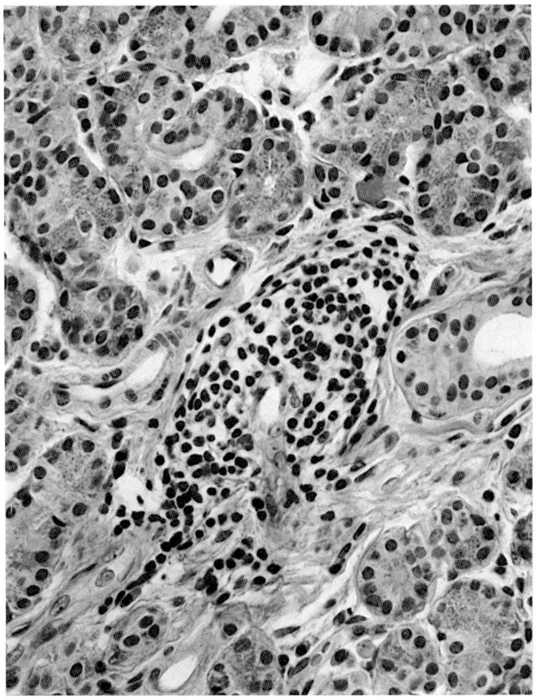

Fig. 1—A small lymphocytic focus in the perivascular area in patient with prostatic carcinoma (grade II). H & E, ×309

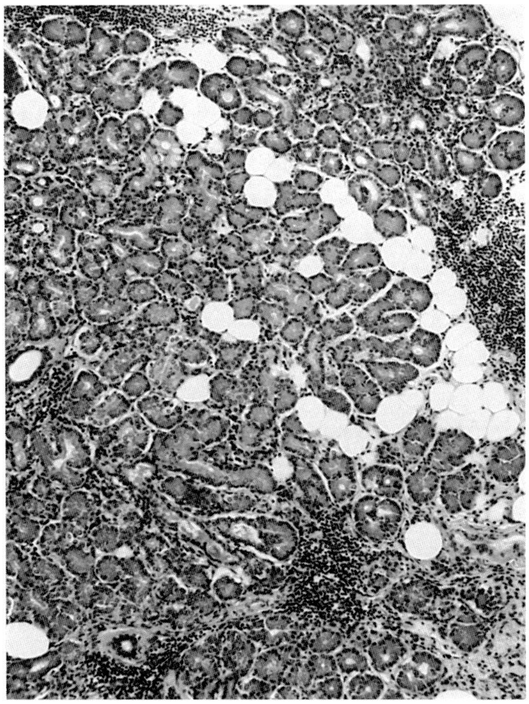

Fig. 2—Many lymphocytic foci in patient with SLE (grade III). H & E, ×69

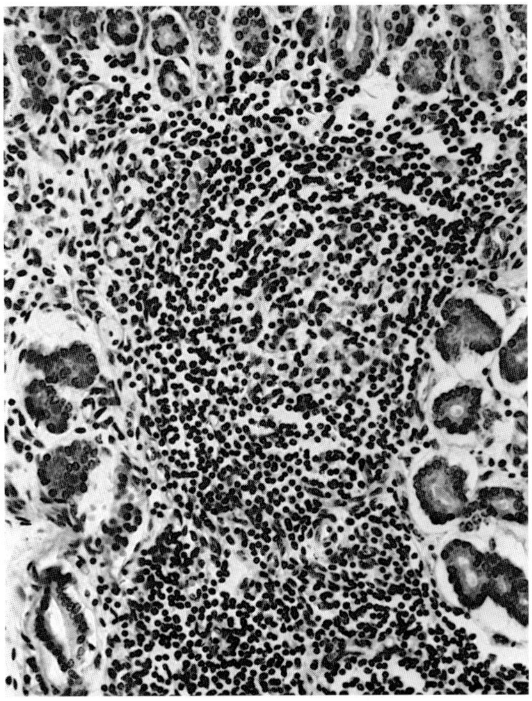

Fig. 3—A large lymphocytic focus with destroyed and atrophied acinar cells in patient with SLE (grade IV). H & E, ×196

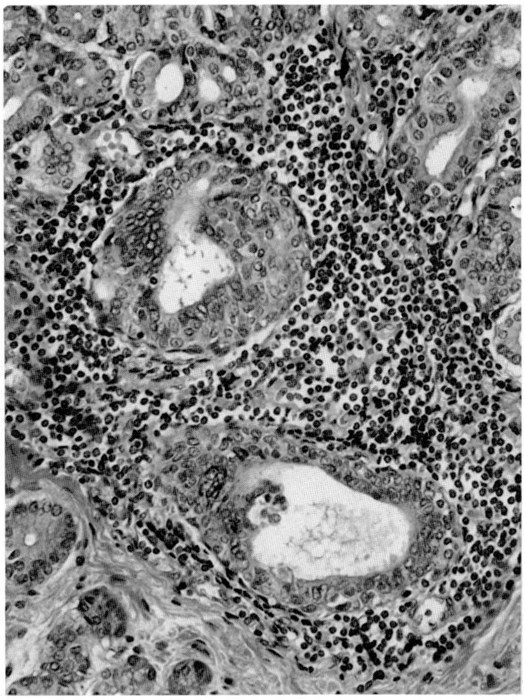

Fig. 5—Hyperplastic change of the ductal epithelium with lymphocytic infiltration in patient with SLE. H & E, ×207

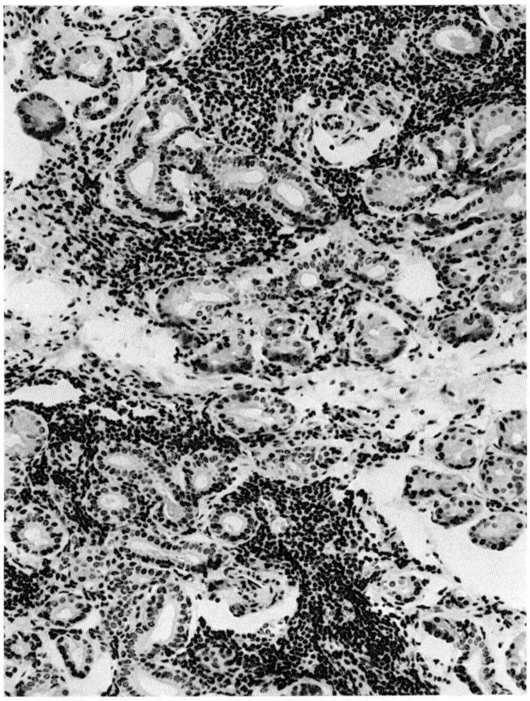

Fig. 4—Diffuse lymphocytic infiltration with destroyed acinar cells in patient with Sjögren's syndrome (grade IV). H & E, ×127

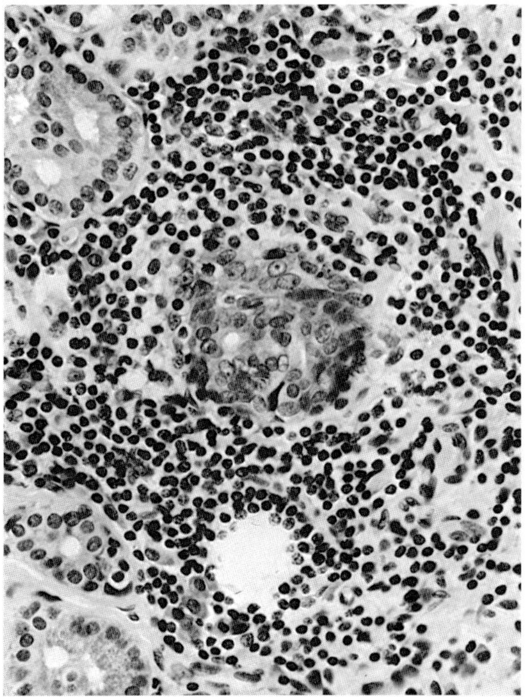

Fig. 6—Epimyoepithelial island with lymphocytic infiltration in patient with Sjögren's syndrome. H & E, ×299

Patients without autoimmune diseases

The relationship between the grade of lymphocytic infiltration, sex and age are shown in Table II. Lymphocytic infiltration was found in 63·9 per cent of the males and in 62·8 per cent of the females. There was no significant sex difference in the prevalence of positive glands. However, lymphocytic infiltration of grade III was seen in 11·6 per cent of the females and in 5·6 per cent of the males. Table II also shows that the prevalence of lymphocytic infiltration was low in younger groups and high in older groups. There was a significant difference between those who were older than 40 and those younger than 40 ($P<0·01$). The underlying diseases in nine cases of grade III consisted of benign nephrosclerosis, hepatic cirrhosis, pulmonary tuberculosis and neoplasms of the breast, brain, maxilla, submaxilla and pharynx. Focal lymphocytic infiltration of grade II or III were seen in all of the patients with hepatic cirrhosis (three cases) and prostatic carcinoma (three cases). A constant relationship between lymphocytic infiltration and underlying disease was not found. However, the frequency of lymphocytic infiltration in patients with cancer was less (36 of the 67 patients, 55·2 per cent) than in those without cancer (36 of the 48, 75 per cent) ($P<0·01$).

Autoimmune diseases

The age of the nine patients with SLE ranged from 22 to 54 years (mean, 34·9 years), while those with RA, from 28 to 76 years (mean, 50·3 years). The male to female ratio was 1:8 in SLE and 1:2 in RA. Lymphocytic infiltration was found in all cases. The glands from patients with SLE showed lymphocytic infiltration of grade IV in one case, of grade III in four, of grade II in three and of grade I in one. In patients with RA, lymphocytic infiltration of grade IV was found in one case, of grade III in one and of grade I in one. The prevalence of total positive glands (grades I–IV) in those with autoimmune diseases was significantly higher than in those without autoimmune diseases ($P<0·01$), and the frequency of grades III and IV combined was more significantly increased ($P<0·001$).

Sjögren's syndrome

The four patients were 35, 35, 45 and 49 years old, and were all females. The lymphocytic infiltration was grade IV in all of them. However, the parenchyma was better preserved than that of the submandibular glands in these patients.[6] Table III summarizes the prevalence of lymphocytic infiltration in various diseases.

Table II—Lymphocytic infiltration of lacrymal gland in non-immune diseases

Age in years	Male: Number with grade of severity 0	I	II	III	IV	Total	Per cent positive	Female: Number with grade of severity 0	I	II	III	IV	Total	Per cent positive
0–39	5	3	0	0	0	8	37·6	6	1	2	0	0	9	33·3
40–49	3	3	1	0	0	7	42·9	2	1	2	1	—	6	66·7
50–59	8	4	4	1	0	17	52·9	2	2	2	1	0	7	71·4
60–69	4	9	4	0	0	17	76·2	6	4	2	3	0	15	60·6
79–79	6	3	6	1	0	16	62·5	0	2	4	0	0	6	100·0
Over 80	0	2	3	2	0	7	100·0	—	—	—	—	0	—	—
Total	26	24	18	4	0	72	63·9	16	10	12	5	0	43	62·8

Table III—Lymphocytic infiltration of lacrymal gland in various diseases

Diseases	Number with grade of severity (per cent) 0	I	II	III	IV	Total	Per cent positive
Non-immune diseases	42 (36·6)	34 (39·6)	30 (30·1)	9 (7·8)	0	115	63·5
SLE	0	1 (11·1)	3 (33·3)	4 (44·4)	1 (11·1)	9	100
RA	0	1 (33·3)	0	1 (33·3)	1 (33·3)	3	100
Sjögren's syndrome	0	0	0	0	4 (100)	4	100

DISCUSSION

The incidence of lymphocytic infiltration was relatively high even in patients without autoimmune disease (male, 63·9 per cent and female, 62·9 per cent) and higher among those older than 40 years. This observation suggests that lymphocytic infiltration in the lacrymal gland can be explained by the ageing process. There was neither a sex difference in the prevalence of lymphocytic infiltration, nor a distinct relationship between lymphocytic infiltration and underlying diseases other than autoimmune diseases. However, the frequency of lymphocytic infiltration was lower in patients with cancer than those without. We are unsure of the reason for this difference, although the effect of oncostatic chemotherapy might be significant. Interestingly, all the three patients with prostatic carcinoma had lymphocytic infiltration, which may be a reflection of female hormone therapy. The action of sex hormones on autoimmunity has been pointed out.[9,10]

In the patients with SLE and RA, focal lymphocytic infiltration of the lacrymal glands was very common, being observed in all the glands examined and was of high grade. Alarcon-Segovia *et al.*[11] indicated that clinical or subclinical evidence of Sjögren's syndrome is found in almost all patients with SLE. Furthermore, the coexistence of RA and Sjögren's syndrome has been reported by many authors.[2,12,13] In the authors' observation of submandibular glands,[6] focal lymphocytic infiltration was found in all 26 patients with collagen diseases, who had showed no clinical signs of Sjögren's syndrome. Lymphocytic infiltration was frequently present and was of severe degree in the submandibular and/or lacrymal glands of the patients affected by collagen diseases who had no clinical signs of Sjögren's syndrome. These findings suggest that these secretory glands show focal immunologic lesions in collagen diseases.

The histologic features were essentially the same regardless of whether or not the patients had autoimmune diseases, including Sjögren's syndrome. A difference in the grade of lymphocytic infiltration can be recognized however. Cellular infiltration seems to occur mostly in periductal and perivascular regions and extend into the interacinar areas; the cells are mainly composed of small lymphocytes and a few plasma cells. Epimyoepithelial islands, which were occasionally present in the submandibular glands of those with collagen diseases or Sjögren's syndrome,[6] were seen in the lacrymal gland of only one patient with Sjögren's syndrome. Whether or not lymphocytic infiltration has the same role in Sjögren's syndrome and other collagen diseases, has not been clarified but the similar microscopic feature among these lesions suggests same common aetiologic factor in pathogenesis.

REFERENCES

1. Morgan WS, Castleman B. A clinicopathologic study of Mikulicz's disease. *Am J Pathol* 1958; **29:** 471.
2. Bloch KJ, Buchanan WW, Wohl MJ, Bunin JJ. Sjögren's syndrome. A clinical, pathological and serological study of sixty-two cases. *Medicine (Baltimore)* 1965; **44:** 187.
3. Waterhouse JP, Doniach I. Post-mortem prevalence of focal lymphocytic adenitis of the submandibular gland. *J Pathol Bacteriol* 1966; **91:** 53.
4. Chisholm DM, Mason DK. Labial salivary gland biopsy in Sjögren's syndrome. *J Clin Pathol* 1969; **21:** 656.
5. Tarpley TM, Anderson LG, White CL. Minor salivary gland involvement in Sjögren's syndrome. *Oral Surg* 1974; **37:** 64.
6. Nasu M. Histological observation of the submandibular gland with special reference to the focal lymphocytic infiltration. *Bull Tokyo Med Dent Univ* 1982; **29:** 139.
7. Waterhouse JP. Focal adenitis in salivary and lacrymal glands. *Proc Roy Soc Med* 1963; **56:** 25.
8. Williamson J, Gibson AAM, Wilson T, Forrester JV, Whaley K, Dick WC. Histology of the lacrymal gland in keratoconjunctivitis sicca. *Brit J Ophthal* 1973; **57:** 852.
9. Malez KA, Reeves JP, Sterinberg AD. Regulation of the expression of autoimmunity in NZBxNZWF$_1$ mice by sex hormones. *J Immunopharmacol* 1978–1979; **1:** 27.
10. Talal N. Systemic lupus erythematosus, autoimmunity, sex and inheritance. *New Eng. J Med* 1978; **301:** 838.
11. Alarcon-Segovia D, Ibanet G, Velazquez-Ferero F, Hermandez-Ortiz J, Gonzalez-Jimenez Y. Sjögren's syndrome in systemic lupus erythematosus. *Ann Inter Med* 1978; **81:** 577.
12. Shearn MA. Sjögren's Syndrome. Philadelphia: W. B. Saunders, Co., 1971: 110.
13. Bencz G, Lokatos L. Relationship of systemic lupus erythematosus to rheumatoid arthritis, discoid erythematosus and Sjögren's syndrome. *Ann Rheumat Dist* 1963; **22:** 273.

JOURNAL OF PATHOLOGY, VOL. **143**: 17–29 (1984)

CYTOSKELETAL CONTROL OF NUCLEAR ARRANGEMENT IN LANGHANS MULTINUCLEATE GIANT CELLS

P. J. RIGBY AND J. M. PAPADIMITRIOU

Department of Pathology, University of Western Australia, Queen Elizabeth II Medical Centre, Nedlands, Western Australia 6009, Australia

Received 8 June 1983
Accepted 28 November 1983

SUMMARY

Examination of the role of the cytoskeleton in macrophage polykarya (multinucleate giant cells) has established that microfilaments and microtubules are interrelated and contractile cytoskeletal components with opposing actions; when critically maintained at equilibrium, they are responsible for maintenance of the highly organized cellular architecture characteristic of Langhans type syncytia. Disruption of the function of these structures by *in vitro* incubation with cytochalasin B and/or colchicine can result in reversion to a cytoarchitecture which is more typical of the 'foreign body' multinucleate giant cell. These observations strongly reinforce previous suggestions that Langhans multinucleate giant cells are special, more highly organized forms than are 'foreign body' multinucleate giant cells.

KEY WORDS—Giant cells, Langhans giant cells, cytoskeleton, microfilaments, microtubules.

INTRODUCTION

In many inflammatory reactions, mononuclear phagocytes fuse to form multinucleate giant cells:[1–3] the factors responsible for their formation and their role in inflamed tissue are unclear. Nuclei of some multinucleate cells assemble into a semicircular arrangement surrounding a common cytocentrum. This arrangement is typical of the Langhans type multinucleate giant cell and distinguishes it from the 'foreign body' type in which the nuclei are apparently randomly aggregated in the central zone of the syncytium.

Several reports and reviews have documented the properties of multinucleate giant cells.[4–6] These syncytia have been shown to be both motile and contractile, with characteristic cellular movements depending on their size.[7,8] A well-developed cytoskeletal system of cytoplasmic filaments and microtubules has been suggested as being implicated in the organellar organization which distinguishes Langhans from 'foreign body' multinucleate giant cells.[6,9,10]

The location, arrangement and anchoring of nuclei in mononuclear cells has been attributed to various components of the cytoskeletal system, especially the microfilamentous networks.[11] Intermediate filaments have similarly been assigned a skeletal and organizing role in nuclear positioning,[12] while nuclear migration has been attributed to the action of both microtubules and microfilaments.[13–15] Although there is much evidence (for review, see Weatherbee[16]) to suggest that microfilaments and microtubules are involved in such motile processes, there is a lack of direct evidence for a cause and effect relationship.[16,17]

It is generally agreed that, *in vivo,* cytochalasin B affects the organization of actin microfilaments which are thought responsible for cell motility,[18] although its exact mode of action is unclear.

0022–3417/84/050017–13$01.30

Molecular studies indicate that it blocks addition of further G-actin monomers to F-actin filaments,[19,20] although it may also arrest direct filament interactions and/or reduce the length of F-actin filaments.[18] These effects would be expected, *in vivo,* to seriously weaken the bulk polymer strength of the network and affect its ability to propagate long-range forces.

Microtubule polymerization, *in vitro,* and under steady state conditions, occurs by net tubulin addition at one end of the polymer, with net tubulin loss at the other end. It has been suggested that this *in vitro* flux of tubulin from one end of the microtubule to the other could represent an *in vivo* molecular 'treadmill' with the potential for doing work.[21] Colchicine is known to interfere with microtubule function in cells, where it has been shown to bind specifically to the 6S tubulin dimer, followed by binding of the colchicine–tubulin complex to the growing end of microtubules, effectively blocking the addition of further tubulin subunits.[21] This results in a net tubulin loss from the polymer and a gradual loss of microtubular structures from within the cell.

The cooperative action of both microfilaments and microtubules in producing and controlling cell movement was the basis of a model formulated by Cheung *et al.*[22] to explain the effects of cytochalasin B and colchicine on macrophage adhesion, spreading and movement. Their model proposed that radially-arranged microtubules and microfilament bundles interacted with each other and controlled cytocortical submembranous microfilament bundles by suppressing and keeping their contractility to a minimum. Regional disruption or breakdown of the radial filamentous structures could result in increased cytocortical microfilament contractility and enhanced movement and membrane ruffling.

Previous studies on the involvement of cytoskeletal systems in movement and orientation of nuclei in multinucleate cells have concentrated on the repositioning and organization of nuclei following fusion of mononuclear cells into pre-existing syncytia.[2,6,10,23–26] These studies establish that the undisturbed coordination of microfilaments, microtubules and centrioles in macrophages and multinucleate giant cells is a necessary prerequisite for fusion, intracellular movements, and regrouping of nuclei. Our report further examines the cytoskeleton of the 'foreign body' and Langhans multinucleate giant cells, and specifically attempts to investigate and elucidate the roles played by microfilaments and microtubules in maintenance of the Langhans multinucleate giant cell morphology.

MATERIALS AND METHODS

Animals

Adult male mice of the C57BL/6J strain were used.

Multinucleate giant cells

These were collected by the subcutaneous implantation of single, 10 mm diameter, sterile glass coverslips in the dorsum of mice under ether anaesthesia. After 4–12 days, mice were killed by cervical dislocation and coverslips were removed, washed briefly in phosphate buffered saline, pH 7·3, and treated as required. These techniques have been previously documented.[27]

Light microscopy

Coverslips were incubated for varying periods in 35 mm Petri dishes containing 5 ml of tissue culture medium composed of HEPES and bicarbonate buffered minimal essential medium, pH 7·3 (Gibco, New York, U.S.A) supplemented with 10 per cent fetal calf serum (Commonwealth Serum Laboratories, Australia), penicillin (250 units/ml) (Crystapen, Glaxo, Australia) and streptomycin sulphate (250 μg/ml) (Glaxo, Australia). All cultures were maintained at 37°C in a humidified atmosphere of 5 per cent carbon dioxide in air. When required, coverslips were removed from the medium and fixed immediately in methanol at 22°C for 10 min, stained with Leishman's stain, mounted and blind coded. Entire coverslips were scanned at ×400 magnification and the number of nuclei in individual multinucleate giant cells was recorded. These syncytia were scored as either foreign body type (with dispersed or randomly organized nuclei) or Langhans type (with concentrically or crescentically arranged nuclei and a clearly defined, eosinophilic cytocentrum) (see Lewis[28] and Mariano and Spector[22]). Binucleate and trinucleate giant cells, which commonly have ill-defined nuclear arrangement patterns and/or poorly-defined cytocentra, were not scored. Results from multiple experiments are represented as the mean±standard deviation. Multinucleate cells were photographed on a Leitz Ortholux II microscope (Leitz Wetzlar, West Germany) with either ×40 or ×63 objectives, on Ilford Pan F (Ilford, England) 35 mm, black and white negative film.

Scanning electron microscopy

Coverslips, after 4 h culture, were fixed immediately at 22°C in 2·5 per cent glutaraldehyde in 0·1 M cacodylate buffer, pH 7·4, 330 mOsm. Following post-fixation in 1·0 per cent osmium tetroxide, cells were dehydrated through graded solutions of ethanol and critical point dried from liquid carbon dioxide in a Polaron critical point drying apparatus. They were coated with platinum to a thickness of 20 nm in a Polaron E5100 sputter coater, and examined in a Philips PSEM 500 scanning electron microscope at 70° tilt, using a modified specimen holder. Ilford FP4 (Ilford, England) black and white negative film was used to record the photographic images. Stereopair photomicrographs were taken at +6° and −6° to the horizontal, and the height of all cells in the field was measured using the technique described by Kristensen and Papadimitriou.[29] The Student's *t*-test was used to estimate the levels of confidence between different treatments.

Drug treatments

Cytochalasin B (Sigma, U.S.A.) and colchicine (Sigma, U.S.A.) were made up as 100 μg/ml stock solutions in culture medium, and added to the cultures to give final concentrations ranging from 0·5 to 10·0 μg/ml. Control samples were run concurrently with all drug treatments.

RESULTS

Light microscopy

Untreated cells—Coverslips, which were not cultured *in vitro,* but fixed immediately after removal from the animal, showed large numbers of firmly adherent mononuclear and multinucleate cells. The number and size of the multinucleate giant cell population (which consisted of both 'foreign body' and Langhans type syncytia) varied with the time the coverslip had been implanted in

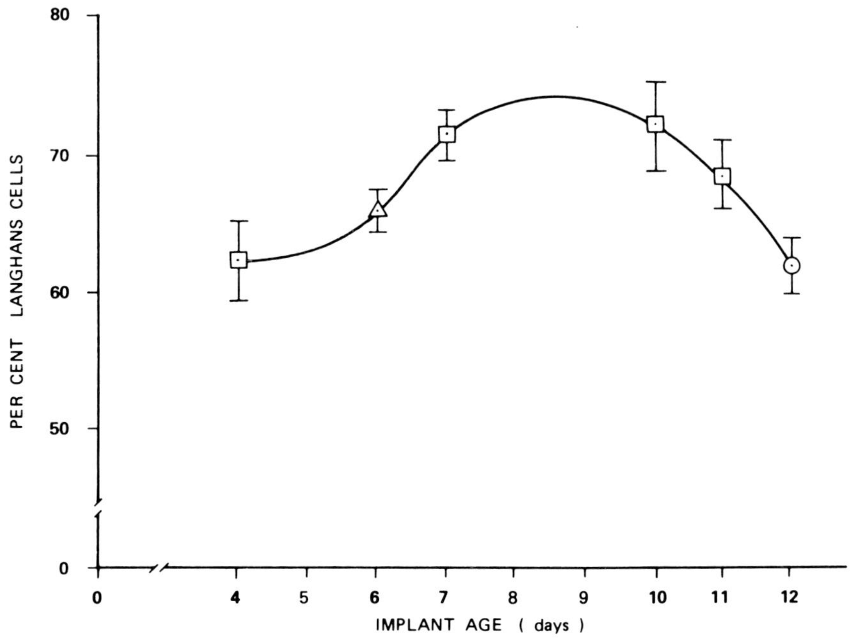

Fig. 1—The influence of the duration of coverslip implantation on the proportion of multinucleate syncytia demonstrating Langhans cytoarchitecture. The total number of multinucleate giant cells scored at each point is given by: □ = 100–500 cells; ○ = 501–1200 cells; △ = 1201–1500 cells. Each point = mean ± standard deviation

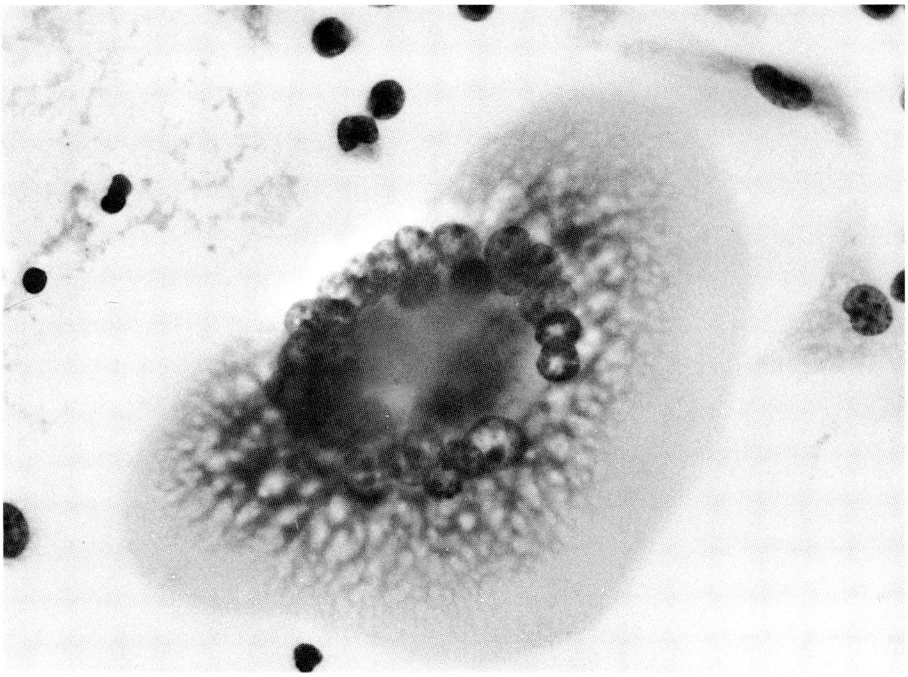

Fig. 2—Light micrograph of a typical Langhans multinucleate giant cell from an *in vitro* control culture. Leishman's stain, ×620

the animal. Four days after implantation, cells on the coverslips were predominantly macrophages with many small (3–4 nuclei) multinucleate cells. Six days after implantation the number and size of the syncytia had greatly increased, while very large (greater than 50 nuclei) multinucleate cells were not seen until 10–14 days after implantation.

Control cells—The proportion of Langhans type multinucleate giant cells in the syncytial population on explanted coverslips which were incubated *in vitro* for 4 h, was found to vary with the age of the implant (Fig. 1). Langhans multinucleate giant cells (Fig. 2) formed 62·3±2·9 per cent of the syncytial population scored at 4 days, and this proportion increased steadily with time to 71·5±2·0 per cent at 7 days. From 72·2±3·6 per cent at 10 days, the proportion of Langhans multinucleate giant cells decreased (62·0±2·0 per cent by day 12) and this drop corresponded with an increased proportion of syncytia containing more than 50 nuclei.

Cytochalasin B and colchicine treatments—The *in vitro* effects of cytochalasin B and colchicine on nuclear arrangement of Langhans type multinucleate giant cells were tested using 6 day coverslip implants. The effects of varying drug concentration and length of time of exposure to the two drugs in tissue culture conditions were also examined.

A shift in the proportion of multinucleate giant cells displaying the Langhans syncytial semilunar or circular array of nuclei was observed when coverslip implants were incubated with cytochalasin B. Following this treatment, an increased proportion of multinucleate giant cells displayed nuclei either dispersed throughout the cytoplasm or tightly clumped in central aggregations (Fig. 3). Such a nuclear arrangement is more typical of the 'foreign body' type multinucleate giant cell. A similar decrease in the ratio of Langhans to 'foreign body' syncytia occurred when cells were incubated with colchicine (Fig. 4). Analysis of the mean number of nuclei in both Langhans and 'foreign body' type multinucleate giant cells indicated that, on 6 day implants, cytochalasin B and colchicine affected equally both large (containing more than seven nuclei) and small multinucleate cells.

Effect of drug concentration and drug combination

The concentration of cytochalasin B and colchi-

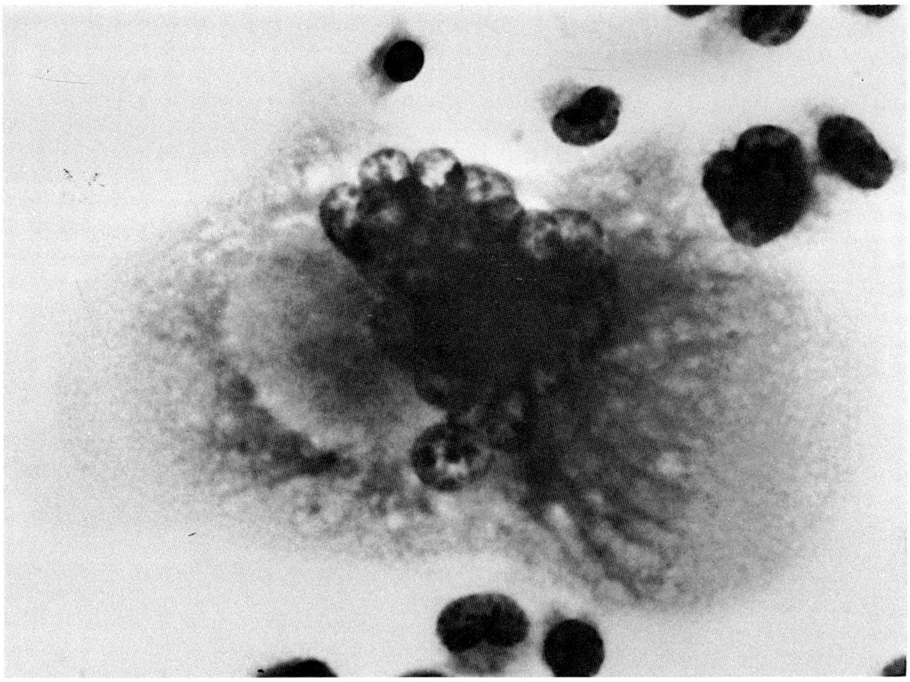

Fig. 3—A multinucleate syncytium following culture in medium containing cytochalasin B ($4 \mu g/ml$). The nuclei are tightly clumped in a central aggregation, which was observed to lie in a focal plane above the base of the cell. Leishman's stain, ×1000

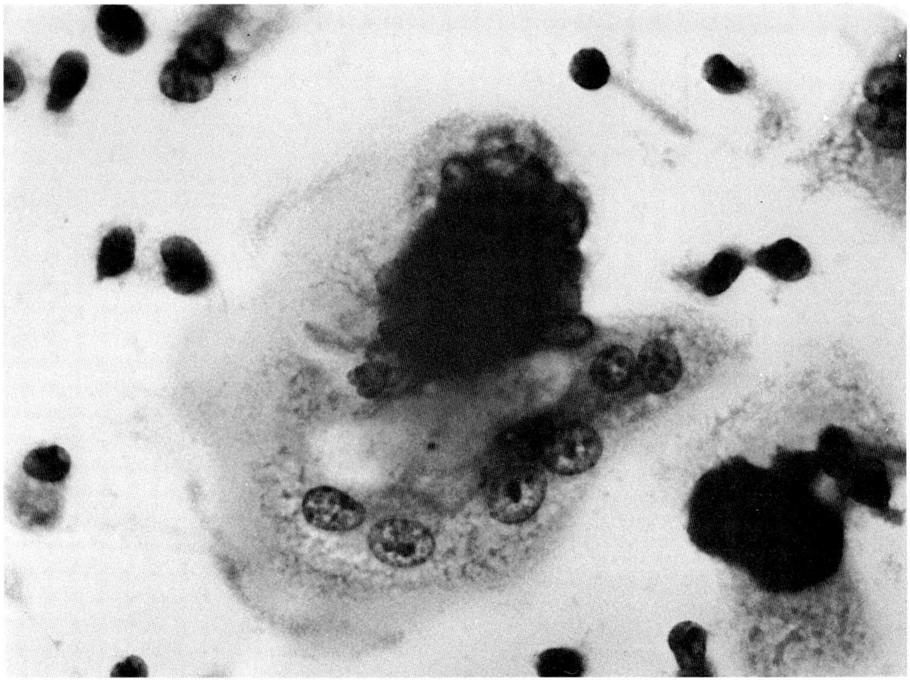

Fig. 4—Nuclear clumping in a multinucleate giant cell cultured in medium containing colchicine ($4 \mu g/ml$). Leishman's stain, ×620

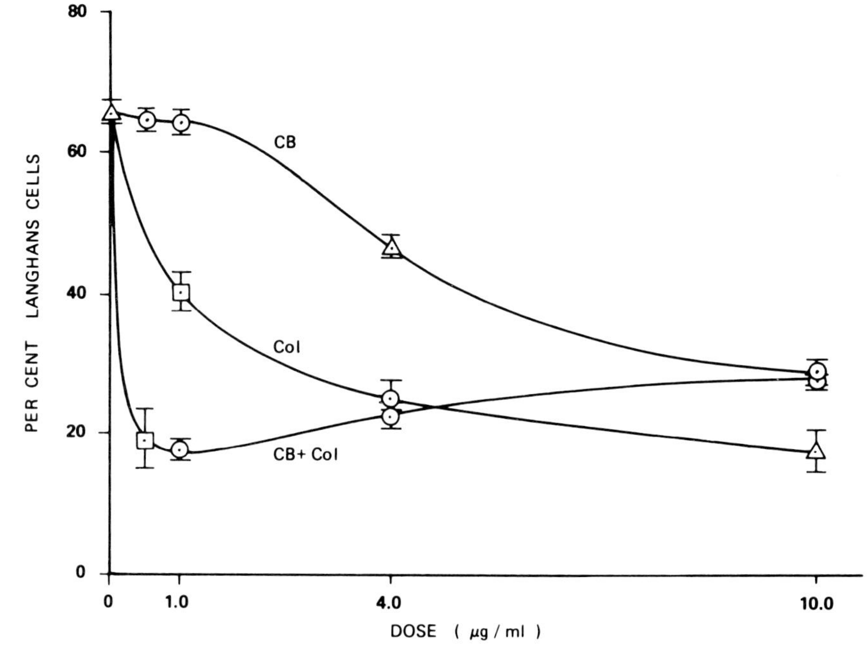

Fig. 5—Graph illustrating changes in the proportion of Langhans syncytia observed on coverslips cultured for 4 h in medium containing varying concentrations of cytochalasin B (CB), colchicine (Col), and cytochalasin B and colchicine combined (CB+Col). See Fig. 1 for symbol legend

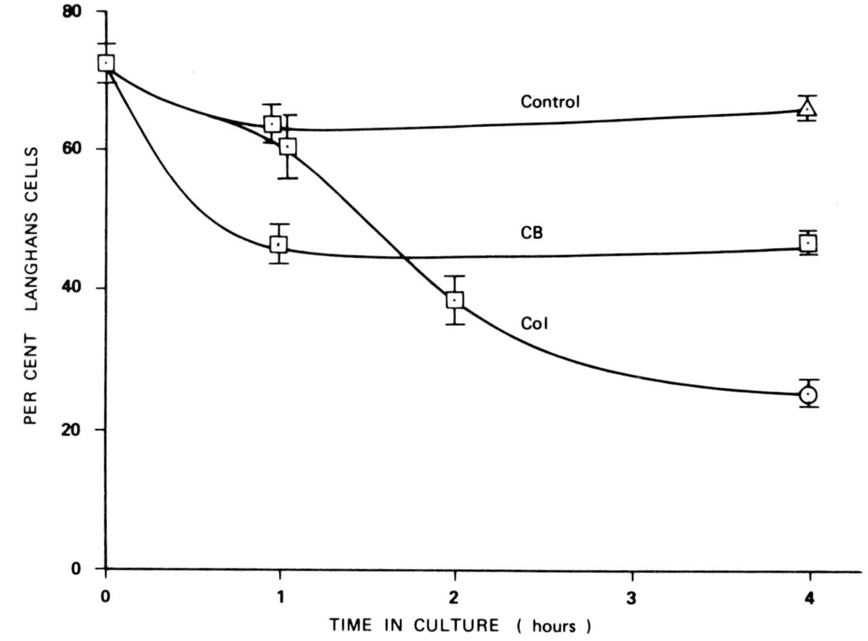

Fig. 6—The duration of *in vitro* culture in media containing 4 μg/ml cytochalasin B (CB) or 4 μg/ml colchicine (Col) influences the percentage of Langhans syncytia seen on coverslip implants. See Fig. 1 for symbol legend

cine in the culture medium influenced the number of multinucleate giant cells which were of the Langhans type on the coverslips (Fig. 5). Cytochalasin B concentrations below 1·0 μg/ml had little effect on the structure of the syncytial population, while low concentrations (1·0 μg/ml) of colchicine, on the other hand, produced disruption of the nuclear organization in more than one-third of the Langhans cells. Higher concentrations (up to 10 μg/ml) of both cytochalasin B and of colchicine further decreased the number of polykarya having Langhans type morphological features. When cytochalasin B and colchicine were combined (1·0 μg/ml of each), 17·7±2·9 per cent of multinucleate giant cells on coverslips had Langhans architecture. Increasing concentrations of combinations of these two drugs, however, resulted in less pronounced effects on the multinucleate cell population and, at 10 μg/ml of each, 28·5±1·9 per cent of the syncytial population consisted of Langhans cells. This figure closely resembled that obtained when cytochalasin B only was used at that concentration.

Effect of incubation time

Incubation in culture medium containing cytochalasin B (4 μg/ml) for 4 h reduced the number of Langhans cells on the explanted coverslips to 46·6±1.3 per cent of the total multinucleate giant cell population, with this reduction occurring mainly in the first hour (Fig. 6). However, culture in medium containing colchicine (4 μg/ml) produced almost no alteration in the percentage of Langhans cells in the syncytial population during the first hour, although incubation for a further 3 h resulted in a decrease in number of Langhans multinucleate giant cells at an approximately constant rate (Fig. 6).

Scanning electron microscopy

Control cells—Scanning electron microscopy of giant cells (presumed to be multinucleate if their diameter exceeded 30 μm) from 6 day implants showed that the syncytia possessed a central, slightly elevated, mass surrounded by a broad, thin peripheral zone, which, in some cells, was divided into a number of distinct and separate lamellipodia. The cell surface overlying the central mass of the syncytium possessed irregular contours and complicated patterns of ridge-like folds and densely packed flaps which varied in width, length

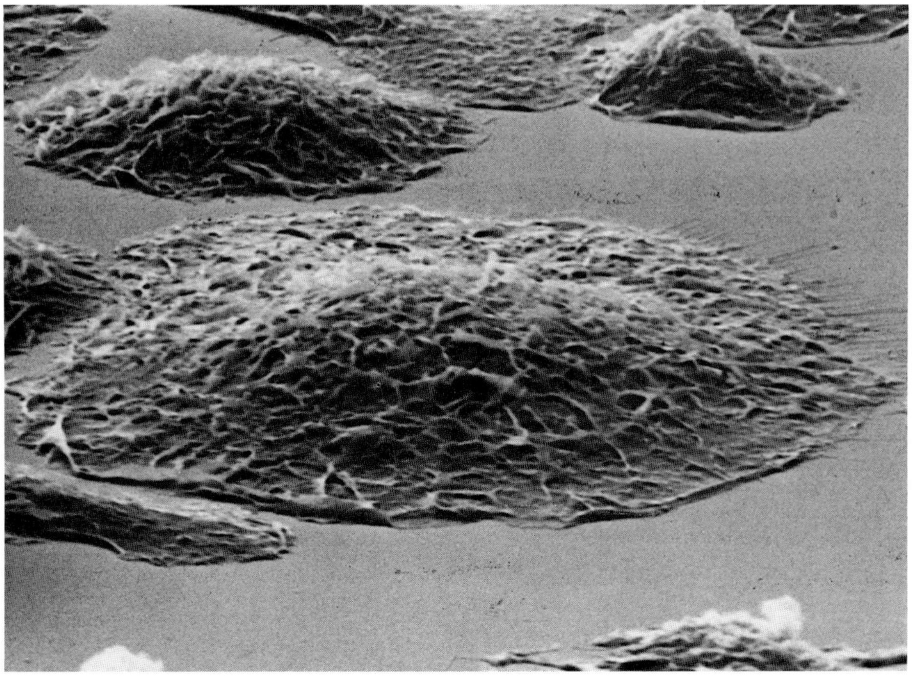

Fig. 7—Scanning electron micrograph of a multinucleate giant cell from an *in vitro* control culture. Note the generally flattened appearance with only a slightly raised central region. ×2400

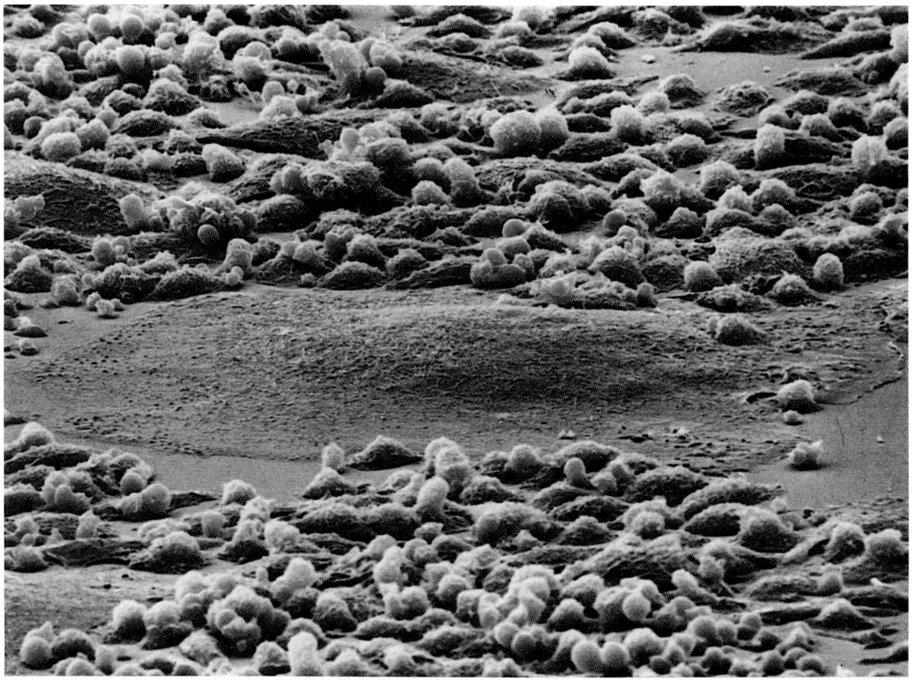

Fig. 8—A very large flattened syncytium without clearly defined lamellipodia. This is typical of many commonly found on coverslip implants. ×600

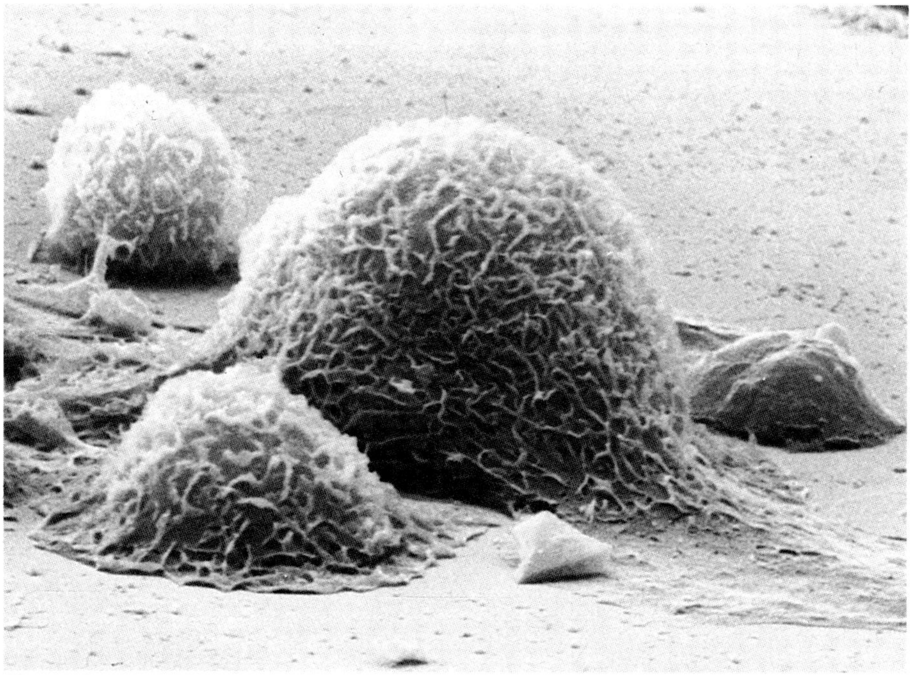

Fig. 9—Scanning electron micrograph of a multinucleate giant cell treated with cytochalasin B (10 μg/ml) for 4 h. The central bulbous region of the syncytium is raised above the rest of the cell. ×3250

and height (Fig. 7). Approximately one-third of the syncytial population did not possess distinct lamellipodia, and in these cells, the peripheral zone was relatively smooth and fine filopodia often projected from the cell extremity. Where distinct lamellipodia were obvious, long, parallel, ridge-like elevations could be seen (though less numerous and densely packed than those which characterized the central region), while surface folds or ruffles near the periphery of the cell were generally observed. Approximately 25 per cent of the multinucleate giant cell population were very large, flattened syncytia which generally did not possess a clearly defined central elevated region. About one-half of these larger multinucleate giant cells did not possess distinct lamellipodia (Fig. 8). Stereoscopic measurement of the height of all giant cells from the 6 day implants in a number of random field micrographs showed the normal multinucleate giant cell population to be 3·2±1·2 μm high (N=397). Incubation for 4 h in normal culture medium produced no discernible alteration to the morphological appearance of the syncytial population.

Cytochalasin B-treated cells—Following 4 h *in vitro* culture with medium containing cytochalasin B at a concentration of 4 μg/ml, the scanning electron microscopic appearance of multinucleate giant cells showed significant changes from control cells. The most distinct morphological feature was development of a central elevated region which was, in most instances, bulbous in shape (Fig. 9). This region was more prominent than the central area seen in control cells. The height of the cytochalasin B-treated cell population was 4·2±1·3 μm (N=107) which was significantly (P<0·001) taller than control cells. The cell surface over this raised region was very densely packed with interwoven ridges of similar size and shape, while the peripheral areas were characterized by smaller ridges and folds. Lamellipodia, which were present on approximately one-half of cytochalasin B-treated syncytia, were generally smooth in appearance, being devoid of most cell surface detail.

Colchicine-treated cells—Colchicine treatment (4 μg/ml for 4 h) altered multinucleate giant cell morphology even more than that seen in the

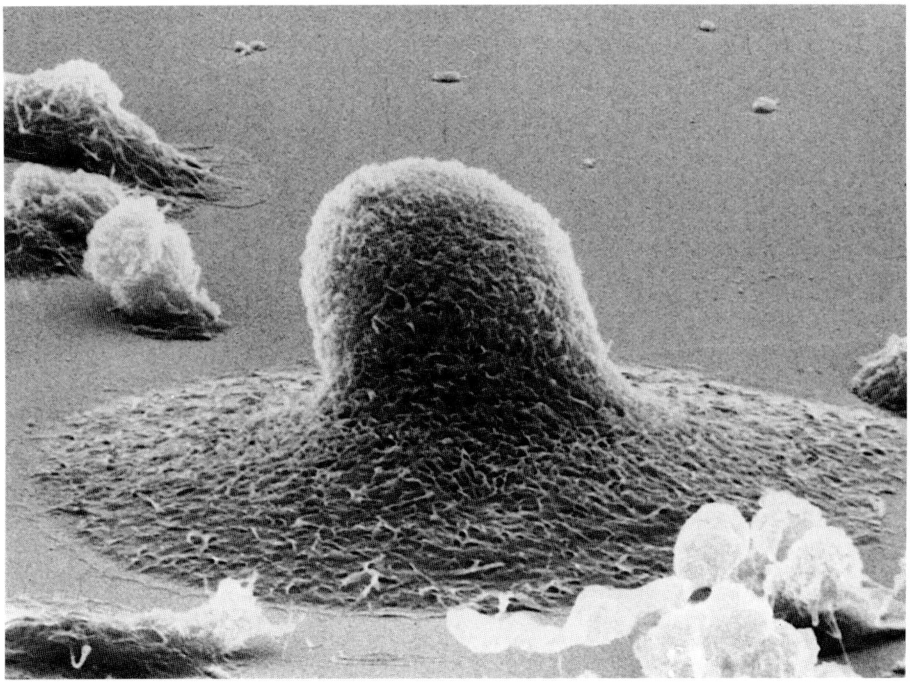

Fig 10—Scanning electron micrograph of a syncytium observed on a coverslip cultured in medium containing 10 μg/ml colchicine. The columnar shaped cell is surrounded by a broad, thin, circumferential process of cytoplasm. This raised central region was typical of the appearance of multinucleate giant cells treated with colchicine. ×2000

cytochalasin B-treated syncytia. A raised central area resulted in a syncytial population with a height of $4{\cdot}6 \pm 1{\cdot}5\,\mu m$ ($N=87$). This was significantly ($P<0.001$) taller than the control cell population. Almost the entire mass of the polykaryon appeared to be concentrated in this elevated region (Fig. 10). The columnar shaped central area was generally supported by a thin circumferential process of cytoplasm which was typically covered with small, fine ridges and undulations. Filopodia were frequently seen, especially in larger giant cells, where they were radially arranged.

DISCUSSION

While cytoskeletons of mononuclear cells have been studied extensively, the role of cytoskeletal structures in multinucleate giant cells has received little attention. In this investigation, the role of microfilaments and microtubules in maintenance of the highly specialized and organized morphology of Langhans multinucleate giant cells, has been examined.

The clumping and aggregation of nuclei observed in cytochalasin B-treated Langhans multinucleate giant cells bears many morphological similarities to the release of nuclei from mononuclear cells during cytochalasin-induced enucleation. Perinuclear microfilamentous meshworks have been suggested as being responsible for the positioning and anchorage of nuclei in mononuclear cells[13,30] and, since they are arranged in a ring-shaped woven network encircling the nuclei in Langhans syncytia,[9,10] weakening of the microfilamentous meshwork by cytochalasin B[11] would allow repositioning of nuclei. Since a highly organized radial arrangement of microtubules, which emanate from a common central pool of centrioles in Langhans syncytia, exists,[6,10] and since nuclear migration is microtubule-associated,[13,5,30] then it is possible that microtubules could provide the motive force for nuclear repositioning in cytochalasin B-treated Langhans multinucleate giant cells, perhaps by a 'treadmilling' or dynein-related transport mechanism (for review, see Margolis and Wilson[21]).

It was also observed that colchicine treatment causes disruption of the nuclear arrangement in Langhans syncytia. In addition to reports of organelle and nuclear movement following microtubule depolymerization,[16,17] microtubules are considered essential for the post-fusion ordering process by which 'foreign-body' type multinucleate giant cells assume the morphological and functional specialization of Langhans syncytia.[2,10] It is clear from results presented in this report that microtubules are also essential in maintaining the organizational state of Langhans multinucleate giant cells and that microtubule disruption can result in reversion to the 'foreign body' form.

The mechanism by which colchicine alters the arrangement of nuclei in Langhans syncytia appears to be related to a contractile function of actin microfilaments. The model of Cheung *et al.*[22] proposes that the contractility of cytocortical submembranous microfilaments can be enhanced by microtubule disruption and that, in normal cells, microtubules regulate membrane ruffling and random movement by suppression of this contractile function. Nuclear repositioning has been attributed to both the cytocortical band of microfilaments[31] and to perinuclear microfilamentous meshworks which are interconnected with radially oriented microfilamentous bundles.[30,32,33] It is perhaps through a combination of both the cytocortical and perinuclear/radial bundle microfilamentous systems that nuclei in Langhans multinucleate giant cells are reorganized. Since skeletal microtubules probably oppose cytoplasmic flow,[14] their depolymerization may be a necessary prerequisite for microfilament-induced nuclear clumping and reorganization in colchicine-treated Langhans syncytia. Due to similarities in the cytoskeletal structures of both multinucleate giant cells and their macrophage precursor cells,[9,10] it may be possible that production of motive force for nuclear movement in Langhans syncytia could occur by a mechanism similar to that of the model proposed by Cheung *et al.*[22]

It was found that concentrations of cytochalasin B below $1{\cdot}0\,\mu g/ml$ were not sufficient to allow nuclear repositioning in Langhans multinucleate giant cells. Despite probable weakening of the radial microfilament bundles, which may be more sensitive to cytochalasin B than cytocortical microfilament bundles,[22] restraining action by cytocortical microfilaments probably inhibits nuclear repositioning. Higher cytochalasin B concentrations weaken the cytocortical microfilament bundles, allowing microtubule-related transport of nuclei into the cytocentral region of the syncytium. Since the radiating array of microtubules originate from, and may be controlled by, microtubule organizing centres,[10,34] of which the centrioles are a part, and since all centriole pairs are grouped together in the cytocentrum of Langhans syncytia,[10,34] it is likely that the intracellular organelle transport and cytocentral clumping of nuclei is peculiar to Langhans multinucleate giant cells.

It is proposed that the movement of nuclei into a centrally aggregated clump in Langhans syncytia following colchicine treatment results from depolymerization of microtubules, followed by contraction of both the radial/perinuclear and cytocortical submembranous microfilament bundles (since the suppression of contractility by microtubules has been removed). Although colchicine binding to microtubular protein is slow, [34] its binding is strong and causes microtubule depolymerization at low concentrations,[22] a finding which agrees with our results (Figs 5, 6).

The behaviour of multinucleate giant cells when incubated with a combination of both cytochalasin B and colchicine in approximately equimolar concentrations, provides further evidence to justify the model of Cheung *et al.*[22] While colchicine at 1·0 μg/ml induces nuclear rearrangement in approximately one-third of all Langhans syncytia, a similar concentration of cytochalasin B only leaves the nuclear array unaffected. However, when both cytochalasin B and colchicine are combined at a concentration of 1·0 μg/ml each, there is enhanced nuclear rearrangement, with approximately 75 per cent of all Langhans syncytia being affected. These results indicate a synergistic action of cytochalasin B and colchicine on Langhans cell structure, which appears to be closely related to: (1) the concentration of both drugs; (2) the filamentous system that is most affected at that concentration; and (3) the time taken for the drug to produce a measurable effect.

As outlined above, cytochalasin B action is rapid, being complete within 30–45 min,[31,36] and destabilizing of radial microfilament bundles probably occurs at concentrations below 1·0 μg/ml. Similar concentrations of colchicine induce microtubule depolymerization although, due to the slow binding of colchicine, there is little microtubule depolymerization during the first hour of incubation. Subsequent combined destabilization of both radially-arranged microfilament bundles and depolymerization of microtubules could make enhanced contraction by cytocortical microfilament bundles possible. This mechanism could account for the increased nuclear rearrangement which occurs, in multinucleate syncytia, to an extent greater than when microtubules only are depolymerized.

In this study the synergistic action of cytochalasin B and colchicine was not evident when concentrations of 10 μg/ml of each were used, and nuclear reorganization in Langhans multinucleate giant cells was equivalent to that seen when 10 μg/ml of only cytochalasin B was used. This is probably due to a loss of contractile and restraining function by both radial and cytocortical microfilamentous bundles. Since colchicine alone has little effect on nuclear arrangement within the first hour, microtubule-related nuclear repositioning probably occurs during this time (similar to cytochalasin B only treatment), with no further nuclear movement taking place once there is sufficient colchicine-induced microtubule depolymerization.

While it is likely that microfilaments and microtubules could provide the motive force for nuclear repositioning, the function of intermediate filaments is not clear in the events reported above. Intermediate filaments of the vimentin type have been described in multinucleate giant cells,[6] and have been assigned a role in nuclear anchoring in fibroblasts.[12] It is most likely that intermediate filaments have a true skeletal role and function as spatial organizers through close structural integration with other cytoskeletal components, and are not directly involved in dynamic force production.[37,38] Evidence for structural interaction comes from demonstration of almost complete colinearity between microtubules and intermediate filaments,[39] and from collapse of the intermediate filament network into perinuclear caps following disruption of cytoplasmic microtubules with antimicrotubule agents.[37] Similarly, microfilament–intermediate filament interaction is suggested in enucleation of fibroblasts, where disruption of the microfilamentous network by cytochalasin B is required prior to nuclear release from the intermediate filament skeleton.[12] Since both colchicine and cytochalasin B have been shown to induce nuclear and intermediate filament reorganization, the possibility that microtubules and microfilaments act through the intermediate filament skeleton to modify cell shape and organization should be considered.

The morphological changes seen with the scanning electron microscope following cytochalasin B or colchicine treatment were consistent with the light microscopical observations. Since the central, slightly elevated, region of normal multinucleate giant cells represents the nuclear region,[10] the bulbous region of cell surface observed in scanning electron micrographs of treated cells reflect the clumping of nuclei in these cells. The bulbous appearance could reflect the natural tendency of the syncytium to assume a thermodynamically more stable, spherical shape, although incomplete extrusion of the nuclear region during mononuclear cell enucleation produces a similar appearance. Alterations to the structure and size of folds, flaps and lamellipodia are consistent with previously reported effects of cytochalasin B on ruffles and lamellipodia.[8,31,36] Cytochalasin B or colchicine-induced alteration of cell surface morphology by interference with control of cytocortical submembranous microfilament bundles and networks (which are responsible, at least partly, for maintenance of cell surface detail—see Henderson and Weber[33]), probably occurs by a mechanism similar to that responsible for nuclear repositioning in Langhans syncytia.

While investigations using cytochalasin B and colchicine provide only indirect evidence for cytoskeletal mediated nuclear repositioning in Langhans multinucleate giant cells, the results presented in this report could be extended by examining the redistribution of nuclei concurrently with changes in cytoskeletal organization. The use of immunostaining techniques with monospecific antibodies to microfilaments, microtubules and vimentin intermediate filaments would be one means of achieving this.

Undisturbed coordination of centrioles, microfilaments and microtubules has previously been shown necessary for transformation of 'foreign body' type multinucleate giant cells into more highly organized Langhans syncytia.[10] The present data indicate that these two filamentous systems maintain the positional integrity of nuclei in Langhans multinucleate giant cells through interrelated contractile cytoskeletal components having opposing actions, which, in the stable state, are critically maintained at equilibrium. Disruption of this equilibrium can cause conversion back to the 'foreign body' type multinucleate giant cell morphology. This strongly reinforces previous suggestions[2,10,27] that Langhans multinucleate giant cells are special, more highly organized forms of 'foreign body' giant cells. The special functional advantages, if any, conferred on the Langhans multinucleate giant cell by its highly ordered cellular architecture await elucidation.

ACKNOWLEDGEMENTS

The authors wish to thank Mr A. R. Murch and Dr M. D. Grounds for their constructive criticisms during the preparation of this manuscript. This work was supported by grants from the National Health and Medical Research Council of Australia and the Cancer Council of Western Australia.

REFERENCES

1. Sutton JS, Weiss L. Transformation of monocytes in tissue culture into macrophages, epithelioid cells, and multinucleated giant cells. An electron microscope study. *J Cell Biol* 1966; **28:** 303.
2. Mariano M, Spector WG. The formation and properties of macrophage polykaryons (inflammatory giant cells). *J Path* 1974; **113:** 1.
3. Murch AR, Grounds Miranda, Marshall C, Papadimitriou JM. Direct evidence that inflammatory multinucleate giant cells form by fusion. *J Path* 1982; **137:** 177.
4. Papadimitriou JM. Macrophage fusion *in vivo* and *in vitro*: a review. In: Poste G, Nicolson GL, eds. Membrane Fusion. Amsterdam: Elsevier/North-Holland, 1978: 181.
5. Papadimitriou JM, Walters MN-I. Macrophage polykarya. *CRC Crit Rev Toxicol* 1979; **6:** 211.
6. Cain H, Kraus B. Cytoskeleton in cells of the mononuclear phagocyte system. Immunofluorescence microscopic and electron microscopic studies. *Virchows Arch B (Cell Pathol)* 1981; **36:** 159.
7. Papadimitriou JM, Archer M. The morphology of murine foreign body multinucleate giant cells. *J Ultrastruct Res* 1974; **49:** 372.
8. Papadimitriou JM, Kingston K.J. The locomotory behaviour of the multinucleate giant cells of foreign body reactions. *J Path* 1977; **121:** 27.
9. Papadimitriou JM, Rigby PJ. The detection of a contractile apparatus in murine multinucleate giant cells. *J Path* 1979; **129:** 91.
10. Cain H, Kraus B, Fringes B, Osborn M, Weber K. Centrioles, microtubules and microfilaments in activated mononuclear and multinucleate macrophages from rat peritoneum: electron-microscopic and immunofluorescence microscopic studies. *J Path* 1981; **133:** 301.
11. Osborn Mary, Weber K. The detergent-resistant cytoskeleton of tissue culture cells includes the nucleus and the microfilament bundles. *Exp Cell Res* 1977; **106:** 339.
12. Laurila P, Virtanen I, Stenman S. Intermediate filaments in enucleation of human fibroblasts. *Exp Cell Res* 1981; **131:** 41.
13. Franke WW. Structure, biochemistry, and functions of the nuclear envelope. *Int Rev Cytol Suppl* 1974; **4:** 71.

14. Wang E, Goldman RD. Functions of cytoplasmic fibers in intracellular movements in BHK-21 cells. *J Cell Biol* 1978; **79:** 708.
15. Tucker JB. Spatial organization of microtubules. In: Roberts K, Hyams JS, eds. Microtubules. London: Academic Press, 1979: 315.
16. Weatherbee JA. Membranes and cell movement: interactions of membranes with the proteins of the cytoskeleton. *Int Rev Cytol Suppl* 1981; **12:** 113.
17. Hyams JS, Stebbings H. Microtubule associated cytoplasmic transport. In: Roberts K, Hyams JS, eds. Microtubules. London: Academic Press, 1979: 487.
18. Painter RG, Whisenand J, McIntosh Ann T. Effects of cytochalasin B on actin and myosin association with particle binding sites in mouse macrophages: implications with regard to the mechanism of action of the cytochalasins. *J Cell Biol* 1981; **91:** 373.
19. Lin DC, Tobin KD, Grumet M, Lin S. Cytochalasins inhibit nuclei-induced actin polymerization by blocking filament elongation. *J Cell Biol* 1980; **84:** 455.
20. Brown Susan S, Spudich JA. Mechanism of action of cytochalasin: evidence that it binds to actin filament ends. *J Cell Biol* 1981; **88:** 487.
21. Margolis RL, Wilson L. Microtubule treadmills—possible molecular machinery. *Nature* 1981; **293:** 705.
22. Cheung HT, Cantarow WD, Sundharadas G. Colchicine and cytochalasin B (CB) effects on random movement, spreading and adhesion of mouse macrophages. *Exp Cell Res* 1978; **111:** 95.
23. Holmes, KV, Choppin, PW. On the role of microtubles in movement and alignment of nuclei in virus-induced syncytia. *J Cell Biol* 1968; **39:** 526.
24. Sapp JP. An ultrastructural study of nuclear and centriolar configurations in multinucleated giant cells. *Lab Invest* 1976; **34:** 109.
25. Wang E, Cross RK, Choppin PW. Involvement of microtubules and 10-nm filaments in the movement and positioning of nuclei in syncytia. *J Cell Biol* 1979; **83:** 320.
26. Wang E, Connolly JA, Kalnins VI, Choppin PW. Relationship between movement and aggregation of centrioles in syncytia and formation of microtubule bundles. *Proc Natl Acad Sci USA* 1979; **76:** 5719.
27. Papadimitriou JM, Spector WG. The origin, properties and fate of epithelioid cells. *J Path* 1971; **105:** 187.
28. Lewis WH. The formation of giant cells in tissue cultures and their similarity to those in tuberculous lesions. *Amer Rev Tuberc* 1927; **15:** 616.
29. Kristensen SEL, Papadimitriou JM. The measurement of cell volume and surface area by SEM photogrammetry. *J Microsc* 1981; **124:** 155.
30. Britch M, Allen TD. Effects of cytochalasin B on the cytoplasmic contractile network revealed by whole-cell transmission electron microscopy. *Exp Cell Res* 1981; **131:** 161.
31. Temmink JHM, Spiele H. Effect of vinblastine and cytochalasin B on the cytoskeletal domains in 3T3 cells. *J Cell Sci* 1981; **48:** 55.
32. Trotter JA, Foerder BA, Keller JM. Intracellular fibres in cultured cells: analysis by scanning and transmission electron microscopy and by SDS-polyacrylamide gel electrophoresis. *J Cell Sci* 1978; **31:** 369.
33. Henderson D, Weber K. Three-dimensional organization of microfilaments and microtubules in the cytoskeleton. Immunoperoxidase labelling and stereo-electron microscopy of detergent-extracted cells. *Exp Cell Res* 1979; **124:** 301.
34. Solomon F. Organizing microtubules in the cytoplasm. *Cell* 1980; **22:** 331.
35. Snyder JA, McIntosh JR. Biochemistry and physiology of microtubules. *Annu Rev Biochem* 1976; **45:** 699.
36. Lin S, Lin DC, Flanagan MD. Specificity of the effects of cytochalasin B on transport and motile processes. *Proc Natl Acad Sci USA* 1978; **75:** 329.
37. Lazarides E. Intermediate filaments as mechanical integrators of cellular space. *Nature* 1980; **283:** 249.
38. Brinkley BR. Summary: organization of the cytoplasm. *Cold Spring Harbor Symp Quant Biol* 1982; **46:** 1029.
39. Singer SJ, Ball EH, Geiger B, Chen W-T. Immunolabeling studies of cytoskeletal associations in cultured cells. *Cold Spring Harbor Symp Quant Biol* 1982; **46:** 303.

JOURNAL OF PATHOLOGY. VOL. **143:** 31–37 (1984)

HISTOMETRICAL INVESTIGATION OF THE PULMONARY ARTERY IN SEVERE HEPATIC DISEASE

O. MATSUBARA, T. NAKAMURA, T. UEHARA AND T. KASUGA

Department of Pathology, Faculty of Medicine, Tokyo Medical and Dental University, Tokyo, Japan

Received 15 September 1983
Accepted 22 September 1983

SUMMARY

Histological changes of the pulmonary vasculature in comparison with that of the portal vein in necropsy cases of severe hepatic injury that had not been associated with clinical pulmonary hypertension were analysed qualitatively and quantitatively. The main changes of the intra-hepatic portal vein were dilatation (88·3 per cent), thickening of the wall (58·5 per cent) and thrombi (22·3 per cent). The changes of the pulmonary vasculature were limited to muscular type arteries, which showed dilatation (31·9 per cent), thickening of the wall (30·9 per cent) and thrombi (10·6 per cent). Association of wall thickening of the portal vein and the small pulmonary artery was observed in 30·9 per cent, these associations being statistically significant. Coincidence of thrombus formation in the portal vein and pulmonary vasculature was observed only in 4·3 per cent, which was not statistically significant. After the circumferences of the internal and external elastic laminae of small pulmonary arteries and the cross-sectional area of the media were measured, the anatomical radius and wall thickness of each artery were calculated according to Furuyama's method. The relations between the anatomical radii and wall thickness of small pulmonary arteries in controls and hepatic cirrhosis groups were investigated by analysis of covariance to compare the equality of the two corresponding regression lines. The wall thickness and the ratio of wall thickness to the anatomical radius of small pulmonary arteries were significantly larger in the cirrhotic group than in the control group. This study suggests that patients with severe hepatic injury are in a state of subclinical pulmonary hypertension and that symptoms of severe pulmonary hypertension may develop progressively or abruptly in some of them. The mechanism of pulmonary hypertension complicating portal hypertension or severe hepatic injury is discussed in reviewing the reported cases.

KEY WORDS—Hepatic injury, portal hypertension, pulmonary vasculature, pulmonary hypertension.

INTRODUCTION

There have been many reports of an association between severe hepatic injury or portal hypertension and pulmonary hypertension.[1–13] Our interest in this problem stemmed from these case reports and our observation that pulmonary arteries in cases of hepatic cirrhosis frequently showed wall thickening. Therefore, we made qualitative and quantitative studies on histological changes of the pulmonary vasculature in necropsy cases of severe hepatic injury that had not been associated with clinical pulmonary hypertension.

MATERIALS AND METHODS

The histology of the blood vessels of the liver and lungs were studied qualitatively in 94 adult cases of severe liver disease including 62 of post-hepatitic cirrhosis, 13 of post-necrotic cirrhosis, seven of biliary cirrhosis, four of sub-massive necrosis, one of fatty cirrhosis and one of haemochromatosis. The mean age of the cases was 61·6 ± 12·0 (S.D.) years (male 78, female 16). The mean weights of the liver, lungs, spleen and heart were 1212·9 ± 427·6 g, 1000·3 ± 370·3 g,

Addressee for correspondence: Dr Osamu Matsubara, Department of Pathology, Faculty of Medicine, Tokyo Medical and Dental University, 1-4-45 Yushima, Bunkyo-ku, Tokyo 113, Japan.

0022–3417/84/050031–07$01.00

234.0 ± 190.6 g and 322.8 ± 88.8 g, respectively. None of the cases had a smoking history, taken drugs toxic to the lungs, or had lived at high altitude. No cases had received a portal-systemic shunt. The causes of death were hepatic coma (41·7 per cent), rupture of oesophageal varices (33·3 per cent), gastro-intestinal bleeding (19·4 per cent) and infection (5·6 per cent). The lungs were taken at necropsy and fixed by trans-bronchial injection of 10 per cent formalin. Sections embedded in paraffin were stained with haematoxylin and eosin, elastic/van Gieson and Masson's trichrome. Histological examinations were mainly concentrated on the figures of the blood vessels, such as dilatation of the lumen, thickening of the wall and thrombus formation. More than 100 arteries and veins per case were examined. Cases in which over 25 per cent of the blood vessels showed changes of dilatation or thickening was classified as positive, those showing 10–25 per cent changes were classified as positive-negative, and those showing under 10 per cent changes as negative.

Quantitative analyses of the pulmonary artery were made on 21 cases of hepatic cirrhosis (mean age; 64.9 ± 8.6 years) and 19 controls (58.6 ± 13.3 years). The 21 cases were chosen at random from the cases which had been studied qualitatively. Using an Image Analysing System (Muto and Canon, Tokyo), histological sections stained by elastic/van Gieson were traced on a screen for morphometry at appropriate magnifications. The outlines of the internal and external elastic laminae were drawn with a light pen and the circumferences of the internal (L) and external elastic laminae were measured. The cross-sectional area of the media (S), defined as the area in between the internal and external elastic laminae including both laminae, was then determined. Using these data two idealized circles, defined as those when the elastic laminae are completely distended, were calculated and the anatomical radius (R) and wall thickness (D) of each artery were determined from the following equations:

$$S = 2\pi R D, \qquad L = 2\pi\left(R - \frac{D}{2}\right)$$

Assuming that the area of the media is constant irrespective of the degree of arterial contraction, the anatomical radius and wall thickness were calculated according to Furuyama's idea[14]:

$$R = \frac{S}{\sqrt{L^2 + 4\pi S} - L}, \qquad D = \frac{\sqrt{L^2 + 4\pi S} - L}{2}$$

The relation between the anatomical radius and the wall thickness was investigated in cases of hepatic cirrhosis and controls.

The chi-square test with Yate's correction and Student's two-tailed test were used to assess the relations of histological changes and measured data. Analysis of covariance was also used to assess the equality of the two corresponding regression lines.

RESULTS

Qualitative study

Histological findings in the pulmonary and intra-hepatic blood vessels are shown in Table I. The main changes of hepatic vasculature were dilatation (88·3 per cent), thickening of the wall (58·5 per cent) and thrombi (22·3 per cent) in the portal vein, and thickening of the wall of the artery (30·9 per cent). Most cases showing wall thickening of the portal vein also showed dilatation of the portal vein. Thrombi consisted of organized ones (16 cases) and fresh ones (five cases). Liver cell carcinoma was a complication in 22 cases (23·4 per cent). Tumour thrombi (three cases; 3·2 per cent) were also seen.

Changes of the pulmonary artery were mainly limited to muscular type arteries, whose inner diameter ranged from 100 to 800 μm, with a few changes of small veins. Small arteries showed dilatation (31·9 per cent), thickening of the wall 30·9 per cent) and thrombi (10·6 per cent). Small veins showed thickening of the wall (28·7 per cent), dilatation (20·2 per cent) and thrombi (2·1 per cent). These hypertrophic changes were mainly observed in arteries of less than 300 μm diameter, corresponding to grade 2.[15] Occasionally small arteries showed plexiform-like lesions, lymphocytic infiltration of the wall and calcium deposition. Coincidence of wall thickening of the portal vein and small pulmonary arteries was observed in 29 cases (30·9 per cent), the relation being statistically significant (chi-square with Yate's correction = 16·214, $P < 0.001$) (Table II). Thrombi in all pulmonary blood vessels were observed in 15 cases (16·0 per cent), which was less than the frequency of portal thrombi (22·3 per cent), and coincidence of the two was observed in only four cases (4·3 per cent), which was not statistically significant (chi-square with Yate's correction = 0·10778, $0.7 < P < 0.8$) (Table III).

Table I—Histological findings in the intra-hepatic and pulmonary blood vessels

		Dilatation of the lumen		Thickening of the wall		Thrombi
		+	±	+	±	+
Liver	Central veins	3	0	2	0	0
	Arteries	0	0	29	9	0
	Portal veins	83	1	55	0	21 (3*)
Lung	Large arteries	0	0	1	0	0
	Middle-sized arteries	4	0	5	0	4
	Small arteries	30	0	29	15	10
	Capillaries	18	0	0	0	2
	Small veins	19	0	27	6	2
	Middle-sized veins	0	0	0	0	0
	Large veins	0	0	0	0	0 (5†)

* Only tumour emboli were observed in three cases.
† Only tumour emboli were observed in the arteries and veins in five cases.

Table II—Wall thickening of the portal vein and small pulmonary arteries*

		Wall thickening of the small pulmonary arteries +	−	Total
Wall thickening of the portal veins	+	29†	26	55
	−	4	35	39
Total		33	61	94

* Numbers of cases showing wall thickening of the portal veins and/or the small pulmonary arteries.
† The coincidence of wall thickening of the portal veins and the small pulmonary arteries is statistically significant (chi-square with Yate's correction = 16·214, $P<0·001$).

Table III—Thrombus formation in the portal veins and pulmonary blood vessels*

		Thrombus formation in pulmonary blood vessels +	−	Total
Thrombus formation in the portal veins	+	4†	15	19
	−	11	64	75
Total		15	79	94

* Numbers of cases with thrombi in the portal veins and/or pulmonary blood vessels.
† The coincidence of thrombus formation in both the portal veins and pulmonary blood vessels is not statistically significant (chi-square with Yate's correction = 0·10778, $0·7<P<0·8$).

Quantitative study

The relations between the anatomical radius and wall thickness of small pulmonary arteries in the control and hepatic cirrhosis groups are shown in Figs 1 and 3. The mean wall thickness in the two groups were $15·3 \pm 7·5$ μm and $21·2 \pm 10·4$ μm, respectively. The relations between the anatomical radius and the ratio of wall thickness to the anatomical radius of small pulmonary arteries in the two groups are shown in Figs 2 and 4. The mean ratios were $0·13 \pm 0·07$ and $0·21 \pm 0·09$, respectively. These measured and calculated data cannot be compared directly, because the radii were different. So, the relations between the anatomical radii and wall thickness in the two groups were examined by analysis of covariance to compare the equality of the two corresponding regression lines. The regression line of the radius and the wall thickness of the pulmonary artery in the cirrhotic group was different from that in the control group ($P<0·005$). The regression line of the radius to the ratio of the wall thickness to the radius of the pulmonary artery in the cirrhotic group was also different from that in the control group ($P<0·005$). Results showed that the wall thickness and the ratio of the wall thickness to the radius of the pulmonary artery were significantly larger in cirrhotic group than in the control group.

DISCUSSION

No histological analysis of the pulmonary vasculature in comparison with that of the portal

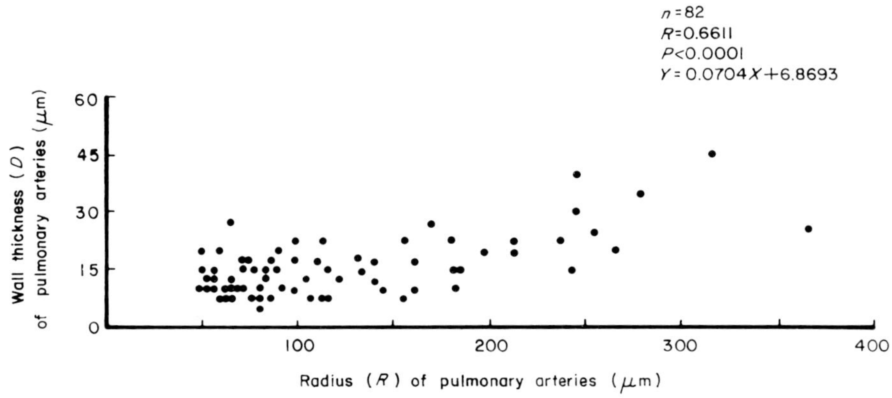

Fig. 1—Relation between the anatomical radii and wall thickness of small pulmonary arteries in the control group

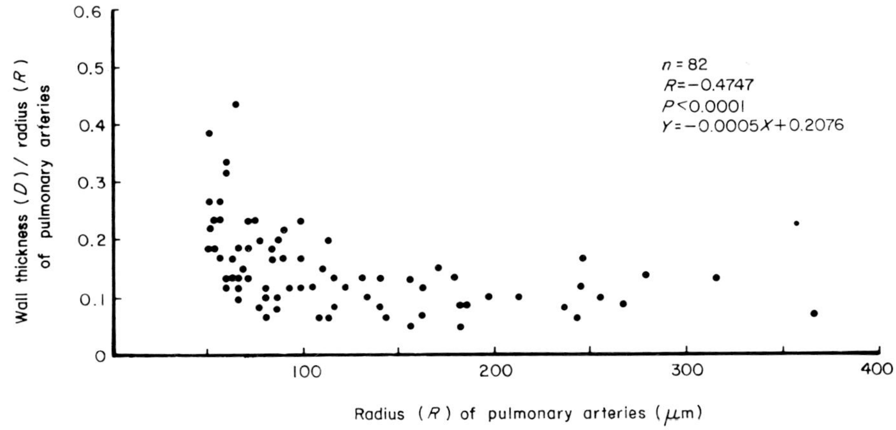

Fig. 2—Relation between the anatomical radii and the ratio of wall thickness to the anatomical radius of small pulmonary arteries in the control group

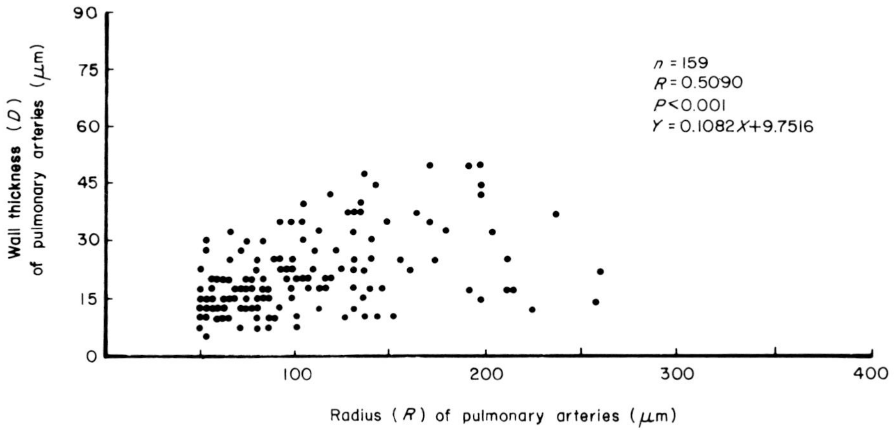

Fig. 3—Relation between the anatomical radii and wall thickness of small pulmonary arteries in the hepatic cirrhosis group

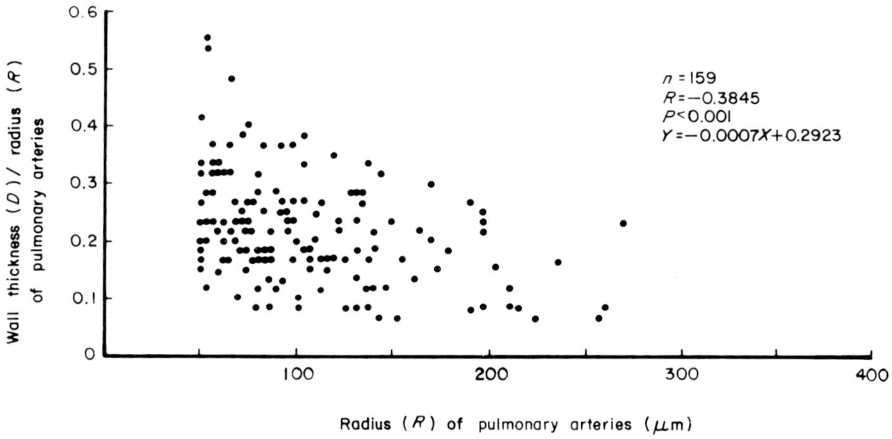

Fig. 4—Relation between the anatomical radii and the ratio of wall thickness to the anatomical radius of small pulmonary arteries in the hepatic cirrhosis group

vein in patients with severe hepatic diseases has been made previously. Our study showed a significant correlation of wall thickening of the portal vein and small pulmonary arteries in cases of hepatic injury. Our results also showed that wall thickness and the ratio of the wall thickness to the radius of the small pulmonary arteries are significantly larger in cases of hepatic cirrhosis than in controls. The increase in wall thickness of the small pulmonary arteries implies an increase in resistance to flow, namely, in blood pressure, according to Wagenvoort *et al.*[16] This study suggests that patients with severe hepatic injury are in a subclinical pulmonary hypertensive state, and that symptoms of severe pulmonary hypertension may develop progressively or abruptly in some of them. Convincing evidence of an association of pulmonary hypertension and portal hypertension is seen in many serial case reports and studies. Pulmonary hypertension can affect patients with portal hypertension of any cause. The high prevalence of cirrhosis in these cases probably reflects the predominance of this cause over other causes of portal hypertension in general.

The bloodstreams of the portal vein and the pulmonary artery seem to have no direct relationship. But, they have the following common physiological relations: they are both in a low-pressure circulatory system, they both have important roles after birth and they keep blood in reserve for the two ventricles of the heart. Thus, they may have some unknown embryological, physiological or haemodynamic relations.

The mechanism of pulmonary hypertension complicating portal hypertension or severe hepatic injury is not fully understood. In many case reports and a review,[17] various mechanisms have been discussed, such as thromboembolism, arterio-venous shunt, vascular spiders, a humoral mechanism, chronic hypoxia, porto-pulmonary anastomosis, an autoimmune mechanism, or iron accumulation. Of 21 reported cases that were necropsied, eight had portal thrombosis, and all six cases of Naeye[2] and two of 11 cases of Senior[5] had massive or multiple thrombi in the pulmonary artery. These findings suggest that thromboembolism from the portal vein was responsible for the pulmonary arterial lesions. Mantz and Craige,[1] Naeye,[2] Senior *et al.*,[5] Lal and Fletcher,[6] Lai *et al.*[8] and Saunders *et al.*[10] all favour this view. But, our study on the coincidence of thrombus formation in the pulmonary vasculature and the portal vein does not support this view.

From angiographical studies Rydell and Hoffbauer,[18] Murray *et al.*,[19] Berthelot *et al.*[20] and Gamal *et al.* [21] considered that multiple A-V shunts in the lungs are responsible for pulmonary hypertension. Since we did not examine the lungs by angiography we cannot comment on this, but we wonder whether A-V shunts are a cause or result of pulmonary hypertension.

The concept of a humoral influence is an attractive alternative. This was proposed by Shorr *et al.*[22] and Segel *et al.*,[7] and supported by the finding that fulvine caused both hepatic necrosis and hypertensive pulmonary vascular disease.[23]

Lebrec *et al.*[11] suggested that pulmonary hypertension resulted from the effect of a vasoconstrictive agent on the small pulmonary artery or of a substance toxic to the walls of these vessels that was produced in the splanchnic territory, destroyed by the liver in normal subjects, and that reached the pulmonary arteries through portal-systemic shunts. It is very interesting that some prostaglandins ($PGF_{2\alpha}$) cause vasoconstriction of both the pulmonary artery and the portal vein of rabbits.[24] Serotonin, aminorex (5-amino-5-phenyloxazoline) and other substances are also thought to be candidates for this effect.

The fact that hypoxia causes the arterial change of the lungs is well known.[25] The relation between liver injury and hypoxia is not direct. Chronic hypoxia in patients with liver injury can be explained by several factors, such as marked ascites, metabolic acidosis or respiratory alkalosis. Since these signs and symptoms occur in the terminal stage of liver disease, chronic hypoxia does not seem to be a possible direct cause.

Porto-pulmonary venous anastomosis was observed by Calabresi and Abelmann,[26] Shaldon *et al.*[27] and Khaliq, Kay and Heath[28] and it may increase as hepatic injury progresses. We consider that it is a highly possible cause of abnormalities, but we did not obtain any evidence for this in this study.

Morrison *et al.*[12] reported that four of five patients with liver disease and pulmonary hypertension had evidence of autoimmune phenomena. Their idea of a relation between these phenomena is very attractive, but further studies are needed to clarify the autoimmune mechanism for these lesions.

Molden and Abraham[13] reported a case of pulmonary hypertension associated with hepatic cirrhosis and iron accumulation. Our qualitative study includes only one case of haemochromatosis, other cases showing no remarkable iron accumulation. Thus, we think that iron accumulation is an extremely rare cause of the association of pulmonary hypertension and portal hypertension.

Several methods have been proposed for morphometry of blood vessels, such as measurement of the lumen-to-wall ratio,[29] lumen-to-diameter ratio,[30] media-to-diameter ratio,[31] quantification of the cross-sectional area of the arterial media[32,33] and the method of Furuyama.[14] We think that irregular contraction and wavy elastic laminae do not allow the precise measurements that are necessary to differentiate between normal and abnormal values, except in Wagenvoort's and Furuyama's methods. Since we considered that the degree of dilatation of alveolar spaces might affect measurements in Wagenvoort's method, we used Furuyama's method.

ACKNOWLEDGEMENTS

The authors are grateful to Mr Y. Ogura, Miss E. Harasawa and Miss T. Mochizuki for their technical assistance. This study was supported in part by a Science Grant-in-aid from the Ministry of Education, Science and Culture of Japan.

REFERENCES

1. Mantz FA Jr, Craige E. Portal axis thrombosis with spontaneous portacaval shunt and resultant cor pulmonale. *AMA Arch Pathol* 1951; **52:** 91.
2. Naeye RL. Primary pulmonary hypertension with coexisting portal hypertension. A retrospective study of six cases. *Circulation* 1960, **22:** 376.
3. Kerbel NC. Pulmonary hypertension and portal hypertension. *Can Med Assoc J* 1962; **87:** 1022.
4. Cohen N, Mendelow H. Concurrent active juvenile cirrhosis and primary pulmonary hypertension. *Am J Med* 1965; **39:** 127.
5. Senior RM, Britton RC, Turino GM, Wood JA, Langer GA, Fishman AP. Pulmonary hypertension associated with cirrhosis of the liver and with portacaval shunts. *Circulation* 1968; **37:** 88.
6. Lal S,, Fletcher E. Pulmonary hypertension and portal venous system thrombosis. *Br Heart J* 1968; **30:** 723.
7. Segel N, Kay JM, Bayley TJ, Paton A. Pulmonary hypertension with hepatic cirrhosis. *Br Heart J* 1968; **30:** 575.
8. Lai KS, McFadzean AJS, Yeung R. Microembolic pulmonary hypertension in pyogenic cholangitis. *Br Med J* 1968; **1:** 22.
9. Levine R, Harris RC, Blanc WA, Mellins B. Progressive pulmonary hypertension in children with portal hypertension. *J Pediatr* 1973; **83:** 964.
10. Saunders JB, Costable TJ, Heath D, Smith P, Paton A. Pulmonary hypertension complicating portal vein thrombosis. *Thorax* 1979; **34:** 281.
11. Lebrec J, Dhumeaux D, Benhamou JP. Pulmonary hypertension complicating portal hypertension. *Am Rev Respir Dis* 1979; **120:** 849.
12. Morrison EB, Gaffney AF, Eigenbrodt EH, Reynolds RC, Buja LM. Severe pulmonary hypertension associated with macronodular (postnecro-

tic) cirrhosis and autoimmune phenomena. *Am J Med* 1980; **69:** 513.
13. Molden D, Abraham JL. Pulmonary hypertension, its association with hepatic cirrhosis and iron accumulation. *Arch Pathol Lab Med* 1982; **106:** 328.
14. Furuyama M. Histometrical investigations of arteries in reference to arterial hypertension. *Tohoku J Exp Med* 1961; **76:** 388.
15. Heath D, Edwards JE. The pathology of hypertensive pulmonary vascular disease. A description of six grades of structural changes in the pulmonary arteries with special references to congenital cardiac septal defects. *Circulation* 1958; **18:** 533.
16. Wagenvoort CA, Nauta J, van der Schaar PJ, Weeda HWH, Wagenvoort N. Effect of flow and pressure on pulmonary vessels. Semiquantitative study based on lung biopsies. *Circulation* 1967; **35:** 1028.
17. Wagenvoort CA, Wagenvoort N. Pathology of Pulmonary Hypertension. New York: John Wiley, 1977: 95.
18. Rydell R, Hoffbauer FW. Multiple pulmonary arteriovenous fistulas in juvenile cirrhosis. *Am J Med* 1956; **21:** 450.
19. Murray JF, Dawson AM, Sherlock S. Circulatory changes in chronic liver disease. *Am J Med* 1958; **24:** 358.
20. Berthelot P, Walker JG, Sherlock S, Reid L. Arterial changes in the lungs in cirrhosis of the liver—lung spider nevi. *N Engl J Med* 1966; **274:** 291.
21. Gamal ME, Stocker JB, Spiers EM, Whitaker W. Cyanosis complicating hepatic cirrhosis. *Am J Cardiol* 1970; **25:** 490.
22. Shorr E, Zweifach BW, Furchgott RF. Hepatorenal factors in circulatory homeostasis. Influence of humoral factors of hepatorenal origin on vascular reactions to hemorrhage. *Ann NY Acad Sci* 1948; **49:** 571.
23. Kay JM, Heath D, Smith P, Bras G, Sammerell J. Fulvine and the pulmonary circulation. *Thorax* 1971; **2:** 249.
24. Kitamura K, Suzuki H, Kuriyama H. Prostaglandin action on the main pulmonary artery and portal vein of the rabbit. *Jap J Physiol* 1976; **26:** 681.
25. Hasleton PS, Heath D, Brewer DB. Hypertensive pulmonary vascular disease in states of chronic hypoxia. *J Path Bact* 1968; **95:** 431.
26. Calabresi P, Abelmann WH. Porto-caval and porto-pulmonary anastomoses in Laennec's cirrhosis and in heart failure. *J Clin Invest* 1957; **36:** 1257.
27. Shaldon S, Caesar J, Chiandussi L, Williams HS, Sheville E, Sherlock S. Demonstration of porta-pulmonary anastomoses in portal cirrhosis with use of radioactive krypton (Kr^{85}). *N Engl J Med* 1961; **265:** 410.
28. Khaliq DU, Kay JM, Heath D. Porta-pulmonary venous anastomoses in experimental cirrhosis of the liver in rats. *J Path* 1972; **107:** 167.
29. Damman JF Jr, Ferencz C. The significance of the pulmonary vascular bed in congenital heart disease. *Am Heart J* 1956; **52:** 7.
30. Rosen L, Bowden DH, Uchida I. Structural changes in pulmonary arteries in first year of life. *Arch Pathol* 1957; **63:** 316.
31. Granston AS. Morphologic alterations of the pulmonary arteries in congenital heart disease. *Proc Inst Med Chic* 1958; **22:** 116.
32. Wagenvoort CA. Vasoconstriction and medial hypertrophy in pulmonary hypertension. *Circulation* 1960; **22:** 535.
33. Takahashi T, Wagenvoort N, Wagenvoort CA. The density of muscularized pulmonary arteries in normal lungs. *Arch Pathol Lab Med* 1983; **107:** 19.

JOURNAL OF PATHOLOGY, VOL. **143:** 39–50 (1984)

THE HISTOCHEMISTRY OF GLYCOSIDASES IN HUMAN BENIGN AND MALIGNANT BREAST TISSUE

ROSEMARY A. WALKER

Department of Pathology, Clinical Sciences Building, Leicester Royal Infirmary, P.O. Box 65, Leicester LE2 7LX, England

Received 20 July 1983
Accepted 7 September 1983

SUMMARY

Histochemical methods for the localization of four glycosidases (β-glucuronidase, β-*N*-acetyl glucosaminidase, β-D-galactosidase and α-mannosidase) have been applied to 40 cases of human normal and hyperplastic breast tissue and 100 human breast carcinomas. All tissues have been fixed in formol–calcium at 4°C and washed in gum sucrose. β-Glucuronidase and β-*N*-acetyl glucosaminidase have consistently been detected in essentially all cells of normal and hyperplastic tissue. A similar distribution has been found for better differentiated carcinomas but the number of cells with detectable enzyme decreases in the more poorly differentiated tumour. β-D-Galactosidase and α-mannosidase have only been demonstrated in very occasional cells in normal breast tissue. The incidence increases in hyperplastic tissue, and in approximately half the carcinomas many cells have detectable enzyme. The localization of β-D-galactosidase has not been related to tumour differentiation but the better differentiated carcinomas tend to have few cells with demonstrable α-mannosidase. Although it has been suggested that glycosidases can have an effect on membrane function no differences have been found between those carcinomas having a few or many cells with detectable enzyme and the presence or absence of axillary lymph node metastasis. Total enzyme activity cannot be detected in fixed tissue, nor can an accurate quantitative assessment be made, but under the conditions of this study it is possible to conclude that there are differences between normal and malignant breast tissue in the localization of glycosidases.

KEY WORDS—Breast disease, breast carcinoma, glycosidases, histochemistry.

INTRODUCTION

Glycosidases are enzymes that catalyse the hydrolysis of glycosidic bonds in simple glycosides, oligosaccharides and polysaccharides, as well as in complex carbohydrates such as glycoproteins and glycolipids.[1] Within the cell they are present in lysosomes although some hydrolases are also located in endoplasmic reticulum[2,3] and in the Golgi complex.[4] Because of their hydrolytic action glycosidases can be involved in the modification of the carbohydrate component of glycoproteins, and they are essential for the synthesis of *N*-linked oligosaccharide chains of glycoproteins.[5]

Glycosidases could be of importance in the development and maintenance of the neoplastic state. Weiss[6] has suggested that lysosomal enzymes could induce modifications of the cell periphery by sub-lethal autolysis, a process in which there is a controlled extracellular release and activation of these enzymes in both physiological and pathological conditions. This process may be important in maintaining the malignant or transformed state. Lysosomal hydrolases have been shown to produce alterations in membrane function, such as differences in lectin agglutination and cell growth[7] and reduction in specificity of cell adhesion. Alterations in these enzymes could be directly or indirectly related to the modifications of oligosaccharide components of glycoproteins which have been described in malignant cells.[9]

Many of the studies concerning glycosidases and neoplasia have been confined to cell lines.

0022–3417/84/050039–12$01.20

Increased levels have been reported in viral-transformed fibroblasts[10, 11] and in rat hepatoma membranes[12] but similar increases were not found in dimethyl nitrosamine-transformed hamster cells.[13] Studies of whole tissues have shown elevations in activity of β-D-glucuronidase in several different types of malignant human neoplasms,[14] and increases in β-D-galactosidase and α-mannosidase in human breast and colonic carcinomas.[15] Homogenization of tissue was required since biochemical assays were performed. The results could have been affected by the presence of macrophages and other inflammatory cells, all of which contain lysosomal enzymes.

In the present study histochemical techniques have been used to demonstrate four lysosomal enzymes, namely β-glucuronidase, β-*N*-acetyl glucosaminidase, β-D-galactosidase and α-mannosidase, in normal, benign and malignant breast tissue. The methods being histological have the advantage of allowing distinction between reactions in breast epithelial cells and inflammatory cells. The staining patterns in the various tissues have been compared, and the findings in the carcinomas related to tumour differentiation and the presence or absence of local lymph node metastasis.

MATERIALS AND METHODS

Tissues

Tissue from 40 individual human benign breast specimens and 100 human breast carcinomas was examined. Samples from each case, not more than 2 mm in thickness, were fixed in 4 per cent formol–calcium solution at 4°C for 24 h, then transferred to Holt's gum sucrose mixture at 4°C. The tissue was then frozen on to chucks using carbon dioxide.

Methods

Sections 8 μm in thickness were cut from the fixed-frozen tissue at −25°C in a cryostat, mounted on chemically clean slides and air-dried. Serial sections from each case were assessed for the presence of the four enzymes by the following methods.

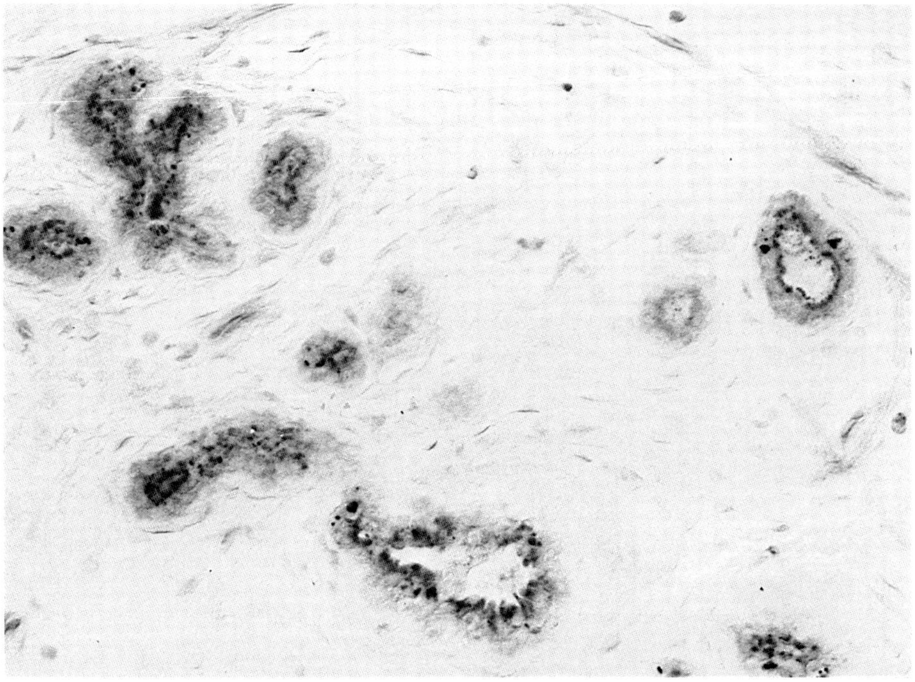

Fig. 1—β-Glucuronidase in normal breast tissue. The epithelial cells have an even reaction which is present in the cytoplasm, between the nucleus and lumen, apart from one acinus where it is in a subluminal position. ×220

(i) β-Glucuronidase—the simultaneous azo-coupling method of Hayashi *et al.*[16] with naphthol-AS-Bl-β-glucuronide as the substrate and an incubation time of 30 min at 37°C.

(ii) β-*N*-Acetyl glucosaminidase—the simultaneous azo-coupling method of Hayashi,[17] naphthol-AS-Bl-β-*N*-acetyl glucosaminide being the substrate with an incubation time of 60 min at 37°C.

(iii) α-Mannosidase—the simultaneous azo-coupling method of Gossrau,[18] with 1-naphthyl-α-mannopyranoside as the substrate and an incubation time of 4 h at 37°C.

(iv) β-D-galactosidase—the indigogenic method of Lojda,[19] 5-bromo-4-chloro-3-indoxyl-β-galactoside being the substrate, with an incubation time of 90 min at 37°C.

Sections were counterstained with 1 per cent aqueous methyl green or nuclear fast red (β-D-galactosidase), dehydrated, cleared and mounted in XAM.

The control for each reaction was the staining of serial sections but with omission of the substrate.

The results were assessed by considering the proportion of cells having a reaction. The categories were: *many* if 70 per cent or more of the tumour cells reacted; *few* if only scattered cells throughout the tumour gave a reaction; and *moderate* for those tumours which fell between the other two grades. Variation in intensity of staining within a given tissue was noted but inter-tissue variation was not assessed.

Histology

Adjacent tissue samples from each case studied by histochemistry was fixed in 4 per cent formaldehyde in 0·15 M sodium chloride solution and routinely processed; haematoxylin and eosin stained sections of this material were examined. The benign breast lesions were divided into two groups: those which were assessed as being relatively normal or showing small foci of mild hyperplastic change and those which had well defined hyperplastic changes (adenosis, epitheliosis, papillomatosis) throughout the samples. Histological differentiation of carcinomas was assessed using the grading criteria of Bloom and Richardson[20] with a modification in that only mitotic figures and not mitotic figures plus hyperchromatic nuclei were considered.[21] The axillary node status was known in 76 of the 100 cases of carcinoma.

RESULTS

Benign breast tissue

Twenty cases were assessed as being relatively normal or showing mild focal hyperplasia, and 20 showed moderate to marked hyperplasia. In none was there definite evidence of atypia.

β-Glucuronidase and β-*N*-acetyl glucosaminidase could be demonstrated in the majority of cells of all acini of all lobules, and in duct epithelium. β-Glucuronidase was localized, in the form of fine rounded granules, to the area of cytoplasm between the nucleus and the luminal periphery of the cells (Fig. 1), but in some instances a subterminal localization, just beneath the luminal cell membrane, was present. β-*N*-Acetyl glucosaminidase could be demonstrated in similar cellular sites but in some lobules was predominantly in the basal parts of the acini (Fig. 2). It was difficult to discern whether the reaction was in myoepithelium or the basal areas of epithelial cells. Variations in intensity of reaction could be seen for both enzymes and was occasionally between acini of an individual lobule but was more frequently between lobules. The reaction was always strong in cells showing apocrine metaplastic change. Acini and ducts showing hyperplastic features generally had a stronger staining for both enzymes than breast epithelium considered to be normal that was present in the same tissue sample.

β-D-Galactosidase and α-mannosidase were either not detectable or only localized in a few acinar cells in all tissues assessed as normal or only showing mild hyperplasia. A similar pattern was found for 11 of the 20 cases which had more prominent hyperplastic change but these were not the same cases for the two enzymes. In those tissues in which these glycosidases were more readily demonstrated the proportion of the epithelium showing a reaction varied from case to case but all were graded no more than moderate. An intra-tissue variation in intensity was often present. Those cells showing a change to apocrine metaplasia consistently gave a strong reaction for both β-D-galactosidase and α-mannosidase. The cellular localization was similar to that described for β-glucuronidase.

There was no evidence of staining in the control sections.

Carcinomas

In most samples examined there were cells

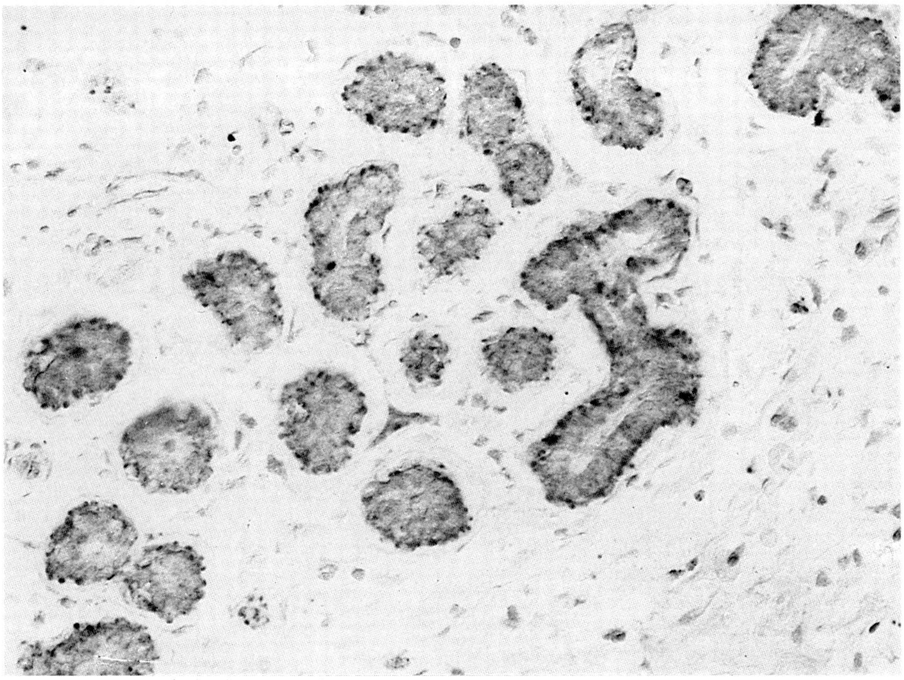

Fig. 2—β-*N*-Acetyl-glucosaminidase in normal breast tissue. The reaction is seen at the base of the epithelial cells and may be present in myoepithelium. ×220

present, either in the stroma or intermingled with tumour cells, that gave a strong reaction for all glycosidases, but in particular β-glucuronidase and β-*N*-acetyl glucosaminidase, and these were clearly macrophages. They could readily be distinguished from tumour cells by the consistency and intensity of their reactions.

Many cells gave a reaction for β-glucuronidase in 76 per cent of carcinomas (Fig. 3), 13 per cent of tumours had a *moderate* number of cells staining and 11 per cent *few* cells reacting. A clearly defined granular reaction could be seen within the cytoplasm of the cells (Fig. 4) with no specific localization apart from some of the better differentiated carcinomas when the reaction could be seen to be between the luminal cell surface and the nucleus in those cells forming tubular structures. In the tumours with *many* cells reacting there was either an even staining intensity or intra-tumour variation, whereas carcinomas with *few* or *moderate* numbers staining tended to show intra-tissue variations in intensity of reaction.

β-*N*-Acetyl glucosaminidase could be demonstrated in *many* cells of 49 per cent of carcinomas. Twenty-seven per cent of tumours had a *moderate* number of cells reacting and 24 per cent a *few* cells. The site and pattern of reaction within the cells was similar to β glucuronidase (Fig. 5) as was the variations in intensity of staining seen.

In contrast to the normal and the hyperplastic tissue 48 per cent of the carcinomas had *many* cells reacting for β-D-galactosidase, and in 52 per cent α-mannosidase was localized to *many* cells. *Moderate* numbers of cells stained for β-D-galactosidase in 21 per cent and for α-mannosidase in 35 per cent, whilst only a *few* cells reacted in 31 per cent (β-D-galactosidase) and 13 per cent (α-mannosidase) of tumours. The numbers concerned are summarized in Table I.

β-D-Galactosidase was seen within tumour cells as a fine granular staining throughout the cytoplasm with, in some cells, the formation of focal dense aggregates (Fig. 6). This appeared to be due to the number of granules in one position rather than staining of a specific cell structure. In a few of the better differentiated carcinomas the reaction was localized to the sub-luminal area of cells related to tubular structures (Fig. 7). Variations in

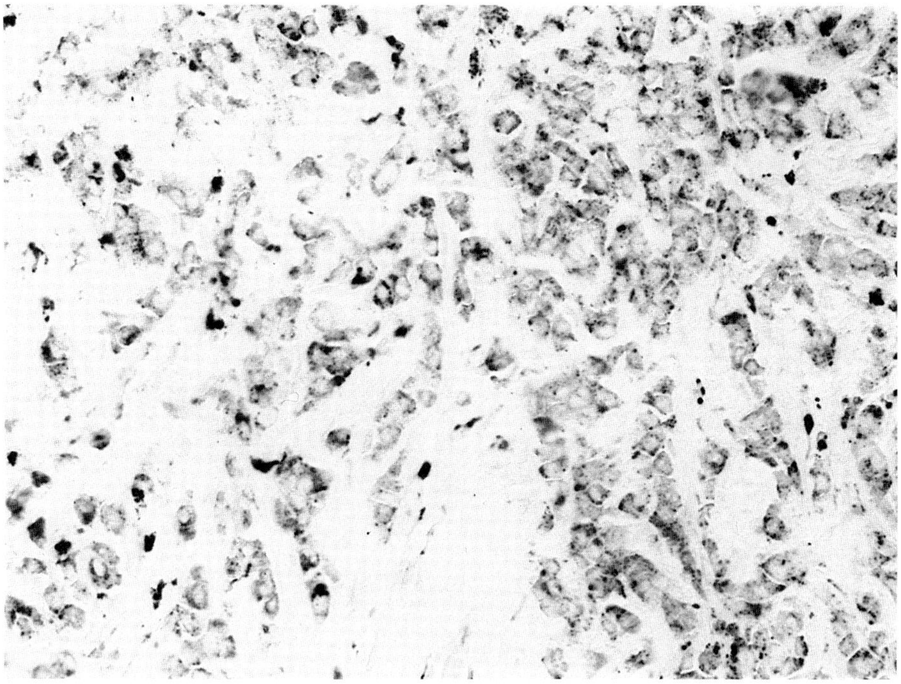

Fig. 3—A moderately differentiated breast carcinoma in which many of the cells give a reaction for β-glucuronidase. ×220

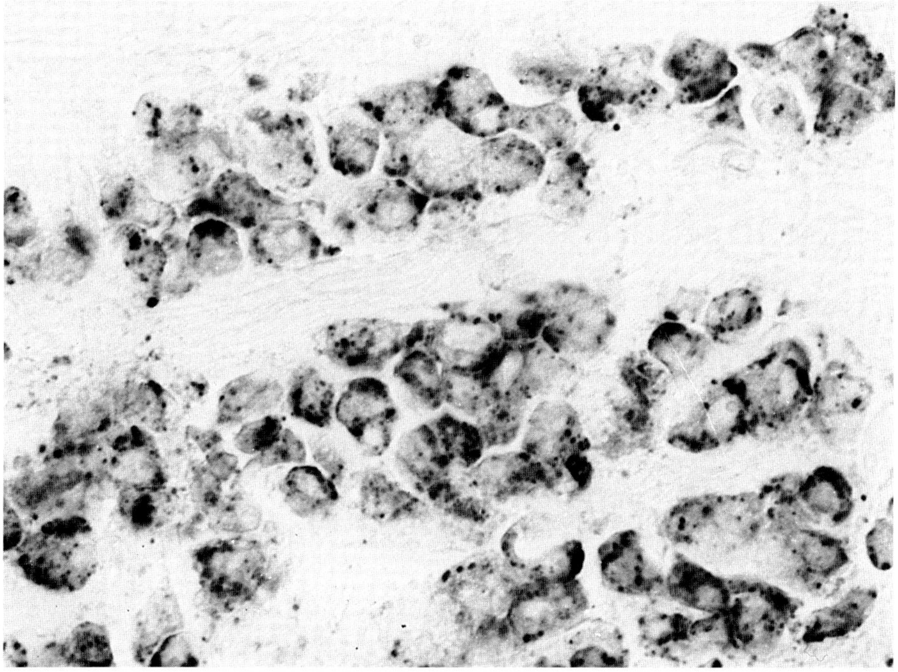

Fig. 4—The same carcinoma as shown in Fig. 3. The reaction is in the form of cytoplasmic granules, presumed lysosomes, of which the numbers vary from cell to cell. ×560

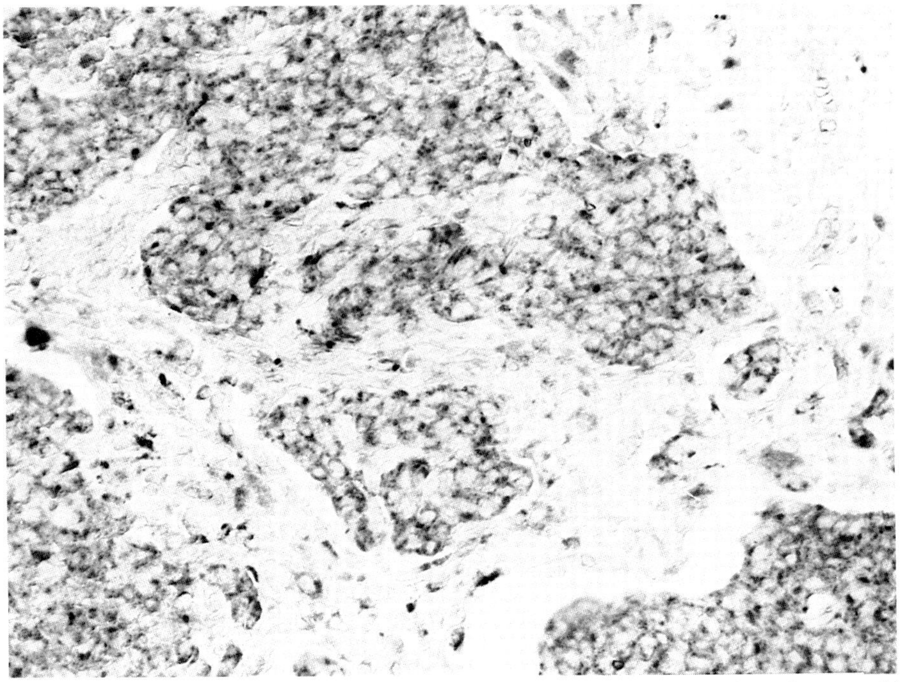

Fig. 5—A moderately differentiated breast carcinoma in which many of the cells have demonstrable β-*N*-acetyl glucosaminidase. ×220

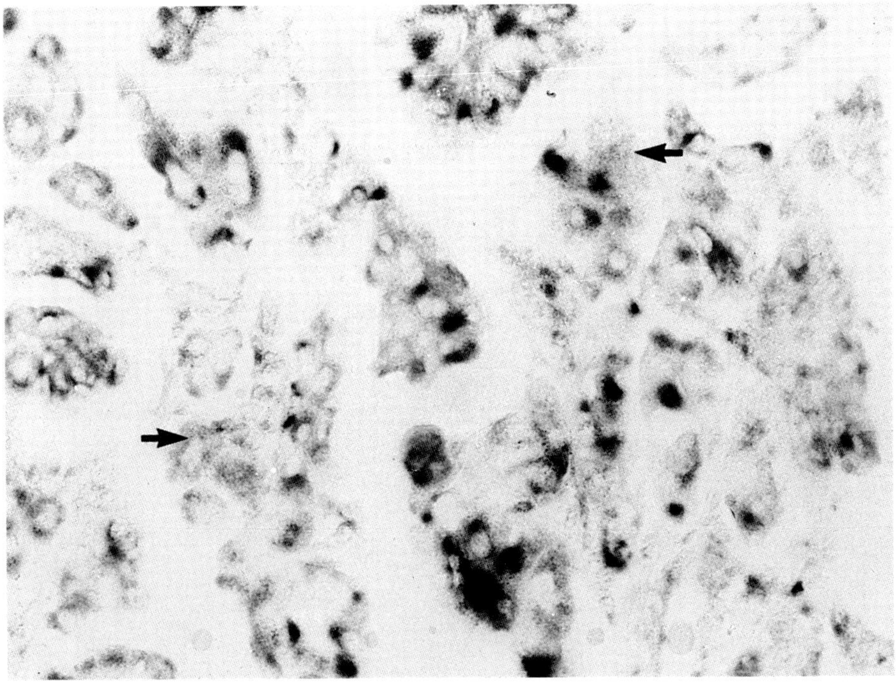

Fig. 6—β-D-Galactosidase within a carcinoma. In some cells the reaction is in the form of discrete small granules (arrowed) whereas in others there is a dense staining product. ×560

Table I—The relationship between the proportion of cells within a carcinoma reacting for each enzyme and histological differentiation

Grade	β-Glucuronidase			β-*N*-Acetyl glucosaminidase			β-D-Galactosidase			α-Mannosidase			Total
	Many	Mod.	Few	Many	Mod.	Few	Many	Mod.	Few	Many	Mod.	Few	
I	7	1	0	8	0	0	5	0	3	1	3	4	8
II	52	7	3	30	17	15	31	14	17	39	20	3	62
III	17	5	8	11	10	9	12	7	12	12	12	6	30
Total	76	13	11	49	17	14	48	21	31	52	35	13	100

Table II—Correlation between the proportion of cells within a tumour reacting for each enzyme and the axillary lymph node status

Axillary lymph node	β-Glucuronidase			β-*N*-Acetyl glucosaminidase			β-D-Galactosidase			α-Mannosidase			Total
	Many	Mod.	Few	Many	Mod.	Few	Many	Mod.	Few	Many	Mod.	Few	
Metastasis	30	5	4	17	14	8	16	8	15	19	16	4	39
Free from tumour	25	5	7	20	7	10	18	7	12	20	10	7	37

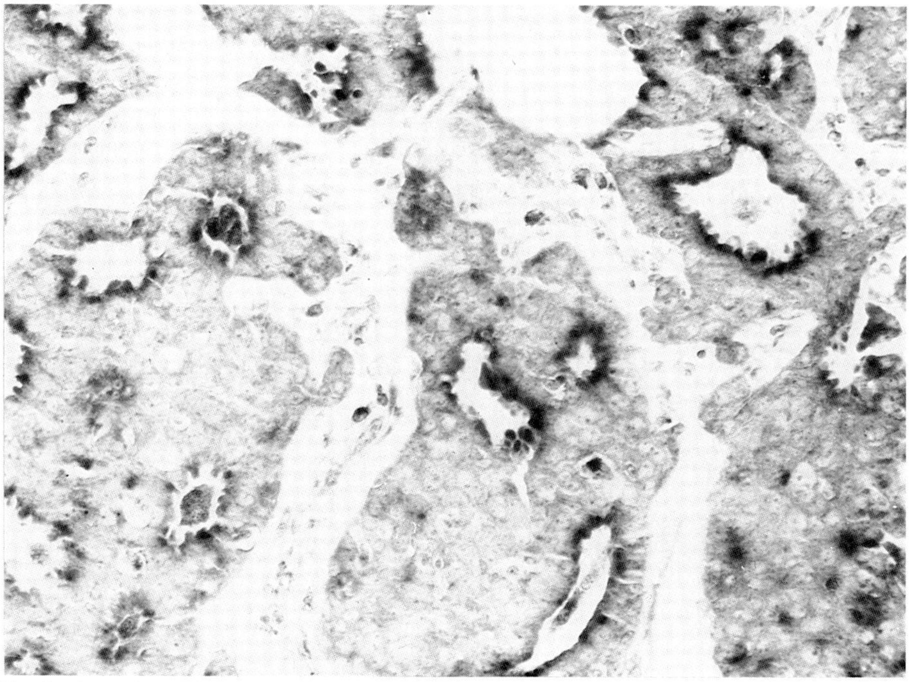

Fig. 7—A carcinoma in which the reaction for β-D-galactosidase is predominantly in cells related to intercytoplasmic lumina, although staining is also seen in the cells of solid aggregates. ×220

intensity could be seen and these seemed to be related to the numbers of granular structures stained within a cell.

Staining for α-mannosidase was in the form of more coarsely granular bodies within tumour cell cytoplasm but the definition of the reaction site was less clear than that seen with the other enzymes. Variations in intensity were noted in most tumours with focal strong staining seen in variable numbers of cells (Fig. 8).

There were 12 carcinomas in which all four enzymes could be demonstrated in *many* of the cells; 10 were moderately differentiated and two poorly differentiated tumours. Comparison of serial sections of individual carcinomas showed that in some instances different enzymes could be identified within the same cells. Four tumours had little evidence of reaction for all glycosidases, with only a *few* cells having detectable enzymes. One was a moderately differentiated carcinoma but the other three poorly differentiated. The other combinations of staining reactions were numerous, and no easily discernible pattern could be found. Although β-D-galactosidase and α-mannosidase were more readily demonstrable in carcinomas than normal and hyperplastic breast there were 16 tumours in which the one enzyme was seen in *few* cells and the other enzyme in *many* cells, and vice versa, and only 29 in which both glycosidases were detected in *many* cells.

The relationship between the proportions of cells within a carcinoma having a reaction for the individual enzyme and the histological differentiation is shown in Table I. There is a significant correlation between the presence of β-glucuronidase ($0{\cdot}02>P>0{\cdot}01$) and β-*N*-acetyl glucosaminidase ($0{\cdot}05>P>0{\cdot}02$) in *many* cells and good histological differentiation. There is no relationship between the proportion of cells with demonstrable β-D-galactosidase and histological differentiation but there is a significant correlation ($0{\cdot}01>P>0{\cdot}001$) between the lack of reactivity for α-mannosidase and better histological differentiation.

The relationship between the staining patterns obtained for each enzyme and lymph node status is shown in Table II. The numbers in each category are fairly equally divided between those carcino-

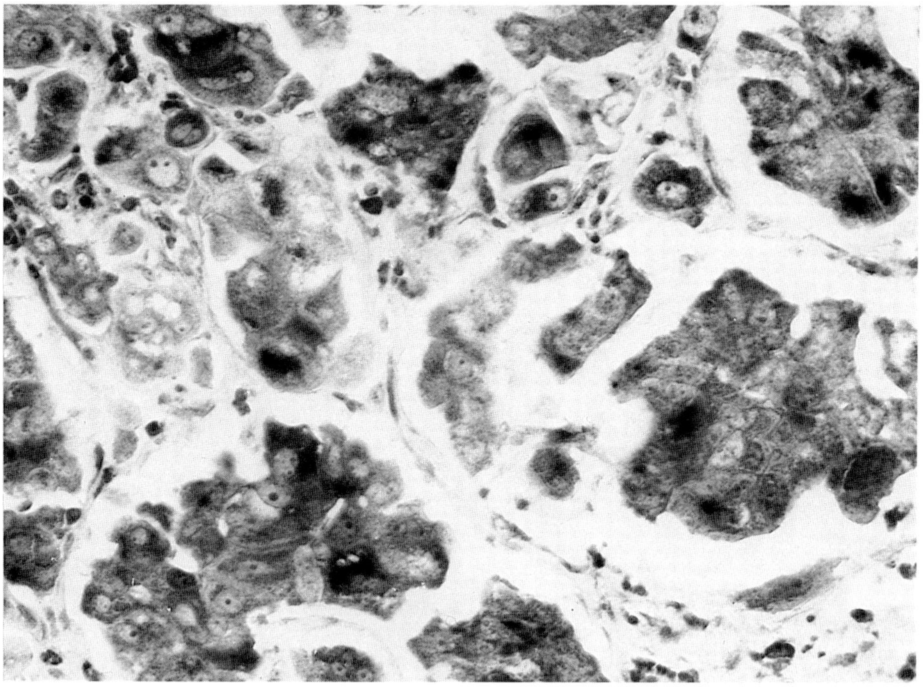

Fig. 8—α-Mannosidase demonstrated in a moderately differentiated carcinoma. The cells have focal dark staining areas of variable sizes. ×560

mas with evidence of axillary lymph node metastasis and those without.

As with the benign breast tissue there was no evidence of staining in control sections.

DISCUSSION

This histochemical study has shown that there are differences between normal, benign and malignant human breast tissue with regard to the detection of four glycosidases; β-*N*-acetyl glucosaminidase and to a lesser extent β-glucuronidase having a decreased incidence of localization in carcinomas, whilst β-D-galactosidase and α-mannosidase are more readily demonstrated in malignant tumours.

All tissue samples studied had been fixed in 4 per cent formol–calcium. Fixation has been shown to lead to a drop in enzyme activity as measured by biochemical assay, with different glycosidases being inactivated to varying degrees.[22] Formaldehyde also alters the enzymes in that they can no longer be solubilized due to having become firmly bound to particles.[23] The use of frozen material could overcome the problem of loss of activity; semi-permeable membranes can be used to prevent the soluble enzymes from diffusing, but even so good localization can be difficult to achieve. For a study in which clear cell definition is required so as to distinguish macrophages from tumour cells a balance between sufficient retention of activity and good localization has to be attained. For the demonstration of lysosomal glycosidases using naphthyl substrates aldehyde fixation is necessary,[24] and so formol–calcium fixation was chosen as the method of tissue preparation for this study, with the proviso that total activity of glycosidases could not be evaluated.

Naphthol AS-BI-β-D-glucuronide is the substrate of choice for the detection of β-glucuronidase since the rate of hydrolysis is high and the low water solubility of the naphthol AS-BI liberated reduces diffusion artefacts.[25,26] Similar criteria apply for naphthol-AS-BI–β-*N*-acetyl glucosaminide.[27] The rate of hydrolysis is, similarly, high for 5-bromo-4-chloro-3-indoxyl-β-*N*-galactoside and the reaction is carried out at the pH optimum for β-D-galactosidase making this the substrate of choice.[19] Although the maximal reaction velocity is higher with the 6-Br-2-naphthyl derivative than with 1-naphthyl-α-D-mannoside it has an uneven binding capacity which can result in poor localization, and so the latter substrate is the one of choice for α-mannosidase.[24]

Quantification was only undertaken in relation to the proportion of cells within a given tissue having evidence of a reaction. Variations in intensity of reaction between tissues were not considered. There are problems in quantifying enzyme activities by histochemical staining techniques. Although a marked drop in activity can occur with fixation, as assessed biochemically, there may be no difference in the density of the coloured reaction product obtained by histochemistry.[23] However, these authors[23] consider that differences in reactions obtained with tissues from the same organ of the same species treated in the same way, as has been done in this study, can be considered to be significant.

β-Glucuronidase and β-*N*-acetyl glucosaminidase were consistently detected in normal and hyperplastic breast tissue but a decrease in localization occurred in carcinomas, which appeared to be related to histological differentiation. Fishman and Anlyan[14] detected increases in β-glucuronidase activity in six breast carcinoma homogenates, using a biochemical assay. Delides *et al.*[28] though, applying a similar approach but on a larger number of cases, found that levels of activity for this enzyme could be elevated, the same, or decreased in comparison to normal tissue. It is difficult to compare biochemical and histochemical results, especially when fixed tissue has been used, but the findings in this study for β-glucuronidase would seem to fit with the results obtained by Delides *et al.*[28]

β-D-Galactosidase and α-mannosidase show the opposite pattern to the other two enzymes, few cells having detectable enzyme in normal breast tissue but with an increase occurring in hyperplastic tissue and approximately half the carcinomas having marked reactivity for the individual enzymes. No discernible relationship between the localization of β-D-galactosidase and histological differentiation could be found but α-mannosidase was less readily demonstrated in the better differentiated tumours, the reverse of what was found for β-glucuronidase and β-*N*-acetyl glucosaminidase. Increased levels of activity for both β-D-galactosidase and α-mannosidase were found on biochemical assay of breast tumour homogenates by Bosmann and Hall.[15] Although these two enzymes are similar in their overall distribution within normal and pathological breast tissue, it does not follow that an alteration in the demonstration of the one enzyme will signify a change for the other since in 32 per cent of carcinomas there was a marked variance in the proportions of cells reacting for the two glycosidases.

One factor that cannot be excluded is that there may be differences in the intracellular localization of the various enzymes between normal and malignant cells, which would not be detected since fixed tissue has been used. For example, α-mannosidase present within the Golgi complex can only be detected by the use of unfixed frozen sections with semi-permeable membranes and therefore the differences found for this enzyme between normal and malignant tissue may reflect a shift in the predominant site of compartmentalization rather than a true increase. However from studies on human skin fibroblasts, it has been proposed that glycosidases are synthesized and processed in the endoplasmic reticulum and Golgi complex and then transported by a complex mechanism to lysosomes,[29] a process that would seem to be more likely to become deranged with neoplastic transformation. Such an alteration in intracellular distribution could account for the differences between normal and neoplastic tissue found for β-glucuronidase and β-*N*-acetyl glucosaminidase but not for β-D-galactosidase and α-mannosidase which have an increased localization in lysosomes.

The significance of the findings in this study are difficult to interpret. Glycosidases have been shown to produce alterations in membrane function[7] and reductions in specificity of cell adhesion[8] but no relationship has been found between increased localization of these enzymes and axillary lymph node metastasis, one possible marker of altered cell–cell contact. Ip and Dao[30] suggested that the increased levels of β-D-galactosidase activity that they found in homogenates of rat mammary tumours could be a function of the tumour growth rate. Graham[31] considered that raised levels of glycosidases in the neoplastic cell may be part of a general increase in degradative enzymes but speculated that such increases could lead to a more effective incorporation of an aberrant transformation-dependent molecule. However, since glycosidases are themselves glycoproteins, any modifications of these enzymes present within neoplastic cells may just be a reflection of the alterations that can occur in such molecules with the malignant process.

ACKNOWLEDGEMENTS

I am grateful to M. E. Eagles and M. E. Allen for excellent technical assistance; Professor F. Walker for helpful criticism of the manuscript; Mrs G. Holmes for secretarial help; and Ms B. Jordan for photographic assistance. Financial assistance was gratefully received from Trent Regional Health Authority.

REFERENCES

1. Flowers HM, Sharon N. Glycosidases—properties and application to the study of complex carbohydrates and cell surfaces. *Adv Enzymol* 1979; **48:** 29.
2. Fishman WH, Goodman SS, DeLellis R. Dual localization of β-glucuronidase in endoplasmic reticulum and in lysosomes. *Nature* 1967; **213:** 457.
3. Grinna LS, Robbins PW. Glycoprotein biosynthesis. Rat liver microsomal glucosidases which process oligo saccharides. *J Biol Chem* 1979; **254:** 8814.
4. Tabas I, Kornfeld S. Purification and characterization of a rat liver Golgi alpha-mannosidase capable of processing asparganine-linked oligosaccharides. *J Biol Chem* 1979; **254:** 11655.
5. Hubbard SC, Ivett RJ. Synthesis and processing of asparganine-linked oligosaccharides. *Annu Rev Biochem* 1981; **50:** 555.
6. Weiss L. The Cell Periphery Metastasis, and Other Contact Phenomena. Amsterdam: North Holland, 1967.
7. Poste G. Changes in susceptibility of normal cells to agglutination by plant lectins following modification of cell coat material. *Exp Cell Res* 1972; **73:** 319.
8. Roth S, McGuire EJ, Roseman S. An assay for intercellular adhesive specificity. *J Cell Biol* 1971; **51:** 525.
9. Warren L, Buck CA. The membrane glycoproteins of the malignant cell. *Clin Biochem* 1980; **13:** 191.
10. Bosmann HB. Glycoprotein degradation: glycosidases in fibroblasts transformed by oncogenic viruses. *Exp Cell Res* 1969; **54:** 217.
11. Bosmann HB, Lockwood T, Morgan HR. Surface biochemical changes accompanying primary infection with Rous sarcoma virus. *Exp Cell Res* 1974; **83:** 25.
12. Blomberg F, Raftell M. Membrane fractions from rat hepatoma II. Immunochemical characterization of detergent-soluble membrane esterases, glycosidases, and leucyl-β-napthylamidase. *Biochim Biophys Acta* 1973; **291:** 431.
13. Sela BA, Lis H, Sharon N, Sachs L. Different locations of carbohydrate containing sites in the surface membrane of normal and transformed mammalian cells. *J Membrane Biol* 1970; **3:** 267.
14. Fishman WH, Anlyan AJ. β-Glucuronidase activity in human tissues some correlations with processes of malignant growth and with the physiology of reproduction. *Cancer Res* 1947; **7:** 808.
15. Bosmann HB, Hall TC. Enzyme activity in invasive tumours of human breast and colon. *Proc Natl Acad Sci USA* 1974; **71:** 1833.
16. Hayashi M, Nakajima Y, Fishman WH. The cytologic demonstration of β-glucuronidase employing naphthol AS-Bl β-glucuronide and hexazonium-P-rosanaline; a preliminary report. *J Histochem Cytochem* 1964; **12:** 293.
17. Hayashi M. Histochemical demonstration of *N*-acetyl-β-glucosaminidase employing naphthol AS-Bl *N*-acetylglucosaminide as a substrate. *J Histochem Cytochem* 1965; **13:** 355.
18. Gossrau R. Uber den histochemischen and mikrochemischen Nachweis der β-glucuronidase, α-galactosidase und α-mannosidase mit l-naphthylglykosiden *Histochemie* 1973; **36:** 367.
19. Lojda Z. Indigogenic methods for glycosidases II. An improved method for β-D-galactosidase and its application to localization studies in the intestine and other tissues. *Histochemie* 1970; **23:** 266.
20. Bloom, HJG, Richardson W. Histological grading and prognosis in breast cancer: a study of 1409 cases of which 359 have been followed for 15 years. *Br J Cancer* 1957; **11:** 359.
21. Walker Rosemary A. The binding of fluorescent-labelled concanavalin-A to human breast tissue—a marker of differentiation. *J Path* 1983; **140:** 255.
22. Janigan DT. Tissue enzyme fixation studies I. The effects of aldehyde fixation on β-glucuronidase, β-galactosidase, *N*-acetyl-β-glucosaminidase, and β-glucosidase in tissue blocks. *Lab Invest* 1964; **13:** 1038.
23. Lake BD, Ellis RB. What do you think you are quantifying? An appraisal of histochemical methods in the measurement of the activities of lysosomal enzymes. *Histochem J* 1976; **8:** 357.
24. Gossrau R. Localization of glycosidases with naphthyl substrates. *Histochem* 1976; **8:** 271.
25. Pearse AGE. Histochemistry: Theoretical and Applied, Vol. 1, 3rd edn. London: Churchill, 1968: 564.
26. Pearse AGE. Histochemistry: Theoretical and Applied, Vol. 2, 3rd edn. London: Churchill, 1972: 816.
27. Lojda Z, Gossrau R, Schiebler TH. Enzyme Histochemistry a Laboratory Manual. Berlin: Springer Verlag, 1969: 159.
28. Delides GS. Tsavaris N, Delides A, Pavlakis E, Lissaios B. The histoenzymological pattern of human breast carcinoma. *Eur J Cancer* 1980; **16:** 1333.
29. Berger EG, Buddecke E, Kamerling JP, Kobata A, Paulson JC, Vliegenthart JFG. Structure, biosynth-

esis and functions of glycoprotein glycans. *Experientia* 1982; **38:** 1129.
30. IP C, Dao TL. Increase in serum and tissue glycosyltransferases and glycosidases in tumor bearing rats. *Cancer Res* 1977; **37:** 3442.
31. Graham JM. In: Hynes RO, ed. Surfaces of Normal and Malignant Cells. Chichester: John Wiley, 1979: 226.

JOURNAL OF PATHOLOGY, VOL. **143**: 51–56 (1984)

ON THE POSSIBLE ORIGIN OF EXTRA-EPITHELIAL ENTEROCHROMAFFIN CELLS BY BUDDING FROM THE CRYPTS OF LIEBERKUHN

PAUL D. MILLIKIN

Department of Pathology, University of Illinois College of Medicine at Peoria, Illinois 61614, U.S.A.

Received 15 September 1983
Accepted 15 December 1983

SUMMARY

This study was undertaken to test Pierre Masson's still unconfirmed theory that extra-epithelial enterochromaffin cells in the gut arise in adult life by budding from the crypts of Lieberkuhn under conditions of low grade inflammation. Appendices (900) were reviewed and 19 were selected for serial section study because in random sections they showed lateral fusion of the crypts, one of the key features described by Masson. Ten specimens without crypt fusion served as controls. Sixteen of the 19 study specimens and one of the control specimens showed budding, averaging one bud in every 88 sections. Most buds were in direct contact with Schwann cells in the adjacent lamina propria and 45 per cent of them contained enterochromaffin cells. There was also histologic evidence linking buds and lateral crypt fusion to low grade inflammation. Masson's ideas are, therefore, confirmed insofar as the existence of buds and their relationship to enterochromaffin cells, Schwann cells, and inflammation is concerned. The actual separation of buds from the crypts to form extra-epithelial enterochromaffin cells has yet to be proved.

KEY WORDS—Enterochromaffin cell, APUD cell, appendix, Schwann cell, neuroendocrine cell.

INTRODUCTION

For many years, enterochromaffin (EC) cells were regarded as a mildly interesting laboratory curiosity, worth studying only in so far as they might give rise to carcinoid tumours. However, recent developments in molecular biology and neurochemistry have aroused the suspicion that they and their neuroendocrine cousins not only have a definite neural function, but may even form a whole new division of the nervous system, perhaps equally as important to bodily functions as the autonomic branch.[1] The magnitude of that possibility has understandably kindled new interest in their behavour.

Originally thought to be purely epithelial, EC cells are now known also to be capable of independent existence in the lamina propria, where they are invariably surrounded by Schwann cells and unmyelinated nerve fibres.[2–4] Whether epithelial EC cells originate from the neural crest or locally from the crypt epithelium has been the subject of much international debate, but relatively few studies have asked where the extraepithelial enterochromaffin (EEEC) cells come from. It is the purpose of this paper to reopen that question.

Perhaps the leading theory on their origin was propounded many years ago by Pierre Masson, who thought that they arise by budding from the crypt epithelium.[5,6] Unfortunately, his idea was given rather short shrift by his colleagues, apparently because of a technical problem.

He was the first to describe the association between EEEC cells and Schwann cells, and one of his criteria for identifying the Schwann cells was that their unmyelinated nerve fibres stained pink with his own trichrome stain. He conceded that they did not stain at all with the silver stains then in common use, but saw no reason to change his mind about their identity. Perhaps understandably, his neuropathologic colleagues would not accept that discrepancy, but regrettably, in rejecting his

Addressee for communications and reprint requests: Paul D. Millikin, M.D., Department of Pathology, Proctor Community Hospital, 5409 North Knoxville, Peoria, Illinois 61614, U.S.A.

0022–3417/84/050051–06$01.00

technique, they apparently rejected his whole theory as well, and it has never been revived.

However, electron microscopy has now vindicated him completely and proved the identity of the Schwann cells beyond doubt,[4] so it seems only just, as well as prudent, to reconsider Masson's ideas and to reopen the whole subject.

In brief, he found thin epithelial buds near the bottoms of the crypts, many of them containing EC cells, and most of them in contact with Schwann cells in the adjacent lamina propria. He thought that inflammation somehow stimulated buds to form, and that as they grew, some of their cells differentiated into enterochromaffin cells which then sought out the neural elements in the lamina propria. Later the buds appeared to constrict at their origins and to separate from the crypts, leaving a cluster of enterochromaffin cells (now EEEC cells) lying free in the lamina propria, surrounded by Schwann cells.

Masson published this rather startling idea only after studying serial sections of 1200 appendices and finding buds in 15 of them (1·25 per cent). Even so, in his prize specimen, where buds were the most numerous, he found them on an average of only once in every 17 sections. Because of the monumental amount of work involved, he noted that 'finding buds is a matter of perseverance', and was unwilling to accept criticism from anyone who had not examined a like amount of material. To date, no one has been willing to do that, although several authors have supported him in part.[7–12]

Fortunately for those of us less persevering than Masson, he left several useful clues. Clinically, most of his budded specimens were removed from young adults with mild appendicitis, and histologically, most of them contained crypts which were fused laterally near their lower ends, forming a previously undescribed histologic pattern.

During a previous study,[4] we found a specimen with fused crypts, and on examining it serially, were rewarded with what appeared to be a bud. We thereupon decided to look for more specimens with fused crypts, hoping to learn conclusively whether Masson was right. The preliminary results are reported here.

METHODS

Surgically removed appendices (900), including those removed for acute appendicitis as well as those removed incidental to other abdominal surgery, were reviewed for lateral crypt fusion and 19 suitable specimens were found (2 per cent). The sections were cut at 5 μm, averaging 244 sections per specimen. All sections were stained by the Fontana–Masson silver procedure and counterstained with haematoxylin and eosin. Schwann cells were identified as previously described.[4]

Sixteen of the 19 appendices (84 per cent) also showed 'acute focal appendicitis' (AFA), with purulent exudate in the lumen but not in the wall.[13] Therefore, for control purposes, the remaining 881 specimens were again reviewed, this time for AFA only, without crypt fusion. Fifty-seven were found (6 per cent), and the 10 best preserved were selected for serial study. By definition, AFA is focal and, therefore, not present in each section on every slide. For that reason, one suitable section with exudate in its lumen was selected from each slide for further study. The corresponding tissue was removed from the original paraffin block, re-embedded singly, and processed like the specimens in the study group.

RESULTS

Lateral crypt fusion was easy to recognize in random sections. Sometimes two crypts were

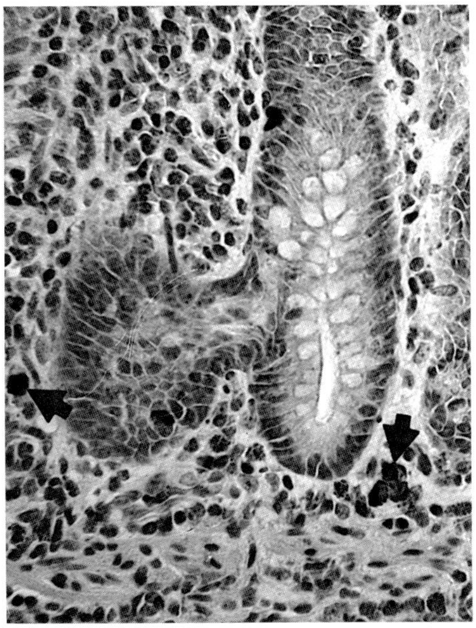

Fig. 1—Laterally fused crypts with common lumen. Note mucosal EC cells (arrows). Fontana–Masson, H & E, ×300

completely fused and had a common lumen (Fig. 1), but more often, fusion was only partial (Fig. 2), creating a pattern aptly labelled by a pathology resident as 'the kissing crypts'. Both patterns were easily distinguished from the more common crypt bifurcation (Fig. 3) which occurs in the reparative phase of inflammatory bowel disease.[14]

Buds were found in 16 of the 19 appendices in the study group (84 per cent), averaging one bud in every 88 sections, and ranging from one in 53 sections to one in 207. Seventeen buds contained EC cells (Figs 4–7), and all abutted on Schwann cells in the adjacent lamina propria. Another 21 buds had no EC cells (Fig. 8) and 18 of them (86 per cent) were in contact with Schwann cells. The number of buds per specimen varied from one to four. These findings and the clinical data are summarized in Table I. Finally, the Schwann cells adjacent to the buds were frequently present in markedly increased numbers, confirming Masson's impression of hyperplasia in the mucous plexus. It was very difficult to photograph Schwann cells by light microscopy (Fig. 6), but electron microscopy left no doubt about their identity.

In the control group, two buds were found, both in the same specimen. Both contained EC cells and

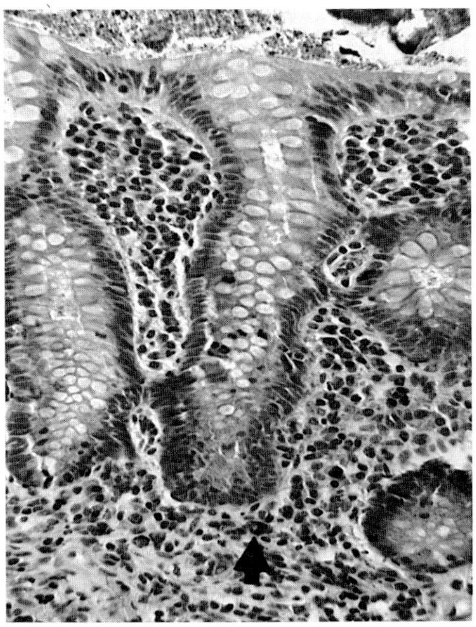

Fig. 2—Crypts with multiple areas of lateral fusion. Note mucosal EC cells (arrows). Fontana–Masson, H & E, ×300

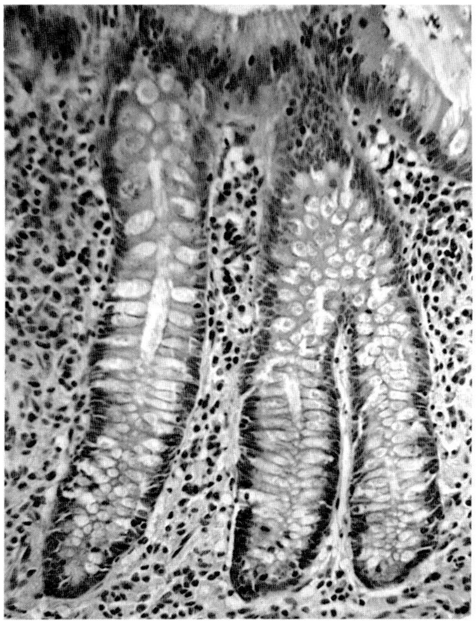

Fig. 3—Crypt bifurcation like that seen in inflammatory bowel disease. Fontana-Masson, H & E, ×300

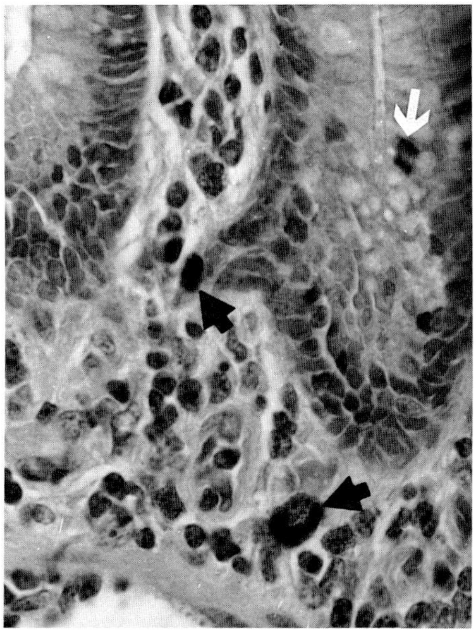

Fig. 4—Bud with a single EC cell in the tip. Black arrows indicate EC cells. White arrow shows a mitotic figure. Fontana–Masson, H & E, ×550

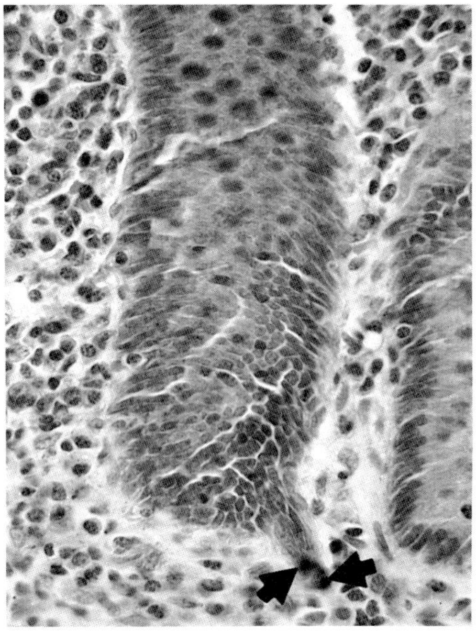

Fig. 5—Bud with two EC cells in the tip (arrows). Fontana–Masson, H & E, ×550

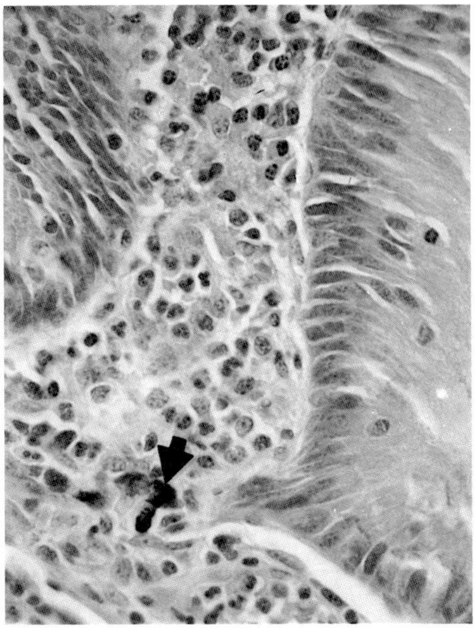

Fig. 7—Bud touching a cluster of mucosal EC cells (arrow). Note the possible line of constriction between the two. Fontana–Masson, H & E, ×550

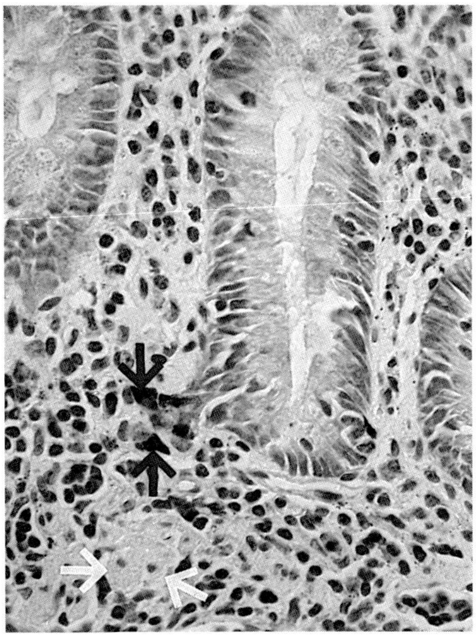

Fig. 6—Bud with a cluster of EC cells in the tip. (Between black arrows.) Schwann cells are just discernible (white arrows). Fontana–Masson, H & E, ×550

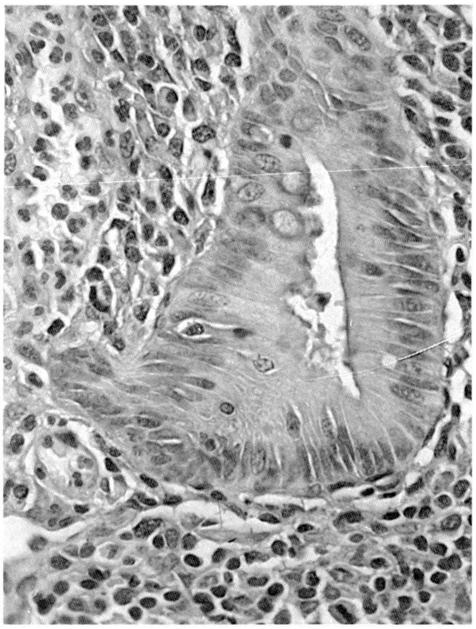

Fig. 8—Bud without EC cells. Fontana–Masson, H & E, ×550

were in contact with Schwann cells. The clinical data for this group are summarized in Table II.

Masson's clinical findings were also corroborated to some extent by this study. Note in Table I that all of the specimens from male patients contained buds and that five of those six patients had primary appendectomies because of appendiceal symptoms. Their average age was 12. The oldest male, aged 36, had an incidental appendectomy during surgery for gallbladder disease.

Table I—Number of buds per specimen—lateral crypt fusion group

Case	Age	Sex	Surgery*	EC† buds	No. EC‡ buds	AFA§
1	5	M	Prim.	0	1	+
2	10	M	Prim.	2	4	+
3	13	M	Prim.	1	0	+
4	13	M	Prim.	1	1	+
5	20	M	Prim.	1	0	+
6	36	M	Incid.	1	0	+
7	18	F	Incid.	1	0	0
8	19	F	Incid.	1	0	0
9	21	F	Incid.	2	0	+
10	22	F	Incid.	2	0	+
11	26	F	Incid.	0	3	+
12	45	F	Incid.	3	1	0
13	45	F	Incid.	0	5	+
14	52	F	Incid.	0	1	+
15	57	F	Incid.	1	5	+
16	61	F	Incid.	1	0	+
17	9	F	Prim.	0	0	+
18	11	F	Prim.	0	0	+
19	32	F	Incid.	0	0	+

* Type of surgery. Primary appendectomy or appendectomy incidental to other abdominal surgery.
† Number of buds containing EC cells.
‡ Number of buds with no EC cells.
§ Presence or absence of acute focal appendicitis.

Table II—Number of buds per specimen—AFA group no lateral crypt fusion

Case	Age	Sex	Surgery*	EC† buds	No. EC‡ buds
1	58	M	Incid.	0	0
2	24	F	Incid.	2	0
3	25	F	Incid.	0	0
4	27	F	Incid.	0	0
5	27	F	Incid.	0	0
6	29	F	Incid.	0	0
7	43	F	Incid.	0	0
8	45	F	Incid.	0	0
9	46	F	Incid.	0	0
10	57	F	Incid.	0	0

* Type of surgery. Primary appendectomy for appendiceal symptoms or incidental appendectomy during other surgery.
† Number of buds with EC cells.
‡ Number of buds with no EC cells.

All the females whose appendices contained buds also had incidental appendectomies during other abdominal surgery. Their average age was 37. No explanation was found for these age and sex differences.

In the control group, the specimen with buds came from a 24 year old woman and was removed incidental to cholecystectomy.

DISCUSSION

This study confirms Masson's claims that epithelial buds do exist, are associated with EC cells, Schwann cells, and inflammation, and are detectable only by means of serial sections or fantastically good luck. However, it does not appear necessary to cut serial sections on 80 different specimens in order to find one bud, as Masson was compelled to do, because he left data which permit screening for a much higher yield.

For example, in the study group with lateral crypt fusion, the yield was 16 out of 19 specimens, or 84 per cent, in contrast to Masson's figure of 15 out of 1200, or 1·25 per cent for all appendices, and to the control (AFA) group figure of one out of 10 or 10 per cent. Therefore, looking for buds has now become a manageable chore if one begins by initially screening the specimens for lateral crypt fusion. If the selected specimens also show AFA and are removed from young males with appendiceal symptoms, then so much the better.

Perhaps now the emphasis can be shifted from whether or not buds exist to what they do. Masson's theory that they give rise to EEEC cells is still the most plausible explanation and is certainly worth pursuing to a definite conclusion. However, even if it proves true, there is still the unsolved problem of the EEEC cells and what *their* function is.

Masson apparently considered them to occur normally in young adults, although their close association with inflammation suggests that they may be pathologic. In this study, they were found in 89 per cent of the specimens with crypt fusion, and 100 per cent of those in the control group. In another series they occurred in at least 50 per cent of random sections through unselected appendices,[4] so they are certainly very common, whether they occur normally in uninflamed appendices or not.

Their constant association with Schwann cells and nerve fibres, the presence of the neurotransmitter substance serotonin in their granules and the presence of neuron-specific enolase in their cytoplasm[3] offer strong circumstantial evidence that they may indeed belong to the nervous system. Certainly their ability to grow without epithelial support suggests that they can no longer be considered purely epithelial.

Finally, both Masson's data and ours indicate that EEEC cells and the two factors of budding and mucous plexus hyperplasia are all closely linked to low grade inflammation in some unknown manner. It has been noted that these phenomena may be associated with the reparative phase of inflammation, when proliferation of cells of all kinds is the rule.[4] That raises the interesting possibility that one or more discoverable growth factors might be released into the exudate to account for the increase in neural elements and EEEC, and perhaps even for buds and 'kissing crypts' as well.

REFERENCES

1. Pearse AGE. The diffuse neuroendocrine system: falsification and verification of a concept. In: Grossman MI, Brazier MAB, Lechago J, eds. Cellular Basis of Chemical Messengers in the Digestive System. New York: Academic Press, 1981: 13–19.
2. Auböck L, Ratzenhofer M. 'Extra-epithelial enterochromaffin cell–nerve fibre complexes' in the normal human appendix and in neurogenic appendicopathy. *J Pathol* 1982; **136:** 217–226.
3. Rode J, Dhillon AP, Papadaki L, Griffiths D. Neurosecretory cells of the lamina propria of the appendix and their possible relationship to carcinoids. *Histopathol* 1982; **6:** 69–79.
4. Millikin PD. Extra-epithelial enterochromaffin cells in the human appendix. *Arch Pathol Lab Med* 1983; **107:** 189–194.
5. Masson P. Carcinoids (argentaffin-cell tumors) and nerve hyperplasia of the appendicular mucosa. *Am J Pathol* 1928; **4:** 181–212.
6. Masson P. Neural proliferations in the vermiform appendix. In: Penfield W, ed. Cytology and Cellular Pathology of the Nervous System. New York: Paul B Hoeber, Inc, Vol. 3, 1932: 1095–1130.
7. Schack L. Über die gelben Zellen im menschlichen Wurmfortsatz. *Beitr Pathol* 1932; **90:** 441–478.
8. Simard LC. On the frequency of nervous lesions of the vermiform appendix: 'neuroappendicopathy'. *Can Med Assoc J* 1935; **33:** 518–521.
9. Lassmann G. Zum Problem der neurogenen Appendizitis, *Mikrosk* 1949; **4:** 277–295.
10. Isaacson NH, Blades B. Neuroappendicopathy. Review of the literature and report on 52 cases. *Arch Surg* 1951; **62:** 455–466.
11. Feyrter F. Über die peripheren endokrinen (parakrinen) Drüsen des Menschen. Wien: Wilhelm Maudrich, 1953.
12. Kazzaz BA. Argentaffin and argyrophil cells in the appendix. *J Pathol* 1971; **104:** 206–209.
13. Schenken JR, Anderson TR, Coleman FC. Acute focal appendicitis. *Am J Clin Pathol* 1956; **26:** 352–359.
14. Yardley JH, Donowitz M. Colo-rectal biopsy in inflammatory bowel disease. In: Yardley JH, Morson BC, Abell MR, eds. The Gastrointestinal Tract. Baltimore: The Williams and Wilkins Co, 1977: 63, 65.

JOURNAL OF PATHOLOGY, VOL. **143**: 57–68 (1984)

ULTRASTRUCTURAL LOCALIZATION OF ANIONIC AND CATIONIC FERRITIN IN THE RAT GLOMERULAR BASEMENT MEMBRANE IN PROTEIN-OVERLOAD PROTEINURIA

D. J. BLISS AND D. B. BREWER

Department of Pathology, Medical School, University of Birmingham, Birmingham B15 2TJ, England

Received 6 December 1983
Accepted 27 January 1984

SUMMARY

The penetration into the glomerular basement membrane of anionic and cationic ferritin has been studied in rats made proteinuric by intraperitoneal administration of bovine serum albumin. In comparison with control animals anionic ferritin penetrated the glomerular basement membrane to a much greater extent in proteinuric rats. Some ferritin particles were observed in small invaginations of the epithelial cell membrane adjacent to the glomerular basement membrane and incorporated in pinocytotic vesicles within the epithelial cell cytoplasm. This was not seen in control animals. Cationic ferritin distribution in the glomerular basement membrane was similar in control and proteinuric rats suggesting that the increased anionic ferritin penetration observed occurs without any reduction in fixed anionic charge.

KEY WORDS—Proteinuria, glomerulus, glomerular basement membrane.

INTRODUCTION

Repeated intraperitoneal administration of heterologous serum albumin has been frequently reported to result in the development of proteinuria.[1–9] In the female Wistar rat, proteinuria induced by intraperitoneal administration of 5 g of bovine serum albumin (BSA) over 5 days is associated with marked changes in glomerular morphology. However, even in rats with very heavy proteinuria (>500 mg/day) only about 80 per cent of the glomeruli are affected, the remainder appearing normal.[6]

Native anionic ferritin and a cationic derivative of ferritin have been used by many authors as electron-opaque particulate tracers in the study of glomerular basement membrane (GBM) charge and permeability, both in normal and diseased states in experimental animals.[10–15] In the present study we have investigated the relationship between ultrastructural damage and glomerular permeability by comparing the degree of penetration of anionic and cationic ferritin into the GBM with the degree of foot process loss following induction of proteinuria.

Addressee for correspondence: D. J. Bliss, Department of Pathology, Medical School, University of Birmingham, Birmingham B15 2TJ, England.

0022–3417/84/050057–12$01.20

MATERIALS AND METHODS

Female Wistar rats (Bantin and Kingman, Hull, U.K.), weight range 166–250 g, were used. The rats were given free access to a standard pellet diet and water throughout the experiment. Eight rats were given an intraperitoneal injection of 0·5 g BSA (Cohn V, Sigma A4503) as a 20 per cent solution in distilled water twice daily for 5 days. Eight control rats received distilled water only. On days 4 and 5 the rats were housed in individual metabolic cages, urine was collected and the total protein excretion per 24 h estimated by the Biuret method following trichloroacetic acid precipitation of protein.

Preparation of ferritin

Anionic (native) horse spleen ferritin in 0·15 M NaCl (Sigma) was twice dialysed against 2000 ml 0·05 M ethylenediaminetetraacetic acid in phosphate buffered saline (pH 7·4) for 24 h at 4°C and then twice dialysed against 2000 ml phosphate buffered saline (pH 7·4) at 4°C for 12 h.[16] The anionic ferritin was used as a 10 per cent solution.

Cationic ferritin was prepared from the anionic ferritin by the method of Danon *et al.*[17] as modified by Kanwar and Farquhar.[15] Briefly, 100 mg of anionic ferritin was reacted with 25 mg of the carboxyl group activator 1-ethyl-3(3-dimethylaminopropyl)carbodiimide and 4 ml of 2 M *N,N*-dimethyl-1,3-propanediamine (a nucleophile) at pH 7·0 for 2 h. After modification the ferritin was purified on a Sephadex G25 column using 0·15 M NaCl as the eluent and then concentrated by negative pressure dialysis.

The isoelectric points (p*I*) of the anionic and cationic ferritin preparations were determined by isoelectric focusing on thin layer agarose plates. The p*I* of anionic ferritin was 4·1–4·6 and that of the cationic ferritin 6·8–7·4.

Ferritin administration

Following 5 days of intraperitoneal administration of BSA or distilled water, rats were anaesthetized with an intraperitoneal injection of Sagatal (sodium pentobarbitone, 6 mg/100 g body weight; May and Baker). Blood pressure was recorded via a carotid cannula which was connected to a pressure transducer (Bell and Howell); the left femoral vein was cannulated for ferritin infusion. Anionic ferritin (100 mg/100 g body weight) or cationic ferritin (50 mg/100 g body weight) was infused over 10 min at a rate of 0·2 ml/min using a constant infusion pump (Sage Instruments, Syringe Pump Model 355). Four BSA-injected and four control rats received anionic ferritin, four BSA-injected and four control rats received cationic ferritin. At 15 min after the completion of the anionic ferritin infusion or 30 min after the completion of the cationic ferritin infusion the left kidney was removed and tissue taken for transmission electron microscopy.

Tissue processing

Samples of renal cortical tissue were fixed in 2·5 per cent glutaraldehyde in 0·1 M sodium cacodylate buffer (pH 7·4) for 1·5 h at 4°C, washed in cacodylate buffer then postfixed in 1 per cent osmium tetroxide for 1·5 h at 4°C. The tissue was dehydrated in alcohol, embedded in Araldite and ultrathin sectioned to give sections with a pale gold interference colour.[18] Grids were either stained with lead citrate or viewed unstained in a JEOL 100S electron microscope at 80 kV.

Morphometry

Morphometric assessment of foot process loss was based on the method of Pinto and Brewer.[19] Ten randomly chosen fields (× 1·4K) from different glomeruli were selected from each animal. The percentage of the GBM covered by normal foot processes was determined by intercept counting on photographic prints at a final magnification of 4·2K. Foot processes wider than 1·07 μm (4·5 mm at this magnification) were considered to be abnormal. Intercept counting was performed over the whole length of the GBM and not just the peripheral basement membrane as in the study by Pinto and Brewer.[19]

Assessment of the degree of penetration of the GBM by anionic and cationic ferritin was performed on unstained sections. Two areas of GBM, not adjacent to mesangium, were randomly chosen from each of the lower power fields described above. These were photographed at 28K and printed at 98K. Ferritin counts were made over a 1·53 μm length of basement membrane (15 cm at this magnification). As it was not possible to clearly delimit the layers of the GBM, the lamina densa was taken to be the central three-fifths of the basement membrane. Total ferritin counts were made in the laminae rarae, the lamina densa and in an area of adjacent capillary lumen equal in size to that of the GBM.

Statistical analysis

The results are expressed as the mean ± S.E.M. The significance of differences between control and experimental group means was assessed by Student's *t*-test.

RESULTS

Proteinuria and glomerular foot process loss

Intraperitoneal administration of BSA over 5 days to female Wistar rats resulted in heavy

Table I—The 24 h urine output and protein excretion on day 5 of injection compared with loss of discrete foot processes

	No. of animals	No. of glomeruli	Urine output ml/24 h	Protein output mg/24 h	Percentage glomerular basement membrane without foot processes
Controls	8	80	6·93 ± 1·15	2·29 ± 0·33	18·99 ± 0·69
BSA-injected	8	80	7·85± 1·36	377·03 ± 112·88	48·60 ± 2·93
P			N.S.	<0·01	<0·001

N.S.—not significant.

proteinuria and marked changes in glomerular ultrastructure. The level of protein excretion in the albumin-injected animals was very variable, the range being 97·23–1087·02 mg/24 h on day 5 of injection. All control animals excreted less than 4 mg protein/24 h. The ultrastructural changes associated with protein-overload proteinuria have been described in detail elsewhere.[6,9,20] Briefly, the glomerular epithelial cells were swollen with many large pale vacuoles and dark protein droplets in their cytoplasm. There was extensive loss of discrete foot processes however no areas were observed where the epithelial cell layer had become detached from the GBM although this has been previously described in protein-overload proteinuria[6,20,21] and in puromycin aminonucleoside nephrosis.[22,23] Even in the most heavily proteinuric animals there were some glomeruli that appeared ultrastructurally normal.

The 24 h urinary output and urinary protein loss on day 5 of injection as well as the degree of foot process loss were not significantly different in control and experimental animals receiving anionic ferritin compared to those receiving cationic ferritin. Therefore, these results for both groups were combined and are presented in Table I.

Blood pressure

The mean arterial blood pressure in all animals used remained above 100 mm Hg for the duration

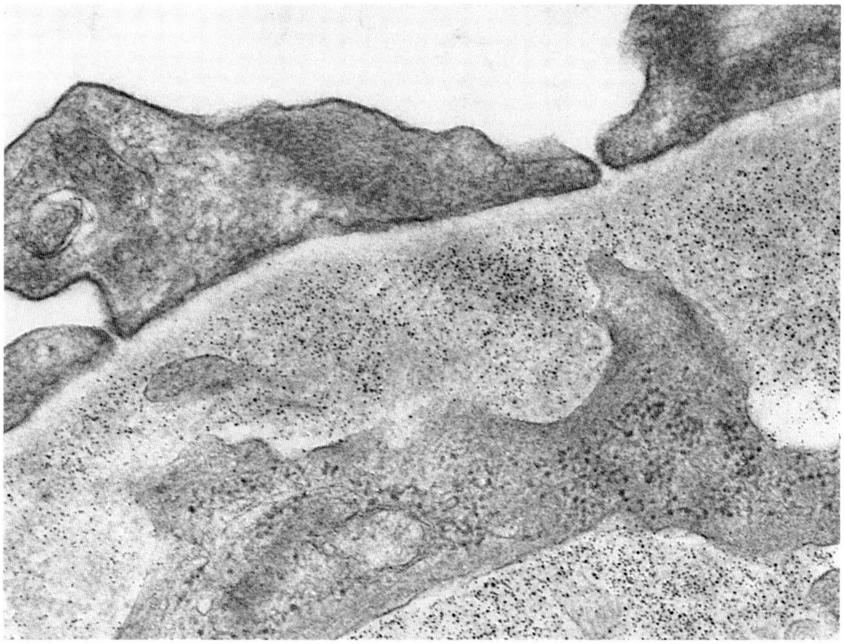

Fig. 1—Anionic ferritin in the mesangial matrix of a proteinuric rat. Lead citrate. × 45 000

of the experiment. Infusion of ferritin (anionic or cationic) occasionally produced a slight fall in blood pressure of 5–10 mm Hg. The blood pressure recovered before the end of the infusion and then remained stable for the rest of the experiment.

Ferritin distribution

Anionic ferritin—Following infusion, large numbers of anionic ferritin particles were found in the capillary lumen of glomeruli from both control and BSA injected rats. The numbers in each group were not significantly different. Particularly large amounts of ferritin were found to accumulate in the mesangial matrix (Fig. 1). There was a very marked gradient in ferritin concentration between the capillary lumen and the lamina rara interna showing that this layer formed a major barrier to the filtration of ferritin. The number of ferritin particles in each of the 3 layers of the GBM is shown in Fig. 2. As can be seen, in control animals most of the anionic ferritin is restricted to the lamina rara interna with very little penetrating as far as the lamina rara externa. In proteinuric animals greater amounts of ferritin penetrate the GBM. There is no longer a gradient between the

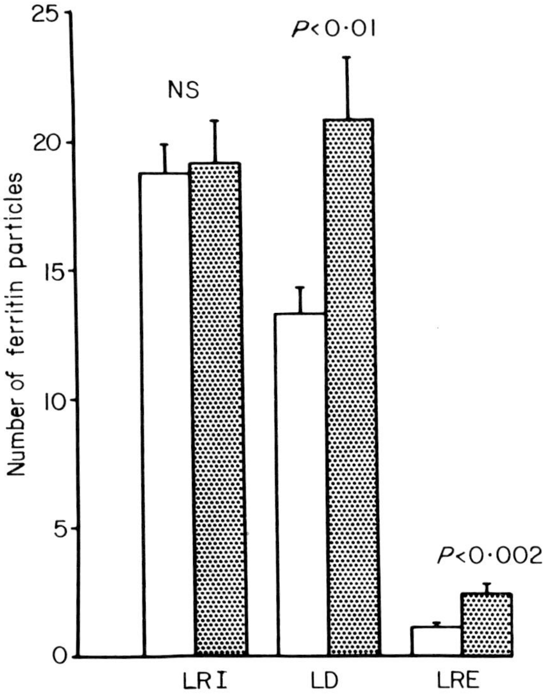

Fig. 2—Distribution of anionic ferritin in GBM from control and proteinuric rats. Controls—open columns; proteinurics—shaded columns. LRI—lamina rara interna; LD—lamina densa; LRE—lamina rara externa. N.S.—not significant

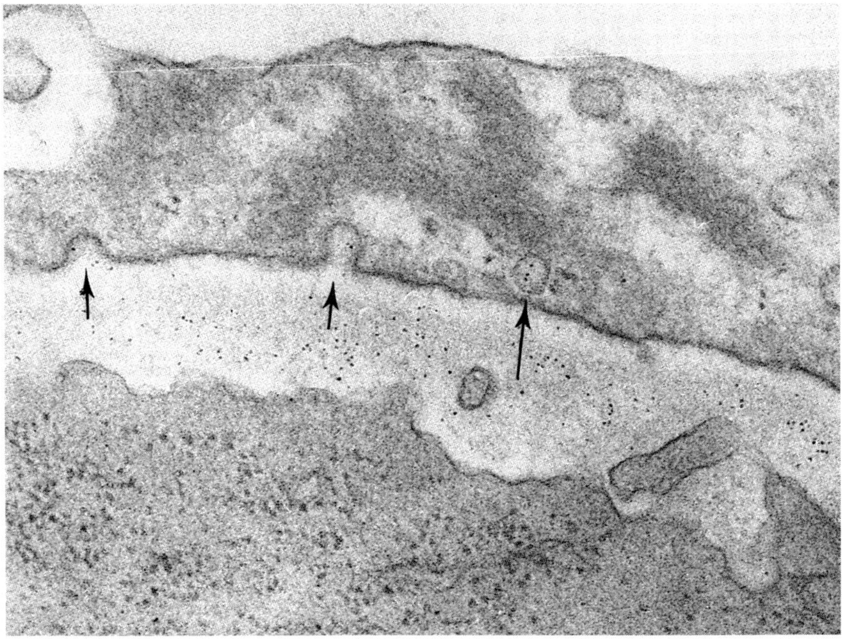

Fig. 3—Epithelial cell from proteinuric rat showing anionic ferritin in small invaginations of the cell membrane (short arrows) and within a small vesicle in the cell cytoplasm (long arrow). Lead citrate. ×63 000

lamina rara interna and lamina densa, and significantly more ferritin is present in the lamina densa and lamina rara externa than in control animals. In proteinuric animals ferritin was found to accumulate in small invaginations of the epithelial cell membrane adjacent to the GBM or within small vesicles present in the epithelial cell cytoplasm (Figs 3, 4). This was not observed in control animals.

The degree of ferritin penetration was not uniform throughout the GBM of proteinuric animals. Greatest penetration was found to occur in regions of the GBM underlying a continuous layer of epithelium (Table IIa, Fig 5a–5c).

Cationic ferritin—As with anionic ferritin, large amounts of cationic ferritin were found to accumulate in the mesangial matrix. However, in contrast, cationic ferritin was found to penetrate the basement membrane to a much greater extent in both control and proteinuric rats than anionic ferritin (compare Figs 2 and 6, note the difference in scales of the ordinates). Cationic ferritin was localized mainly in the lamina rara interna and externa often appearing in clumps with a separation of 50–70 nm (Fig. 7). Cationic ferritin in the lamina densa appeared to be randomly distributed. Ferritin was also found in small invaginations and vesicles of the epithelial cells with a greater frequency than observed following administration of anionic ferritin to proteinuric animals.

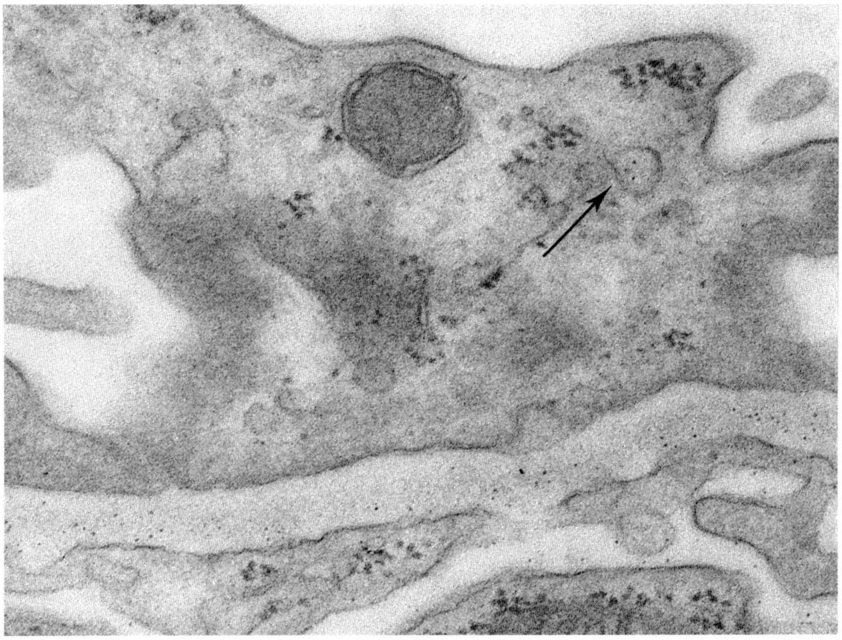

Fig. 4—Anionic ferritin in epithelial cell vesicle (arrow) of proteinuric rat. Lead citrate. ×63 000

It was of interest to see whether the basement membrane permeability to ferritin was different in the ultrastructurally damaged glomeruli compared to glomeruli with a normal appearance in BSA-treated rats. Damaged glomeruli were taken to be those where less than 60 per cent of the GBM was covered by discrete foot processes.[6] These results are shown in Table IIb. There were no significant differences in ferritin numbers between the two groups in any of the basement membrane layers.

The distribution of cationic ferritin in basement membranes from control and experimental animals was not significantly different. Furthermore, the distribution of cationic ferritin was not affected by the presence or absence of discrete foot processes overlying the GBM (Table IIIa, Fig. 8a and b), nor was any difference in distribution

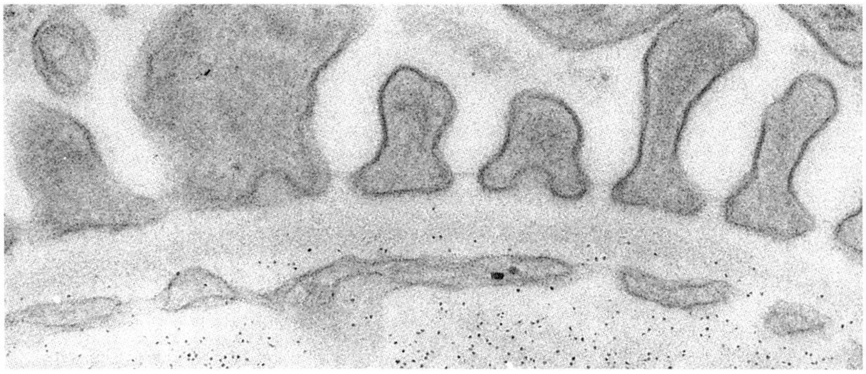

(a)

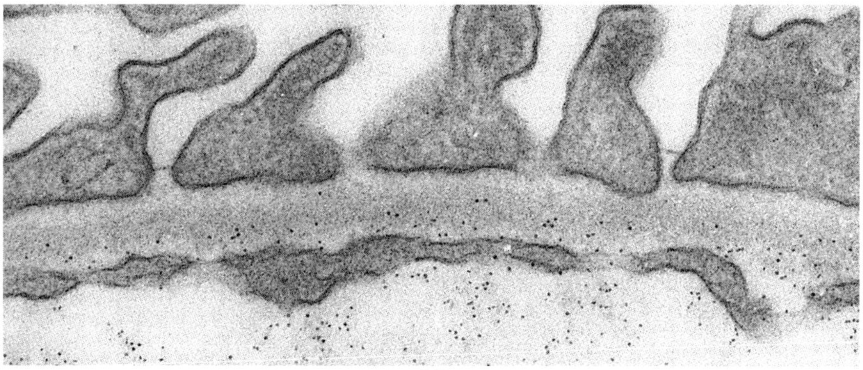

(b)

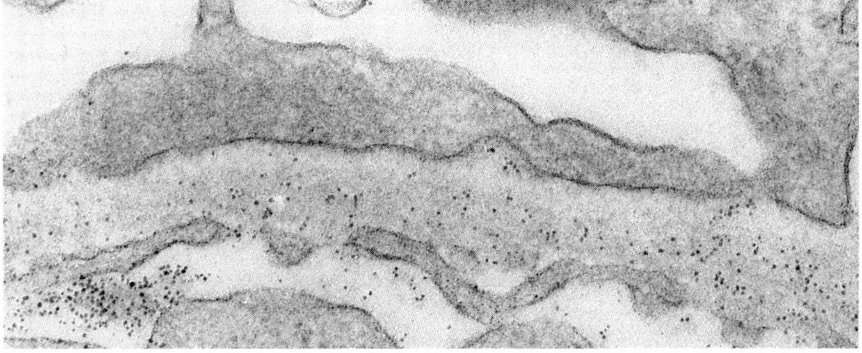

(c)

Fig. 5—Anionic ferritin in GBM from control rat (a) and proteinuric rats in the presence (b) or absence (c) of discrete foot processes. Lead citrate. ×63 000

Table IIa—Distribution of anionic ferritin in the GBM of proteinuric rats in the presence or absence of discrete foot processes

		Number of ferritin particles in:		
	n	LRI	LD	LRE
Discrete foot processes	44	18·45 ± 1·56	17·89 ± 2·26	1·36 ± 0·19
No discrete foot processes	36	18·22 ± 2·18	24·22 ± 3·47	3·19 ± 0·54
P		N.S.	N.S.	<0·01

n = number of GBM segments examined; LRI—lamina rara interna; LD—lamina densa; LRE—lamina rara externa; N.S.—not significant.

Table IIb—Distribution of anionic ferritin in the GBM of ultrastructurally normal and abnormal glomeruli from proteinuric rats

		Number of ferritin particles in:		
	n	LRI	LD	LRE
≤60% discrete foot processes	22	18·82 ± 2·34	21·91 ± 3·69	2·50 ± 0·52
>60% discrete foot processes	18	19·50 ± 2·27	19·83 ± 3·00	2·28 ± 0·44
P		N.S.	N.S.	N.S.

n = number of glomeruli; LRI—lamina rara interna; LD—lamina densa; LRE—lamina rara externa; N.S.—not significant.

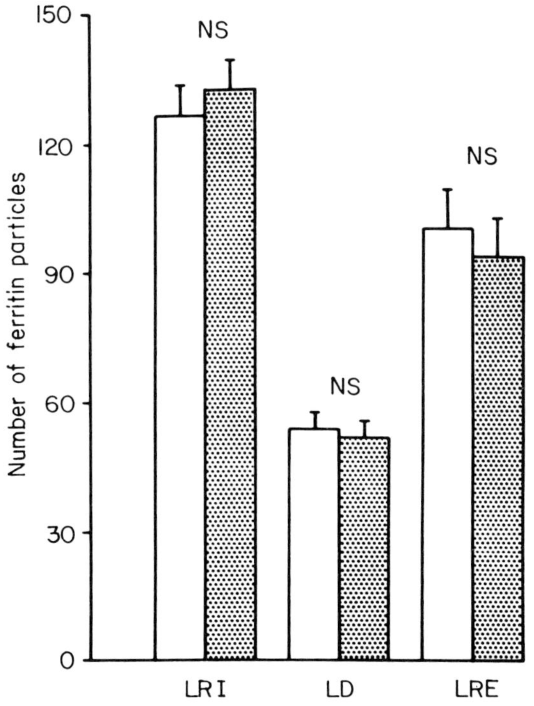

Fig. 6—Distribution of cationic ferritin in GBM from control and proteinuric rats. Note that the ordinate scale is greater than for Fig. 2. Controls—open columns; proteinurics—shaded columns. LRI—lamina rara interna; LD—lamina densa; LRE—lamina rara externa. N.S.—not significant

found when comparing ultrastructurally normal and abnormal glomeruli from BSA-treated rats (Table IIIb).

DISCUSSION

Following 5 days of intraperitoneal administration of BSA all animals developed proteinuria, in most cases in excess of 200 mg/day. This proteinuria has been shown to consist mainly of rat and bovine serum albumin.[6,24] The proteinuria was accompanied by a marked loss of discrete foot processes with over half the glomeruli examined having only 60 per cent or less of the GBM covered by foot processes. Lawrence and Brewer[20] have shown that proteinuria following protein-overload precedes loss of foot processes suggesting, therefore, that foot process loss is not the cause but possibly a result of proteinuria.

Anionic ferritin distribution in the GBM of control animals was similar to that described previously.[11,12,14,25] The ferritin particles were mainly restricted to the lamina rara interna with very few penetrating the whole depth of the GBM. In proteinuric animals, far greater numbers of ferritin particles were seen in the lamina densa and lamina rara externa. Also ferritin was seen in small

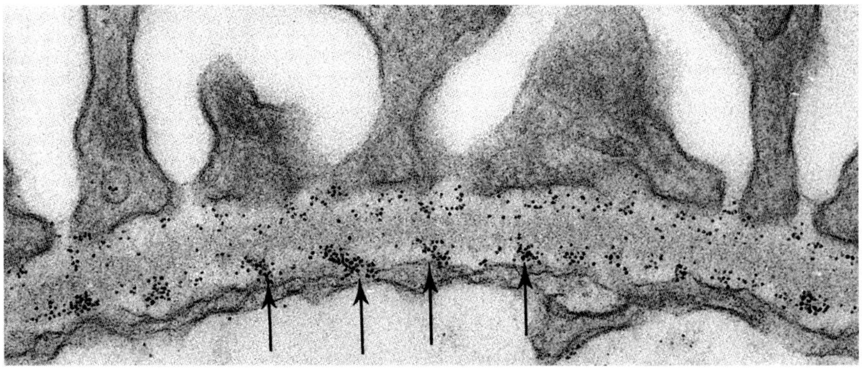

Fig. 7—Cationic ferritin in GBM from control rat showing discrete clusters of ferritin in the lamina rara interna (arrows)

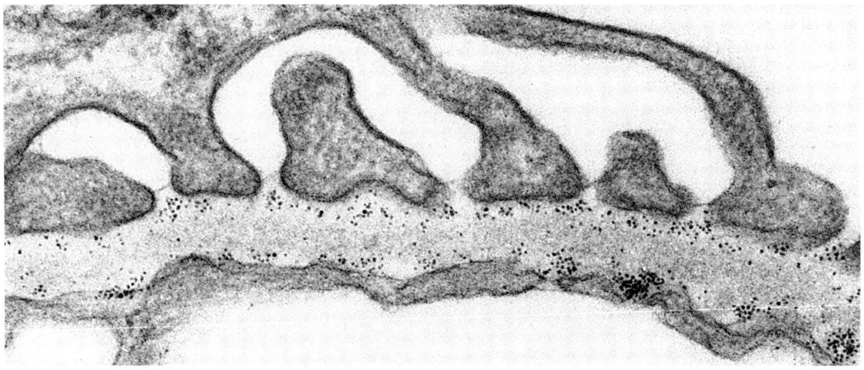

(a)

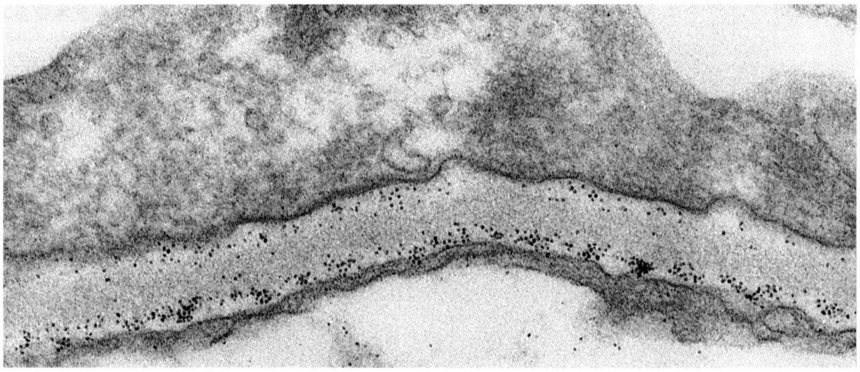

(b)

Fig. 8—Cationic ferritin in GBM from proteinuric rats in the presence (a) or absence (b) of discrete foot processes. Lead citrate. ×63 000

Table IIIa—Distribution of cationic ferritin in the GBM of proteinuric rats in the presence or absence of discrete foot processes

	n	Number of ferritin particles in: LRI	LD	LRE
Discrete foot processes	38	154·84 ± 7·36	51·88 ± 4·72	127·53 ± 6·17
No discrete foot processes	42	147·07 ± 9·39	63·43 ± 8·53	109·54 ± 7·88
P		N.S.	N.S.	N.S.

n = number of GBM segments examined; LRI—lamina rara interna; LD—lamina densa; LRE—lamina rara externa; N.S.—not significant.

Table IIIb—Distribution of cationic ferritin in the GBM of ultrastructurally normal and abnormal glomeruli from proteinuric rats

	n	Number of ferritin particles in: LRI	LD	LRE
≤60% discrete foot processes	20	146·42 ± 11·25	57·08 ± 12·83	114·92 ± 10·36
>60% discrete foot processes	20	155·00 ± 7·11	59·17 ± 4·85	122·33 ± 7·40
P		N.S.	N.S.	N.S.

n = number of glomeruli; LRI—lamina rara interna; LD—lamina densa; LRE—lamina rara externa; N.S.—not significant.

invaginations of the epithelial cell membrane adjacent to the GBM and in pinocytotic vesicles within the epithelial cell cytoplasm in proteinuric but not in control rats. No preferred channels for ferritin passage across the GBM were detected. This distribution of ferritin in proteinuric animals is similar to that described in puromycin aminonucleoside nephrotic rats.[10, 26] Interestingly, in our study it was found that the greatest GBM penetration occurred in areas where discrete foot processes were lost.

Increased anionic ferritin penetration of the GBM may represent a partial loss of charge in the glomerular filtration barrier. In support of this possibility, increased anionic ferritin penetration of the GBM has been observed following neutralization of the charge barrier with protamine.[13] We investigated the possibility that the increased anionic ferritin penetration observed in proteinuric animals could be due to a reduction in the glomerular charge barrier using a cationic derivative of ferritin. The binding of this cationic molecule to the GBM anionic sites is ionic in nature.[15]

Following infusion into control animals, cationic ferritin was found to be mainly localized in the lamina rara interna and externa often in discrete clusters with a separation of 50–70 nm, as has been described by Kanwar and Farquhar.[15] This distribution was not altered in proteinuric animals supporting the recent study by Rollason and Brewer [27] who were unable to demonstrate any alteration in GBM binding of a range of cationic probes in protein-overload proteinuria.

The possibility of a defect in the charge selective barrier in proteinuria induced by puromycin aminonucleoside is suggested by clearance studies using the anionic molecules, dextran sulphate[28] and succinylated horseradish peroxidase.[29] The renal clearance of both these substances is increased in puromycin aminonucleoside nephrosis whereas the clearance of their neutral equivalents is either decreased (dextran) or increased but to a lesser extent (horseradish peroxidase). Light microscopic studies using colloidal iron (a stain for the sialic acid component of the epithelial cell coat) tended to support this idea showing a reduction in staining with the onset of proteinuria.[30] However, it is thought that this decrease in staining seen at the light microscopic level merely represents a reduction of the cell surface area available for colloidal iron binding in epithelial cells that have lost many foot processes.[31–33] Electron microscopic studies with colloidal iron have either shown no change in binding[33] or where a reduction in the thickness of cell coat staining was observed this seemed unrelated to the increase in GBM permeability.[34] The use of other cationic probes, cationized cytochrome *c* and cationic ferritin, in puromycin aminonucleoside nephrosis has failed to demonstrate any reduction in fixed anionic charge in the GBM.[29,35]

These ultrastructural studies, therefore, suggest that a reduction in fixed anionic charge is not necessary for proteinuria following puromycin aminonucleoside or protein-overload. However, Caulfield and Farquhar[36] have been able to demonstrate a reduction, progressing to a complete loss of anionic staining with developing proteinuria in puromycin aminonucleoside nephrosis using the small cationic molecule lysozyme. The reason for this discrepancy with studies using other cationic probes is unclear. Possibly lysozyme binding is more sensitive to slight reductions in glomerular charge, alternatively the lysozyme may be staining a different component of the GBM and epithelial cell coat. Thus, it is possible that a slight reduction in the glomerular electrostatic barrier could occur in proteinuria which would not be detected by the cationic ferritin used in the present study. Lysozyme binding in protein-overload proteinuria needs to be investigated.

In puromycin aminonucleoside nephrosis, areas where the epithelial cells have become detached from the GBM, so-called bare areas, are frequently seen.[24] These areas have been implicated as the sites of protein leakage. Marked anionic ferritin penetration has been observed at the sites of detachment.[22,29,34] Also plasma proteins and immunoglobulin G have been shown to cross the GBM and reach Bowman's space at these sites.[37] Staining of anionic sites in the GBM is normal in these regions.[33,35] The importance of epithelial cell detachment in the early stages of proteinuria is unclear. It has been reported that epithelial detachment is first seen about 10 days after the start of administration of puromycin whereas proteinuria starts 3–4 days earlier.[23] However in a previous study Ryan and Karnovsky[22] found that the onset of proteinuria and epithelial detachment occurred at the same time. This discrepancy may be due to the different protocols adopted for induction of aminonucleoside nephrosis by the two groups. Ryan and Karnovsky[22] used a single large dose of puromycin (15 mg/100 g body weight) whereas Caulfield *et al.*[23] administered daily subcutaneous injections (1·67 mg/100 g body weight) over the experimental period.

In the present study and that of Rollason and Brewer[9] protein-overload proteinuria was not associated with epithelial cell detachment. Where epithelial detachment has been reported in this condition it has been an infrequent finding occurring in animals with heavy proteinuria[20] or where epithelial cell degeneration had become particularly advanced some days after completion of BSA administration.[6] Thus focal detachment of the epithelial cells is unlikely to be a significant cause of the urinary protein loss in protein-overload.

Following interruption of renal blood flow prior to fixation of the kidney, immunoglobulin G, catalase and serum albumin are found to penetrate the GBM to a greater extent than when fixation is performed without interference with the renal blood vessels.[38,39] The possibility that haemodynamic alterations could be responsible for the increase in anionic ferritin penetration in protein-overload proteinuric animals is unlikely as Rennke and Venkatachalam[14] have shown that the distribution of anionic ferritin in the GBM was unaffected when fixation was performed during reduced renal perfusion pressure or following a period of renal ischaemia.

In summary, in protein-overload proteinuria there is a general increase in glomerular basement membrane permeability as evidenced by an increased penetration by anionic ferritin. This penetration is particularly marked in areas of the glomerular basement membrane where discrete foot processes have been lost. This increased permeability occurs without any demonstrable reduction in fixed anionic charge. Anionic ferritin particles were found incorporated in pinocytotic vesicles within the epithelial cell cytoplasm in proteinuric rats. Such an appearance has also been described in puromycin aminonucleoside nephrotic rats by Farquhar and Palade[26] who suggested that this may represent transcellular passage of protein which could contribute to the proteinuria.

ACKNOWLEDGEMENTS

We wish to thank Mrs Jill Sparke and Mrs Ann Logan for their excellent technical assistance; the Immunodiagnostic Research Laboratory, University of Birmingham, for their help with the isoelectric focusing and Miss Jane Melhuish for typing the manuscript. This work was supported by a grant from the Medical Research Council.

REFERENCES

1. Lippman RW. Mechanism of proteinuria. Effect of parenteral protein injections on haemoglobin excretion in the rat. *Am J Physiol* 1948; **154:** 532.
2. Anderson MS, Recant L. Fine structural alterations in rat kidney following intraperitoneal bovine serum albumin. *Am J Path* 1962; **40:** 555.
3. Lannigan R, McQueen EG. The effect on the renal glomerular epithelial cells of proteinuria induced by infusions of human serum albumin in rabbits and rats. *Br J Exp Path* 1962; **43:** 549.
4. Karl IE, Garcia P, White WL, Recant L, Kissane JM. Proteinuria induced by albumin injection: effect on kidney and liver enzymes in the rat. *Lab Invest* 1964; **13:** 1600.
5. Brewer DB, Filip O. The morphometry of the glomerular epithelial cell and its foot processes after the injection of bovine serum albumin or egg albumin. *J Path* 1976; **120:** 209.
6. Davies DJ, Brewer DB, Hardwicke J. Urinary proteins and glomerular morphometry in protein overload proteinuria. *Lab Invest* 1978; **38:** 232.
7. Lawrence Gillian M, Brewer DB. Normal urinary protein composition in the female Wistar rat and its relationship to the proteinuria induced by intraperitoneal bovine albumin. *Clin Sci* 1981; **60:** 693.
8. Lawrence Gillian M, Brewer DB. The effect of strain and sex on the induction of hyperalbuminaemic proteinuria in the rat. *Clin Sci* 1981; **61:** 751.
9. Rollason TP, Brewer DB. A scanning and transmission electron microscopic study of glomerular damage in the rat following heterologous serum albumin overload. *J Path* 1981; **134:** 39.
10. Farquhar Marilyn G, Palade GE. Glomerular permeability. II. Ferritin transfer across the glomerular capillary wall in nephrotic rats. *J Exp Med* 1961; **114:** 699.
11. Farquhar Marilyn G, Wissig SL, Palade GE. Glomerular permeability. I. Ferritin transfer across the normal glomerular capillary wall. *J Exp Med* 1961; **113:** 47.
12. Kelley Vicki E, Cavallo T. Glomerular permeability: ultrastructural studies in New Zealand Black/White mice using polyanionic ferritin as a molecular probe. *Lab Invest* 1977; **37:** 265.
13. Kelley Vicki E, Cavallo T. Glomerular permeability, transfer of native ferritin in glomeruli with decreased anionic sites. *Lab Invest* 1978; **39:** 547.
14. Rennke HG, Venkatachalam MA. Glomerular permeability: *in vivo* tracer studies with polyanionic and polycationic ferritins. *Kidney Int* 1977; **11:** 44.
15. Kanwar YS, Farquhar Marilyn G. Anionic sites in the glomerular basement membrane. *In vivo* and *in vitro* localization to the laminae rarae by cationic probes. *J Cell Biol* 1979; **81:** 137.
16. Spall RD, Ainsworth SK. Serum histamine levels following administration of ultrastructural tracers in three strains of rats. *Agents Actions* 1978; **8:** 206.
17. Danon D, Goldstein T, Marikovsky Y, Skutelsky E. Use of cationized ferritin as a label for negative charges on cell surfaces. *J Ultrastruc Res* 1972; **38:** 500.
18. Peachy LD. Thin sections. I. A study of section thickness and physical distortion produced during microtomy. *J Biophys Biochem Cytol* 1958; **4:** 233.
19. Pinto JA, Brewer DB. Glomerular morphometry: combined light and electron microscope studies in normal rats. *Lab Invest* 1974; **30:** 657.
20. Lawrence Gillian M, Brewer DB. Studies on the relationship between proteinuria and glomerular ultrastructural change in hyperalbuminaemic female Wistar rats. *J Path* 1982; **138:** 365.
21. Davies DJ, Brewer DB. Irreversible glomerular damage following heterologous serum albumin overload. *J Path* 1977; **123:** 45.
22. Ryan GB, Karnovsky MJ. An ultrastructural study of the mechanisms of proteinuria in aminonucleoside nephrosis. *Kidney Int* 1975; **8:** 219.
23. Caulfield JP, Reid Joanne, Farquhar Marilyn G. Alterations of the glomerular epithelium in aminonucleoside nephrosis. Evidence for formation of occluding junctions and epithelial cell detachment. *Lab Invest* 1976; **34:** 43.
24. Lawrence Gillian M, Brewer DB. A morphometric, biochemical and histochemical comparison of puromycin aminonucleoside and hyperalbuminaemic induced proteinurias in the female Wistar rat. *J Path* 1983; **139:** 115.
25. Kanwar YS, Linker A, Farquhar Marilyn G. Increased permeability of the glomerular basement membrane to ferritin after removal of glycosaminoglycans (heparan sulfate) by enzyme digestion. *J Cell Biol* 1980; **86:** 688.
26. Farquhar Marilyn G, Palade GE. Segregation of ferritin in glomerular protein absorption droplets. *J Biophys Biochem Cytol* 1960; **7:** 297.
27. Rollason TP, Brewer DB. A study of glomerular basement membrane anionic sites and glomerular visceral epithelial cell coat in protein overload proteinuria in the rat. *J. Path* 1984; **142:** 301–316.
28. Bohrer MP, Baylis Christine, Robertson CR, Brenner BM. Mechanisms of the puromycin-induced defects in the transglomerular passage of water and macromolecules. *J Clin Invest* 1977; **60:** 152.
29. Olson JL, Rennke HG, Venkatachalam MA. Alterations in the charge and size selectivity barrier of the glomerular filter in aminonucleoside nephrosis in rats. *Lab Invest* 1981; **44:** 271.

30. Michael AF, Blau EB, Vernier RL. Glomerular polyanion-alterations in aminonucleoside nephrosis. *Lab Invest* 1970; **23:** 649.
31. Faraggiana T, Grishman E. Behaviour of anionic charges of podocytes in nephrotic subjects. *Kidney Int* 1979; **16:** 861.
32. Latta H. In: Maunsbach AB, Olsen TS, Christensen EI, eds Functional Ultrastructure of the Kidney. London: Academic Press, 1980: 3.
33. Alcorn Diane, Ryan GB. Distribution of anionic groups in the glomerular capillary wall in rat nephrotoxic nephritis and aminonucleoside nephrosis. *Pathology* 1981; **13:** 37.
34. Kanwar YS, Rosenzweig LJ. Altered glomerular permeability as a result of focal detachment of the visceral epithelium. *Kidney Int* 1982; **21:** 565.
35. Kanwar YS, Rosenzweig LJ, Kerjaschki DI. Glycosaminoglycans of the glomerular basement membrane in normal and nephrotic states. *Renal Physiol* 1981; **4:** 121.
36. Caulfield JP, Farquhar Marilyn G. Loss of anionic sites from the glomerular basement membrane in aminonucleoside nephrosis. *Lab Invest* 1978; **39:** 505.
37. Ryan GB, Hein SJ, Karnovsky MJ. The distribution of albumin and immunoglobulin G in the glomerular capillary wall in aminonucleoside nephrosis. *Pathology* 1978; **10:** 335.
38. Ryan GB, Karnovsky MJ. Distribution of endogenous albumin in the rat glomerulus. Role of hemodynamic factors in glomerular barrier function. *Kidney Int* 1976; **9:** 36.
39. Ryan GB, Hein SJ, Karnovsky MJ. Glomerular permeability to protein. Effect of hemodynamic factors on the distribution of endogenous immunoglobulin G and exogenous catalase in the rat glomerulus. *Lab Invest* 1976; **34:** 415.

Pathological Society of Great Britain and Ireland

Dutch Pathological Society

Norwegian Pathological Society

Joint Meeting, 24–25 May 1984

at

University of Bergen, Haukeland Hospital, Bergen, Norway

SYNOPSES OF PAPERS

Papers and posters presented at the meeting have not been refereed or reviewed in the *Journal of Pathology*.

PROGNOSTIC FACTORS IN OVARIAN CARCINOMA

J. P. A. Baak

Pathological Institute, Free University Hospital, De Boelelaan 1117 1007 MB Amsterdam, The Netherlands

ccording to the literature, the prognosis of patients with ovarian cancer depends on any factors, such as therapy, FIGO stage, size of residual tumour prior to treatment, arnofsky index, age, histological type, nuclear and histological grade. However, histo- id cyto-pathological criteria are usually not included in the therapeutic decision- aking process. Thus, it seems that, in comparison with other features, their prognostic gnificance is regarded as too weak or the assessment as not reliable enough. To ercome this problem, adequate sampling of the primary tumour is essential. Secondly, tra- and inter-observer disagreement in grading and typing should be studied, and, if ssible, minimized. Quantitative microscopical techniques, when selectively used by a illed pathologist, can be helpful for this purpose.

ANEUPLOIDY IN HUMAN ENDOMETRIAL AND OVARIAN CANCERS MEASURED BY FLOW CYTOMETRY

O. E. Iversen

Kvinneklinikken, 5016 Haukeland Sykehus, Norway

esh tumor specimens from endometrial and ovarian cancers have been homogenized physiological saline before fixation in ethanol at −20°C. Cytoplasm was removed by psin treatment and the nuclei stained with ethidium bromide/mithramycin. Relative llular DNA content was measured on an Ortho ICP 22 flow cytometer. In general high solution DNA-histograms with a coefficient of variation (CV) 2–5% based on easurements of 10,000–100,000 cells could be obtained. No particular DNA-pattern stinguished endometrial from ovarian carcinomas. The tumors were characterized by degree of DNA-abberation as expressed by the DNA-index. The distribution of cells S- and G_2-phase reflects the tumor growth rate. Aneuploid stemlines and mixed oidies were a frequent finding. Correlations to clinical findings have been made. onclusion: a close comparison between DNA-abberations, hormone receptor status d clinical features may enable the division into subgroups of patients with differing nical courses and severity of disease.

DIAGNOSIS OF ENDOMETRIAL MALIGNANCY

Elsa Skaarland

Department of Pathology, N-5016 Haukeland Hospital, Bergen, Norway

nical signs or symptoms leading to D & C with histological analysis of tissue from the dometrium is the traditional procedure behind the diagnosis of endometrial malig- ncy. Search for less resource-demanding methods has focused interest on cytology mplers. Three different samplers have been tested as to their clinical applications and gnostic accuracy versus conventional histological analysis in 3 series of 200 patients m our hospital. Cytological results are promising as there is no difference in detection malignancy compared to histology. Problems arise with the diagnosis of adenomatous perplasia. The cytological material which is quite different in appearance to ditional exfoliated cells will be presented. Morphometric analysis of benign and lignant epithelial cells has been carried out and results will be related to diagnostic eria for malignancy. The cytology samplers are accepted by the gynaecologists in our ion and are in routine use. Criteria for use will be discussed. Endometrial cytological mpling now replaces more than 70% of diagnostic curettings in our region.

BASIC BIOLOGY OF TERATOMAS

H. Fox

Department of Pathology, University of Manchester, Stopford Building, Manchester M13 9PT, England

Two animal models for the development of gonadal teratomas have been studied, both being in highly inbred mouse strains. Ovarian teratomas develop in a high proportion of LT/Sv mice and it can be shown that such neoplasms originate from ovarian oocytes which have completed the first meiotic division and are showing pathogenetic development. Testicular teratoma arise with considerable frequency in 129/Sv-*ter* mice and such tumours arise during fetal life from germ cells within the seminiferous tubules of the fetal testis. In both ovarian and testicular teratomas the early stages of development mimic closely those of normal early embryogenesis. Teratomas can be experimentally induced either by embryo transplantation or by genital ridge transplantation: induction of teratomas by these techniques is highly time and temperature dependant. Cells from transplantable malignant teratomas can be inserted into a normal blastocyst and a chimera will result, some tissues and organs being derived from tumour cells: by selective inbreeding it is possible to produce an animal which is derived totally from cells which were originally a component of a transplantable malignant teratoma. Cells from such an animal can be converted back to a malignant teratoma. The significance of these findings in respect to teratomas occurring in humans is discussed.

USE OF INTERMEDIATE FILAMENT ANTIBODIES IN DIFFERENTIAL DIAGNOSIS OF GYNAECOLOGICAL NEOPLASIA

G. P. Vooijs, J. J. G. Puts and F. C. S. Ramaekers

Pathology Department, St. Radboudziekenhuis, Geert Grootaplein Zuid 24, 6525 GA Nijmegen, The Netherlands

Intermediate-sized filaments form an essential part of the intracellular matrix. The protein composition of these cytoplasmic 10 nm filaments is tissue specific. Polyclonal antibodies to cytokeratin, vimentin, desmin, neurofilaments and GFAP can be used to distinguish between epithelial, mesenchymal, myogenic, neuronal and glial cells respectively by means of immuno-histochemical methods. Monoclonal antibodies to cytokeratin subsets allow the distinction between different kinds of epithelia. In general the tissue specific intermediate filament pattern is retained when cells become neoplastic. Therefore these antibodies are valuable tools for diagnostic purposes in histo- and cyto-pathology. They can also be used in histogenetic studies. Applications in the differential diagnosis of several types of gynaecological tumors and in a study dealing with the histogenesis of premalignant lesions of the uterine cervix will be discussed.

HUMAN PAPILLOMAVIRUSES AND CERVICAL CANCER

Dulcie V. Coleman

Department of Pathology, St. Mary's Hospital, London W2 1PG, England

Morphological changes characteristic of papillomavirus infection are frequently seen in squamous epithelial cells in cervical biopsy material, and papillomavirus structural antigens and papillomavirus particles have been demonstrated in dysplastic cervical epithelium. Biochemical studies have revealed the presence of human papillomavirus DNA in both premalignant and malignant lesions of the cervix. These findings suggest that there may be an association between wart virus infection and cervical cancer. DNA sequences homologous with HPV-6 have been found most frequently in biopsies showing the changes of cervical intraepithelial neoplasia whereas HPV-16 and 18 have been detected in over 70% of invasive cervical cancers. In addition HPV-18 has been found in several cell lines derived from cervical carcinomas including HeLa cells. The preferential association of HPV-16 and 18 with invasive cancer has led to the suggestion that the human papillomaviruses present in the cervix may vary in their pathological potential and that the viruses may play a part in tumourgenesis. The evidence for this is discussed and a model for testing this hypothesis is described.

HYDATIDIFORM MOLE: MORPHOLOGICAL CHARACTERISTICS AND hCG-VALUES

Ellen Risse, H. Franke, P. Kenemans, P. Hous, H. Stolk and P. Vooijs

Departments of Pathology, Universities of Nijmegen and Groningen; Departments of Obstetrics and Gynecology, Universities of Nijmegen and Amsterdam (Free University), Geert Grooteplein zuid 24, 6525 GA Nijmegen, The Netherlands

On review of endometrial curettings in 377 patients with a diagnosis of hydatidiform mole or partial mole, in 18% (69) of these patients the histopathological diagnosis was changed to hydropic degeneration of chorionic villi. In 283 patients the review diagnosis was 'hydatidiform mole' and in 25 patients 'partial mole'. Clinical follow-up findings and hCG-values correlated with the review diagnoses. The regression rate of hCG-values in patients with hydatidiform mole differed significantly from the regression rate of hCG-values in patients with partial moles or hydropic degeneration of chorionic villi. In one patient with a diagnosis of partial mole (confirmed on review) 75 days after primary evacuation an invasive mole was diagnosed. In the other patients with a review diagnosis of hydatidiform mole and partial mole on follow-up there were no signs of persistent trophoblastic disease. To avoid unnecessary follow-up and long term contraception it is recommended to apply only strictly defined histopathological criteria in the diagnosis of hydatidiform mole. It is further recommended to maintain a national registry of hydatidiform mole diagnoses and to concentrate serological testing and review of histopathological specimens in specialised laboratories.

CYTOSKELETAL CHANGES INDUCED BY RETINOIDS IN CULTURED CERVICAL CARCINOMA CELLS

J. Halgunset and T. Espevik

Department of Pathology and Institute of Cancer Research, University of Trondheim, Regionsykehuset, N-7000 Trondheim, Norway

Retinoids, analogues of vitamin A, have a profound influence on the direction and degree of differentiation in various cell types, and may also promote the differentiation in some transformed cells. Retinoic acid provokes a striking reorganization of the intermediate filaments in NHIK 3025, a cervical carcinoma cell line, *in vitro*, inducing a more elaborate and well-organized pattern of cytokeratin fibres as revealed by immunofluorescence microscopy. The cytokeratins, a family of closely related proteins, constitute an important part of the cytoskeletal framework of epithelial cells. Intermediate filaments seem to be involved in the maintenance of cell morphology and in some types of cell-to-cell interaction. The ability to modify the pattern of cytokeratin expression in transformed cells may lead to a better understanding of the role played by the cytoskeleton in cell differentiation and neoplasia.

USING POSTAL CODE FOR EPIDEMIOLOGIC STUDIES ON CYTOLOGICALLY DETECTED CERVICAL INFECTIONS, CIN, AND THEIR INTERRELATION

Josephine J. M. Alons-van Kordelaar and Mathilde E. Boon

Leids Cytologisch Laboratorium, Groenesteeg 7, 2312 SP Leiden, Oude Delft 153B, 2611 HA Delft, The Netherlands

It is a well known fact that certain cervical infections are more frequent in urban than in rural areas, and so is cervical intra-epithelial neoplasia (CIN). In the Netherlands, the postal code is highly refined, and thus from it can be deduced whether a person lives in a rural area, small city, large city or metropolis. Using the postal codes, we analysed the rate of cases cytologically classified as containing signs of Trichomonads, fungi, Actinomyces, Herpes, Condyloma and Chlamydia. The analysis was performed on 47,000 cytologically negative and 1,295 positive (containing CIN) smears. Trichomonads and Actinomyces were more frequent in positive smears, but these differences disappeared when the data were corrected for age and urbanisation. In contrast, the highly significant differences of the frequencies of Condyloma and Chlamydia, both higher in positive smears, did not disappear after correction for age and urbanisation. This investigation is an example how the Dutch postal code can be used for epidemiologic studies.

CLASSIFICATION OF LYMPHOID CELLS IN PARAFFIN SECTIONS USING MONOCLONAL ANTIBODIES

C. S. Holgate, P. Jackson and C. C. Bird

Department of Pathology, University of Leeds, Leeds LS2 9JT, England

The identification of subpopulations of lymphoid cells in tissue sections using monoclonal antibodies has gained considerable importance in the diagnosis and classificatio of lymphoproliferative disorders. However, using conventional immunostaining proce dures the majority of these antibodies are only applicable to frozen tissue sections. Thi is a considerable disadvantage and severely limits the use of these reagents. In this pape we report the application of a number of these monoclonal antibodies for the first tim to paraffin sections of human lymphoid tissue using the immunogold-silver stainin (IGSS) method. The IGSS method is a novel and highly sensitive immunohistologica staining procedure which we have previously reported to this Society.

NUMERICAL TAXONOMY OF NON-HODGKIN'S LYMPHOMA

J. M. Skinner and L. R. Jarvis

Department of Pathology, Flinders University, Bedford Park 5042, South Australia

Tissues from 83 cases of non-Hodgkin's lymphoma have been examined usin computerised image analysis. 1μ sections of araldite resin embedded material wer examined and data derived for the perimeter, area, shape factor for cell, nucleus an nucleoli. For each case the variation in area, shape (and number per cell in the case o nucleoli) were established. Statistical analysis of the derived data has been performe using discriminant function analysis comparing the numerical data with the Kiel an other subjective classifications. The significant variables defining each category ar nuclear shape, number of cells per unit area, N/C ratio and the skewness of the N/ ratio. The correlation between subjective and numerical analysis is of the order of 80 and it can be argued that the discrepancy is due to errors in subjective analysis Furthermore using a plot of the bivariate distribution of the two most powerful function the decision boundaries between classifications have been determined at the 95 tolerance levels. The measured features of the centroblastic category overlap immuno blastic and centrocytic/centroblastic to a significant degree giving weight to the assertio that errors of classification involving the boundaries with centroblastic lymphoma ar inevitable.

LARGE-CELL LYMPHOMAS; DIFFERENTIAL DIAGNOSIS OF CENTROBLASTIC AND B-IMMUNOBLASTIC SUBTYPES BY MORPHOMETRY ON HISTOLOGICAL AND CYTOLOGICAL PREPARATIONS

C. J. L. M. Meijer, P. van der Valk, Penny Ball and J. Lindeman

Pathologisch Instituut V.U., de Boelelaan 1117, 1007 MB Amsterdam, The Netherland

33 Large-cell lymphomas, 18 centroblastic or large non-cleaved follicle centre ce lymphomas and 15 B-immunoblastic lymphomas, diagnosed by morphology and marke studies were studied with morphometry. The parameters studied were: nuclear an nucleolar area, nuclear shape, cytoplasm to nucleus ratio, number of nucleoli pe nuclear cross-section, location of the nucleolus within the nucleus, as expressed by th relative nucleolar eccentricity (rNE), and the percentage of morphometrically define immunoblasts. Mean values and standard deviations were calculated and statisticall analyzed. The groups differed significantly in their nucleolar area (mean and SD) cytoplasm to nucleus ratio (mean), number of nucleoli per nuclear cross-section (mea and SD), rNE (mean) and percentage of immunoblasts. Using non-linear discriminan analysis, the possibility was investigated of classifying individual cases with the studie parameters. 29 cases were reliably classified (88%), 3 were classified correctly, bu below a 95% certainty, 1 case was misclassified. A comparison with the results of similar study on cytological preparations from the same patients demonstrated tha morphological measurements on these two types of material are not interchangeable but in general the same conclusions were reached by morphometry on histological an cytological specimens. The results indicate a spectrum ranging from centroblastic to B immunoblastic lymphoma. Transition forms occur and can be accurately defined wit morphometry.

COMPARISON OF POINT COUNTING AND ELECTRONIC PLANAR ANALYSIS IN LYMPH NODE STEREOLOGY

A. O. Myking and L. M. Cruz-Orive

The Gade Institute, Department of Pathology, University of Bergen, and Department of Anatomy, University of Bern, N-5014 University of Bergen, Norway

In the recent 5–6 yr, electronic equipment for planar and linear analysis have bee increasingly popular in stereological work. These instruments are characterized by high precision for individual measurements and by a high cost in money. However, bein of great value where a high precision of individual measurements is required, the significance in biological research has been questioned. For further evaluation of th problem, the accuracy and efficiency of electronic planar analysis was compared wit simple point counting in lymph node stereology. The material consists of equispace step-sections from the whole lymph node thickness in 40 mice and 30 guinea pig lymp nodes, totalling over 1100 sections drawn on tracing paper at 40× magnification. Poir counting was performed by using a double lattice test grid with an average of 16 te points within each lymph node section in mice, and 70 in guinea pigs. Planar analysis wa performed by a MOP-AM 03 (Kontron). Volume fractions were virtually the same wit the two methods. However, the cost in time units was on average 3.2 times higher usin the electronic equipment.

MALLORY BODIES AND HEPATIC INTERMEDIATE FILAMENT COMPONENTS ARE CHEMOTACTIC FOR POLYMORPHS

J. A. Morton and J. O'D. McGee

University of Oxford, Nuffield Department of Pathology, John Radcliffe Hospital, Oxford, OX3 9DU, England

ne mechanism underlying the accumulation of polymorphonuclear leucocytes in flammatory reactions, is their positive response to chemotactic factors. In alcoholic epatitis, inflammatory cells including polymorphs accumulate around Mallory body MB)-containing and other hepatocytes. This paper addresses itself to the question: are MBs and the organellar system from which they are derived, viz., intermediate laments, chemotactic for polymorphs? MBs and liver intermediate filaments were urified from alcoholic and normal liver respectively. Both were pure as assessed by ectron microscopy and SDS-PAGE gels. Both MBs and intermediate filaments have ssociated with them a water-soluble component(s) which is markedly chemotactic for olymorphs in an *in vitro* assay. The component(s) derived from MBs has a molecular eight <500 daltons. It is not derived from, or dependent on the complement system for s activity. It is evident, therefore, that the accumulation of polymorphs in alcoholic epatitis may be due to the release of chemotactic factors which are associated with MBs nd intermediate filaments of hepatocytes. In addition, it has been found that termediate filaments from sources other than liver (e.g. neurofilament) also possess olymorph chemotactic activity. Polymorph chemotactic activity, therefore, may be an tribute of all intermediate filaments.

DISTRIBUTION OF HLA CLASS II (DR) ANTIGENS IN HUMAN LIVER USING A MONOCLONAL ANTIBODY

Calypso Barbatis and J. Greveson

Department of Histopathology, Lewisham Hospital, London SE13 6LH, England

fresh needle diagnostic liver biopsies were studied with a monoclonal antibody to LA-DR antigens and two monoclonal common-leucocyte antibodies by an indirect mmunoperoxidase technique. In 14 normal livers, HLA-DR antigens were strongly xpressed in portal spindle cells, in mononuclear cells scattered in the bile duct pithelium and in sinusoidal cells of the reticuloendothelial system. All hepatocytes, the le duct epithelium and endothelium of all blood vessels were negative. In 40 cases of arious liver deseases HLA-DR distribution was similar to normal liver with the xception of 2/6 cases of primary biliary cirrhosis where HLA-DR was demonstrated in e endothelium of portal blood vessels. Positive bile duct epithelium was observed in 4 ses including 1/6 cases of primary biliary cirrhosis, two cases of resolving non-B viral epatitis, one case of nonspecific reactive hepatitis associated with pyrexia of unknown igin and 1/4 cases of idiopathic active cirrhosis. The HLA-DR positive spindle cells in e portal tracts although they resemble fibroblasts expressed common-leucocyte ntigens on their surface. In view of the function of HLA-DR antigens as immune-sponse regulators, the significance of HLA-DR distribution in the liver will be scussed.

PREHEPATIC PORTAL HYPERTENSION: A CASE REPORT AND EXPERIMENTAL STUDIES

Andreas O. Myking and Jan F. Halvorsen

The Gade Institute, Department of Pathology, and Institute of Surgery, N-5014 University of Bergen, Norway

utopsy study of a 20-year-old man revealed old, partially recanalized thrombi of the ain portal vein branches at their entry into the liver parenchyma. The main finding was enormous dilatation of the cystic vein, functioning as a bypass for the obstructed rtal vein. A separate study of the venous drainage from the gallbladder in human aterial, showed that the presence of a cystic vein in its classical sense, exists in only %. These findings initiated a series of experiements in rats where the main results are: development of a simple and highly reproducible model for chronic prehepatic portal pertension by controlled mechanical stenosis of the portal vein; 2) successful creation portohepatic vascular bypass by transposition of various splancnically drained organs o the liver parenchyma. The methods may prove to be of value in the surgical eatment of selected paediatric patients who, for reason of age or previous surgery have suitable veins for direct portosystemic anastomosis.

LECTIN HISTOCHEMISTRY OF NORMAL HUMAN GASTROINTESTINAL MUCOSA AND GASTRIC INTESTINAL METAPLASIA

M. Wells, Monique J. Taylor and M. F. Dixon

Department of Pathology, University of Leeds, Leeds LS2 9JT, England

ectins are potentially useful tools in histopathology for the identification of carbohyd-te moieties in glycoproteins. The lectin histochemistry of gastric intestinal metaplasia 27 formalin fixed gastrectomy specimens for benign (15) and malignant (12) disease as been compared with: (a) lectin histochemistry of normal gastrointestinal mucosa, nd (b) conventional mucin histochemistry. Both direct methods (using peanut, heatgerm and soybean lectins conjugated to horseradish peroxidase) and indirect ethods (using labelled antibodies to peanut and soybean lectins) have been employed he sugar specificities of these lectins are: peanut: terminal β-D-galactosyl residues and 3 N acetyl-D-galactosamine; wheatgerm: D-N acetylglucosamine and N-acetyl euraminic (sialic) acid; soybean: D-N acetyl galactosamine. Appropriate blocking gars were used to confirm the specificity of binding. Indirect methods seem to provide increased sensitivity as do prior trypsinisation and neuraminidase (with peanut) treatment of sections. The following results are of particular interest: firstly, some metaplastic cells are reactive for peanut lectin although neither normal small nor large intestine react. Secondly, intense reactivity is obtained with soybean lectin in incomplete (Type IIb) metaplasia and gastric dysplasia. Thirdly, gastric adenocarcinomata show a heterogeneous reactivity pattern from area to area of the same tumour. These and other findings and their possible significance will be presented.

HISTOPATHOLOGIC FINDINGS IN INFLAMMATORY BOWEL DISEASE IN HLA-B27 POSITIVE (REACTIVE) ARTHRITIS

C. Cuvelier, M. Devos, H. Mielants, H. Roels and E. Veys

Department of Pathology, State University of Ghent, Belgium

HLA-B27 positive individuals are predisposed to peripheral and axial joint inflammation. The relation between HLA-B27 and ankylosing spondylitis (AS), IBD, Reiter's syndrome and reactive arthritis secondary to bacterial infections is well documented. 20% of the patients with Crohn's disease can develop reactive asymmetrical polyarthritis with enteropathies, without presence of HLA-B27. Ileocoloscopy with biopsy was performed on patients with B27 reactive arthritis. Only four patients had gastrointestinal symptoms. Routine gastrointestinal investigation revealed no signs of IBD. Half of these patients had no macroscopic lesions and biopsies were taken blindly. All patients examined until now had signs of inflammation and three types of inflammatory pattern could be recognised: a) lymphoid hyperplasia, oedema, increased intra-epithelial lymphocytic infiltration; b) increased inflammatory cell content in the lamina propria with striking contents of eosinophils, crypt cell hyperplasia and villous atrophy; and c) aphtoid ulceration, crypt abcess and microgranuloma formation. In nine patients with juvenile chronic arthritis, rheumatoid arthritis or A.S. without arthritis, serving as controls, there were no macroscopic or microscopic signs of IBD.

ULTRASTRUCTURAL ASPECTS OF ANTERIOR CRUCIATE LIGAMENT DIVISION MODEL OF OSTEOARTHROSIS

Constance R. Orford, D. L. Gardner and Patricia O'Connor

Department of Histopathology, University Hospital of South Manchester, Nell Lane, Withington, Manchester M20 8LR, England

Fifteen beagle dogs aged 9 to 20 mth underwent closed surgical division of the left anterior cruciate ligament. The right stifle joints served as sham-operated controls. Animals were sacrificed at intervals between 3 days and 24 wk after operation. Conspicuous alterations in chondrocyte morphology and matrix organisation were observed by transmission electron microscopy in femoral condylar cartilage from operated limbs when compared with cartilage from sham-operated limbs and from 3 non-operated dogs. Chondrocytes in Zone 1 lost their flattened shape and became rounded, cells in zones I and II occurred in pairs more often than usual, developed an extensive endoplasmic reticulum and were situated in enlarged electron lucent lacunae. These changes are suggestive of increased synthesis of matrix components. Associated with altered cell function, the extracellular matrix became disordered; collagen fibrils were widely separated and disorientated giving an appearance consistent with increased hydration of the matrix. It is possible that the disorder is primarily one of inappropriate cell function.

CHARACTERIZATION OF HISTIOCYTIC CELLS IN MALIGNANT FIBROUS HISTIOCYTOMAS

P. Roholl, J. Kleyne and J. A. M. van Unnik

Institute for Pathology, Pasteurstraat 2, Utrecht, The Netherlands

Malignant fibrous histiocytomas (MFH) manifest a fibroblastic and also a histiocytic morphology. The origin of the histiocytic tumorcells is not yet clear. From culture and electron microscopical studies it has been proposed that they could originate from undifferentiated or fibroblastic cells. On the other hand the histiocytic cells share many characteristics with monocytes, so that also a monocytic origin has been suggested. The purpose of this study was to characterize soft tissue tumors (STT) and malignant histiocytosis (MH) with several monoclonal antibodies and antisera on frozen and deparaffinized sections. None of the STT cells express monocyte specific determinants, whereas MH tumor cells were prominently positive. All of the MFH tumors express fibroblast specific determinants. HLA-Dr/Ia antigens were present on all MH, on 50% of the MFH, but not on other STT. Peanut and soya bean agglutinin binding sites are present on MH and on a small part of the MFH cases. MH and MFH express both α_1-antitrypsis (AT) and α_1-antichymotrypsin (ACT) antigens. Therefore we propose that the MFH tumor cells do not originate from monocytic cells but from (undifferentiated) fibroblastic cells. During transformation into histiocyte-like cells these cells can express several characteristics, which they share with tissue macrophages, including HLA-Dr/Ia, AT or ACT antigens.

NEPHROBLASTOMAS WITH FAVOURABLE – NORMAL – UNFAVOURABLE PROGNOSIS; A SIOP MORPHOLOGICAL STUDY

J. F. M. Delemarre, B. Sandstedt, D. Harms and Marie F. Tournade

Antoni van Leeuwenhoek Ziekenhuis, Plesmanlaan 121, 1066 CX Amsterdam, The Netherlands

On the basis of a study of 889 cases of mephroblastomas from the files of the SIOP

(International Society of Paediatric Oncology) it was possible to recognize histological subtypes with favourable, normal and unfavourable prognosis. A histological description with follow-up of these types will be presented. Favourable types are: the multicystic type (27 cases), the tubular type (21 cases) and nephroblastoma with fibroadenomatouslike structures (23 cases). Unfavourable types are: nephroblastomas with anaplasia (20 cases), the clearcell type c.q. bone metastasizing tumour of the kidney in children (19 cases) and the rhabdomyosarcomatous type (5 cases). All other cases are classified as nephroblastomas with normal prognosis. A short survey of the results of the SIOP Nephroblastomas from 1972 till now will be presented.

DEVELOPMENT OF IMMUNE REACTION AGAINST TUMOURS

W. Den Otter, H. F. J. Dullens, H. Van Loveren and R. A. De Weger

Pathologisch Instituut, Division of Experimental Pathology, Pasteurstraat 2, 3511 HX Utrecht, The Netherlands

This paper will give a review of data concerning reactions of the immune system against antigens on tumour cells and against simple haptens, and a hypothesis on antitumour immune reactions based on these data. Antigens on tumour cells can be recognized directly by T-cells. This enables T-cells to react with the release of specific factors. One of these factors can attach to monocytes/macrophages. Another factor (or the same factor?) can attach to mast cells. These specific factors can function as a bridge between tumour cells and macrophages or mast cells. This contact induces the release of factors by macrophages and mast cells. The macrophage factors cause killing of tumour cells. This will be followed by phagocytosis of tumour cell debris and antigen presentation. This will lead to the induction of helper T-cells and consequently the further development of the immune response. Mast cell factors that play a role are probably vasoactive compounds that enable the entry of lymphocytes and macrophages in the tumour. These cells are potentially cytotoxic.

EFFECT OF CHEMOTHERAPY ON HISTOLOGICAL APPEARANCES OF TESTICULAR TERATOMA METASTATIC TO LUNG; CORRELATION WITH PATIENT SURVIVAL

B. Corrin, P. Goldstraw, Marie Madden and M. J. Peckham

Brompton and Royal Marsden Hospitals, London SW3, England

We report on 20 patients with teratoma of the testis metastatic to the lungs who underwent surgical enucleation of the pulmonary metastases. Seven patients showed predominantly undifferentiated tumour in the pulmonary metastases: six of these died within 26 mth whilst the seventh was lost to follow up. Four patients showed only scarring or total necrosis of their pulmonary lesions: these patients all received full courses of chemotherapy prior to surgery and are alive and well with no evidence of recurrence up to four years after diagnosis. In nine patients the pulmonary nodules consisted of mature differentiated tissues, sometimes resembling primary pulmonary adenochondromas: these patients also received full courses of chemotherapy prior to surgery: one died of disseminated disease but the other eight are all alive and well with survival intervals of up to 14 yr after presentation. These findings demonstrate that following chemotherapy, necrosis and maturation of teratomatous pulmonary metastases signify a good prognosis.

VINCRISTINE-RESISTANCE, ASSESSED BY THE POST-METAPHASE INDEX

P. G. Ince, Karen J. Finney, J. P. Sunter, D. R. Appleton and A. J. Watson

Department of Histopathology, Royal Victoria Infirmary, Newcastle upon Tyne, England

Stathmokinetic studies on human colonic adenocarcinoma, grown in our laboratory in a short-term organ culture system, have indicated a resistance to vincristine of tumour cells compared to mucosal cells. Similar resistance has been demonstrated in human tumour cell lines, and in therapy; the underlying biochemical mechanisms are under investigation. This paper describes the preliminary findings of a study of the mechanisms of resistance to chemotherapeutic drugs, using a morphological method based on the stathmokinetic properties of the Vinca alkaloids. A dose-response experiment using 1,2-dimethylhydrazine (DMH)-treated rats was performed to compare the amount of escape from metaphase in carcinogen-induced intestinal neoplasms, carcinogen-treated mucosa, and normal mucosa, at five doses of vincristine. Groups of 25 control, and 50 experimental rats (yielding 27 tumours from 17 animals) were used. Counts of histological preparations of tumours and mucosae were performed to calculate the proportion of unequivocal post-metaphase mitotic figures to all mitotic figures (the post-metaphase index, PMI). Significant differences in dose-response relationship were found between different tissues, indicating more escape from metaphase, particularly at high doses, in the DMH-treated tissue. The PMI may be useful in screening agents thought capable of enhancing the effects of chemotherapeutic drugs.

HISTOLOGICAL STUDY OF EFFECTS OF CHEMOTHERAPY IN MICE WITH ESTABLISHED HERPES SIMPLEX VIRUS (HSV) ENCEPHALITIS

Janice R. Anderson and H. J. Field

Department of Histopathology, Addenbrooke's Hospital, Cambridge CB2 2QQ and Division of Virology, University of Cambridge, England

Mice are highly susceptible to HSV infection and provide a suitable animal model fo studying the efficacy of chemotherapy in encephalitis and the extent of tissue damage i survivors. Murine encephalitis was produced by intra-nasal inoculation of a type 1 strai of HSV. The onset of chemotherapy was delayed until infection was definitel established in the central nervous system (CNS). Mice received regular treatment wit one of three different nucleoside analogues; acyclovir (ACV), bromovinyldeoxyuridin (BVDU) or dihydroxypropoxymethyl guanine (DHPG). The animals were killed a frequent intervals and the CNS was examined microscopically, using an immunoperoxid ase technique to map the distribution of HSV antigen. Untreated animals, and likewis those receiving BDVU, died with florid encephalitis and numerous virus infected cells i the brain. In contrast, the majority of animals treated with ACV and all of thos receiving DHPG survived. During the recovery phase virus antigen gradually disap peared from all infected regions of the CNS. In later survivors there were foci c inflammation and myelin degeneration, but no virus infected cells were detected. Thes experiments show that certain chemotherapeutic agents can halt progression of acut herpetic encephalitis and apparently eliminate infectious virus from the CNS, howeve the residual tissue damage may be considerable.

THE INVERSE EXPERIMENT IN TWO STAGE SKIN CARCINOGENESIS IS NOT AS INNOCUOUS AS GENERALLY BELIEVED

O. H. Iversen

Institute of Pathology, Rikshospitalet, Oslo 1, Norway

One of the corollaries of the two stage theory of skin carcinogenesis is that if promotio is given first, and initiation thereafter, no tumours occur. It seems possible to explai this as a result of the experimental set up. The lack of tumour yield may be due to ce kinetic changes and increased cellular resistance. Hairless mice have been give promoting treatment for 18 wk with twice weekly applications of 10 nmole 12-(tetradecanoylphorbol-13-acetate and then been initiated with 7,12-dimethylbenz(anthracene at various dose levels, using skin application and intraperitoneal injectior The results show that when the inverse experiment is performed such as to compensat for cell kinetic alterations and increased resistance, the inverse experiment is nc innocuous at all, but results in a tumour yield characterized by 50% tumour-bearir animals and several malignant tumours.

NEW FREEZING METHOD FOR X-RAY MICROANALYSIS OF CULTURED CELLS IN STUDY OF INTRACELLULAR ION SHIFTS RELATED TO CELL DIFFERENTIATION

K. E. Tvedt, J. Halgunset, G. Kopstad and O. A. Haugen

Department of Pathology and Institute of Cancer Research, University of Trondheim, Regionsykehuset i Trondheim, 7000 Trondheim, Norway

X-ray microanalysis of cultured cells can provide new insight into the mechanisms whic regulate fundamental biological processes, like cell division and differentiation, ar thereby contribute to the understanding of neoplasia. Cell monolayers may be grow directly on formvar covering a central hole (15 mm in diameter) in round polystyrer plates which are placed in ordinary culture wells. For fixation the formvar film is rapid covered by a polyvinyl pyrrolidone solution on both sides, thereby expelling residues the culture medium, and plunged into supercooled Freon 22. With this new techniqu monolayers may be prepared in less than 20 sec with a minimal risk of causir redistribution of water and solutes. Numerous vertical cryosections are obtained wi the cells still anchored to the substratum. The method is simple and the necessa equipment is easily made from inexpensive and readily available materials. Furth processing and freeze-drying of the thin cryosections is routinely performed with a lo elemental support and a transportable section press. Agents which interfere with cc proliferation and differentiation cause intracellular ion shifts in prostatic carcinoma ce cultured *in vitro*.

GYNAECOLOGICAL PATHOLOGY – Slide Seminar

H. Fox

Department of Pathology, University of Manchester, Stopford Building, Manchester, England

The sections from a series of cases will be available for study throughout the meetir The main features will be presented and discussed during this session.

SPONTANEOUS AND CHOLESTEROL INDUCED ATHEROMA IN PIGEONS

P. J. Gallagher, Aud. Svindland and L. Walløe

Department of Pathology, University of Southampton, Southampton, England and Departments of Pathology and Informatics, University of Oslo, Norway

The White Carneau pigeon is a unique experimental model of atherosclerosis for, li man, it develops aortic disease spontaneously at comparatively low serum cholester concentrations and prematurely under the stress of cholesterol supplemented diets. T purpose of this study is to compare these two types of lesions and to evaluate the role haemodynamic factors in their development. Control birds (mean serum cholester concentration 8.8, range 7.2–16.8 mmol/l) were fed a mixed grain diet throughout life and killed at 3.5 yr. A large atheromatous plaque was invariably present around the first major abdominal aortic branch and small lesions were often identified in the large calibre innominate and subclavian artery supplying the wing. The chief histological features were fibrous, intimal thickening and foam cell accumulation. In general terms these appearances were a fair representation of early human atherosclerosis. A second set of birds aged 6 wk to 14 mth were fed cholesterol coated grain for 6 mth. The degree of supplementation was adjusted to maintain mean serum cholesterol values of 15 mmol/l (range c. 8–20 mmol/l). The histological features of the two types of lesions will be contrasted and the distribution of plaques as assessed by computerized topography will be presented.

FREQUENCY OF LUNG CANCER IN IRAN; A COMPARISON OF SURGICAL HISTOLOGY AND AUTOPSY FINDINGS

M. Bahadori and N. P. Bahadori

Department of Pathology, Sina Hospital, Emam Khomeini Ave., Teheran 11164, Iran

With regard to the incidence of lung cancer in Iran we have performed studies on four different category of cases. Category I: 30,417 identified cancer cases proved on the basis of histopathology during 1956–1971; Category II: 5,160 cases of randomly performed autopsies during the same period; Category III: 5,141 identified cases of malignant tumours during 1975–1980; Category IV: 375 autopsies performed during 1975–1980. Our study showed that: 1) Though carcinoma of the lung is not as common as it is in western countries it is much more common than present statistics would suggest. 2) Many patients do not receive medical or surgical treatment. Only those patients who seemed clinically manageable or for exploration underwent surgery. 3) In many autopsy cases the disease was clinically diagnosed as either tuberculosis, suppurated granulomatous infection, pulmonary abscess or metastastic carcinoma; sometimes it was found as an incidental autopsy finding. 4) The percentage of lung cancer is much higher than current statistics suggest and is at least the third commonest cancer in Iran. 5) The incidence of lung cancer is increasing in our country. 6) The findings show that the male/female ratio is 4:1 and the greatest incidence is at 50–65 yr of age. 7) Over 60% of patients are recorded as cigarette smokers. 8) The incidence of lung cancer is now estimated to be 2 per 100,000 of population.

ASBESTOSIS: THE LUNG ASBESTOS FIBRE CONTENT AND PATHOLOGICAL CHANGES OF CURRENT CASES IN THE U.K.

A. W. Jones

Departments of Pathology, Manchester University and Hope Hospital, Salford, England

Although the industrial use of asbestos has increased, there have been strenuous efforts to control asbestos exposure in the work place. With this in mind, the severity of asbestosis and degree of asbestos fibre exposure as measured by lung fibre counts have been assessed in 206 cases with a variable occupational history of asbestos exposure. The lifelong asbestos fibre exposure was assessed using a potassium hydroxide digest method with phase contrast microscopy on two samples from the left lung. Coated and uncoated fibres were counted and expressed as total fibres per gram of dried lung. Sixty-five (32%) of the 206 exposed cases had asbestosis, 25 cases occurred alone, 10 occurred in cases of mesothelioma and 30 had an accompanying bronchial carcinoma. The asbestos fibre count of control non-exposed urban lungs was between 0–191,000 fibres (mean: 25,000, n–30) but in the majority of these (93%) the count was below 50,000. In 60 (92%) of the asbestosis cases the fibre count was over one million fibres (range 1–1051 million) and in only one case was it below 500,000. In order for asbestosis, of even microscopic extent to occur, there has to be substantial fibre exposure. The relationship between lung fibre counts and the severity of the fibrosis will be discussed. In 38% of the 65 cases the asbestosis was of microscopic extent only. Of the 25 cases of solitary asbestosis without an associated malignancy, only 3 cases were sufficiently severe to produce fatal respiratory failure, whilst in 12 cases (48%) the asbestosis was one of the contributing factors in causing death and in the remaining 10 cases (40%) asbestosis was an incidental finding only. These findings indicate that whilst substantial cases of asbestosis still occur, only a minority are of a severe extent.

SOME NEW MECHANISMS IN FOETAL LUNG DISEASE

M. S. Kearney and Tone Sparr

Department of Pathology, University Hospital, Tromsø and Department of Medicine, Kirkenes Hospital, Kirkenes, Norway

The pathological findings in a 12 hr-old, 33 wk gestation, premature baby with congenital rubella and intrauterine embolisation from a dead co-twin are described. There was massive aspiration of amniotic fluid causing intrauterine lung rupture with leakage of amniotic fluid into the pleural cavities and interstitial tissues. Degenerate squames were found on the surface of the pleura, and in interstitial tissues, lymphatics and hilar lymph nodes. There were multiple old pale cystic lung infarcts which were partly organised, containing calcium and haemosiderin. Many peripheral pulmonary arteries (diameter 250–100μ) showed severe medial hypertrophy, with circumferential or eccentric intimal fibrosis, often with complete luminal occlusion. Recanalisation was seen and the intimal fibrous tissue often contained haemosiderin. A single fresh thrombus was found. Numerous peripheral pulmonary arteries showed massive sub-involution, some had almost disappeared, represented only by coarse clumps or slender threads of elastin. Micro-thrombi were found in some glomeruli and the spleen contained scars with calcium and haemosiderin. The brain showed severe hydrancephaly with massive necrosis and focal calcification. The pathogenesis and possible significance of these findings are discussed.

RELAPSING RAPIDLY PROGRESSIVE GLOMERULONEPHRITIS SUCCESSFULLY TREATED BY PLASMA EXCHANGE

J. Christensen, Y. Willassen and I. Morild

Gade Institute, Department of Pathology, 5016 Haukeland Hospital, and Medical Department, 5016 Haukeland Hospital, Norway

A 30-yr-old man was admitted to Haukeland Hospital, Bergen, Norway on 9th July 1982 after 1½ mth with slight fever and tenderness in joints and muscles. On admittance he had acute renal failure with serum creatinine 400/μmol/l. Serum complement and AST were normal, ANF was negative. There had been no hemoptysis. Renal biopsy showed a pronounced mesangial proliferation and newly formed crescents in all glomeruli. Following treatment with Prednisone, Imurel and 10 plasma exchanges the renal function returned to normal. In the repeat biopsy 3 mth later, only old cresents were found. After treatment with Prednisone and Imurel was stopped, the renal function was still normal in October 1983. The urine was free of protein. One month later the patient was admitted to the medical department again with the same symptoms as in 1982: acute renal failure and proteinuria. Renal biopsy now showed newly formed crescents together with old crescents in more than 80% of the glomeruli. The patient was treated in the same way as in 1982; responded well and has at present normal renal function. We conclude that the course of the glomerulo-nephritis was decisively influenced by the plasma exchanges.

RENAL CORTICAL INTERSTITIUM AND ITS IMPORTANCE FOR RENAL FUNCTION

A. Bohle

Institute of Pathology, University of Tübingen, Federal Republic of Germany

Studies made to correlate structure and function in inflammatory and non-inflammatory glomerular diseases resulted in: 1) a significant correlation between the level of serum creatinine and the width of the renal cortical interstitium in endocapillary, mesangio-proliferative, membranous and membranoproliferative glomerulonephritis; 2) in membranous and membranoproliferative glomerulonephritis with normal creatinine in serum (60–128μmol/l) there was a significant negative correlation between the creatinine clearance and the width of the renal cortical interstitium; 3) in glomerular amyloidosis and diabetic glomerulosclerosis the level of serum creatinine was not correlated to the degree of glomerular changes but to the extent of cortical interstitial fibrosis; 4) in chronic sclerosing nephristis as well, the level of serum creatinine was correlated to the cortical interstitial fibrosis; 5) with increasing cortical interstitial fibrosis there was a significant decrease in number and total area of postglomerular capillaries and increasing atrophy of tubuli. From these findings we conclude, that the elimination of waste products in the kidney is not primarily dependent of the morphological changes in the glomeruli as the filtration organ, but on the condition of the postglomerular capillaries. It follows that with increasing cortical interstitial fibrosis the glomerular blood flow and hence filtration is reduced. This in turn causes an elevation of the serum creatinine.

SEASONALITY OF BREAST CANCER

N. Kirkham, D. Machin, D. W. K. Cotton and J. M. Pike

Departments of Pathology and Community Medicine, Faculty of Medicine, University of Southampton, Southampton SO9 4XY, England

In Bergen breast cancer shows a variation in size and stage that is related to the side of the tumour and the season of presentation. To see if this is a purely Nordic phenomenon, we have conducted a retrospective analysis of data relating to breast cancer in Southampton. Over 400 biopsies of primary breast cancer were submitted to the laboratory between September 1975 and August 1981. We retrieved cases from the SNOP index and for each one recorded the date of biopsy, the patient's date of birth, the side, size, histological type and axillary lymph node status associated with the tumour. Our analysis shows a strong seasonal variation in the time of presentation of tumours, with the peak in June. The relationship between this seasonality and the other factors analysed will be discussed.

HISTOLOGY AND PROGNOSIS IN BREAST CANCER

T. J. Anderson, J. M. Dixon, R. A. Elton, D. L. Page, S. W. Duffy and D. Lee

University Departments of Pathology, Clinical Surgery and Medical Computing and Statistics, Edinburgh, Scotland

From a histological review of breast cancer in Edinburgh 246 patients treated during the first four years of the review were followed to 1980 or death. Ten histological parameters for each tumour were analysed to determine the relation to survival, with particular reference to the short term (0–5 yr) and the long term (0–20 yr). In addition, the analysis examined the value of these same parameters in judging the probability of survival in the period following the first 5 yr (5–20 yr). Two factors remained significant discriminants in all analyses (0–5, 0–20, 5–20 yr) and these were histological type and histological grade. Discrimination against survival was given by vascular and lymphocytic invasion, necrosis and multifocality with a maximum effect in the first 5 yr. The importance of such information for treatment decisions is apparent. However, different factors are related to short and long term survival and thus a single prognostic index is unlikely to be satisfactory in the evaluation of all patients at the time of first diagnosis.

PROGNOSTIC INDEX BASED ON NODE POSITIVE BREAST CANCER PATIENTS

B. Mæhle, R. Skjærven and F. Hartveit

Department of Pathology, University of Bergen, 5000 – Bergen, Norway

This study includes 112 axillary lymph node positive breast carcinoma patients treated by modified radical mastectomy between 1970–1972. The most important prognostic variables for these patients were whether the efferent nodal vessels (EVI) contained tumour cells or not, the size of the primary tumour and the area of the tumour cell nuclei. Combination of these variables using regression statistics gave a prognostic index predicting the patient survival at 60 and 98 mth after surgery correctly in 83 and 80% of the patients respectively. Other possible combinations of variables are discussed.

ULTRASTRUCTURE OF SCLEROSING LESIONS OF HUMAN BREAST

Sharon Battersby and T. J. Anderson

Department of Pathology, University of Edinburgh, Teviot Place, Edinburgh, Scotland

The human breast can be affected by a range of distinctive but interrelated sclerosing changes, such as sclerosing adenosis and radial scars, in addition to physiologically sclerosing lobules. We have examined 50 sclerosing lesions including two examples of obliterative mastitis to identify features that are common and those that are distinctive. The radial scar is unique in displaying central elastosis, associated with large numbers of myofibroblasts. Sclerosing adenosis and physiological sclerosis also show focal elastosis, but this is relatively sparse in extent and distribution. Study of early, active stellate scars shows that myofibroblasts are seen initially surrounding central ductules, which show epithelial degradative change. Loss of basement membrane is a prominent feature. This is unlike physiologically sclerosing lobules or sclerosing adenosis in which reduplication and thickening of the basement membrane are often outstanding. The myofibroblast activity is similar to obliterative mastitis, where there is pronounced collagen and elastin synthesis accompanied by obliteration of the ductal lumen.

QUANTITATION OF MACROPHAGES IN HUMAN BREAST CANCER USING MONOCLONAL ANTIBODY (EBM/11) TO HUMAN MACROPHAGES

E. Bliss, M. Naien, J. Burns, K. Bell and J. O'D. McGee

University of Oxford, Nuffield Department of Pathology, John Radcliffe Hospital, Oxford OX3 9DU, England

A monoclonal antibody (EBM/11) has been raised against isolated human lung macrophages. Immunohistochemically this antibody reacts with fresh acetone fixed blood monocytes and mononuclear cells (presumptive macrophages) of lung, skin, stomach, small and large bowel, pancreas, spleen and tonsil, peritubular and mesangial cells in kidney, placenta, liver, gall bladder, heart, thyroid, pituitary and brain (microglial cells). It does not react with any other cell type in the tissues screened except the epithelium of renal proximal tubules. It also reacts with mononuclear stromal cells in invasive mammary cancer. By comparison with non-neoplastic breast there is a great increase in the number of EBM/11 positive cells per unit area in breast cancer.

Posters and Demonstrations

MYOCARDIAL INFARCTION IN CHILDREN

D. W. K. Cotton, P. J. Gallagher and R. A. Sleet

Department of Pathology and Accident and Emergency Unit, Southampton University General Hospital, Southampton SO9 4XY, England

Subendocardial infarction, like other forms of myocardial infarction, is strongly associated with coronary artery disease. Consequently it is a rare event in children. Two cases of subendocardial infarction occurring in boys aged 12 and 14 are described. Both had collapsed unexpectedly, one following an epileptic fit, the other after an unexplained incident at a fairground. Each received some form of cardiopulmonary resuscitation before being transferred to intensive care for ventilation. One child died three days later after a cardiac arrest, the other was declared dead on brain death criteria after six days. In both cases there was extensive subendocardial infarction in the left ventricle, but apart from cerebral and pulmonary oedema no other significant changes. We interpret these findings as being secondary to an episode of inadequate coronary perfusion. This is probably a relatively common event in patients who collapse with episodes of cardiac arrhythmias. However it will only become apparent if the patient survives, or is kept alive long enough, for the gross and histological signs to develop.

MONOCLONAL ANTIBODIES TO CYTOKERATINS IN STUDY OF PREMALIGNANT LESIONS OF UTERINE CERVIX

J. Puts, O. Moesker, Anita Huysmans, P. Vooijs and F. Ramaekers

St. Radboud University Hospital, Department of Pathology, Geert Grooteplein Zuid 24, 6525 GA Nijmegen, The Netherlands

Cytokeratins are intermediate filament proteins that occur specifically in epithelial cells. Using antibodies to these proteins epithelial cells can be detected specifically by immunohistochemical methods. Thus, using a polyclonal rabbit keratin antiserum in the indirect immunofluorescence technique on frozen tissue sections from normal cervix, both ectocervical stratified squamous epithelium and endocervical glandular epithelium show a positive staining reaction. A monoclonal antibody, raised against a HeLa-cell cytokeratin specifically and exclusively recognizes glandular epithelial cells. This type of cytokeratin is no longer detectable in endocervical squamous metaplastic and dysplastic epithelial cells. A second monoclonal antibody specifically stains keratinizing cells in stratified squamous, metaplastic and dysplastic epithelium. These data indicate that alterations in cytokeratin expression occur in premalignant lesions of the uterine cervix.

JOURNAL OF PATHOLOGY, VOL. **143:** 69–80 (1984)

MORPHOMETRIC AND RELATED QUANTITATIVE TECHNIQUES IN THE STUDY OF LYMPHOID NEOPLASMS. A REVIEW

J. CROCKER

Department of Histopathology, East Birmingham Hospital, Bordesley Green East, Birmingham B9 5ST, U.K.

Received 7 July 1983
Accepted 22 September 1983

KEY WORDS—Malignant lymphoma, non-Hodgkin's lymphoma, Hodgkin's disease, morphometry.

EQUIPMENT AND TECHNIQUES

Most morphometric studies of lymphoid tissue have been carried out in the last ten years and consequently many have involved the use of various computer-assisted or controlled image analysers. However, earlier investigations, particularly those dependent upon ultrastructural analysis, made use of 'conventional' manual point-counting methods. It is not appropriate in this review to describe such techniques in detail but the reader is referred to the two excellent accounts by Steer[1] and by Aherne and Dunnill.[2] Manual point-counting methods are slow and sometimes cumbersome and more recently image-analysing machines have been introduced in many biological and medical fields to rapidly and accurately acquire many more morphometric data than is possible by manual means.

Fully automatic image-analysers (such as the Zeiss Microvideomat and Cambridge Quantimet 720) have, in the past, suffered from severe limitations in the investigation of lymphomas because they are generally very poorly suited to the examination of sections of lymphoid tissues. Most fully-automatic image-analysers operate on the basis of pre-adjusted 'grey scales' by virtue of which the user assigns a 'grey-level' to a feature of interest (for example, a cell nucleus) which is then discriminated by the machine. An image is generated by a 'television' camera, such as a Plumbicon tube and is relayed to further processors, memory stores and visual display consoles. With sections cut at conventional thickness or even with 'thin' plastic-embedded sections, there is considerable overlap or contact between cells or nuclei. Thus, cell clusters are 'read' by the machines as single, large, features. In some instances this can be overcome by light-pen-editing but this is tiresome and not always accurate. Thus, although many data are very rapidly acquired by such equipment, the results may be inaccurate. The problems of setting up such devices, the use of grey-scales and the modification of discrimination by automatic image-analysers is very well surveyed by Bradbury.[3]

Much better suited to the study of lymphoid tissue are the semi-automatic planimeter-type machines which incorporate a 'graphic tablet' or digitizer, linked to a microprocessor mini-computer. These systems may be hard- or soft-wired, the latter being more flexible and allowing the measurement of larger ranges of features. Examples of such image-analysers are the Reichert-Jung (Kontron) MOP series of machines, the Leitz ASM and the PDP 11/10-graphic tablet system. Micrographs may be placed on the graphic tablet and features of interest outlined by a sensitive pen coupled to the microprocessor. More directly, a *camera lucida* drawing system may be used with a conventional microscope; a light-emitting diode in the sensitive pen tip is then seen superimposed on the image of the section being studied. This can be traced accordingly over the digitizing pad. (Of course, the use of micrographs on the pad with pen-outlining is

0022-3417/84/060069-12$01.20

necessary for ultrastructural investigations.) By this means, the problems of cell or nuclear overlap or contact, which so severely limit the use of fully automatic analysers, are overcome, since the user selects features of interest and outlines them. However, two disadvantages result. Firstly, the process is much slower than that with fully automatic devices; nonetheless, with experience, the operator can accurately and quite quickly generate many data, which are sufficient to be of statistical value. Secondly, and of more importance, a problem of randomization arises. Great care must be taken (using, for example, eyepiece grid graticules) to measure all of the examples of features of interest in each field; similarly, fields themselves must be chosen, as far as is possible, at random.

The advent of a novel generation of automatic image-analysers, which 'recognize' overlapping or contiguous features by a process of 'erosion-dilatation' may revolutionize morphometric studies of a variety of tissues and enable the very rapid generation of many and complex data. Such a machine is the Reichert-Jung (Kontron) IBAS II system.

NORMAL CELLS AND TISSUES

Lymphoid cells have been morphometrically or stereologically described in several studies, mainly as free cells, as such analysis offers the possibility of comparison with biochemical data and because cell suspensions may readily be 'handled' or cultured. In addition, phenomena such as blast transformation may be morphometrically studied. Thus, Biberfield[4] used histometric methods in a study of morphogenesis in blood lymphocytes stimulated by phytohaemagglutinin. Similarly, Douglas *et al.*[5] later performed planimetry on electron micrographs of mitogen-stimulated normal and chronic lymphocytic leukaemic lymphocytes. More recently, Petrzilka *et al.*[6] used 'manual' point-counting techniques to quantify cell size and various ultrastructural components of human peripheral blood T-lymphocytes. The mean volume of a small, 'resting' cell was 103·8 μm^3, with a mean nuclear and cytoplasmic volume of 47·5 and 55·9 μm^3, respectively. The mean numbers of mitochondria and free ribosomes were also counted and the cisternae of the rough endoplasmic reticulum and Golgi apparatus measured. It was admitted that although the system for cell preparation yielded a fairly pure cell population, small numbers of T-cell subtypes may have been present. The data were, in general, in accord with those of Biberfield[4] and of Douglas *et al.*[5]

In an attempt to differentiate human T- and B-lymphocytes from the peripheral blood, Renau-Piqueras *et al.*[7] applied morphometric analysis to electron micrographs of these cells. The cells were identified by sheep erythrocyte rosetting or by immunoperoxidase conjugate labelling. Numerous measurements were made and differences between T- and B-lymphocytes were found with regard to nuclear eccentricity, the relative surface area occupied by peripheral and condensed chromatin, the mean number of central chromatin clumps and the number of perichromatin granules in relation to the area of nuclear surface. In addition, the cell surface area of B-lymphocytes was significantly greater than that of T-lymphocytes. Previous, qualitative transmission electron microscopy had revealed no differences between human B- and T-lymphocytes[8] and the value of a painstaking morphometric study is evident. A careful morphometric analysis of chromatin distribution and perichromatin granule density by Miragall and Renau-Piqueras[9] also revealed distinct differences between small cortical and medullary thymocytes in the rat. This study, concerned specifically with nuclear/chromatin structures, extends previous studies by Abe and Ito[10] and Matter[11] who demonstrated quantitative differences between the two cell types.

Some kinetic studies of lymphocytes are worthy of note, although a comprehensive account of such research is not within the scope of this review. Stewart and Ingram[12] isolated nuclei from canine lymphocytes (in culture) and measured their size distribution using an electronic particle counter. Subsequently, Stewart *et al.*[13] extended this study to the measurement of human lymphocyte nuclei; in both studies the cells were, in effect, examined in the S-phase of growth. Phytohaemagglutinin-stimulation was used by Takahashi,[14] who used a fully automatic image-analyser, the Quantimet 720, to measure volume changes in Feulgen(DNA)-stained lymphocyte nuclei. It was found that a significant amount of nuclear enlargement was not seen until day 2 *in vitro*. In an attempt to clarify the effects of mitogen-stimulation upon lymphocytes, Brown *et al.*[15] used a Quantimet 720 to examine the size-distribution of lymphocytes after phytohaemagglutinin stimulation. As the Quantimet 720 uses a Plumbicon tube for analysis, cells were widely spread in the examined preparations to avoid cell–cell contact problems. It was found that the percentage of cells undergoing growth in size was consistent with the mathematics of cell growth up to an initial mitosis and the authors suggested that this technique could have general application to studies of cell growth in culture.

In addition to the morphometric examination of individual lymphoid cells, there have been occasional studies of normal lymphoid tissues, using quantitative methodology. These have principally been aimed at the measurement of zones (such as T- and B-dependent areas) in normal lymph nodes or in those responding to various stimuli. Meyer *et al.*,[16] for example, used point-counting techniques in an attempt to define 'normal' values for the proportions of T- and B-areas of lymph nodes, in BALB/c mice. T-regions were demonstrated by virtue of punctate cytoplasmic acid α-naphthyl acetate esterase (ANAE) activity within lymphocytes and B-areas were shown by means of the immunohistochemical technique for intracytoplasmic immunoglobulins. Several tissue compartments were defined and measured, namely, the non-follicular outer cortex, primary follicles plus lymphocyte cuffs of secondary follicles, germinal centres, medullary cords, paracortical area and capsule and sinuses. Two groups of mice, matched with respect to age and strain were examined. Most interestingly, it was found that the proportion of B cell areas varied significantly with environmental conditions, whereas the proportion of T cell areas remained constant. The two groups of animals had been sacrificed and studied at different times of the year and the authors suggested that some environmental factor of unknown nature provoked differences in the sizes of B cell areas between the groups. In an extension of this work, Meyer and Grundmann[17] investigated the response of nodes to Bacillus Calmette-Guerin (BCG), the response to which is known to be of a cell mediated (T) nature. Thus, a means to affect the T-compartment of lymph nodes was sought. BALB/c mice were challenged with BCG and subsequently the B- and T-areas of nodes measured (by point counting) using the previous criteria of Meyer *et al.*[16] After BCG stimulation there was a profound increase in the nodal T-area together with lymphocytic hyperplasia (which was also supported by autoradiographic data). Thymic-dependent areas in the spleen were also measured; these showed a transient involution, apparently the result of the release of T-cells into the circulation. Subsequently, there was recovery and hyperplasia of these areas in the spleen. None of these changes was observable subjectively and the authors stress the value of histomorphometry in such studies.

The latter results are of interest when compared with those of a previous analysis of immune lymph node responses to transplantable neoplasms by Van de Velde *et al.*[18] Immunogenic and non-immunogenic tumours were inoculated into C57Bl/Ka and CBA/Rij mice and subsequently nodes from several regions were sectioned in semiseries. Morphometric analysis was performed on the cortex and paracortex and the summated values of these areas correlated well with the nodal weight. Apart from these regional nodes, those from non-regional sites were also examined and in this instance, unlike that in the regional group, it was found that the immunogenicity of the injected neoplasm could not be related to the evoked morphometric nodal changes. The conclusion was reached that caution was needed in the interpretation of morphological changes in lymph nodes apparently responding to transplanted tumours. Whether similar care should also be exercised in the case of non-neoplastic stimuli is conjectural.

The human palatine tonsil has been studied by various workers with regard to morphology and immunohistology and provides a useful 'control' organ for many investigations; (see, for example, Curran and Jones;[19] Brandtzaeg *et al.*;[20] Crocker.[21]) Some of these studies have semi-quantitatively measured B-cell numbers in different regions of the tonsil or have adopted a qualitative architectural approach. However, a most painstaking recent paper by Si *et al.*[22] has quantified the numbers and distribution of T-lymphocyte subsets in human tonsils. Monoclonal antisera to total, helper and suppressor T-cells were applied and the biotin–avidin–peroxidase technique used. It was found that 14·2±1·7 per cent of cells in the periphery of germinal centres of secondary follicles were T-cells and in the most central area, T-lymphocytes accounted for 2·4±0·7 per cent of all cells. Seven per cent of cells in the 'mantle zone' were of the T variety. Only 1 per cent of the lymphocytes in these areas were of suppressor subtype. The majority of interfollicular cells were T-lymphocytes; again, suppressor cells were in the minority. This confirms subjective assessments of T-lymphocyte numbers in these regions by Crocker,[21] using the acid α-naphthyl acetate esterase technique, which has been shown to stain Tμ lymphocytes in a punctate fashion by, for example, Zicca *et al.*[23] The potential value of quantitative studies of T-cell subsets in lymphoid tissue could be considerable, perhaps particularly in relation to the investigation of lymph nodes with dermatopathic change or early mycosis fungoides.

MYCOSIS FUNGOIDES AND SÉZARY'S SYNDROME

A frequent diagnostic problem arises from the interpretation of lymphoid infiltrates of the skin. This difficulty has stimulated certain workers to apply morphometric analysis to such specimens, in the hope of arriving at measurements which can usefully distinguish between benign and malignant infiltrates. The feature which has mostly been investigated is the high degree of nuclear convolution which is so prominent in the cells of mycosis fungoides (MF) and Sézary's syndrome (SS). The presence of such 'cerebriform' nuclei has been used, qualitatively, to diagnose MF and SS but it was not until the study by Litovitz and Lutzner[24] that an objective measurement of nuclear convolution was performed. These authors made use of a shape-describing parameter, the nuclear contour index (NCI) which is independent of size. The NCI value of a structure is given by the relationship

$$\mathrm{NCI} = \frac{\text{perimeter}}{\sqrt{\text{area}}}$$

and was first derived by Schrek.[25] A perfect circle has a value of 3·54 ($2/\sqrt{\pi}$) and increasing indentation or convolution results in higher NCI values. Schrek demonstrated by this means that the nuclei of the cells of chronic lymphocytic leukaemia had highly rounded, non-irregular nuclei.

Meijer *et al.*[26] showed, by means of NCI measurements, that early MF infiltrates in the skin could be differentiated from chronic benign skin infiltrates, the MF cells having much higher values for NCI than the benign, infiltrating cells.

Subsequently, van der Loo *et al.*[27] investigated the possibility of diagnosing early MF and SS by performing morphometry on the nuclei of cells isolated from inguinal lymph nodes removed as part of the staging procedure for these conditions. DNA cytophotometry was also performed, as this technique had previously been shown to be of value in the diagnosis of MF by van Vloten *et al.*[29] The morphometric study involved the use of electron micrographs of the isolated cells; at least 75 nuclei were outlined using a graphic digitizer interfaced to a microcomputer, which calculated the nuclear perimeter, area and NCI. A group of nodes showing dermatopathic lymphadenopathy (DL) were also included and non-linear discriminant analysis was applied to the data to differentiate NCI values for cells in nodes with DL from those in nodes with DL and MF. 'Training sets' of lymph nodes involved by cutaneous T cell lymphomas and of nodes removed from patients with other diseases were examined and the mean and standard deviation of NCI were found to be the most useful measurements, with a 90 per cent probability of correct diagnostic assignation. The authors concluded that the diagnosis of early MF involvement of lymph nodes can be aided by measurement of the NCI of isolated cells. Van der Loo *et al.*[28] extended the previous study of mycosis fungoides by combining membrane marker evaluation with morphometric data. A series of 26 patients with MF were studied. The type and extent of their skin disease and the percentage of convoluted cells, and T and B lymphocytes in the peripheral blood and lymph node suspensions were quantified. These data were correlated with the clinical course of the disease and with malignant involvement of regional nodes. Raised levels of circulating cells with convoluted nuclei (i.e. >20 per cent) were found in 9 of 11 patients with MF involving the regional lymph nodes, compared with normal numbers of such cells (2–18 per cent) in patients with MF in the absence of nodal infiltration. Examination of lymph node cell suspensions from 9 of 10 MF patients with node involvement revealed increased levels (>15 per cent) of convoluted cells but two of three MF patients whose lymph nodes were not infiltrated had normal numbers (4 and 7 per cent) of convoluted cells in such preparations. 'Normal' T and B lymphocytes were demonstrated in the peripheral blood of MF patients by virtue of erythrocyte rosetting. A decreased number of normal T cells (≤55 per cent) was found mainly in patients with lymph node involvement but T cell levels were normal in the absence of nodal infiltration. The lymph node cell suspensions showed no significant differences in the numbers of B and T cells between patients whose nodes were or were not involved.

In a further paper by van der Loo *et al.*,[29] an attempt was made to differentiate infiltrates of MF and SS from those of benign lymphoid infiltrates in the skin. Electron micrographs of dermal lesions from 20 patients with MF/SS and 14 with chronic benign lymphoid infiltrates were studied. In addition, 20 patients with suspected MF/SS were included. As before, the mean NCI was measured for each specimen, using a graphic digitizer and microcomputer. Histograms of the NCI measurements for each case were analysed, assuming that a 'cerebriform' cell was one with an NCI of $\geq 6{\cdot}5$. Non-linear discriminant analysis showed that, for known cases of MF/SS or benign infiltration, classification criteria were derived such that all patients could be grouped correctly with high probability (≥ 95 per cent). Of the 34 patients of known diagnosis, only one was classified with low probability (71 per cent). The morphometric criteria arrived at were the presence of cerebriform cells (with an NCI $\geq 11{\cdot}5$) and the frequency distribution of cerebriform cells expressed as the 25th and 70th percentiles of the NCI histograms. The predictive value of these studies was tested on the 29 patients with suspected MF/SS. On the basis of morphometric criteria, 20 were classified as malignant; in the 4-year follow-up period, 17 developed MF, one probably developed MF and two had lymphomatoid papulosis. Eight of the remaining nine patients classified as having benign skin infiltration were proven to have benign skin disease (including psoriasis, Jessner's disease and atopic dermatitis) and one developed MF. The application of these morphometric techniques was felt to be of greater diagnostic accuracy and value than DNA cytophotometry.

Apparently simultaneously, studies independent to those of the above Dutch group were published by McNutt and Crain[31] in the U.S.A. In this paper, electron micrographs of lymphoid cells in MF and benign dermal infiltrates were examined, using a graphic digitizer coupled to a programmable calculator. The nuclear perimeters were outlined and the NCI calculated. Specimens from 77 patients with benign infiltrates, 16 with early MF and 16 with uncertain lesions were studied. The group mean NCI for the MF cases was 6·1, compared with a group mean of 4·6–5·4 for the benign infiltrates, these values being significantly different. The authors suggested that a morphometric ultrastructural diagnosis of MF required two criteria, namely, a mean NCI of $\geq 6{\cdot}1$ and at least 6 per cent of cells with an NCI of $\geq 9{\cdot}0$. Nonetheless, a false positive rate of 3 per cent was observed in benign infiltrates using these requirements. Indeed, a 50 per cent false negative rate was observed in early MF case. It was noted that lymphocytes with an NCI of ≥ 16 are the only absolute reliable criterion for MF but unfortunately such cells were not always present. McNutt *et al.*[32] also investigated the usefulness of nuclear profile perimeter and area (as well as NCI) but found the former two measurements of little value in differentiating MF and benign lesions. However, a combination of a mean NCI of $\geq 7{\cdot}0$ and the proportion of cells with a mean nuclear area of $\geq 30\ \mu m^2$ was useful in this respect.

Most recently, Caorsi *et al.*[33] used planimeter-based morphometry to measure cell area, nucleus to cell size ratio and NCI on electron micrographs of skin biopsies infiltrated by proven MF. As a result of this study, the authors were able to identify 2 main cell lineages, namely, lymphoid cells (including lymphoblastic-like cells, lymphocytes and MF cells) and Langerhans' cells (LC). A zinc–iodide–osmium technique to demonstrate LC showed that they had moved from the epidermis to the dermis and it was proposed that they may 'organize' the disease. Accordingly, contacts between LC and the lymphoid cells were prominent and the suggestion was put forward that the malignant clones may occur primarily in the dermis rather than the epidermis.

NON-HODGKIN'S LYMPHOMAS

The potential value of an accurate and reproducible means of measuring cell and/or nuclear size in non-Hodgkin lymphomas (NHL) is considerable. Modern morphological classifications make use of nuclear size and shape and these are, of course, usually subjectively assessed. Accurate subclassification is essential in NHL, as prognosis and therapy are closely related to the histological subtype. In the classifications of Bennett *et al.*[34] and of Lukes and Collins,[35] cells with large or small nuclei are described, forming, to some extent, a basis of the classifications. In these systems, tumours composed principally of large cells tend to be of higher malignancy than those composed of small cells. The Kiel classification of Gerard-Marchant *et al.*,[36] modified by Lennert[37] makes use of terms such as, for example, 'centroblasts' and 'immunoblasts', whose nuclei are large;

conversely, 'centrocytes' and lymphocytes have small nuclei.

Again, the predominance of such cells in a particular lymphoma and its consequent classification may lead to grouping into high- or low-grade malignancy. Such observations have stimulated several studies of cell and nuclear size in lymphoid tissue, whose aim has been to arrive at objective data and to investigate the diagnostic value of such procedures.

Perhaps the first detailed study of nuclear sizes in lymphomas was that of Crocker and Curran.[33] In this study, 28 lymph nodes were examined, including specimens of Hodgkin's disease (HD), NHL and reactive benign nodes. Eight palatine tonsils were also studied. A fully-automatic image analyser, the Zeiss 'Microvideomat' was used. The proximity and overlap of nuclei in conventional histological sections of the specimens precluded their use and imprint preparations, giving well-separated nuclei, were resorted to. Nuclei were discriminated by their 'grey level' and their horizontal diameter automatically measured. The results gave histograms and mean nuclear diameters for all but 2 of the specimens (which were 'uncountable'). Disappointingly, the scatter of these measurements was considerable and there was much 'overlap' between the disease groups, although 'reactive' nodes and tonsil preparations tended to have lower mean diameters than those from HD and NHL. It was also not possible to correlate the mean nuclear diameter in the NHL group with the subtype of the particular specimen. The limitations of this technique are self-evident for, although many data are rapidly produced, the operator is dependent upon fresh biopsy material as histological sections cannot be used. In addition, some cells may stick to glass more readily than others during imprint preparation.

Subsequently, Abbott *et al.*[39] performed morphometric analysis on a small series of specimens (10) of NHL, using histological sections with an automated (Quantimet 720) and user-controlled, interactive machine (the Kontron MOP-AMO_3). The specimens were classified according to the scheme of Bennett *et al.*[34] and both nuclear area itself and nuclear area correlated with frequency per unit field were measured. These corresponded well with the morphological classification for all specimens, in contrast to the findings of Crocker and Curran with the Zeiss Microvideomat (no doubt as a result of different specimen preparation). The automatic image-analyser was far from satisfactory, much light pen-editing proving necessary, whereas the MOP-AMO_3 was satisfactory in all ten cases. Section thickness correction was performed by the Saltykov method.[40]

Crocker *et al.*[41] used an interactive graphic digitizer–microprocessor, the Kontron MOP-AMO_3, to study the nuclear maximum diameter (D_{Max}) in 21 specimens of NHL, classified according to the Kiel system. The mean D_{Max} values of high-grade lymphomas were considerably higher than in those of low-grade malignancy, although there was considerable overlap of the ranges. The immunoblastic lymphomas had the largest values for D_{Max}. The authors compared the value of the MOP-AMO_3 favourably with that of fully-automatic image analysers. Section thickness correction was performed using Weibel curves as described by Steer[1] and use was made of the simple but powerful technique of probability curve analysis to demonstrate at least two populations of cells (by virtue of their nuclear D_{Max}) in each specimen. The probability curves also showed a small population of giant cells in the specimens of immunoblastic lymphoma.

Most neoplasms designated in the past as 'histiocytic lymphomas' are now known to be of B-cell lineage and include, for example, immunoblastic lymphoma. In an attempt to further characterize such 'large-cell lymphomas', van der Valk *et al.*[42] combined cell surface and cytoplasm marker studies with morphometry. Plastic-embedded thin sections of the tissues from 28 large-cell NHL were used, to give optimal nuclear and nucleolar morphology and morphometric measurements were performed with an MOP-AMO_3 or related image-analyser. The Lukes and Collins classification was used. Nuclear size and shape (by NCI), cytoplasmic area, cytoplasm: nucleus ratio and the size, number and eccentricity of nucleoli were measured. It was found, statistically, that the NCI could differentiate between true histiocytic lymphoma and large noncleaved follicle centre cell tumours or B-immunoblastic lymphomas, the NCI being much greater in the foremost. Large non-cleaved follicle centre cell lymphoma also possessed more nucleoli per nuclear profile and more eccentrically-placed nucleoli than did B-immunoblastic lymphoma. The cytoplasm: nucleus area ratio was of value only in distinguishing true histiocytic lymphoma from large noncleaved follicle centre cell lymphomas. These results were in accord with those of a previous study by van der Valk *et al.*[43] of 10 cases of genuine histiocytic lymphoma. These specimens were characterized morphologically, ultrastructurally, immunologically and cytochemically. The nuclear NCI was measured in sections from each of the 10 cases and was compared with that of five other lymphomas. The latter comprised three specimens of B-immunoblastic lymphoma, one T-lymphoblastic lymphoma and one specimen of 'large cleaved follicle centre cell' lymphoma. In all cases, the histiocytic lymphomas had higher values for NCI than the other NHL.

In an extension of the former study, van der Valk *et al.*[44] performed nuclear morphometry on four cases of proposed dendritic reticulum cell sarcoma. These specimens differed from true histiocytic lymphoma or other B- or T-cell lymphomas as morphometry revealed interdigitations between the constituent cells, monoclonal immunoglobulins or T-cell antigen were absent, as were muramidase, α_1-antitrypsin and α_1-antichymotrypsin. Also, 5′-nucleotidase (a dendritic reticulum cell surface marker) was present in three of the specimens, but acid phosphatase (a macrophage marker) was absent. Ia-like antigens were present on the tumour cells in all four cases. A graphic digitizer–microprocessor system was used for morphometric measurement of the NCI, using photographs of plastic-embedded thin sections. The tumour could be differentiated from true histiocytic lymphomas by virtue of NCI, the percentage of cells with an NCI of $>5{\cdot}5$ being much higher in the latter than in these possible cases of dendritic reticulum cell sarcoma. Thus, a novel form of lymphoma may have been described and partly characterized by morphometry.

A paper by Crocker *et al.*,[45] using the MOP-AMO_3, attempted to find morphometric means to differentiate the subtypes of low- and high-grade NHL and to distinguish these from benign, 'reactive' lymph nodes. Thirty specimens of NHL (classified by the Kiel system) and 10 reactive nodes were examined and for each the mean nuclear D_{Max} and area were measured. In addition, the mean nuclear form factor (*FF*) was quantified as a representation of nuclear irregularity. The *FF* of a structure is given by the simple relationship:

$$FF = \frac{4\pi \text{ Area}}{\text{Perimeter}^2}$$

For a perfect circle, $FF=1{\cdot}0$. Deviations from this lead to values approaching 0·1. Thus, highly irregular, infolded or lobulate nuclei have values away from unity, whilst a truly round nuclear cross-section has an *FF* value of 1·0. The specimens of high-grade lymphoma (immunoblastic, lymphoblastic, centroblastic and unclassifiable) had much higher values for mean nuclear area and D_{Max} than did the low-grade (centrocytic and centroblastic–centrocytic) specimens. Unfortunately, neither mean nuclear area of D_{Max} was able to distinguish between reactive lymph node and low-grade NHL. The values obtained were, in general, larger than those of other workers; this is readily accounted for, as the MOP-AMO_3 was programmed here to exclude nuclei with a D_{Max} of <5 μm or area of <50 μm^2 in an attempt to reduce the problem of non-equatorial sectioning. In addition, paraffin sections cut at approximately 4 μm thickness were used, unlike the 1 μm plastic sections of other studies. Furthermore, Weibel techniques were applied as a means of section thickness correction. There was good correlation between mean nuclear area and D_{Max} for all specimens, being particularly so for reactive nodes and low-grade NHL. This would be expected, as a perfect circle should exhibit a linear relationship between D_{Max} and area. The high-grade lymphomas showed rather less close correlation between D_{Max} and area, suggesting more irregularly-shaped nuclei in these specimens. This conclusion was supported by the measurements of mean nuclear *FF*, which was in general lower in high-grade NHL than in low-grade NHL or reactive nodes.

An elegant and complex study of 52 specimens of B-cell NHL by van der Valk *et al.*[46] made use of morphometry on plastic-embedded sections of the tissue, which had been characterized by immunological, histochemical and ultrastructural means. Methyl-methacrylate was preferred to paraffin wax for tissue embedding by the authors, supposedly causing less shrinkage. The specimens comprised cases of chronic lymphocytic leukaemia, lymphoplasmacytoid and polymorphic immunocytoma, centrocytic, centroblastic–centrocytic, centroblastic, immunoblastic and lymphoblastic lymphoma. In addition, five specimens of so-called 'intermediate' lymphocytic lymphoma were included. Several parameters were measured, being those measured in a previous study.[42] In the case of centroblastic and immunoblastic lymphomas, no useful differences were found with regard to nuclear or cytoplasmic area or with NCI. A high standard error of mean (SEM) of nuclear size was noted and reflected the admixture of small and large (blast) cells present. A somewhat higher mean cytoplasm: nucleus ratio was seen in immunoblastic than in centroblastic tumours and nucleolar eccentricity and number were distinctly different between the two groups. For the small-cell lymphomas, distinction between each type could be made on the basis of the SEM of nuclear area, cytoplasm to nucleus ratio and NCI. Lymphoblastic lymphomas had a range of measured features closer to the large-cell (centroblastic and immunoblastic) group than the small-cell tumours; however, their SEM for nuclear size was less than those of the former, reflecting a smaller degree of pleomorphism.

Macrophages or 'histiocytic reticulum cells'[37] are an ubiquitous component of lymphoid tissues and lymphoma but may be less than ideally demonstrated in conventional haematoxylin–eosin stained paraffin sections. However, by means of techniques using frozen sections of fixed tissue and the demonstration of certain hydrolytic enzymes, macrophages are clearly defined (see, for example, Crocker[21]). Crocker *et al.*[47] counted the numbers of such cells, containing α-naphthyl acetate esterase (ANAE), using the MOP-AMO$_3$, in a series of 20 specimens of NHL and 10 reactive lymph nodes. The counts of such cells (which are mainly macrophages, although true dendritic reticulum cells may be weakly ANAE-positive) were performed from random microscopic fields, and were absolute, the positive cell numbers being expressed as a percentage of the 500 total cells enumerated. Tμ lymphocytes, which contain 'dot-like' ANAE-activity[23] were not counted as macrophages. In follicular lesions (reactive or lymphomatous) fields from both follicle centres and interfollicular areas were included in the counting procedure. Striking results were arrived at, ANAE-positive macrophages being much higher in number (10·8–20·5 per cent of total cells) in high-grade NHL than in low-grade lymphoma (range 1·4–4·1 per cent of total cells). Reactive lymph nodes contained a similar number of positive cells (1·4–3·2 per cent) to low-grade NHL. The latter observation was disappointing, as a problem frequently encountered in routine diagnosis lies in the distinction between reactive follicular hyperplasia (RFH) and follicular (low-grade) NHL. (It is of interest to note that Katz[48] using *in vitro* methods, had observed a higher yield of glass-adherent cells, presumably mainly including macrophages, in high-grade NHL than in low-grade lymphomas.) These results were confirmed by Crocker,[49] using acid phosphatase as a macrophage marker. It was suggested that the great number of macrophages in high-grade lymphomas might represent a response to a high individual malignant cell death rate (apoptosis) and/or tissue necrosis. As an extension of this study, Crocker[49] counted ANAE- and acid phosphatase-positive macrophages purely in the centre of reactive and malignant (centroblastic–centrocytic) follicles but, again, no significant differences were noted between the absolute counts in either group of conditions. This is in contrast to subjective impressions gained from the assessment of haematoxylin–eosin stained preparations where, in the past, some authors have regarded the presence of many macrophages as being evidence for benign changes in lymphoid follicles (see, for example, Rappaport[50]). Lennert[37] had previously, subjectively, assessed the numbers of epithelioid cells in immunoblastic lymphomas. 'Moderate' numbers were present in 22·4 per cent of the specimens and the cells were 'very numerous' in 4·3 per cent. However, this assessment appears to have been carried out in Giemsa or haematoxylin–eosin stained preparations, using morphological criteria for epithelioid cells rather than macrophages in general.

A further morphometric difference between high- and low-grade NHL was observed by Crocker *et al.*[51] in a study of the *FF* of ANAE-positive cells (other than Tμ lymphocytes). A consistent finding was that of a much higher mean value of *FF* for these cells in high-grade lymphomas than in those of low-grade histology. Thus, in the 15 high-grade tumours, the mean *FF* was 0·8–0·9 (an excess of rounded cells); whereas in 15 low-grade lymphomas, the mean *FF* was 0·4–0·5 (implying a predominance of branching or irregular cells). Ten reactive nodes were also examined and these had identical *FF* values to those of the low-grade specimens. Hence, again, morphometric differentiation between RFH and low-grade NHL was not possible. Probability curve analysis was performed and showed at least two populations of ANAE-positive cells by virtue of mean *FF* for each specimen. These findings were empirical but the authors discussed previous observations where rounded macrophage-type cells (demonstrated by their metalophilia) were predominant in the lower, centroblast-rich part of reactive follicles. In contrast, higher in the follicle where centrocytes predominate and mitoses are few, metalophil branching cells predominated.[19,52] It was, therefore, suggested that 'microenvironmental' features might, in some unknown fashion, influence macrophage shape in follicles.

Returning again to the problem of the distinction between follicular (usually centroblastic–centrocytic) lymphomas and RFH, Crocker *et al.*[53] have applied morphometric analysis to whole follicles, rather than cells or nuclei. An MOP-AMO_3 image-analyser was used to study the area and *FF* of follicles in 20 specimens of follicular (centroblastic–centrocytic) lymphoma, 15 lymph nodes showing reactive follicular hyperplasia and 10 palatine tonsils. In all specimens, where possible, the whole follicles (including the 'mantle zone' of small lymphocytes) and the follicle centres were measured. In only three of the 20 lymphomas was this possible, 'mantle zones' being absent from the remaining 17. However, in all of the reactive follicles, 'mantle zones' were conspicuous, accounting for up to 65·5 per cent of the mean total follicle area. Reactive lymph nodes had larger mean follicle areas than the specimens of FL and the areas of the reactive follicles showed much greater variation than their malignant counterparts. The mean *FF* was much the same for all types of specimen; however, the SEM of *FF* was significantly greater for RFH than FL. Thus, from this study, it appeared that follicle size is greater with a wider range in RFH than in FL and the shape of follicles is of a wider scatter in the former compared with the latter. An absence of 'mantle zones' is also suggestive of FL rather than RFH. It is of interest that, in one subjective study, the size of the 'parafollicular' zone of small lymphocytes in FL was found to be of prognostic significance.[54] A finding worthy of note is that Lennert,[37] in a study of 77 cases of centroblastic–centrocytic lymphoma, was unable to correlate the numbers of centroblasts present with the mean follicle diameter. The latter appeared not to have correlated with prognosis. In an attempt to further clarify the distinction between FL and RFH, Crocker *et al.*[55] studied the mean nuclear D_{Max} and area from a standard area in the follicle centre only. As in the previous study of follicle size, specimens were selected from proven cases of FL or RFH, to avoid tautology. The technique of selecting follicle centre nuclei only was chosen to avoid the possibility that 'mantle zone' or interfollicular cells (which may or may not be malignant) could alter the mean measurements significantly.[45] It was found that both follicle centre nuclear D_{Max} and area could clearly discriminate between FL and RFH, the former having significantly lower mean sizes than the latter. Also, the standard deviation (SD) was greater for nuclear D_{Max} and area in RFH than in FL, confirming subjective impressions of greater pleomorphism in the former.

HODGKIN'S DISEASE

The extreme pleomorphism of cell types observed in Hodgkin's disease (HD) has probably been instrumental in the paucity of quantitative and morphometric studies of this condition. The admixture of cell types, which form the basis of the Rye classification[56] include lymphocytes, histiocytes, 'Hodgkin' and Reed–Sternberg cells and eosinophils. The relative proportions, of, for example, lymphocytes and 'Hodgkin cells' are assessed by histopathologists and enable, in most instances, fairly accurate 'typing'. However, this is a subjective procedure and a recent study by Holman *et al.*[57] of inter-observer variation showed that whilst the nodular sclerosis (NS) type was readily identified, poorer agreement was attained for lymphocyte predominance (LP), mixed cellularity (MC) and lymphocyte depletion (LD) forms. The latter problem was largely the result of problems in assessing relative numbers of cell types present. Coppleson *et al.*[58] had previously shown that the NS subtype was readily recognized but demonstrated considerable inter-observer disagreement in the LD variety. It appears, therefore, that there is a need for quantitative studies of HD, since accurate Rye subclassification is of prognostic and therapeutic importance. Livesey *et al.*[59] performed differential cell counts on nine specimens of diffuse HD; these comprised two nodes showing the LP type, four of MC type and three with lymphocyte depletion. Surprisingly lymphocytes were found to comprise a higher proportion of the total cell count in LD than in MC specimens. Also, 'mononuclear cells' (including macrophage-series cells and fibroblasts) were more frequent in the MC type than in the other varieties. Thus, the Rye classification was generally supported, although some discrepancies were revealed. Specimens of the NS variant of HD were not included.

It would be expected that diagnostic difficulties might arise in HD of the LP variety where numerous 'reactive' histiocytes or epithelioid cells are present (the 'L and H' subtype of Lukes and

Butler[60]). Such a specimen was examined by Sutherland *et al.*,[61] who performed differential cell counts and found an admixture of cell types much closer to that in MC in the study by Livesey *et al.*[59] However, unlike the latter type of specimen, in this one node most of the 'histiocytes' were epithelioid cells.

Approaching the question of macrophage content of HD from a novel angle, Katz[62] separated macrophages from involved and non-involved nodes and spleen from 44 patients with HD. All subtypes (LP, NS, MC and LD) were included. Macrophages were characterized by means of glass adherence, phagocytosis of latex and anti-body-coated erythrocytes, and their content of acid phosphatase, peroxidase and non-specific esterase. Electron microscopy was also performed. The yield of glass adherent cells from normal, involved and non-involved tissues had mean values at 1·03, 0·92 and $1{\cdot}08\times10^{9}$/dl·g of tissue respectively. Although, of course, cell loss could be great and as a means of quantification this technique is relatively crude, the lower numbers of adherent cells in the involved tissues is of interest. Many of the cells isolated from the HD tissue showed abnormal ultrastructural features and it may be that 'Hodgkin cells' are relatively non-adherent (indeed, abnormal cells were present in the non-adherent fraction).

In an attempt to accurately measure the macrophage content of HD, Crocker *et al.*[63] used a graphic digitizer to rapidly count macrophages by virtue of their content of ANAE. Thirty-two specimens of HD were counted, comprising 12 of the LP, eight of the NS, seven of the MC and five of the LD subtype. Two specimens of true histiocytic lymphoma were also included. Striking and consistent results were obtained; the numbers of ANAE-positive cells ranging from 1·8–16 per cent of all cells in the LP group, 13·6–22·1 per cent in the NS group and 6·5–14·6 per cent in the specimens of MC HD. The specimens of LD HD contained the greatest number of esterase-positive cells, ranging from 39·8–47·7 per cent of all cells. Thus, macrophages form a much larger compartment of cells than do lymphocytes in LD; this is in some conflict with the results of Livesey *et al.*[59] Within the LP group, two 'clusters' of values (from 1·8–5·2 per cent and 12·5–16 per cent) were obtained and the authors concluded that the latter cluster might represent 'L and H' LP disease. The importance of performing absolute cell counts rather than counts of cells per unit area was also stressed. The two specimens of histiocytic lymphoma (whose cells showed phagocytosis and lobulate nuclei) contained 95·2 and 97·5 per cent of ANAE-positive cells, respectively, thus lying well away from the range of LD HD. These data were subsequently confirmed by Crocker[49] using acid phosphatase rather than ANAE as a macrophage marker.

It can be concluded that, while not yet being of diagnostic value, the use of differential cell counts may lead us to re-consider some aspects of the cellular basis of the Rye classification. The different approaches to the techniques of cell enumeration may, in part, account for the somewhat conflicting results.

ACKNOWLEDGEMENTS

The author is grateful to Professor R. C. Curran for proposing the idea of this review. Miss Angela Wright and Mrs Ruth Fry supplied invaluable secretarial assistance.

REFERENCES

1. Steer MW. Understanding Cell Structure. Cambridge: C.U.P., 1981.
2. Aherne WA, Dunnill MS. Morphometry. London: Edward Arnold, 1982.
3. Bradbury S. Microscopical image analysis: problems and approaches. *J Microsc* 1979; **115:** 137.
4. Biberfield P. Morphogenesis in blood lymphocytes stimulated with phytohaemagglutinin. A light and electron microscopic study. *Acta Path Microbiol Scand* 1971; 223 (suppl.).
5. Douglas StD, Cohen G, Brittinger G. Ultrastructural comparison between phytomitogen transformed normal and chronic lymphocytic leukaemia lymphocytes. *J Ultrastruct Res* 1973; **44:** 11.
6. Petrzilka GE, Graf-De Beer M, Schroeder HE. Stereological model system for free cells and base-line data for human peripheral blood-derived small T-lymphocytes. *Cell Tiss Res* 1978; **192:** 121.
7. Renau-Piqueras J, Cerdan F, Barbera E, Cervera J. Electron microscopic morphometric analysis of human T and B peripheral blood lymphocytes. *Virchows Arch B Cell Path* 1978; **28:** 47.
8. Bentwich Z, Douglas SD, Siegal FP, Kunkel HG. Human lymphocyte–sheep erythrocyte rosette formation. Some characteristics of the interaction. *Clin Immunol Immunopathol* 1973; **1:** 511.
9. Miragall F, Renau-Piqueras J. Electron microscopic morphometric analysis of small cortical and medullary thymocytes from the rat. *Virchows Arch B Cell Path* 1979; **30:** 53.

10. Abe K, Ito T. Fine structure of small lymphocytes in the thymus of the mouse: qualitative and quantitative analysis by electron microscopy. *Z Zellforsch* 1970; **110:** 321.
11. Matter A. Morphological definition of thymocyte subpopulations. *Cell Tiss Res* 1975; **158:** 319.
12. Stewart CC, Ingram M. A method for counting phytohemagglutinin-stimulated lymphocytes. *Blood* 1967; **29:** 628.
13. Stewart CC, Cramer SF, Stewart PG. The response of human peripheral blood lymphocytes to phytohaemagglutinin: determination of cell numbers. *Cell Immunol* 1975; **16:** 237.
14. Takahashi K. Karyometric and cytophotometric studies on nucleic acids in the culture of human lymphocytes with phytohaemagglutinin. *Virchows Arch B Cell Path* 1976; **21:** 299.
15. Brown RA, McWalter R, Slidders W, Gibbs J, Swanson Beck J. Measurement by Quantimet 720 of the proportion of actively growing cells in tissue cultures of human lymphocytes. *J Microsc* 1979; **115:** 51.
16. Meyer EM, Schlake W, Grundmann E. Comparative histologic, histochemical and histomorphometric studies of T and B cell areas in peripheral lymphoid organs of normal young adult BALB/c mice. *Path Res Pract* 1979; **164:** 141.
17. Meyer EM, Grundmann E. BCG-induced changes in size of thymic cortex and thymus-dependent areas in spleen and lymph nodes of mice. *Clin Exp Immunol* 1980; **39:** 60.
18. Van de Velde CJH, Meijer CJLM, Cornelisse CJ, van der Velde EA, van Putten LM, Zwaveling A. A morphometric analysis of lymph node responses to tumors of different immunogenicity. *Cancer Res* 1978; **38:** 661.
19. Curran RC, Jones EL. Immunoglobulin-containing cells in human tonsils as demonstrated by immunohistochemistry. *Clin Exp Immunol* 1977; **28:** 103.
20. Brandtzaeg P, Surjan L, Berdal P. Immune systems of human tonsils. I. Control subjects of various ages: quantification of Ig-producing cells, tonsillar morphometry and serum Ig concentrations. *Clin Exp Immunol* 1978; **31:** 367.
21. Crocker J. The enzyme histochemistry of lymphoid and non-lymphoid cells of the human palatine tonsil: a basis for the study of lymphomas. *J Path* 1981; **134:** 81.
22. Si L, Roscoe G, Whiteside TL. Selective distribution and quantitation of T-lymphocyte subsets in germinal centers of human tonsils. Definition by use of monoclonal antibodies. *Arch Path Lab Med* 1983; **107:** 228.
23. Zicca A, Leprini A, Cadoni A, Franzi AT, Ferrarini M, Grossi CE. Ultrastructural localisation of alpha-naphthyl acid esterase in human T_M lymphocytes. *Am J Pathol* 1981; **105:** 40.
24. Litovitz TL, Lutzner MA. Quantitative measurements of blood lymphocytes from patients with chronic lymphocytic leukemia and the Sézary's syndrome. *J Natl Cancer Inst* 1974; **53:** 75.
25. Schrek R. Ultrastructure of blood lymphocytes from chronic lymphocytic and lymphosarcoma cell leukemia. *J Natl Cancer Inst* 1972; **48:** 51.
26. Meijer CJLM, van der Loo EM, van Vloten WA, van der Velde EA, Scheffer E, Cornelisse CJ. Early diagnosis of mycosis fungoides and Sézary's syndrome by morphometric analysis of lymphoid cells in the skin. *Cancer* 1980; **45:** 2864.
27. Van der Loo EM, Cornelisse CJ, van Vloten WA, van der Velde EA, Scheffer E, Meijer CJLM. Diagnostic morphometry of isolated lymph node cells from patients with mycosis fungoides and Sézary's syndrome. *Virchows Arch B Cell Path* 1980; **33:** 107.
28. Van der Loo EM, Meijer CJ, Scheffer E, van Vloten WA. The prognostic value of membrane markers and morphometric characteristics of lymphoid cells in blood and lymph nodes from patients with mycosis fungoides. *Cancer* 1981; **48:** 738.
29. Van der Loo EM, van Vloten WA, Cornelisse CJ, Scheffer E, Meijer CJLM. The relevance of morphometry in the differential diagnosis of cutaneous T cell lymphomas. *Br J Dermatol* 1981; **104:** 257.
30. Van Vloten WA, van Duijn P, Schaberg A. Cytodiagnostic use of Feulgen-DNA measurements in cell imprints from the skin of patients with mycosis fungoides. *Br J Dermatol* 1974; **91:** 365.
31. McNutt NS, Crain WR. Quantitative electron microscopic comparison of lymphocyte nuclear contours in mycosis fungoides and in benign infiltrates in skin. *Cancer* 1981; **47:** 698.
32. McNutt NS, Heilbron DC, Crain WR. Mycosis fungoides: diagnostic criteria based on quantitative electron microscopy. *Lab Invest* 1981; **44:** 466.
33. Caorsi I, Figueroa CD, Rodriguez EM. Morphologic and morphometric study of the two main cell lineages involved in mycosis fungoides: the lymphoid cells and the Langerhans cells. *Ultrastruct Pathol* 1982; **3:** 119.
34. Bennett MH, Farrer-Brown G, Henry K, Jelliffe AM. Classification of non-Hodgkin's lymphomas. *Lancet* 1974; **i:** 405.
35. Lukes RJ, Collins RD. New approaches to the classification of the lymphomata. *Brit J Cancer* 1975; **31: (ii)** (suppl.): 1.
36. Gerard-Marchant R, Hamlin I, Lennert K, Rilke F, Stansfeld AG, van Unnik JAM. Classification of non-Hodgkin's lymphomas. *Lancet* 1974; **ii:** 406.
37. Lennert K. Malignant Lymphomas Other Than Hodgkin's Disease. Berlin, Heidelberg, New York: Springer, 1978.
38. Crocker J, Curran RC. A study of nuclear diameters in lymph node imprints using the Zeiss Microvideomat. *J Clin Pathol* 1979; **32:** 670.

39. Abbott CR, Blewitt RW, Bird CC. Quantitative analysis of non-Hodgkin's lymphoma. *J Clin Pathol* 1982; **35:** 135.
40. Underwood EE. Particle-size distribution. In: Dettoff RT, Rhines FN, eds. Quantitative Microscopy, New York, 1968: 149.
41. Crocker J, Jones EL, Curran RC. Study of nuclear diameters in non-Hodgkin's lymphomas. *J Clin Pathol* 1982; **35:** 954.
42. Van der Valk P, Hermans J, Brand R, Cornelisse CJ, Spaander PJ, Meijer CJLM. Morphometric characterisation of diffuse large-cell (histiocytic) lymphomas. *Am J Pathol* 1982; **107:** 327.
43. Van der Valk P, Te Velde J, Jansen J, Ruiter DJ, Spaander PJ, Cornelisse CJ, Meijer CJLM. Malignant lymphoma of true histiocytic origin: histiocytic sarcoma. A morphological, ultrastructural, immunological, cytochemical and clinical study of 10 cases. *Virchows Arch A Pathol Anat* 1981; **391:** 249.
44. Van der Valk P, Ruiter DJ, Den Otto Lander GJ, Te Velde J, Spaander PJ, Meijer CJLM. Dendritic reticulum cell sarcoma? Four cases of a lymphoma probably derived from dendritic reticulum cells of the follicular compartment. *Histopath* 1982; **6:** 269.
45. Crocker J, Jones EL, Curran RC. A comparative study of nuclear form factor, area and diameter in non-Hodgkin's lymphomas and reactive lymph nodes. *J Clin Pathol* 1983; **36:** 298.
46. Van der Valk P, Mosch A, Kurver PJ, Meijer CJLM. Morphometric characterisation of 52 B cell non-Hodgkin's lymphomas. *J Clin Pathol* 1983; **36:** 289.
47 Crocker J, Jones EL, Curran RC. A quantitative study of α-naphthyl acetate esterase-positive cells in non-Hodgkin's lymphomas and reactive lymph nodes. *J Clin Pathol* 1982; **35:** 1066.
48. Katz DR. Macrophages in non-Hodgkin lymphomas and hairy cell leukaemia. *J Path* 1981; **134:** 117.
49. Crocker J. The enzyme histochemistry of lymphomas. MD Thesis, University of Cambridge, 1983.
50. Rappaport H. Tumors of the hematopoietic system. Atlas of Tumor Pathology. Section III, Fascicle 8. Washington DC: Armed Forces Institute of Pathology, 426.
51. Crocker J, Jones EL, Curran RC. The form factor of alpha-naphthyl acetate esterase-positive cells in non-Hodgkin's lymphomas and reactive lymph nodes. *J Clin Pathol* 1983; **36:** 303.
52. Curran RC, Gregory J, Jones EL. The distribution of immunoglobulin and other plasma proteins in human reactive lymph nodes. *J Pathol* 1982; **136:** 307.
53. Crocker J, Jones EL, Curran RC. A quantitative study of the size of benign and malignant lymphoid follicles. *J Clin Pathol* 1983; **36:** 1055.
54. Ree HJ, Leone LA. Prognostic significance of parafollicular small lymphocytes in follocular lymphoma. *Cancer* 1978; **41:** 1500.
55. Crocker J, Jones EL, Curran RC. Study of nuclear sizes in the centres of malignant and benign lymphoid follicles. *J Clin Pathol* 1983; **36:** 1332.
56. Lukes RJ, Craver LF, Hall TC, Rappaport H, Ruben P. Report of the nomenclature committee. In: Symposium on obstacles to the control of Hodgkin's disease. *Cancer Res* 1966; **26:** 1311.
57. Holman CDJ, Matz LR, Finlay-Jones LR, Waters ED, Blackwell JB, Joyce PR, Kelsall GRH, Shilkin KB, Cullity GJ, Williams KE, Matthews MLV, Armstrong BK. Inter-observer variation in the histopathological reporting of Hodgkin's disease: and analysis of diagnostic subcomponents using Kappa statistics. *Histopath* 1983; **7:** 399.
58. Coppleson LW, Factor RM, Strum SB, Graff PW, Rappaport H. Observer disagreement in the classification and histology of Hodgkin's disease. *J Natl Cancer Inst* 1970; **50:** 1429.
59. Livesey EA, Sutherland FI, Brown RA, Beck JS, MacGillivray JB, Slidders W. Cytological basis of histological typing of diffuse Hodgkin's disease. Demonstration of an implied misnomer in the terminology of the Rye classification. *J Clin Pathol* 1978; **31:** 551.
60. Lukcs RJ, Butlcr JJ. Thc pathology and nomenclature of Hodgkin's disease. *Cancer Res* 1966; **26:** 1063.
61. Sutherland FI, MacGillivray JB, Brown RA, Beck JS. Differential cell counts in the histiocytic variant of lymphocyte predominance subtype of Hodgkin's disease. *J Clin Pathol* 1978; **34:** 1234.
62. Katz DR. The macrophage in Hodgkin's disease. *J Path* 1981; **133:** 145.
63. Crocker J, Jones EL, Curran RC. A quantitative study of α-naphthyl acetate esterase-positive cells in Hodgkin's disease. *J Clin Pathol* 1982; **35:** 1301.

JOURNAL OF PATHOLOGY, VOL. **143:** 81–92 (1984)

PATHOLOGICAL ASPECTS OF DIFFUSE NODULAR HYPERPLASIA OF THE LIVER

K. WEINBREN AND S. S. MUTUM*
Royal Postgraduate Medical School, DuCane Road, London W12 0HS, U.K.

Received 3 August 1983
Accepted 22 September 1983

SUMMARY

The microscopical features in specimens of liver tissue from 14 patients considered to be suffering from Diffuse Nodular Hyperplasia (DNH) were compared with the changes found in livers from five other groups of patients. The diagnoses in these groups were macronodular cirrhosis, hepatic venous occlusion, congestive cardiac failure, compensatory hyperplasia after destruction of part of the liver and chronic biliary disease respectively. In all these groups the formation of thick hepatocyte plates, thought to represent cell proliferation, was a constant and striking feature. Such plate thickening in the periportal regions was associated with congestive cardiac failure and with hepatic venous occlusion. The diffuse involvement of almost all plates formed part of the changes in DNH, cirrhosis, compensatory hyperplasia and chronic biliary disease. Normal vascular relations were retained in the patients with compensatory hyperplasia and chronic biliary disease and lost in cirrhosis and, in some parts, in DNH. The nodules were small in DNH and larger in cirrhosis, where they were surrounded by fibrous tissue. DNH appeared to be recognizable in needle biopsy specimens.

KEY WORDS—Liver, diffuse nodular hyperplasia, cirrhosis of the liver.

INTRODUCTION

Hepatocyte plates in adults are normally one-cell thick, but a striking thickening of individual plates has been frequently reported in several forms of chronic liver disease, notably cirrhosis.[1,2] It is described also in the condition referred to as 'Diffuse Nodular Hyperplasia' or 'Diffuse Nodular Regenerative Hyperplasia' (DNH). The cause and the pathogenesis of this disease are not yet elucidated but the morphological descriptions are generally concordant, provided specimens for examination are of reasonable size. Difficulties are acknowledged, however, about the interpretation of needle biopsy specimens, some authors indicating that such small fragments are probably unreliable for diagnosis.[3–6]

The main clinical features are related either to accompanying systemic abnormalities[3] or to an increased level of portal venous pressure[4] the latter noted to be similar to the changes observed in other conditions associated with portal hypertension, such as cirrhosis. Differences in management of these conditions suggest the need for more confident diagnostic identification even on the most commonly available type of specimen, that derived from the needle biopsy procedure.

Most authors regard the lesions as representing hyperplasia or the result of proliferation by cell division of hepatocytes.[5,7] Early experimental studies by Ponfick[8] and Von Meister[9] led to the view that the process of rapid hepatocyte proliferation represents a compensatory phenomenon and most subsequent animal experiments and observations in human livers were defined and studied from this standpoint.[10–13] For many years, in fact, the convex pale hepatic nodules found so consistently in cirrhosis were referred to as 'regeneration nodules'.[2] The assumption that all nodules or irregular masses of non-neoplastic liver parenchymal cells represent a process stimulated by loss of similar tissue ('compensatory hyperplasia' or 'regeneration') is challenged, however, by the

* Present address: Pathology Department, Regional Medical College, Manipur, India.

0022-3417/84/060081-12$01.20

numbers of reports of nodular changes in liver tissue in which there was no evidence of previous damage extensive enough to have provoked a recognizable compensatory cellular proliferation.[4,5,14,15]

The common observation on which pathogenetic hypotheses are based, is the replacement of normal one-cell thick hepatocyte plates[16] by plates consisting of two juxtaposed layers of hepatocytes between sinusoids. Thus the finding of a high incidence of patients suffering from congestive cardiac failure in the series described by Steiner[7] and the suggestion that the condition may be associated with deprivation of portal blood flow[15] are both related to an interpretation of the changes as compensatory hyperplasia, the structural counterpart of which is the presence of thickened hepatocyte plates.

We have, therefore, compared the microscopical changes in liver tissue from 14 patients in whom the diagnosis of DNH was considered on histological and clinical grounds to be the most appropriate, with the findings in several other groups of patients in whom hepatic plates were strikingly thicker than normal and where confusion seemed to be possible. The groups which made up the series for comparison were derived from patients suffering from the following conditions:

(1) Congestive cardiac failure (12 patients), (patients 15–26).
(2) Macronodular cirrhosis (12), (patients 27–38).
(3) Hepatic venous occlusion (10), (patients 39–48).
(4) Post-resection or post-destruction liver cell proliferation (10), (patients 49–58).
(5) Chronic biliary disease (10), (patients 59–68).

An attempt has been made to assess the reliability of needle biopsy specimens in the diagnosis of DNH.

The clinical conditions associated with DNH in this group of patients were:

(1) Felty's syndrome (rheumatoid arthritis) 6 patients, (patients 1–6).
(2) Polycythaemia vera 1, (patient 7).
(3) Metastatic carcinoma 1, (patient 8).
(4) Hepatocarcinoma 1, (patient 9).
(5) Renal transplant and pulmonary tuberculosis 1, (patient 10).
(6) Chronic granulocytic leukaemia 1, (patient 11).
(7) Pulmonary tuberculosis 1, (patient 12).
(8) Coeliac disease 1, (patient 13).
(9) Chronic lymphocytic leukaemia and adenocarcinoma of colon 1, (patient 14).

MATERIAL AND METHODS

The hepatic tissue consisted of samples resected at surgical operations or by needle biopsy procedures or autopsy specimens. The microscopical changes were noted in all the sections and macroscopical features when suitable specimens were retained. Apart from three patients with Felty's syndrome, all diagnoses were validated at surgical exploration or at autopsy. The tissues available for study are listed in Table I, the total number diagnosed as DNH amounting to 24 specimens from 14 patients and 74 specimens from 54 patients with diseases other than DNH.

Table I—Specimens according to diagnosis

Condition	Total patients	Needle	Wedge	Resection	Autopsy
DNH	14	12 (10 patients)	5 (4 patients)	0	7
Macronodular cirrhosis	12	9 (6 patients)	9 (7 patients)	0	4
CCF	12	0		0	12
HVO	10	9 (8 patients)	3	0	3
Postresection or tumour replacement	10	3 (2 patients)	0	11 (10 patients)	1
Chronic biliary disease	10	10	0	0	0
	68	43	17	11	27

RESULTS

The inclusion of tissues in this investigation rested to a large extent on the identification of liver plates which consisted of two cells in thickness. Based on the analysis of Elias[16] normal adult hepatocyte plates were regarded as consisting of a single layer of hepatocytes with sinusoidal spaces on 2 faces of the cells. The recognition of two-cell thick plates was not difficult and morphological observations were reproducible. Apart from two nuclei being found between two sinusoids, pericanalicular lysosomes usually delineated the junction between adjacent cells arranged longitudinally in the plate.

The changes observed in sections from the various groups involved the following: (1) Alterations in plate thickness; (2) fibrosis; (3) sinusoidal thickening; (4) atrophy of single-cell thick plates; (5) atrophy of 2-cell-thick plates; (6) accumulation of sinusoidal and extra-sinusoidal erythrocytes; (7) replacement of liver tissue by tumours, necrosis or fibrosis or the changes after recent partial hepatic resection.

Alterations in plate thickness

Thick plates, two cells in width, were found either throughout the tissue section examined or were present predominantly in periportal regions. In wedge resections or autopsy sections, the nuclei were usually found to be situated adjacent to the sinusoidal surface of the cell, but this change in nuclear position was not noted in needle biopsy specimens (Figs 1, 2). The term 'diffuse' was reserved for the situation in which almost every plate encountered was two cells thick. In these circumstances, even when cells showed evidence of atrophy, mainly adjacent to definite nodules, atrophic cells were still arranged in two-cell-thick plates (Fig. 3).

When diffuse plate change was identified the relationship of portal tracts (parenchymal parts—Matsumoto *et al.*[17]) to hepatic venous radicles was considered. If normal distances between, and normal frequency of occurrence of, these structures were defined, the lobular or acinar[18] structure was considered to be retained and the term 'lobule' was applied. When foci were noted in

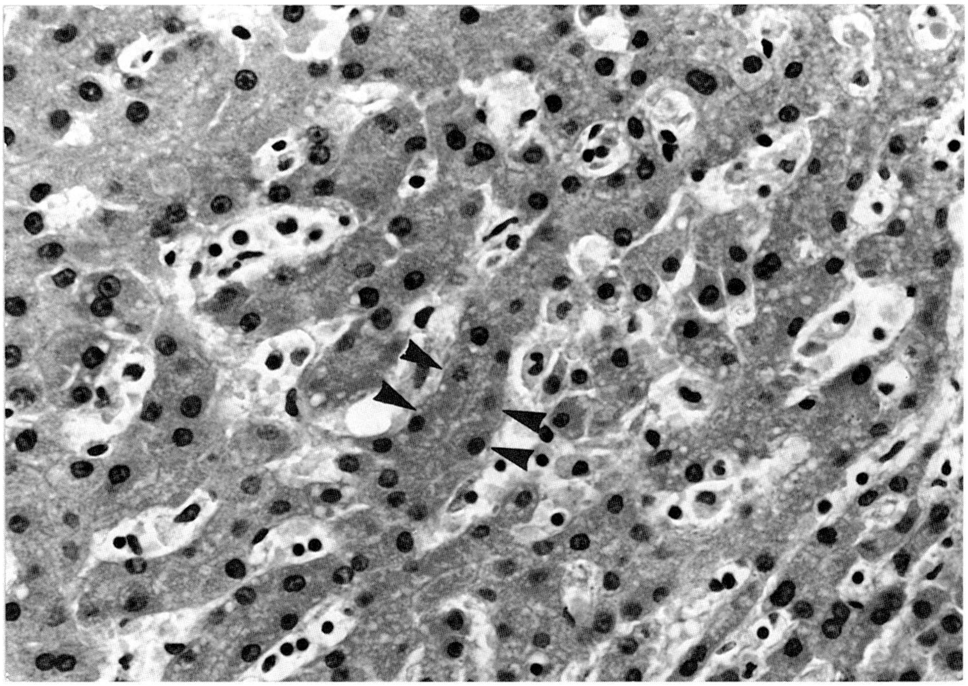

Fig. 1—Autopsy section from patient 7 with DNH, showing nuclei at sinusoidal surface of cells of two-cell-thick plates (arrows). H & E, ×400

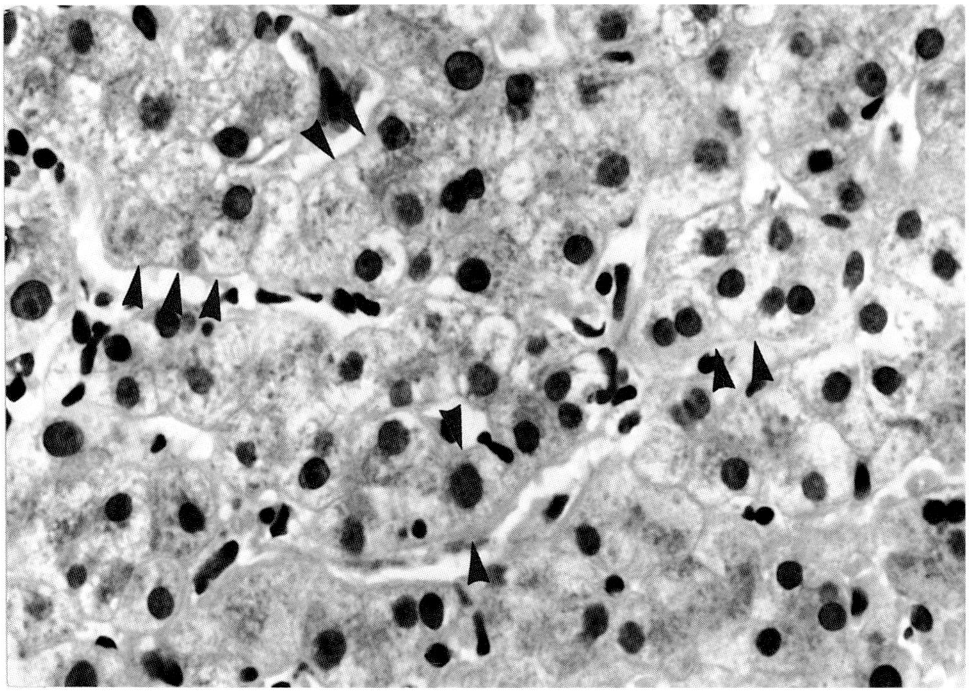

Fig. 2—Needle biopsy section from same patient (7) with DNH showing central position of nuclei in thick plates (arrows). H & E, ×600

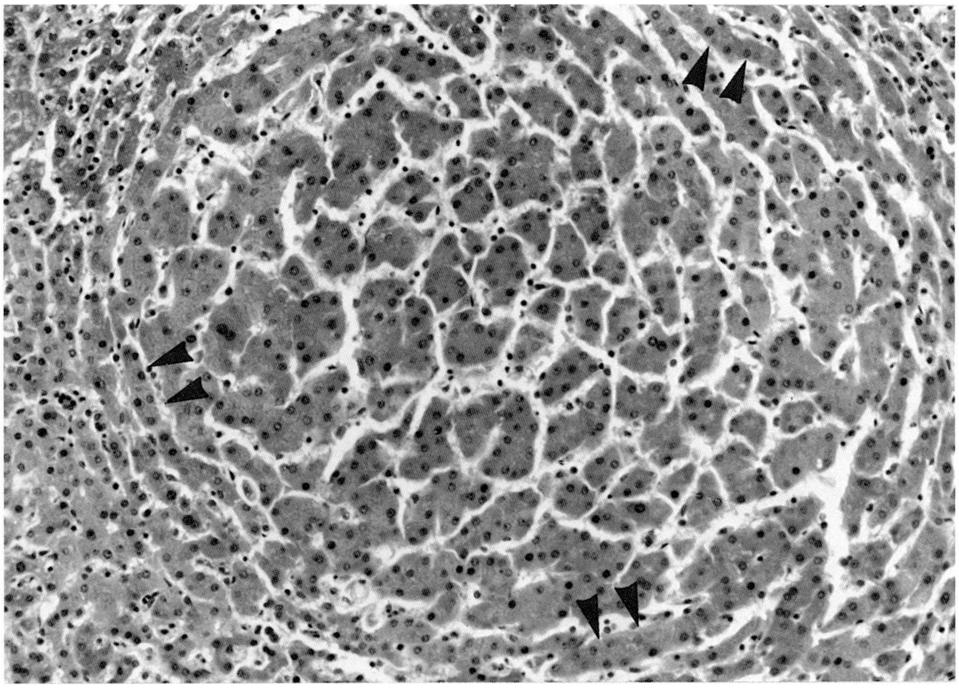

Fig. 3—Autopsy section from patient 2 with DNH showing atrophy of two-cell-thick plates (arrows) at periphery of nodule. H & E, ×150

Table II—Morphological findings in tissues from patients with thick hepatocyte plates

Condition	No. of patients	Thick plates Diffuse	Thick plates Zonal	Structure Lobule	Structure Nodule	Sinusoidal thickening	Fibrosis	Atrophy Single plates	Atrophy Thick plates
DNH	14	14	0	14	14	0	0	0	14
Macronodular cirrhosis	12	12	0	0	12	0	12	0	0
CCF	12	0	12	12	1	12	2	12	1
HVO	10	0	10	10	0	10	6	10	1
Postresection or tumour replacement	10	10	0	10	0	0	0	0	0
Chronic biliary disease	10	10	0	10	0	0	3	0	0

which normal vascular relationships were not identified, whether such foci were larger or smaller than normal lobules, the term 'nodule' was used. In sum, therefore, in this report two-cell-thick hepatocyte plates represent either a diffuse change or a zonal periportal change and if diffuse, the change is either nodular or lobular depending on the identification of normal vascular relationships.

Several other microscopical changes were encountered in the hepatic tissues taken from the different groups of patients and their incidence is listed in the various conditions (Table II). Nodule formation was not found in patients in whom there was evidence of destruction of part of the liver (Fig. 4), and not in our patients with chronic bile duct disease (Fig. 5) in both of which conditions hepatic venous radicles were usually easily identified. Substantial parts of the section in all patients with DNH showed retention of vascular relations, together with interspersed nodules (Fig. 6) a

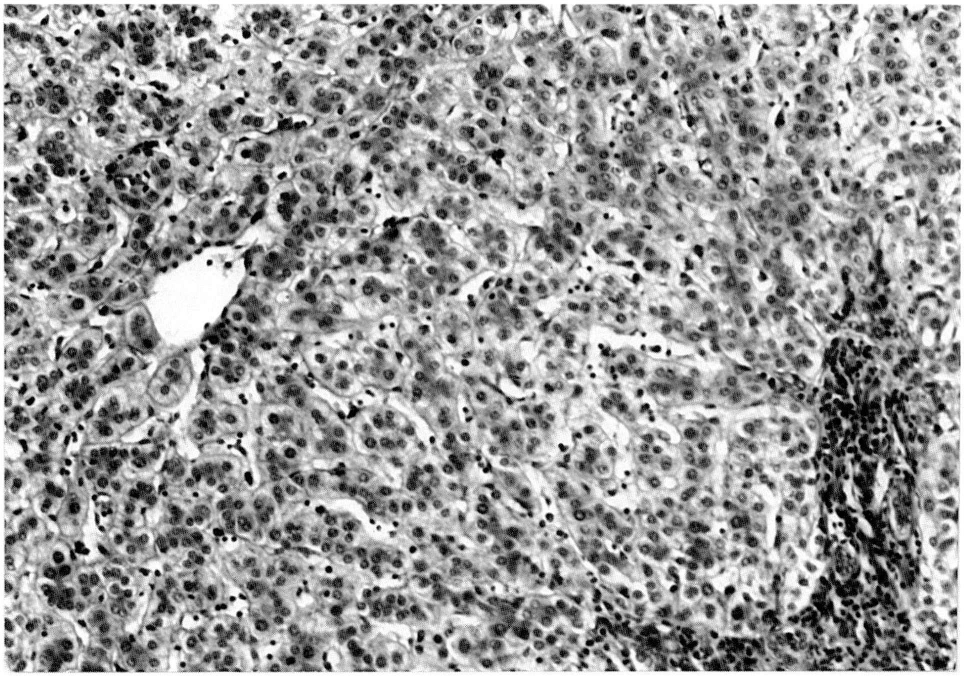

Fig. 4—Wedge resection from patient 51 after major hepatic resection for trauma showing thick plates with retained hepatic vein radicle and portal tract. H & E, ×150

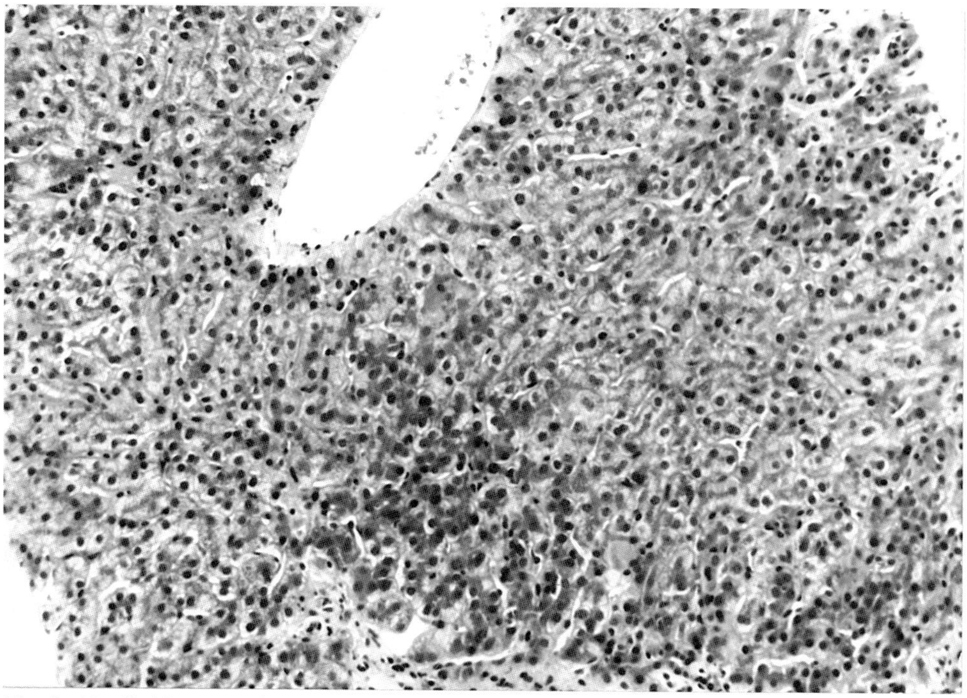

Fig. 5—Needle biopsy specimen from patient 59, suffering from long-standing biliary disease showing diffuse plate thickening with retained vascular relations. H & E, ×150

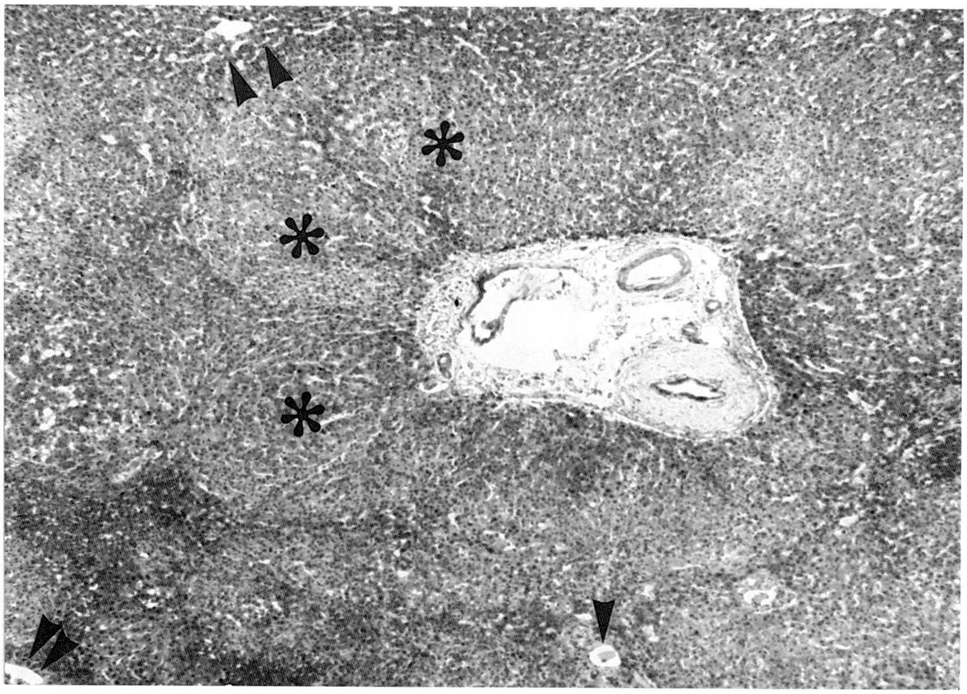

Fig. 6—Wedge resection from patient 10 with DNH, showing diffuse plate thickening with both retention of hepatic venous radicles (lobules) (arrows) and nodules (without veins) (asterisks). H & E, ×60

mixture not encountered in the compensatory lobular hyperplasia associated with loss of hepatic parenchyma. The thickened plates forming nodules generally were arranged neither around portal tracts nor around hepatic venous radicles and usually appeared to compress surrounding parenchymal cells. The nodules varied in diameter from less than the distance between a normal portal tract and hepatic vein radicle to structures several times larger than individual lobules or acini. These were found in all specimens bearing the diagnosis of DNH and from patients with cirrhosis. The nodules in DNH were at the small end of the range (Fig. 7) and those in the patients with cirrhosis much larger (Fig. 8). In one patient with long-standing congestive cardiac failure, in whom the dominant microscopical appearance was periportal thick plates and atrophy and loss of perivenous hepatocytes, a single focus of periportal hepatocytes assumed the appearance of a small nodule, but this was exceptional.

Fibrosis

Substantial fibrosis usually surrounding every nodule was found in some patients with cirrhosis, but in three instances, the fibrosis did not always completely encompass each nodule. In these circumstances of incomplete septal cirrhosis[1] the nodules varied in size, but all were larger than normal lobules and the fibrosis, which often extended intranodularly and sometimes ended bluntly, none the less was strikingly increased over normal (Fig. 8). Although an occasional nodule was not completely surrounded by fibrous tissue, the majority were, and there was close apposition between fibrous bands and nodular parenchyma. Fibrosis was found also in two of 10 patients with congestive cardiac failure. This was particularly marked in a perisinusoidal position usually in relation to hepatic venous radicles, a similar lesion noted in six of 10 patients with hepatic venous occlusion (Fig. 9). This fibrosis was striking but clearly not in any sense perinodular and was not confused with the more abundant fibrosis observed in the examples of cirrhosis.

Sinusoidal thickening

The appearance of a thickened sinusoidal reticulin was noted in different regions of most specimens with one or other of the varieties of

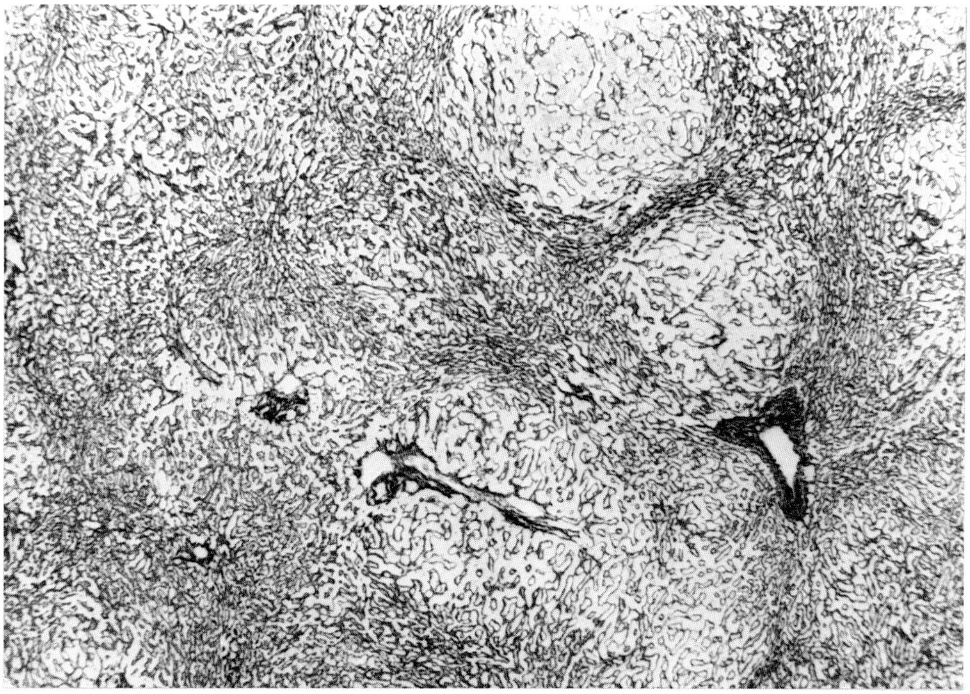

Fig. 7—Autopsy section from patient 2 with DNH showing multiple small nodules. Gordon and Sweet reticulin impregnation, ×40

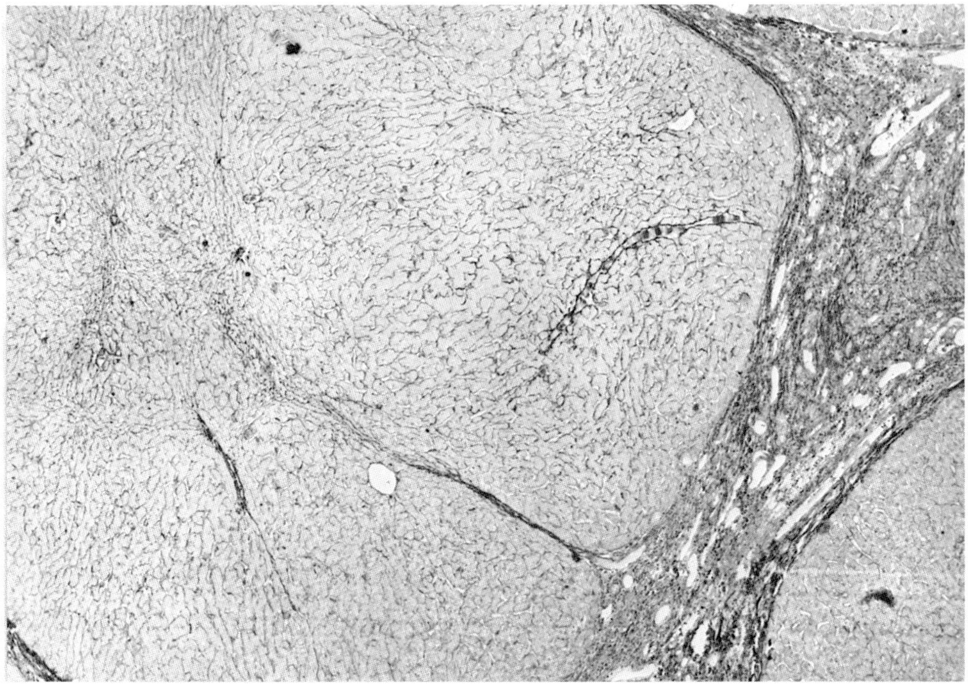

Fig. 8—Wedge resection from patient 33 suffering from macronodular cirrhosis showing large nodules surrounded by abundant fibrous tissue. Gordon and Sweet reticulin impregnation, ×40

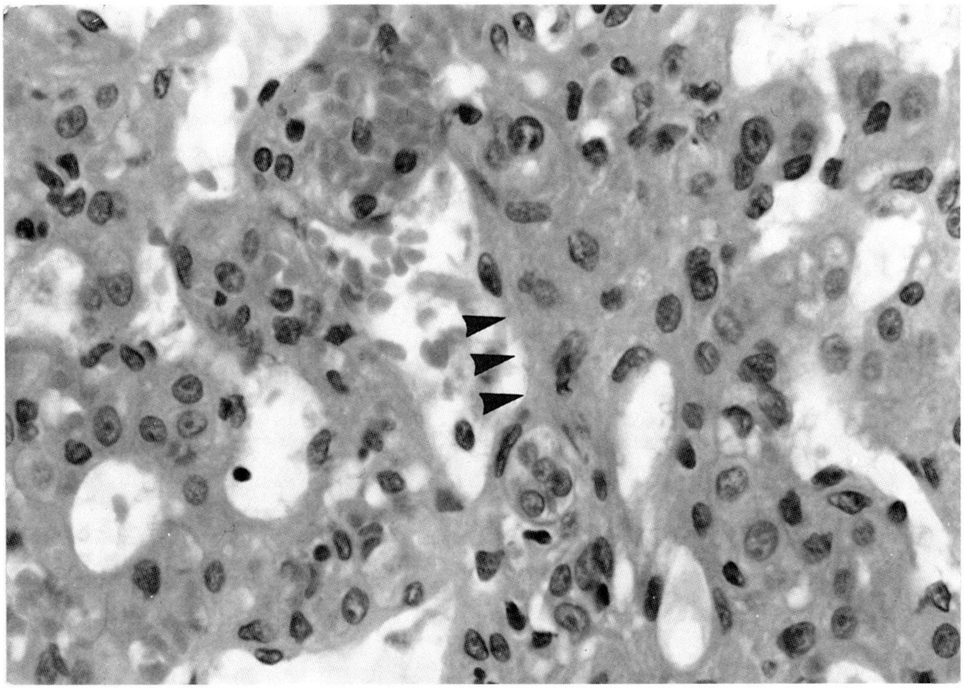

Fig. 9—Needle biopsy specimen from patient 41 with hepatic venous occlusion showing fibrous replacement of liver plates (arrows) and sinusoids containing erythrocytes. This fibrous change was not seen in DNH. H & E, ×600

chronic liver disease examined. The disposition of this change however differed in the different categories. In the 14 patients with DNH there was no discernible change in reticulin thickness within nodules but the direction and contour of the sinusoids were altered. Thickened reticulin was noted only in areas in which hepatocyte plates appeared to be compressed by adjacent nodules. Sinusoidal reticulin thickening was a constant finding in all patients with hepatic venous occlusion and with congestive cardiac failure. It was not a feature in macronodular cirrhosis although there was excessive reticulin between nodules.

Atrophy

The recognition of atrophic cells with attendant reduction in relative protein content depended on the presence of hepatocytes in which the cytoplasm is much reduced in volume and the nucleus is in close proximity to opposite surfaces of the cell. Such atrophy may be observed in cells forming single-cell thick plates and also in cells which make up plates which are two cells thick (Fig. 2). Atrophied cells were found usually adjacent to foci of thick plates and were distributed in different regions in different conditions. A compressed band of atrophied cells was present on the edges of the nodules in all instances of DNH and in each case, substantial numbers of these atrophied plates were two cells thick. Atrophied single-cell-thick plates were observed for the most part in hepatic venous occlusion and in congestive cardiac failure, although in patients with long-standing disease, two-cell-thick plates also were found to be atrophic. Atrophic plates were not encountered in the two patients with incomplete septal macronodular cirrhosis except for occasional attenuated remnants enmeshed in fibrous tissue.

Accumulation of erythrocytes

Intra-sinusoidal erythrocytes were noted to a greater or lesser degree in 15 of the 17 biopsy specimens from patients with DNH and in one of these there was substantial replacement of hepatocyte plates by erythrocytes and occasional collections within the perisinusoidal spaces. Such findings were not seen in biopsy specimens from patients with post-destruction compensatory hyperplasia or in specimens from patients with chronic biliary disease. There were no biopsy specimens from patients with congestive cardiac failure and the accumulation of erythrocytes in autopsy specimens is complicated by post-mortem changes.

The changes noted in needle biopsy specimens only are summarized in Table III. Essentially micronodules were identified in all 12 specimens from patients with DNH and in only 3 of 9 patients with cirrhosis. Substantial fibrosis surrounded nodules in eight specimens of cirrhosis and none was seen in DNH. Erythrocytes accumulated in great excess in one of 12 needle biopsy specimens from patients with DNH and to some degree in all but two, but this was a constant finding in hepatic venous occlusion.

Table III—Distinguishing features on needle biopsy specimens

Condition	No. of specimens	Thick plates: Diffuse	Thick plates: Periportal	Micronodules	Fibrosis	Reticulin thickening	Erythrocytes: In sinusoids	Erythrocytes: In perisinusoidal spaces
DNH	12	12	0	12	0	0	10	1
Macronodular cirrhosis	9	9	0	3	8	0	0	0
HVO	9	0	9	0	5	9	9	9
Postresection or tumour replacement	3	3	0	0	0	0	0	0
Chronic biliary disease	10	10	0	0	3	0	0	0

DISCUSSION

The findings confirm the observation that two-cell-thick hepatocyte plates may be present in different disease entities, instead of the normal arrangement based on walls or plates of one-cell thickness.[16,19]

It seems relevant to question whether the consensus interpretation of thick plates as an indication of hyperplasia of liver cells is reasonable, before conclusions are drawn as to possible pathogenetic mechanisms and causes in these diseases. The evidence on which the hypothesis that macroscopical nodules in cirrhosis are the result of hyperplasia rests, is the analysis by Turnbull and Worthington in 1908[10] and the correlation of such foci with recovery phases after severe toxicity or viral infection.[21] The composition of hyperplastic or cirrhotic nodules had not at first been identified on the basis of specific arrangement of hepatocyte plates although an illustration in a paper by Turnbull and Worthington[20] shows characteristic thick plates in a cirrhotic nodule.

Thick plates have been recognized subsequently in post-necrotic states[21] alcoholic cirrhosis,[22] as a proliferative effect from anabolic hormone administration[23] and post hepatic venous occlusion.[24] It is accepted that hyperplasia is common to all these states and the use of the term for the rearrangement into two-cell-thick plates seems justified in these circumstances. It may be that neoplastic transformation also includes thickening of plates, but this is not a consideration in this series. The plate changes encountered in these groups of patients with some form of chronic liver disease are extensive and all parts of the livers are generally affected. An occasional exception may be expected on theoretical grounds, in circumstances of severe atrophy of part of the liver with hyperplasia of the remaining liver still enjoying a reasonable blood flow. In this series similar changes have been observed as involving either the plates confined to periportal regions only or all plates including those remote from portal tracts.

Periportal hyperplasia has been encountered in those conditions in which there has been substantial unequivocal necrosis or atrophy of hepatocytes situated mainly in perivenous regions and the conclusion is generally drawn that the periportal cell hyperplasia represents a cellular proliferation compensatory to the primary destruction. This is the case in congestive cardiac failure and hepatic venous occlusion, where atrophy and necrosis in variable proportions are clearly represented. The almost complete transformation to two-cell-thick plates, by contrast, is a diffuse change and was a frequent finding in several forms of chronic liver disease. The circumstances in which the vascular relations were identified as normal were present in three main forms of disease. First, in patients in whom there was evidence of severe loss of hepatic parenchyma, for example from trauma, surgical resection or replacement by tumour, the predominant arrangement was lobular as both hepatic venous radicles and portal tracts were easily identifiable and the term 'diffuse lobular hyperplasia' seems appropriate. Secondly, retention of normal vascular relations was found in some parts of the liver accompanying nodule formation in the examples of DNH. Whereas the nodule was defined as not bearing normally arranged hepatic venous radicles and portal tracts, substantial parts of the liver in such patients show a diffuse plate thickening with lobular retention. The foci which show an absence of vascular relations are generally smaller than normal lobules in DNH although macroscopical changes are easily observed. The macroscopical foci, with their pallor and distinct edges are usually a complex of lobules and nodules both consisting of thick plates (Fig. 10). Finally all our patients in this group with long-standing biliary disease showed a diffuse lobular hyperplasia with hepatic venous radicles recognizable among the thick plates with an appropriate relationship to fibrosed portal tracts.

On the other hand, almost complete replacement by hyperplastic nodules without survival of lobules was found in our patients with cirrhosis with its attendant striking fibrosis. The nodules in cirrhosis were always larger than the half-lobule or so diameter nodule of DNH and usually comprised tissue greater than several lobules. Within the cirrhotic nodules, thin-walled veins were sometimes found but the overall distortion of the parenchyma and abundant extranodular and sometimes intranodular fibrosis served to distinguish cirrhosis from DNH.

Periportal hyperplasia as found in our patients with congestive cardiac failure was not confused with DNH although in one series a higher incidence of CCF in DNH was reported.[7]

Hepatic venous occlusion was difficult to distinguish on the basis of exclusive criteria and this was confusing in one specimen from a patient with DNH. The main problem lay in the high

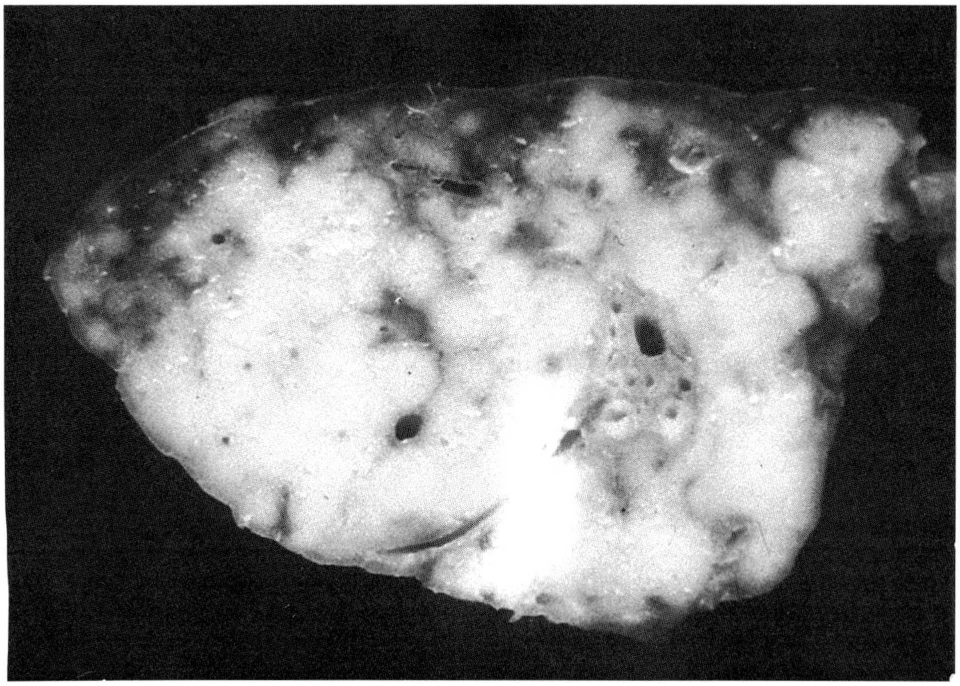

Fig. 10—Wedge resection of liver showing white lobules and nodules with juxtaposed congested subcapsular region. Patient 6. Macrophotograph, ×9

incidence of retained erythrocytes within sinusoids of biopsy specimens from patients with DNH. The erythrocytes accumulated sometimes within small nodules and sometimes in the parenchyma surrounding the nodules but these were not usually associated with necrosis or atrophy of hepatocytes, or with fibrosis. In none of the instances of DNH was there evidence of ostial or large hepatic vein occlusion or veno occlusive disease. It seemed possible that the nodules themselves compressed thin-walled veins.

The adequacy of the needle biopsy specimen for reaching the diagnosis of DNH is supported by the finding in Table III which shows that the micronodules of DNH were clearly delineated in all 12 specimens. The small nodules were usually not confused with the larger cirrhotic nodules bounded by thin septae of fibrous tissue although there was some difficulty if a fragmented biopsy specimen did not include fibrous tissue in a patient with cirrhosis. Differentiation from hepatic venous occlusion usually depended on the degree of erythrocyte accumulation in sinusoids which was more severe in venous occlusion, more frequently involved perisinusoidal spaces and more frequently associated with hepatocyte atrophy or necrosis. However, for reasons which are not clear, in one instance the needle biopsy specimen was dominated by accumulated erythrocytes with hepatocyte loss and the subsequent autopsy did not confirm hepatic venous occlusion but showed the lesions of DNH, albeit with abundant congested, haemorrhagic and necrotic foci. We have not encountered references to these changes in other reports. Nodules are well demonstrated by silver impregnation because of the sparse reticulin between thick plates and because of periportal condensation.

The associated abnormalities were similar to those in other series and we could draw no conclusions as to cause from these. So far as pathogenesis is concerned, this is still unknown, but there is no evidence so far to suggest that this is a form of compensatory hyperplasia following loss of or damage to parenchymal cells. The hypothesis, generally accepted, that the changes encountered in this condition represent some form of cellular proliferation is not seriously challenged by the observations in our patients. It is remarked, however, that the basis for the view that thick hepatocyte plates represent hyperplasia rests on the assumption that the livers in question had already undergone the remodelling process at about 6 years of age which had converted thick childhood plates[19] into single-cell-thick plates, the normal arrangement in adults. There is no reason to suspect that a failure in development might play some part in those conditions in which primary cellular damage or loss is evident, as is probably agreed in the instances of cirrhosis, cardiac failure, venous lesions, destruction of liver or bilary disease, but such pathogenetic pointers are not evident in DNH. There is so far, also no evidence to support this view in DNH from serial examinations of liver structure during the evolution of this disease, but the possibility of failure in development and remodelling of the liver although remote, is not excluded at present.

ACKNOWLEDGEMENTS

We thank the Cancer Research Campaign for providing a generous grant to K.W. Professor N. A. Wright kindly allowed us access to material in the Histopathology Department, Margaret Blount, BSc prepared many microscopical sections and William F. Hinkes many photomicrographs. Agnes Gorrissen undertook macrophotography, some photomicrography and helped to prepare the manuscript. To all these our thanks are due.

REFERENCES

1. Popper H. Pathologic aspects of cirrhosis. *Am J Path* 1977; **87:** 228.
2. Scheuer PJ. Cirrhosis. In: MacSween RNM, Anthony PP, Scheuer PJ, eds. Pathology of the Liver. Edinburgh: Churchill Livingstone, 1979: 258.
3. Blendis LM, Parkinson MC, Shilkin KB, Williams R. Nodular regenerative hyperplasia of the liver in Felty's syndrome. *Q J Med New Series* 1974; **43:** 25.
4. Rougier P, Degott C, Rueff B, Benhamou J. Nodular regenerative hyperplasia of the liver. *Gastroenterology* 1978; **75:** 69.
5. Stromeyer FW, Ishak KG. Nodular transformation (nodular 'regenerative' hyperplasia) of the liver. *Human Path* 1981; **12:** 60.
6. Reubner BH, Montgomery CK. Fibrosis, nodules and cirrhosis. In: Pathology of the Liver and Biliary Tract. New York, Chichester, Brisbane, Toronto and Singapore: Wiley, 1982: 228.
7. Steiner PE. Nodular regenerative hyperplasia of the liver. *Am J Path* 1959; **35:** 943.
8. Ponfick E. Experimentelle Beitrage zur Pathologie der Leber. *Virchows Arch* 1890; **119:** 193.
9. Von Meister V. 'Recreation des lebergewebes nach Abtragung ganzer Leberlappen'. *Ziegler's Beitrage* 1894; **15:** 1.
10. Turnbull HM, Worthington R. Regeneration of the liver. *Arch Path Inst Lond Hosp* 1908; **2:** 35.
11. Mann FC. Restoration and pathologic reactions of the liver. *J Mt Sinai Hosp* 1944; **11:** 65.
12. Starzl TE, Francavilla A, Porter KA, Benichou J, Jones AF. The effect of splanchnic viscera removal upon canine liver regeneration. *Surg Gynecol Obstet* 1978; **147:** 193.
13. Leffert HL, Koch KS, Lad PJ, Skelly H, de Hemptine B. Hepatocyte regeneration, replication and differentiation. In: Arias I, Popper H, Schachter D, Shafritz DA, eds. The Liver: Biology and Pathobiology. New York: Raven Press, 1982: 601.
14. Ranstrom S. Miliary hepatocellular adenomatosis. *Acta Pathol Microbiol Scand* 1953; **33:** 225.
15. Wanless IR, Godwin TA, Allen F, Feder A. Nodular regenerative hyperplasia of the liver in haematologic disorders: a possible response to obliterative portal venopathy. *Medicine* 1980; **59:** 367.
16. Elias H. A re-examination of the structure of the mammalian liver. I. Parenchymal architecture. *Am J Anat* 1949; **84:** 311.
17. Matsumoto T, Komori R, Magara T, Ui T, Kawakami M, Tokuda T, Takasaki S, Hayashi H, Jo K, Hano H, Fujino H, Tanaka H. A study on the normal structure of the human liver, with special reference to its angioarchitecture. *Jikeikai Med J* 1979; **26:** 1.
18. Rappaport AM, Borowy ZJ, Longheed WM, Lotto WN. Subdivision of hexagonal liver lobules into a structural and functional unit; role in hepatic physiology and pathology. *Anat Rec* 1954; **119:** 11.
19. Morgan JD, Hartroft WS. Juvenile liver. *Arch Path* 1961; **71:** 81.
20. Turnbull HM, Worthington R. Three cases illustrating the transition from regeneration to carcinoma in cirrhosis of the liver. *Arch Path Inst Lond Hosp* 1908; **2:** 59.
21. Peters RL. Viral hepatitis: a pathologic spectrum. *Am J Med Sci* 1975; **270:** 17.
22. Rubin E, Lieber CS. Fatty liver, alcoholic hepatitis and cirrhosis produced by alcohol in primates. *N Eng J Med* 1974; **290:** 128.
23. Paradinas FJ, Bull TB, Westaby D, Murray-Lyon IM. Hyperplasia and prolapse of hepatocytes into hepatic veins during longterm methyltestosterone therapy: possible relationship of these changes to the development of peliosis hepatis and liver tumours. *Histopathology* 1977; **1:** 225.
24. Parker RGF. Occlusion of the hepatic veins in man. *Medicine* 1959; **38:** 396.

JOURNAL OF PATHOLOGY, VOL. **143:** 93–101 (1984)

DAMAGE AND HEALING IN THE CONDUCTING TISSUE OF THE HEART (AN EXPERIMENTAL STUDY IN DOGS INFECTED WITH *TRYPANOSOMA CRUZI*)

ZILTON A. ANDRADE, SONIA G. ANDRADE AND MOYSÉS SADIGURSKY
Gonçalo Moniz Research Center (FIOCRUZ/UFBa), Salvador, Bahia, Brazil

Received 14 November 1983
Accepted 8 December 1983

SUMMARY

The consequences of acute inflammatory damage and chronic repair in the conducting system of the canine heart were observed after experimental *Trypanosoma cruzi* infection of young dogs. Acute infection lasted for 18–25 days and caused hyaline and lytic necrosis of the atrio-ventricular conducting fibres, the sinus node and the neurons in the cardiac para-sympathetic ganglia. Dogs that survived acute disease were examined after periods from 8 months to 3 years. Three main types of healing were found in the conducting system: fibrosis (diffuse and/or focal), sclero-atrophy and fatty infiltration. No signs of active chronic inflammation were present, although small focal residual accumulations of mononuclear cells were present in some animals. No evident electrocardiographic alterations were elicited by the presence of such cicatricial lesions. The animal model appears worthwhile for the study of the healing process in conducting tissue of the heart and for the better understanding of the asymptomatic phase of *T. cruzi* infection in man.

KEY WORDS—Conducting tissue, Chagas' disease, myocarditis.

INTRODUCTION

The specialized tissue of the heart for the formation and conduction of the electric stimuli for contraction is composed of the sinus node (the normal pacemaker), internodal tracts, atrio-ventricular node, His bundle and its branches and the Purkinje fibres. This important system can be damaged by disease and arrhythmias of several types and severity may appear therefrom.[1] It is generally assumed that the myo-neural cells of this system are unable to regenerate and that destructive lesions are followed by scarring. However, no direct experimental evidence is so far available to indicate how the specialized tissues of the heart undergo repair. Thus, several end-stage types of lesions seen in human conducting tissue have been variously interpreted as of degenerative, inflammatory or vascular origins.[2] It seems that a better understanding of the pathological changes would be gained if one could have an experimental model for a controlled study of the process of repair within the conducting tissues of the heart.

During experimental studies with *Trypanosoma cruzi* infection in young dogs it became apparent that the severe myocarditis present extended into the conducting tissue, sometimes causing extensive damage to it.[3] Furthermore, such myocarditis eventually subsided almost completely permitting the healing process to take place.[4] Thus, it was apparent that *T. cruzi* infection in dogs could offer for the first time a suitable model for the controlled study of damage and repair in delicate and peculiar structures such as those of the conduction system of the heart.

The present study describes the morphological changes which appear in the conducting system during acute *T. cruzi* myocarditis in dogs and its aftermath 8 months to 3 years following clinical cure.

Supported by Grant No. 2222.8.175/80 from the Brazilian Research Council (CNPq).

0022–3417/84/060093–09$01.00

MATERIAL AND METHODS

Fifty mongrel dogs of both sexes, 2–5 months old, were inoculated intraperitoneally with citrated mouse blood containing $4-6 \times 10^5$ *T. cruzi* trypomastigotes per kg body weight, of the strains 12 SF (São Felipe-Bahia) or Colombian strain.[5]

They all developed positive parasitaemias at approximately 5–7 days after inoculation and showed evident signs of disease (loss of appetite, dyspnoea) around day 15.

There was high mortality from day 19 to 23. Thirteen animals that died or were sacrificed in the height of the acute phase were selected for special study of the conduction system of the heart (see Table I). Nine dogs survived acute infection and started to recover by day 30 on. Three of them were treated during the acute phase with a nitrofuranic drug, Bayer's nifurtimox[6] and six recovered spontaneously. Although parasitaemia became negative, xenodiagnosis and/or the complement fixation test remained positive for all animals. Serological titres ranged from 1:16 to 1:128. These animals appeared healthy and had repeated electrocardiograms within normal limits. They were sacrificed after 8 months to 3 years following inoculation (see Table II).

During the acute and chronic stages of these experiments several electrocardiograms (ECG) were recorded from each animal and compared with their pre-infection ECGs. A one single channel apparatus was used, all 12 classical leads were taken with small metallic needles placed under the skin serving as electrodes.

Autopsies were performed as soon as possible after death. The heart was fixed *in totum*. A 10 per cent buffered formalin solution was injected into the cardiac chambers with the vessels ligated. The heart was gently distended in a diastolic position and placed in formalin for 2–4 days before opening. The sinus node was studied according to Hudson.[7] The atrio-ventricular node, His bundle and proximal portions of its branches as well as the internodal approaches to the AV node, were studied by the Lev's method.[8] The serial sections obtained were mounted on continuous transparent plastic tapes according to the technique described by Pickett and Sommers.[9] After staining with the Masson's trichrome method the sections were examined with a special device adapted to the microscope. An average of 600 sections from the SA node and 3000 from the atrio-ventricular system were examined for each case. Selected sections from every case were taken apart, mounted on glass slides and stained with haematoxylin and eosin, Weigert-Van Gieson method for collagen and elastic fibres, periodic acid-Schiff (PAS) and Gomori's silver method for reticulum. Seven dogs, two males and five females, were not infected and served as normal controls for

Table I—General data on 13 dogs with acute experimental *Trypansoma cruzi** infection used to study changes in the conducting tissue of the heart

Dog No.	Age (months)	Sex	Initial weight (kg)	Parasitaemia (50 fields, 400×) Min.	Parasitaemia (50 fields, 400×) Max.	Duration of infection (days)
1	3	F	2·25	2	22	19
2	3	F	1·75	1	47	22
3	3	F	1·60	5	70	23
4	3	F	1·35	1	25	21
5	3	F	1·50	1	26	22
15	2	M	2·00	7	79	26
24	2	F	1·08	19	388	24
26	2	F	1·11	2	87	25
29	2·5	F	2·17	3	15	25
33	2·5	F	1·72	2	7	23
36	2	F	1·40	8	55	19
39	2	F	2·20	1	33	20
40	2	F	2·00	1	8	29

* Strain: 12-SF (Bahia), except dog 15 (Colombian strain).

serological, electrocardiographic and morphological comparison.

RESULTS

During the acute phase of the infection all the dogs exhibited severe myocarditis. Electrocardiographic examination showed alterations from day 7 on. These included atrial fibrillation, nodal rhythm, wandering pacemaker, inverted T waves, alterations of ST segments and, later on, complete right bundle branch block with or without anterior or posterior left hemiblock. At autopsy the hearts appeared soft and dilated. Examination of the animals on the days 18–22 after inoculation showed a diffuse and intense mononuclear cell infiltration in the myocardium, with *T. cruzi* amastigotes present within some myocardial cells. This inflammation also involved the conducting

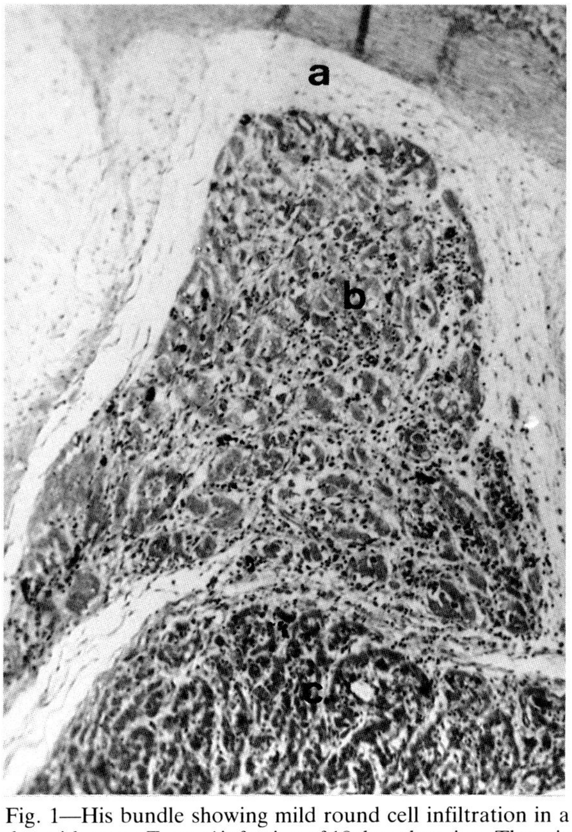

Fig. 1—His bundle showing mild round cell infiltration in a dog with acute *T. cruzi* infection of 18 days duration. There is dissociation of specific fibres and disappearance of some others (lytic necrosis). a = Central fibrous body; b = bundle of His; c = septal myocardium. Masson's trichrome stain, ×120

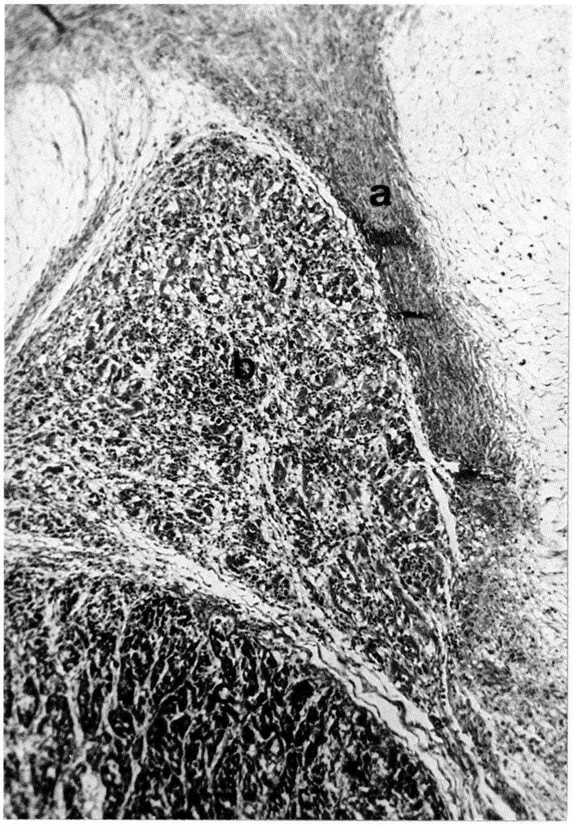

Fig. 2—Acute *T. cruzi* myocarditis involving the main bundle of His in a dog inoculated 22 days previously. Besides the mononuclear cell infiltration there are many clear spaces among the fibres representing areas of lytic necrosis. See Fig. 1 legend for key. Masson's trichrome stain, ×100

system. Figs 1–3 show three degrees of changes in the His main bundle. Similar changes were present throughout the conducting system and in the sinus node. This latter structure was so infiltrated by inflammatory cells that its histological identification was difficult. Sometimes it appeared to be totally effaced with only the nodal artery and a scanty amount of the peculiar nodal stroma around it being tentatively identified. Within the mononuclear infiltration of the myocardial specific tissues there occurred lytic and hyaline necrosis of the fibres. This caused considerable loss of specialized tissue, with the appearance of vacuolated and empty spaces which were followed by collapse of the supporting stroma. Intracellular parasites could be detected in some of these lesions.

Surviving animals showed disappearance of acute electrocardiographic alterations by 2 months after inoculation and soon recovered appetite and became active again. During intervals from 8 months to 3 years (Table II) they were sacrificed.

The hearts were grossly within normal limits. Microscopical changes in the myocardium included patchy areas of fibrosis, focal atrophy of fibres and minute sparse collections of lymphocytes and macrophages. No evidence of chronic active inflammation could be seen in any case.

The sinus node showed considerable fatty infiltration in its surroundings and rarely in the nodal tissue proper. The fibrous stroma showed diffuse condensation and there were small focal areas of dense fibrosis. The nodal artery was little altered. There was focal intimal fibrosis and slight fibrosis and hypertrophy of the media.

The lesions in the conducting tissue were represented by foci of fibrous tissue, fatty infiltration and sclero-atrophy, occasionally with little focal mononuclear cell infiltration (Fig. 4). The AV node and the distal portion of the main bundle and the right bundle branch were the main areas involved. Several areas of fibrous (cicatricial) tissue appeared in the interventricular septum especially involving the right portion of it. Fatty infiltration was prominent in two cases. It appeared in the penetrating part of the main bundle in one case and in the half portion of the distal main bundle in another case. This latter animal had been treated with Nifurtimox (Bayer) plus corticoid (Fig. 5). Fatty tissue was also present in the AV node, and in one instance, it interrupted almost 70 per cent of the right bundle branch (Fig. 6), just in its beginning from the main bundle. Sclero-atrophy was represented by an extreme degree of atrophy of specific fibres while the

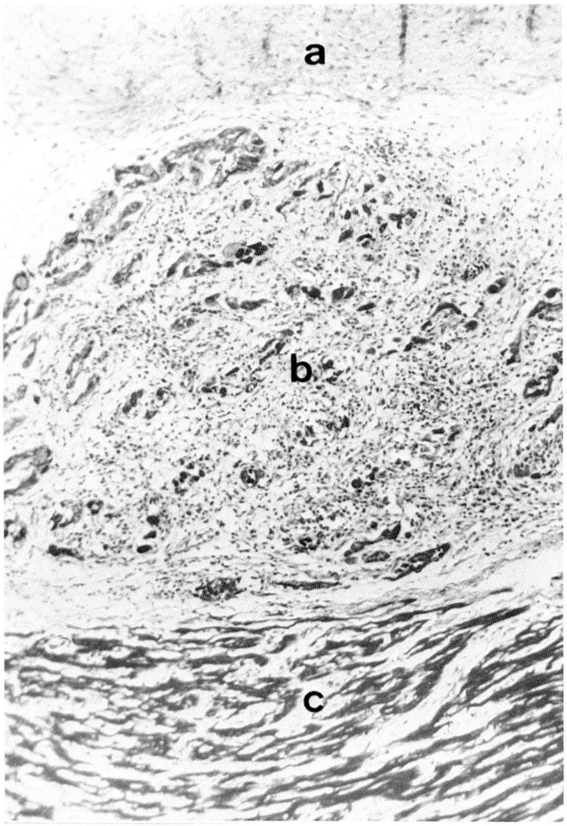

Fig. 3—Considerable inflammatory destruction of the His bundle in a dog with a 20 day old infection by *T. cruzi*. Almost 80 per cent of the conducting fibres have been destroyed. See Fig. 1 legend for key. Masson's trichrome stain, ×120

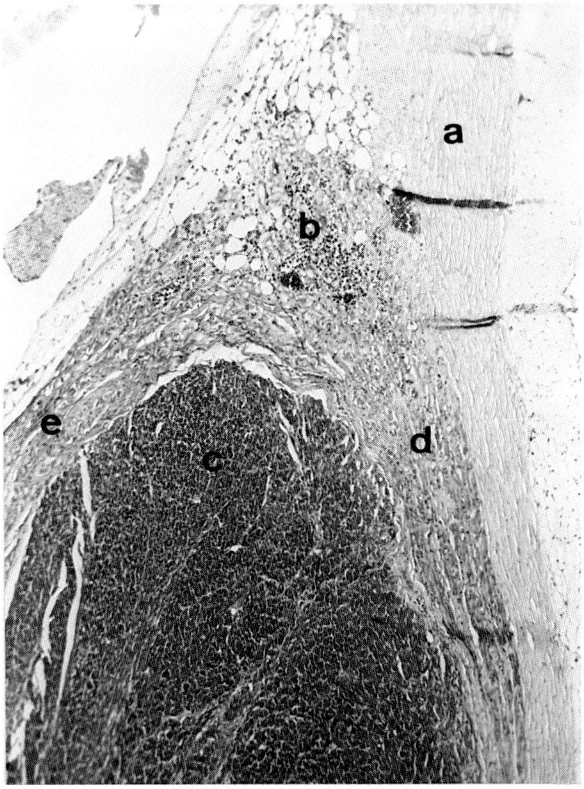

Fig. 4—Diffuse fibrosis, some patchy areas of mononuclear cell accumulations and focal fatty infiltration are present in the conducting tissue of a dog that had acute *T. cruzi* infection 3 years ago. a = Central fibrous body; b = His bundle; c = septal myocardium; d = right bundle branch; e = left bundle branch (anterior division). ECG showed transient sinus arrhythmia only. Haematoxylin and eosin, ×70

Table II—General data on dogs which survived acute infection with *Trypanosoma cruzi* and were later utilized to study the pathology of the conducting tissue of the heart

Dog No.	Initial age (months)	Sex	Initial weight (kg)	Duration of infection (months)	*T. cruzi* strain
12	5	M	8·00	36	12 SF
14	5	M	5·00	36	12 SF
16	2	M	2·00	19	Colombian
18	2	F	1·20	8	12 SF
21	2	M	1·20	28	12 SF
38	2·5	F	2·35	18	12 SF
47	2·5	F	2·40	9	Colombian
49	2·5	F	2·60	9	Colombian
50	2·5	F	2·60	9	Colombian

stroma appeared undisturbed, although partially collapsed. Such change was seen more often in the bundle branches especially in the right side (Fig. 7).

Fibrous scarring was seen as a prominent change twice in the AV node, three times in the main bundle and once in the right bundle branch. A frequent finding was a diffuse interstitial fibrous thickening better seen at the AV node (Fig. 8). Changes in the 12 lead electrocardiograms, during the period of observation were not marked. Five animals developed a prolongation in PR interval,

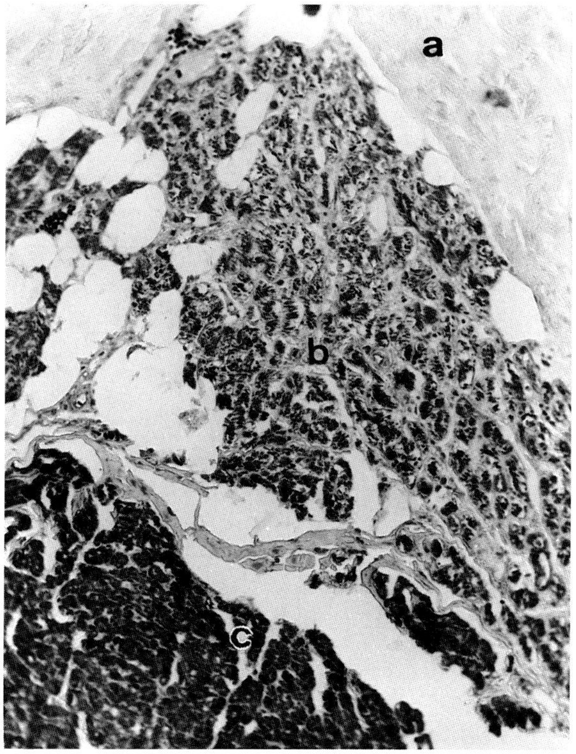

Fig. 5—Bundle of His presenting areas of fatty infiltration and a fine and diffuse interstitial fibrosis. There is no inflammation. Specimen is from a dog that recovered from acute *T. cruzi* myocarditis 9 months ago. See Fig. 4 legend for key. Masson's trichrome stain, ×150

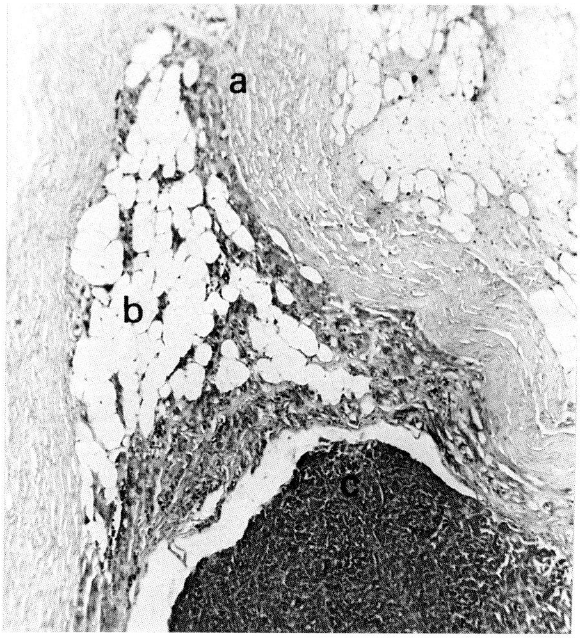

Fig. 6—Marked fatty infiltration replacing the His bundle in a dog that recovered from acute *T. cruzi* infection after treatment with a nitrofuranic drug and corticoid and remained apparently healthy for 18 months when it was sacrificed. Serial sectioning showed that about 70 per cent of the bundle was replaced by fat in that area. ECG did not show cardiac block. See Fig. 4 legend for key. Haematoxylin and eosin, ×120

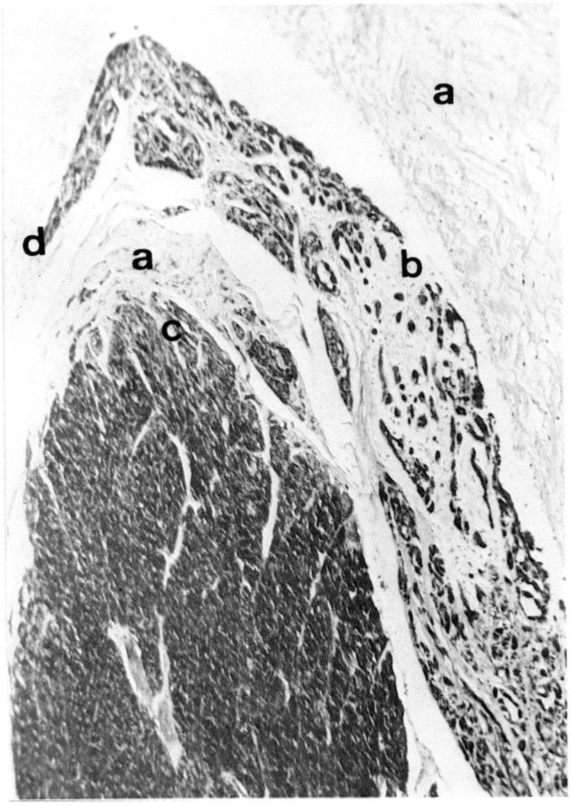

Fig. 7—Areas of sclero-atrophy in the right bundle branch. Dog had acute *T. cruzi* infection 8 months ago. ECG showed morphology of incomplete right bundle branch block. a = Central fibrous body; b = right bundle branch; c = septal myocardium; d – left bundle branch. Masson's trichrome stain, ×100

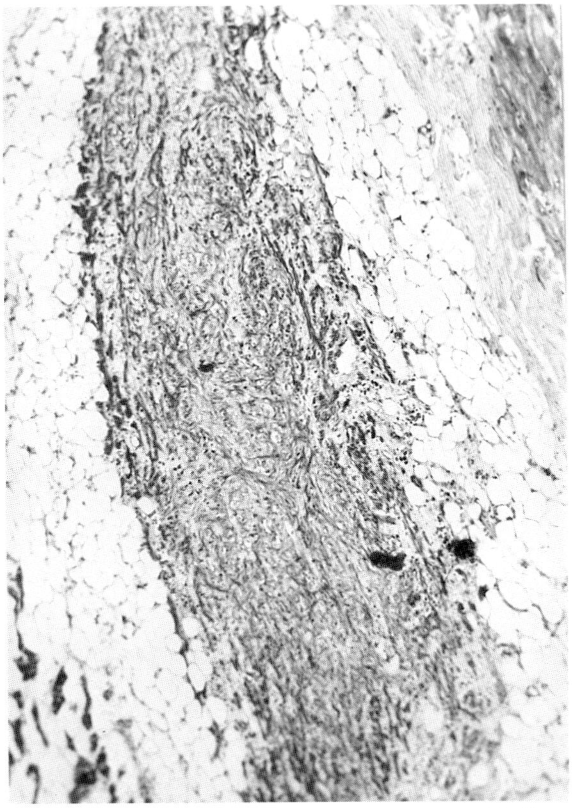

Fig. 8—Diffuse interstitial fibrosis, atrophy of specific fibres and mild residual round cell infiltration present in the atrio-ventricular node. This dog had acute *T. cruzi* infection 3 years ago. Masson's trichrome stain, ×120

although in the majority of them, heart rates had dropped considerably. In one case electrocardiographic changes, compatible with right bundle branch block, which were not present during the acute phase, appeared after 260 days of inoculation. In this case the right bundle branch and the right hemi-portion of the main bundle were replaced by fibrous tissue.

Similar changes as described above were also seen in the autonomic nerve ganglia present in the epicardium and inter-atrial septum. During acute infection there were mononuclear cell infiltration and neuronal destruction (Fig. 9) and during the recovering stage, when inflammation had subsided, there appeared fibrous replacement (Fig. 10).

The tissues around the atrio-ventricular node (approaching tracts to the AV node) also showed severe inflammatory changes during the acute infection and late fibrous replacement and fatty infiltration.

DISCUSSION

An experimental study of the healing process within the conducting system of the heart has not been reported probably due to the lack of an appropriate model. The infection of young dogs with *T. cruzi,* followed by severe acute disease and by clinical cure appears to be a promising model. Dogs have a conducting system similar to that of man,[10–13] can be easily infected with *T. cruzi*[13] and the severe myocarditis which develops during acute infection can be suppressed with drugs at any time.[6]

Acute *T. cruzi* myocarditis is known to involve the conducting tissue of both man[14] and dog[13] causing lytic and hyaline necrosis of specific fibres.

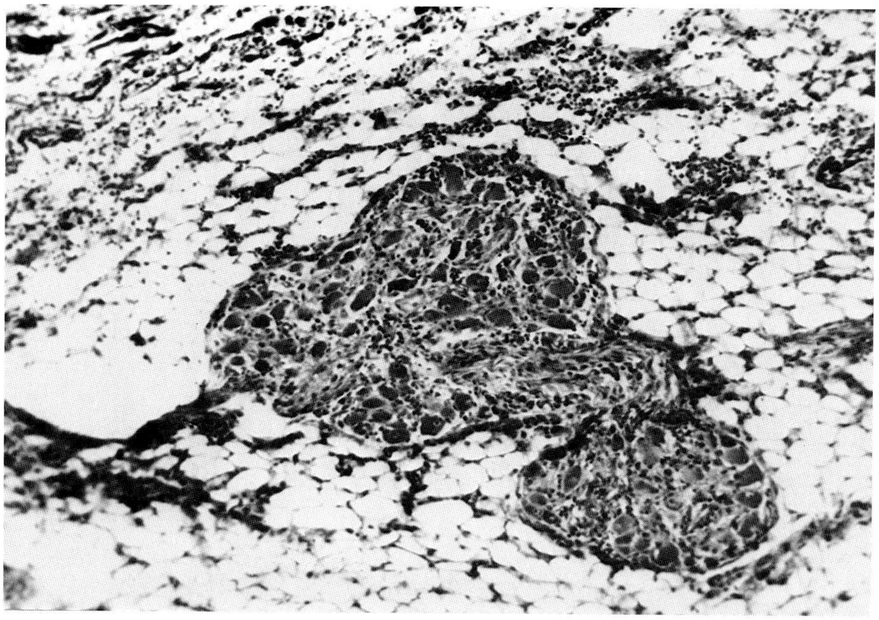

Fig. 9—Sub-epicardial autonomic nervous ganglia of a dog with acute *T. cruzi* infection. There are diffuse mononuclear cell infiltration, interstitial edema, and neuronal degeneration and necrosis. Haematoxylin and eosin, ×100

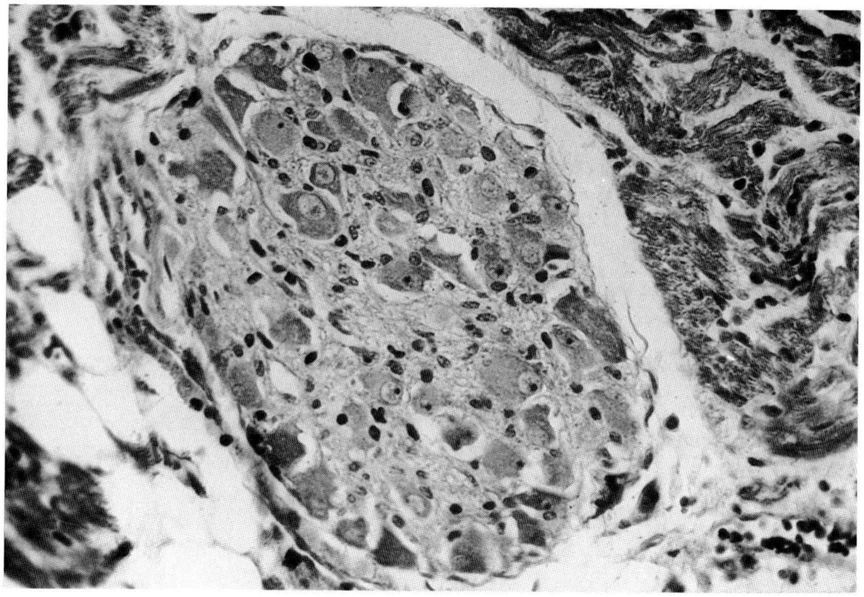

Fig. 10—Interstitial fibrosis, diminution of the number of neurons seen in a nerve ganglion near the right atrial wall. Dog 8 months after the acute phase of *T. cruzi* infection. Haematoxylin and eosin, ×150

The cause of such necrosis in non-parasitized cells remains obscure at present. The possibility of toxic, anoxic or metabolic injury cannot be ruled out. Ribeiro dos Santos and Hudson[15] have presented evidence from *in vitro* studies that *T. cruzi* antigen sensitization of cell membrane could be followed by cellular and/or humoral immune-mediated lysis.

The findings in the present study revealed that three main forms of healing can result from the acute necrotic-inflammatory injury to the canine conducting tissue: fibrosis, sclero-atrophy and fatty infiltration. Fibrosis is a quite common and stereotyped form of repair anywhere and needs no further comment. Sclero-atrophy occurs frequently in the conducting system of man and represents a main lesion found in cases of idiopathic atrio-ventricular block.[16] It is characterized by the presence of considerable atrophy of the conducting fibres while the normal stroma persists as a loose connective framework. It can sometimes collapse and become a dense acellular fibrous tract. Sclero-atrophy has been thought to result from progressive vascular ischaemia[17] although this has been disputed by others.[18] No important vascular involvement was apparent in the present material.

Fatty replacement is also frequently observed in lesions affecting the conducting tissue of man[1,19] and sometimes appears as a sole and prominent lesion in complete atrio-ventricular block.[20] It has been correlated with obesity and aging, and is usually considered as a primary degenerative process rather than a peculiar process of repair within the conducting tissue. It is a curious and paradoxical 'healing' process, since fatty tissue is the least conducting of all living tissues, probably due to its low electrolyte content.[21]

Similar mechanisms of damage and defective repair during *T. cruzi* infection were also observed in the para-sympathetic nervous ganglia of the heart. Loss of neurons in the autonomic nervous system is an important feature of Chagas' disease. Its pathogenesis and significance are controversial. Damage during acute infection seems to be an important mechanism of neuronal loss, as suggested by Köberle.[22]

Another important aspect observed in the present material is that several large or patchy cicatricial areas within the conducting tissue can exist without eliciting alterations in the classical electrocardiogram. This has considerable implications regarding the problem of Chagas' disease in man. It is well known that people who recover from acute Chagas' disease may remain asymptomatic for years or even for a lifetime, although they do not eliminate the infection. Refined methods of cardiac examination may detect conduction disturbances in these individuals.[23] To the cardiologists these findings serve to unmask early cardiac signs of chronic progressive Chagas' myocarditis, which means an ominous prognosis. The administration of conduction depressing drugs, such as ajmaline[24,25] can even make the disturbances detectable by routine electrocardiography. However, there is a possibility that the results of some of these functional studies may depend on the presence of cicatricial areas rather than active lesions in the conducting tissue of asymptomatic subjects with *T. cruzi* infection, as observed in the present study.

REFERENCES

1. Davies MJ. Pathology of Conducting Tissue of the Heart. London: Butterworth, 1971.
2. Lev M, Bharati S. Lesions of the conduction system and their functional significance. In: Pathology Annual. New York: Appleton-Century-Crofts, 1974: 157–207.
3. Andrade ZA, Andrade SG, Sadigursky M, Lima JAC. Doença de Chagas experimental no cão. Relação morfológica e electrocardiográfica na fase aguda da infecção. *Arq Bras Cardiol* 1980; **35:** 485.
4. Andrade ZA, Andrade SG, Sadigursky M, Maguire JH. Experimental Chagas' disease in dogs. A pathologic and ECG study of the chronic indeterminate phase of the infection. *Arch Path Lab Med* 1981; **105:** 460.
5. Federici EE, Abelmann WB, Neva FA. Chronic and progressive myocarditis and myositis in C3H mice infected with *Trypanosoma cruzi. Am J Trop Med Hyg* 1964; **13:** 272.
6. Andrade SG, Andrade ZA, Sadigursky M. Combined treatment with a nitrofuranic and a corticoid in experimental Chagas' disease in the dog. *Am J Trop Med Hyg* 1980; **29:** 766.
7. Hudson REB. The human pacemaker and its pathology. *Brit Heart J* 1960; **22:** 153.
8. Lev, M. The normal anatomy of the conduction system in man and its pathology in atrioventricular block. *Ann New York Acad Sci* 1964; **3:** 817.
9. Pickett P, Sommer JR. Thirty-five mm film as mounting base and plastic spray as cover glass for histologic sections. *Arch Path* 1960; **69:** 239.
10. Lumb G, Shacklett RS, Dawkins WA. The cardiac conduction tissue and its blood supply in the dog. *Am J Path* **35:** 467.
11. James TN. Anatomy of the sinus node of the dog. *Anat Rec* 1962; **143:** 251.
12. Isaacson R, Boucek RJ. The atrioventricular conduction tissue of the dog. Histochemical properties; influence of electric shock. *Am Heart J* 1968; **75:** 206.
13. Andrade ZA, Andrade SG. A patologia da doença de Chagas experimental no cão. *Mem Inst Oswaldo Cruz* 1980; **75:** 77.

14. Andrade ZA, Miziara HL. Alteraçoes do sistema de gênese e condução do estimulo cardíaco na fase aguda da doença de Chagas humana. *Arq Bras Cardiol* 1983; **40:** 233.
15. Ribeiro dos Santos R, Hudson L. Denervation and the immune response in mice infected with *Trypanosoma cruzi. Clin Exp Immunol* 1981; **44:** 349.
16. Lenègre J. Etiology and pathology of bilateral bundle branch block in relation to complete heart block. *Prog Cardiovasc Dis* 1964; **6:** 409.
17. Hudson REB. Cardiovascular Pathology, Vol. 1, Chapter 2, London: E. Arnold, 1965: 53–145.
18. Davies MJ, Harris A. Pathological basis of primary heart block. *Brit Heart J* 1969; **31:** 219.
19. Andrade ZA, Andrade SG, Oliveira GB, Alonso DR. Histopathology of the conducting tissue of the heart in Chagas' myocarditis. *Am Heart J* 1978; **93:** 316.
20. Spain DM, Cathcart RT. Heart block caused by fat infiltration of the interventricular septum (*cor adiposum*). *Am Heart J* 1946; **32:** 659.
21. Schwan HP, Kay CF. The conductivity of living tissues. *Ann New York Acad Sci* 1957; **65:** 1007.
22. Köberle F. Pathogenesis of Chagas' disease. In: Trypanosomiasis and Leishmaniasis with Special Reference to Chagas' Disease. Ciba Foundation Symposium 20. Amsterdam: Associated Scientific Publs, 1974: 137–158.
23. Pimenta J, Miranda M, Pereira CB. Electrophysiologic findings in long-term asymptomatic chagasic individuals. *Am Heart J* 1983; **106:** 374.
24. Chiale PA, Przybylsky J, Laino RA, Halpern MS, Sanchez RA, Gabrieli A, Elizari MV, Rosenbaum MB. Electrocardiographic changes evoked by ajmaline in chronic Chagas' disease without manifest myocarditis. *Am J Cardiol* 1982; **49:** 14.
25. Moleiro F, Mendoza I, Octavio JA, Anselmi A, Castellanos A. Los transtornos de conducción intraventricular y la prueba de ajmalina en pacientes con infección chagásica. *Rev Lat Cardiol* 1982; **3:** 414.

JOURNAL OF PATHOLOGY, VOL. **143:** 103–116 (1984)

THE SUBCELLULAR BASIS OF DAMAGE TO THE HUMAN URINARY BLADDER INDUCED BY IRRADIATION

G. N. ANTONAKOPOULOS*, R. M. HICKS AND R. J. BERRY

School of Pathology and Department of Oncology, The Middlesex Hospital Medical School, London W1, U.K.

Received 21 June 1983
Accepted 4 October 1983

SUMMARY

The effects of x-irradiation on the subcellular structure of the human urinary bladder were investigated by electron microscopic examination of biopsies taken during check cystoscopies from 25 patients between 1 month and 22 years after completion of a course of therapeutic radiation. All tissues of the bladder wall were damaged to some extent by the treatment. In the urothelium this was reflected by the development of more than the usual numbers of lysosomes and autophagic vacuoles in all cell layers. In the bladder wall, large often binucleate or multinucleate fibroblasts were prominent and persistent in all specimens and were associated with the development of progressive fibrosis. The vasculature and the muscle coats of the bladder wall were also damaged. In the blood vessels many endothelial cells were oedematous or necrotic and some intravascular coagulation was also observed. Smooth muscle cells became oedematous soon after irradiation, and after longer time intervals there was focal death and loss of individual muscle cells. The observed degeneration and extensive necrosis of the bladder wall, which involved severe destruction and disorganization of the muscular layers, is sufficient to explain the clinical sequelae of bladder irradiation, namely loss of elasticity, reduced capacity and incomplete micturition with residual urine.

KEY WORDS—Urinary bladder, x-irradiation.

INTRODUCTION

Irradiation of the human urinary bladder is not an uncommon event for radiotherapy is currently used for pre-operative, therapeutic and palliative treatment of urinary bladder cancer and, furthermore, the bladder is often included in the irradiation field during treatment of tumours of neighbouring organs. Although it is regarded as a relatively radio-resistant organ,[1] numerous clinical symptoms and pathological changes in the bladder have been recorded following irradiation and the histopathological changes have been arbitrarily categorized into acute, sub-acute and late-phase damage.[2–15]

Acute damage which may develop within 4–6 weeks after the initiation of therapy, can include injury to the urothelium, endothelial oedema and degeneration, and inflammation and degeneration of smooth muscle cells. In the sub-acute phase, 6 months to 2 years after irradiation, the urothelium may become either focally atrophic or hyperplastic, many vessels in the bladder wall appear telangiectatic or obliterated and fibrosis becomes a problem. Chronic and late effects may be observed many years after irradiation, and can include ulceration and the development of fissures and fistulas. Fibrosis is a major complication of late-stage damage and may lead to induration of the bladder wall and a reduction in the capacity of the organ.

The present study was undertaken in order to determine the ultrastructural changes which underlie the clinical sequelae following irradiation of the human bladder. An account of irradiation-induced changes in the rat urinary bladder,

* Present address: Department of Histology, University of Athens Medical School, Athens, Greece.
Addressee for correspondence: Professor R. M. Hicks, School of Pathology, The Middlesex Hospital Medical School, Riding House Street, London W1P 7LD, U.K.

0022–3417/84/060103–14$01.40

Table I—Human material: pathology of the bladder wall. Thirty specimens were taken from 25 patients, 5 of whom were cystoscopied twice within a few months. The muscular coat was not always included in the biopsy material

No.	Sex	Age	History	Dose of irradiation (cGy)	Time after irradiation	Damage to the urothelium	Fibrosis	Damage to endothelial cells	Damage to the muscular coat*	Damage to the nerves*	Other findings or concurrent diseases
1	♀	69	TCC	4000	1 month	++	+	++	+	+	—
2	♂	66	TCC	3840	1 month	++	+	++		+	Acute cystitis—cystitis cystica
3	♂	70	TCC	3840	1 month	+	+	+		+	—
4	♂	73	TCC	6720	4 months	++	++	++		+	Cystitis cystica—
5	♂	74	TCC	6000	4 months	++	++	++	++	+	—
6	♂	61	TCC	6620	4 months	+	++	++	+++	+	—
7	♂	64	TCC	6240	4 months	+	++	++	++	+	—
8	♂	65	TCC	2400	7 months	+	+	+		—	—
9	Patient	No. 3	TCC	6720	8 months	+	++	+		+	—
10	♀	70	TCC	6240	8 months	++	++	+++	+++	+	—
11	♀	71	TCC	5760	10 months	+	+++	++	++	++	—
12	♂	83	TCC	6040	10 months	++	++	++	+++	++	—
13	♂	70	Prostatic carcinoma. Small TCC of the bladder	4500	10 months	++	++	++	++	+	—
14	♀	34	Carcinoma of the cervix uterus	4840†	13 months	+	++	+++		+	Hepatitis B
15	♂	74	TCC	6420	15 months	+	++	++		+	—
16	Patient	No. 5			16 months	++	++	++	++	+	—
17	♂	58	TCC of ureter—(lower part)	5760	16 months	++	++	++	++	+	Diabetes
18	♂	52	TCC	5760	17 months	+	++	++	++	+	—
19	Patient	No. 11			20 months	++	++	++		+	—
20	♂	69	TCC	5760	21 months	++	++	++	+++	++	—
21	Patient	No. 15			21 months	+	+++	++	++	+	—
22	♂	59	Prostatic carcinoma	6500	22 months	++	+++	++		++	—
23	♀	75	TCC	5840	22 months	+	+++	++	++	+	Rheumatoid arthritis
24	♀	66	Ovarian carcinoma	6000	3 years	+	+++	++		++	—
25	♀	59	TCC	6000	4 years	++	+++	++	+++	++	—
26	♀	68	Carcinoma of the cervix uterus	6000	7 years	+	+++	++		++	Ca of breast
27	♂	82	TCC	6000	8 years	++	+++	++		++	—
28	Patient	No. 27		6000	8½ years	++	+++	++		++	—
29	♂	59	TCC	5500	9 years	+	+++	++	++	++	—
30	♀	65	Carcinoma of the cervix uterus	4405†	15 years	+	+++	+		++	—

* Where neither the presence or absence of damage is indicated in smooth muscle cells or nerves, the structures were not included in the biopsy material examined.

† Plus intracavitary radiation to uterus, with negligible dose to bladder.

+ = Mild damage; ++ = moderate damage; +++ = severe damage.

TCC = Transitional cell carcinoma of the urinary bladder.

including the induction of urothelial carcinoma, has been published elsewhere.[16]

MATERIALS AND METHODS

Thirty biopsies were taken during check cystoscopies of 25 patients at time intervals varying between 1 month and 22 years after completion of their irradiation. Five patients were cystoscoped a second time after an interval of a few months. The age and sex of the patients, diagnosis before irradiation, dose of irradiation, time after treatment and the pathology of the bladder wall are summarized in Table I.

The purpose of the present study was to investigate the subcellular effects of irradiation on normal urinary bladder rather than on tumours and the urologists, therefore, made every effort to obtain biopsies from normal-looking areas. Nevertheless, since most biopsies came from bladder cancer patients, some specimens were found to have obvious pre-neoplastic or neoplastic histology. All such specimens were excluded from the study. In patients irradiated for carcinoma of the cervix, the biopsy material was taken from the trigone area of the bladder; in patients irradiated for prostatic cancer, the neck of the bladder was biopsied. All specimens included urothelium and lamina propria and in 17 part of the muscular coat was also present. Control biopsies were also taken from the bladders of five 'normal' non-irradiated patients, either with a history of urethral strictures or mild prostatic enlargement.

All biopsies were immediately placed in ice-cold cacodylate-buffered 1 per cent osmium tetroxide. After sectioning into small cubes, the pieces were fixed in the same fixative for a further 1·5 h at 4°C. They were then dehydrated through graded ethanols and embedded in Spurr resin. Sections 1 μm thick were stained with toluidine blue for histology, and thin sections (60–90 nm) were contrast-stained with saturated alcoholic uranyl acetate and Reynold's lead citrate before examination in a Jeol 100B transmission electron microscope.

RESULTS

In this study, neoplastic change was observed in some biopsies from patients with a history of bladder cancer. It was not possible to determine whether the changes in these patients were attributable to irradiation *per se* (*cf.* the effect of irradiation in the rat[16]) or were due to previous carcinogen-induced changes in cell differentiation. All neoplastic specimens were, therefore, discarded and only specimens with normal or simple hyperplastic urothelia were examined.

Urothelial changes

Changes were observed both in histologically normal-looking and in hyperplastic urothelia from irradiated patients. The changes were approximately the same irrespective of the growth pattern of the urothelium, even when that included Brunn's nests. The most obvious change, found in all specimens was the presence in all cell layers of numerous lysosomes, phagosomes and lipid droplets (Fig. 1). Normally, lysosomes are only seen in the superficial cells of the urothelium but especially in the first few months post-irradiation they were abundant in the basal and intermediate cell layers also.

Other regular changes observed in the urothelium included the development of nuclear pleomorphism and, during the first few post-irradiation months, the occurrence of darkly-staining cells with coarsely granular, condensed cytoplasm in the basal and intermediate cell layers (Fig. 2). Intra-cytoplasmic cysts which did not connect either with the bladder lumen or with extracellular spaces, were observed in a few intermediate cells (Fig. 3). These cysts contained small vesicles and amorphous material. Of the 30 specimens 12 (40 per cent) were lined by apparently normal, asymmetric luminal membrane, such as is found on the luminal face of normal urothelium, but the remainder had numerous microvilli projecting into the lumina, which were limited by a thinner, symmetrical unit membrane covered by a glycocalyx.

The basal lamina separating the urothelium from the lamina propria was usually thickened and frequently multilamellate in these irradiated tissues.

Connective tissue changes

Fibroblasts were prominent in all irradiated specimens and were noticeable by virtue of the increased amounts of rough surfaced endoplasmic reticulum (rer) and Golgi elements in their cytoplasm. Their nuclei were generally irregular,

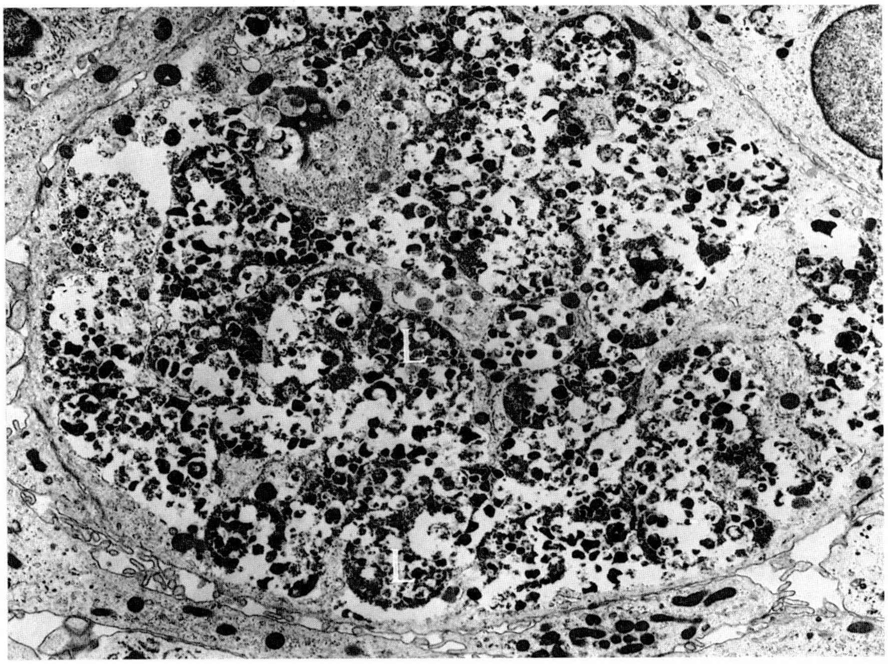

Fig 1—An intermediate urothelial cell filled with lysosomes (L). Specimen taken from a 70-year-old man 1 month after the irradiation. ×5415

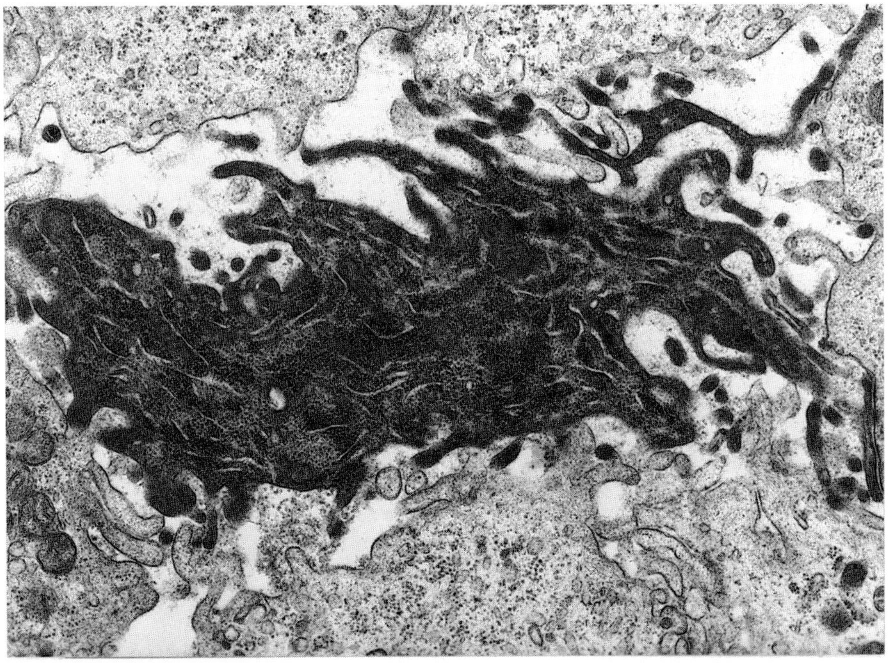

Fig. 2—A condensed, necrotic cell in the intermediate cell layer of the urothelium. Specimen taken from a 69-year-old woman 1 month after irradiation. ×16 150

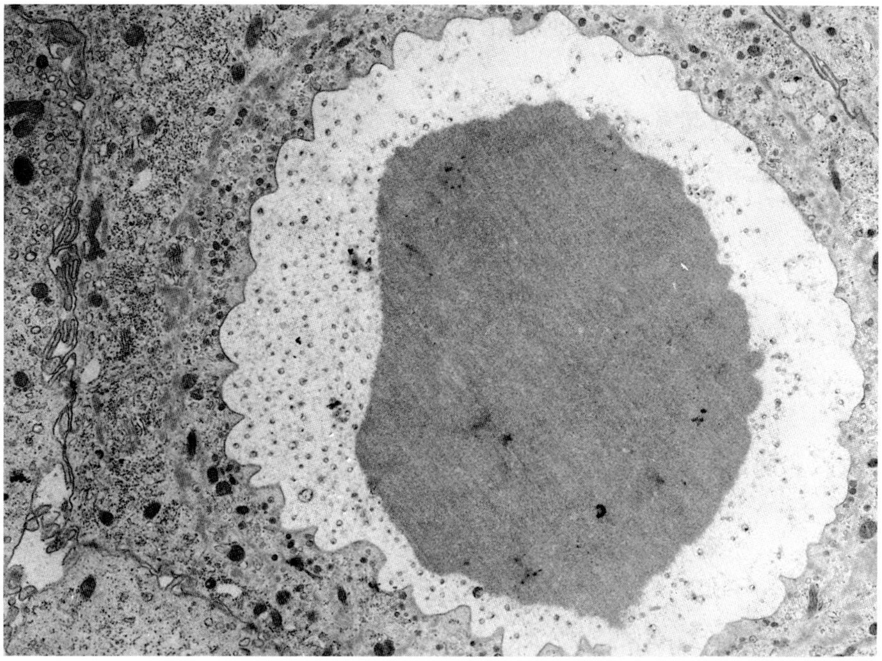

Fig. 3—An intracytoplasmic cyst in an intermediate urothelial cell. The luminal edge is limited by membrane with the characteristic structure of normally differentiated superficial cell luminal membrane. Specimen taken from a 74-year-old man 4 months after irradiation. ×6650

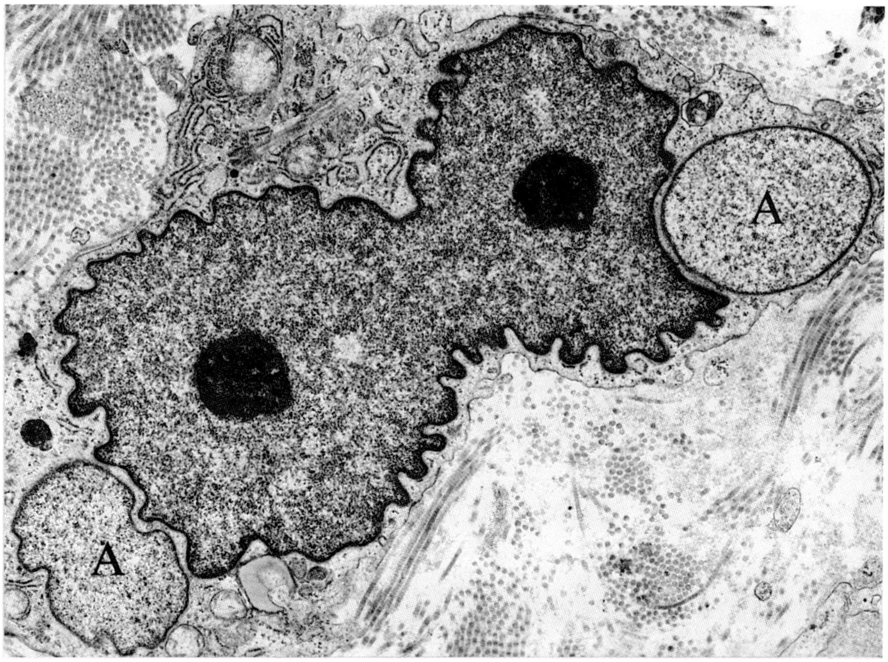

Fig. 4—A large fibroblast with two accessory nuclei (A) in a specimen taken from a 70-year-old woman 8 months after irradiation. ×8550

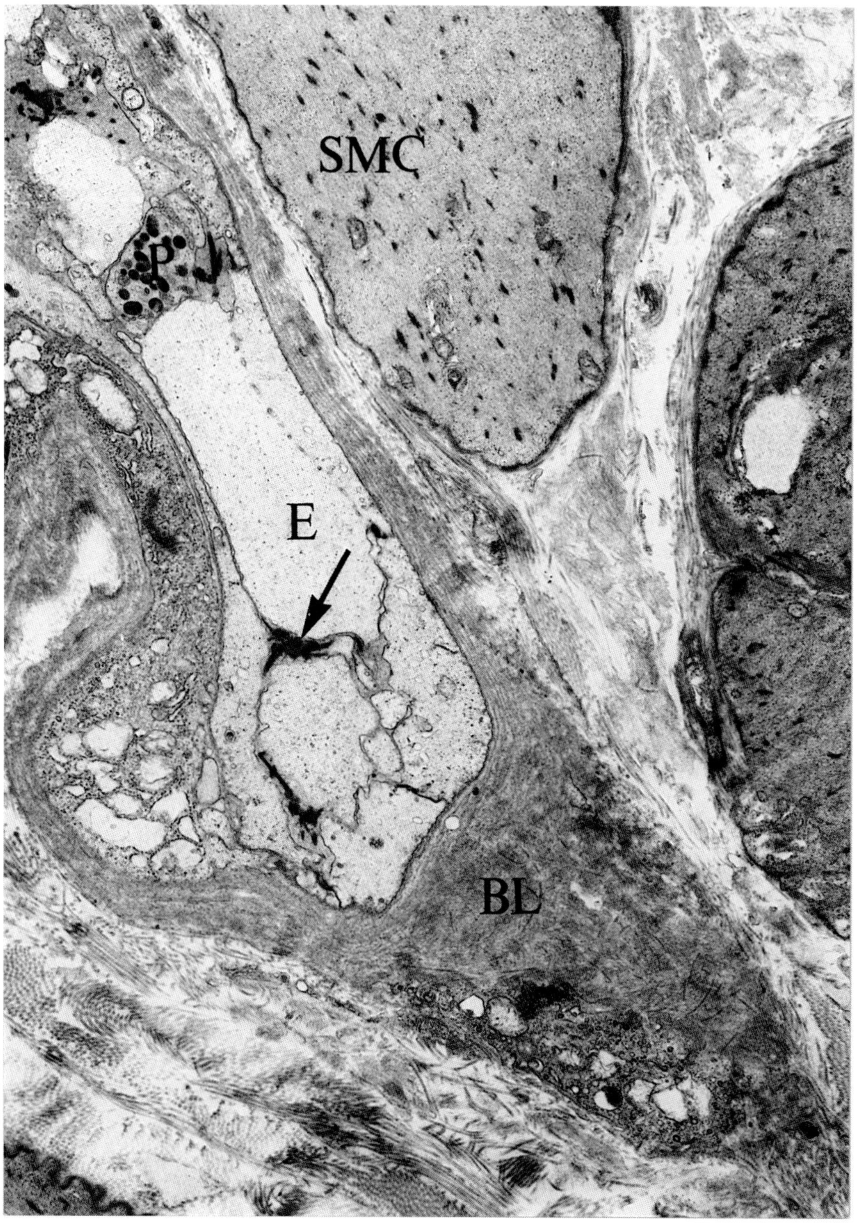

Fig. 5—A blood capillary in the muscular coat of a bladder biopsy from a 58-year-old man 16 months after the irradiation. The endothelial cells (E) are oedematous and swollen to the point where they almost obstruct the lumen. The presence of fibrin in the lumen (arrow) indicates intravascular coagulation. The basal lamina (BL) around the capillary is excessively thickened. P = platelet, SMC = smooth muscle cell. × 6500

but some fibroblasts were binucleated with the two nuclei occupying opposite poles of the cell. Some cells contained accessory nuclei which were round or oval in shape, surrounded by nuclear envelope, and contained finely dispersed chromatin whose pattern was different from the pattern of chromatin in the main nucleus (Fig. 4). In many instances nucleoli and nuclear bodies were found in these accessory nuclei. Such accessory nuclei, although closely adjacent to the main nucleus, were not seen to be in direct contact with it. In these irradiated tissues, accessory nuclei were also found in endothelial cells, pericytes, Schwann cells and occasionally in smooth muscle cells, but they were not observed in the urothelium.

Collagen was also abundant in these specimens in increasing amounts as the time after irradiation increased. This resulted in progressive fibrosis which was particularly prominent around the blood vessels, nerves and bundles of smooth muscle cells. Where there was bullous oedema, the bundles of collagen were separated by lakes of lightly-staining amorphous substance. Where necrosis had occurred, the bladder wall contained a mixture of inflammatory cells, predominantly polymorphonucleocytes and macrophages, cell debris, collagen fibres and a network of fibrin. In many biopsies, a few multinucleated macrophages with plentiful cytoplasmic organelles were observed in the lamina propria.

Changes to the blood vessels

In blood vessels, the endothelial cells were frequently oedematous and partially occluded the vessel lumen (Fig. 5). There appeared to be considerable reduplication of nuclear material in both endothelial cells and in pericytes, with deeply infolded nuclei, numerous binucleate or multinucleate cells and the presence of nuclear bodies and accessory nuclei (Fig. 6).

In some capillaries, the endothelial cells were completely destroyed by radiation to leave a denuded underlying basal lamina. Platelets adhered to the exposed basal lamina and intravascular coagulation was observed in some of these areas (Fig. 7). In addition, ghosts (plasmallemas) of erythrocytes were often found in the lumen of the capillaries.

The basal lamina of the endothelium, especially around capillaries, was frequently multilamellate. In the smooth muscle cells of the vascular wall the sarcoplasmic reticulum was often dilated and their basal laminae were thickened and fibrillar.

Post-irradiation damage to the muscular wall

In the normal bladder, the muscular wall is composed of a complex system of circular and longitudinally arranged detrusor muscles.[17] Each muscle consists of numerous bundles of smooth muscle cells separated by loose connective tissue. The individual muscle cells are closely apposed and form many nexuses and attachment plaques

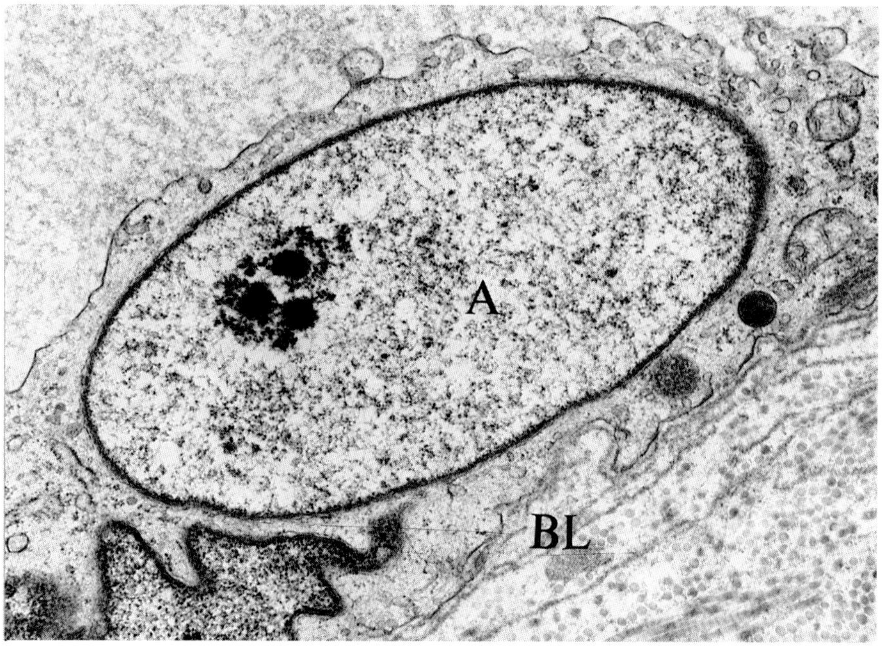

Fig. 6—Part of a capillary in the lamina propria of the same patient as Figs 4, 7, 9. The endothelial cell contains an accessory nucleus (A) with a nucleolus. The chromatin pattern in the accessory nucleus differs from that of the main nucleus. The basal lamina (BL) around this capillary is multilamellate. × 19 000

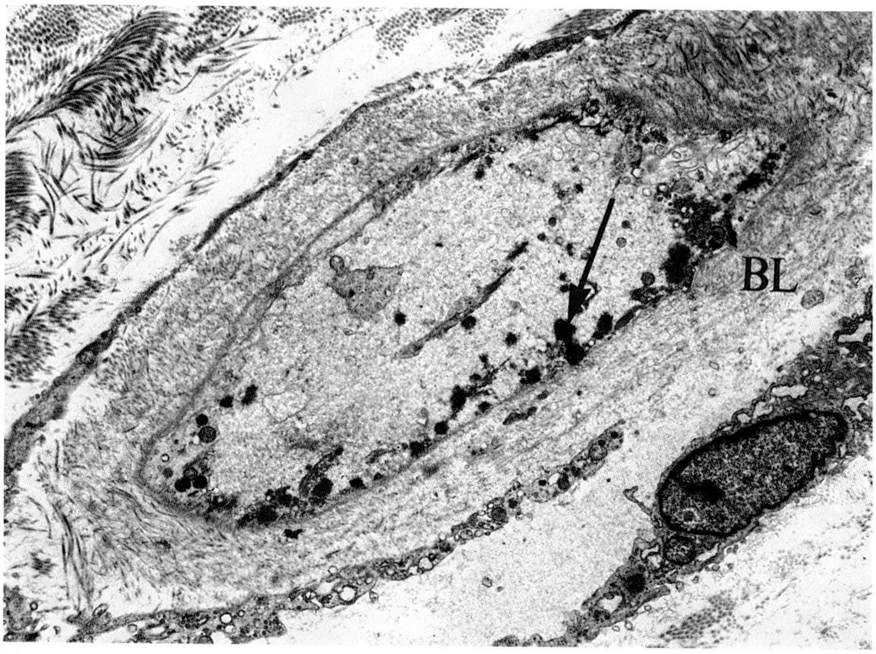

Fig. 7—An occluded capillary in the lamina propria of the same 70-year-old patient as Figs 4, 6, 9. All the endothelial cells have disappeared and fibrin adheres to the denuded basal lamina (arrow). The capillary lumen is filled with fibrin, cell debris and plasma and the basal lamina (BL) is both thick and fragmented. ×4275

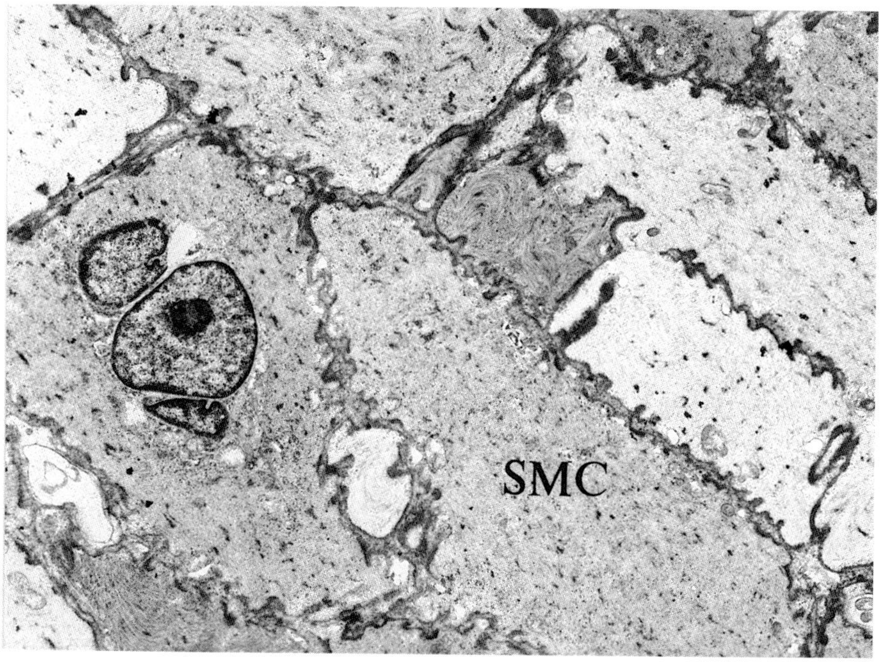

Fig. 8—The subcellular appearance of 'normal' muscle taken from a 69-year-old man, free of bladder symptoms, 2 years after a transurethral prostatectomy. The smooth muscle cells (SMC) contain abundant myofilaments and are closely apposed to each other. ×5320

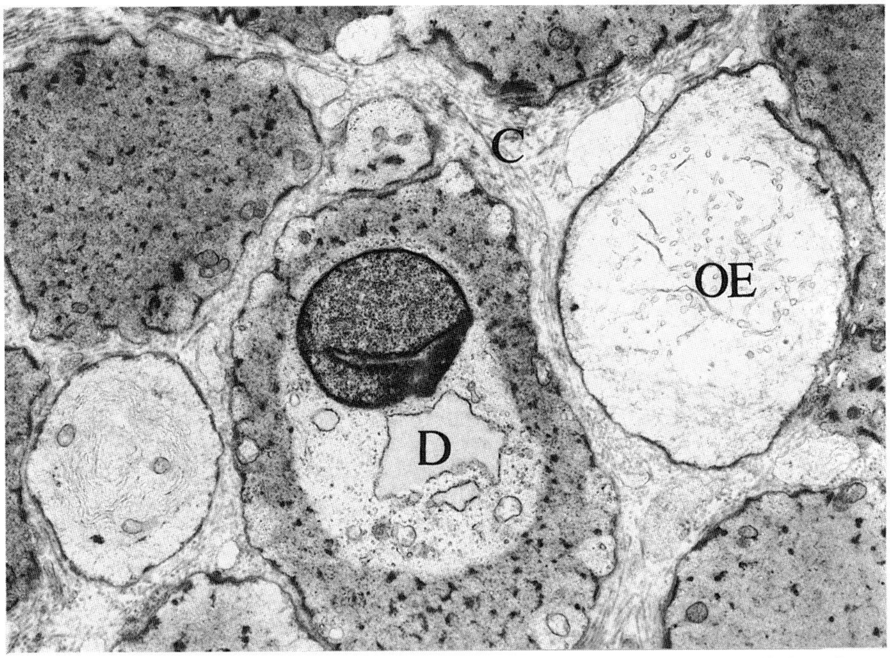

Fig. 9—Muscle in the bladder wall of a 70-year-old patient 8 months after irradiation. Some individual muscle cells are grossly oedematous (OE) and others contain distended cisternae of sarcoplasmic reticulum (D). Collagen fibres (C) separate the cells. ×6650

(Fig. 8) which facilitate co-ordinated contraction of the normal muscle. In irradiated specimens, even after the shortest time period examined, many smooth muscle cells were oedematous with widely separated myofibrils. After longer periods of time, increasing numbers of smooth muscle cells were found to be severely oedematous or degenerate (Figs 9, 10). Such damage was very local so that normal and oedematous cells were often adjacent. In many muscle cells, the nuclei were irregular in shape and some were deeply indented to form a deep groove filled with cytoplasmic organelles, parallel to the long axis of the cell. In a few cells the cytoplasm was packed with lysosomes (Fig. 11) while in many others, blebs of sarcoplasm containing glycogen granules and sarcoplasmic reticulum protruded into the extracellular space through gaps in the basal lamina (Fig. 12). Macrophages were observed both engulfing such blebs and also within the muscular coat having phagocytosed dead smooth muscle cells.

Some years after irradiation, individual surviving smooth muscle cells appeared morphologically near normal, but by contrast, the fibrosis of the muscular coat was more marked (Fig. 13).

Mitoses in the smooth muscle cells of the muscular coat were never observed but very occasionally mitoses were observed in smooth muscle cells of the vascular wall.

Damage to nervous tissue

In post-irradiation biopsies, some damage was also seen in the nerve cells in the bladder wall. Many Schwann cells contained lysosomes and lipofuscin granules and the number of these granules increased with time post-irradiation. The basal laminae of the Schwann cells were fuzzy and thickened. Some of the unmyelinated neuraxones looked oedematous. Collagen deposition both within and around nerve fibre bundles appeared to increase with time post-irradiation.

DISCUSSION

Despite numerous clinical reports of complications arising in the bladder following irradiation of the pelvis, the urinary bladder is generally regarded as a relatively radio-resistant organ.[1] This is largely because most pathological sequelae develop many years after irradiation, whereas in

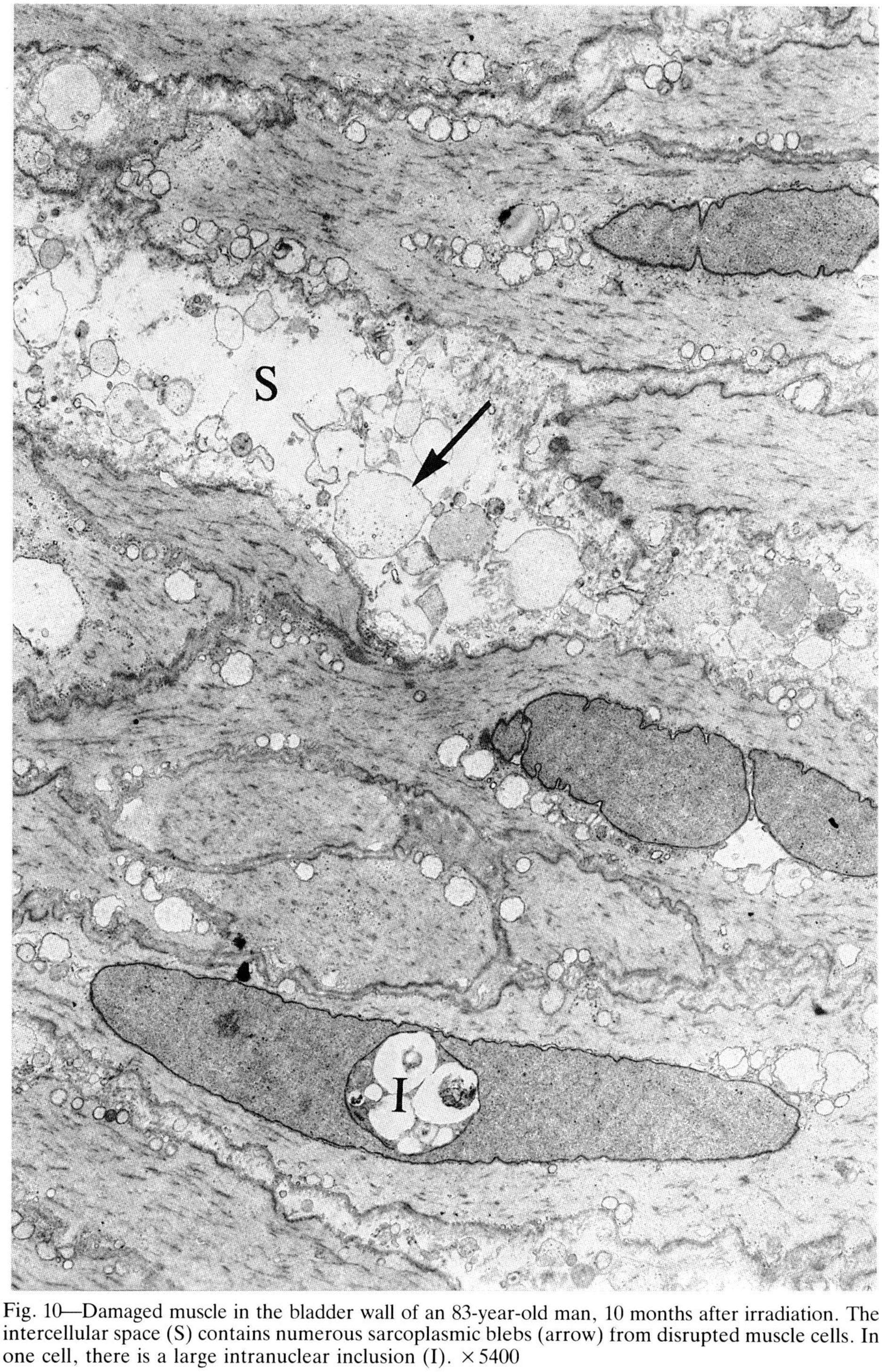

Fig. 10—Damaged muscle in the bladder wall of an 83-year-old man, 10 months after irradiation. The intercellular space (S) contains numerous sarcoplasmic blebs (arrow) from disrupted muscle cells. In one cell, there is a large intranuclear inclusion (I). ×5400

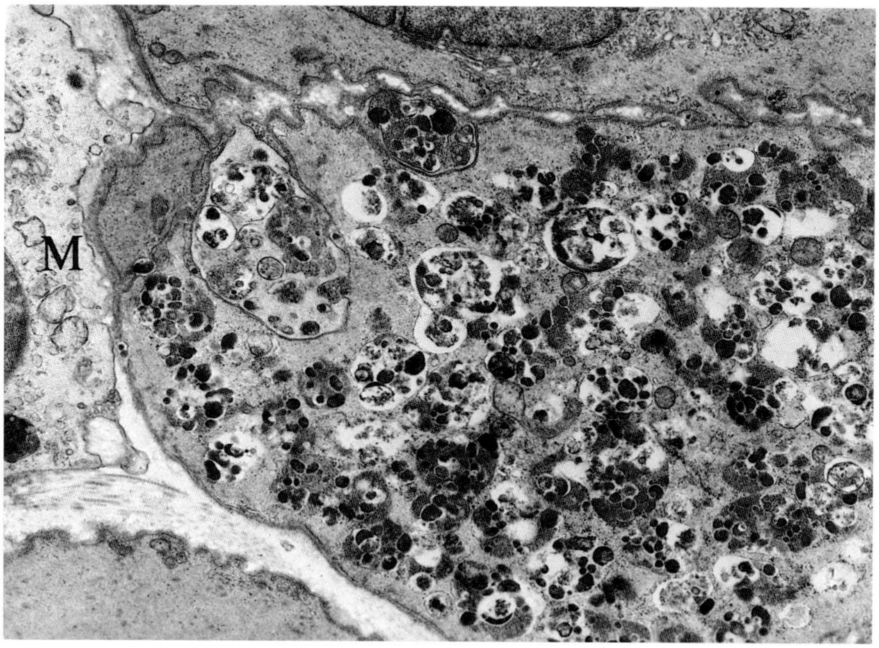

Fig. 11—A muscle cell filled with phagosomes and large lysosomes in the bladder wall of a 75-year-old woman, 22 months after irradiation. Adjacent to the damaged muscle cell is a macrophage (M). ×8170

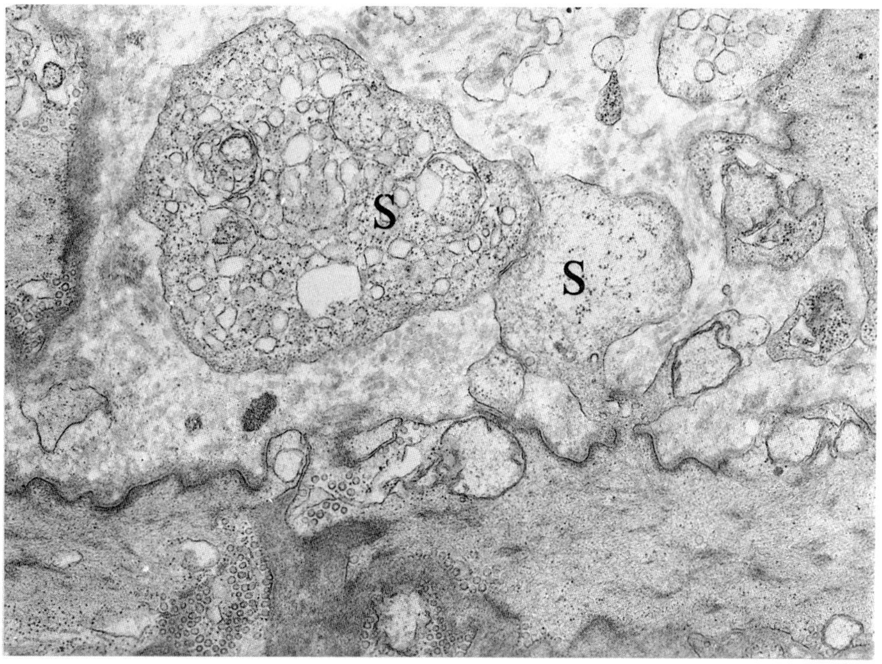

Fig. 12—An area of muscle in the bladder wall of an 83-year-old man, 10 months after irradiation. Sarcoplasmic blebs (S) rich in sarcoplasmic reticulum protrude from a damaged muscle cell through the basal lamina into the intercellular space. ×14 250

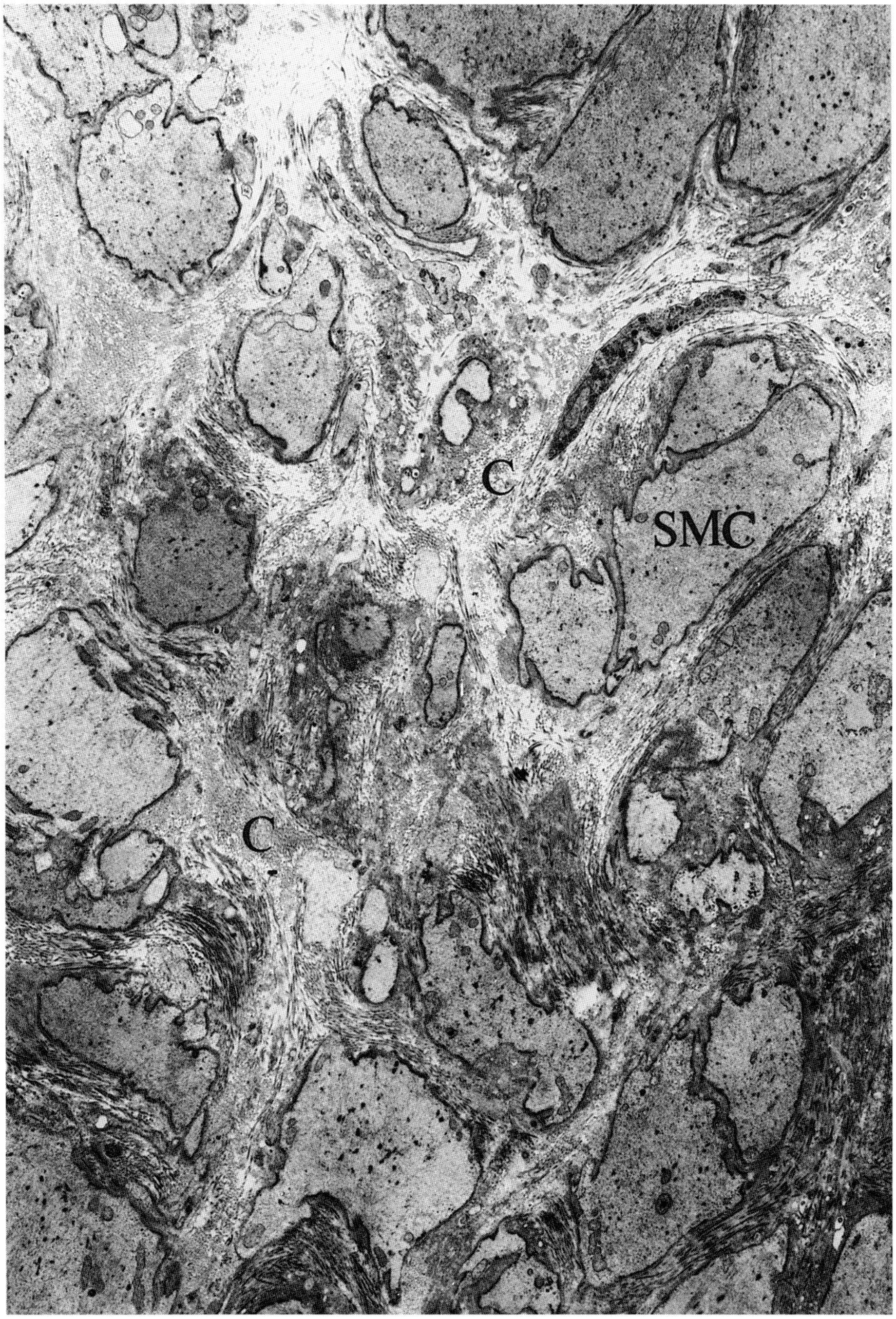

Fig. 13—Severe fibrosis of muscle in the bladder wall of a 59-year-old man, 9 years after irradiation. The smooth muscle cells (SMC) are distorted and widely separated by deposits of collagen fibres (C). ×5000

the immediate post-treatment stage, relatively little functional damage is usually experienced by the patient.

The apparent early resistance of the urothelium to radiation has been attributed to the low turnover rate and very long life-span of the urothelial cells.[18,19] However, the subcellular structure is undoubtedly damaged by radiation as is demonstrated in the current study by the rapid development of large numbers of autophagic lysosomes in all cell layers in the urothelium. This observation parallels reports of increased numbers of lysosomes in other irradiated epithelia.[20] The intracellular cysts seen in a few urothelial cells in biopsies from irradiated bladders are not necessarily a sign of irradiation damage for we have observed them also in normal unirradiated human bladder biopsies maintained in organ culture. The nature of the membrane limiting the space within these cysts varies from normal luminal-type membrane to membrane more characteristic of that seen on the luminal face of pre-neoplastic urothelia. The thickening and layering of the basal lamina in these specimens was probably also the result of radiation damage (*cf.* the perivascular changes) for, although it is common in invasive urothelial carcinoma, it is usually a late-developing phenomenon and not associated with pre-neoplastic change.

In common with other irradiated organs[5,8,10,21] bizarre fibroblasts were a prominent and persistent feature of the irradiated bladders; these have been referred to in other tissues as 'irradiation fibroblasts' or 'giant fibroblasts'. The current study has shown these fibroblasts to be characterized by increased amounts of both cytoplasm and nuclear material and both binucleate cells and cells with accessory nuclei were common. Staining patterns indicated that the overall amount of both condensed and dispersed chromatin was increased in these irradiated fibroblasts by contrast with normal tissue. There was a parallel and sustained increase in the amounts of collagen deposited in the bladder wall, consistent with the observed progressive development of post-irradiation fibrosis.

Fibrosis was not confined to the sub-epithelial lamina propria, but occurred throughout the bladder wall. Thus perivascular fibrosis was seen at all levels and in addition, collagen deposits between bundles of smooth muscle cells caused disruption and fibrosis within the muscular coats. It has been reported previously that irradiation increases the histohaematic barrier in the bladder wall.[10,22] The observed perivascular fibrosis, thickened and multi-layered basal laminae around blood vessels and endothelial damage must all contribute to this phenomenon. In particular, the irradiation-induced oedema of endothelial cells observed here will lead to partial obstruction and reduced oxygenation of the bladder tissues, as has been reported elsewhere in other irradiated organs.[23–25] Where coagulation occurs with complete arrest of the circulation (see Fig. 7), local ischaemia and necrosis are inevitable consequences.

Later complications of irradiating the urinary bladder include uncoordinated micturition and spasm of the muscles in the bladder wall.[26] The sporadic loss of muscle cells observed here is consistent with the clinical findings, for the gaps must inevitably lead to interruption and disruption of the uniform spread of contraction in the various parts of the detrusor muscle. There was no evidence of cell division, nor regeneration in the muscular layers of the bladder wall, and the damage was progressive with time. Muscle cell death is probably attributable both to the direct effects of radiation on the cells and also to ischaemia following vascular damage for perivascular smooth muscle cells, which were presumably better oxygenated, were much less affected than muscle cells deep in the bladder wall at some distance from blood vessels.

This study confirms previous histological observations on the irradiated human bladder and enables clinical findings to be interpreted in terms of subcellular damage to the various tissues in the bladder wall. It indicates that primary damage to the endothelial cells of the blood vessels leads to stasis and ischaemia, that permanent alteration and stimulation of fibroblasts is the underlying cause of the fibrosis and that there is damage and loss of individual muscle cells. These factors are all important in initiating the progressive deterioration of bladder function in the years following irradiation.

ACKNOWLEDGEMENTS

We are grateful to the Republic of Greece for supporting Dr G. Antonakopoulos through their State Scholarship Foundation. We also wish to thank Mr R. Wright for technical assistance. This study formed part of a more extensive research programme into the effects of radiation on the human and rodent bladder which is reported in the Ph.D. thesis of Dr Antonakopoulos, lodged with the University of London.

REFERENCES

1. Strickland P. Radiotherapy. Complications of radiotherapy. *Br J Hosp Med* 1980; **23:** 552–565.
2. Dean AL. Ulceration of the urinary bladder as a late effect of radium applications to uterus. *JAMA* 1927; **89:** 1121–1124.
3. Dean AL. Injury of the urinary bladder following irradiation of the uterus. *J Urol* **29:** 559–570.
4. Watson EM, Herger CC, Sauer HR. Irradiation reactions in the bladder: their occurrence and clinical course following the use of X-ray and radium in the treatment of female pelvic disease. *J Urol* 1947; **57:** 1038–1053.
5. Friedman NB, Ash JE. Tumors of the urinary bladder. Atlas of Tumor Pathology, Section VIII—Fascicle 31a. Washington DC: Armed Forces Institute of Pathology, 1959.
6. Bloom HJG. Treatment of carcinoma of the bladder. *Br J Radiol* 1960; **33:** 471–490.
7. Cox R. Treatment of Carcinoma of the Bladder: A Symposium. II. Treatment by 2 MeV X-Rays. A contribution to the symposium on 'Treatment of Carcinoma of the Bladder' at the British Institute of Radiology, 14 Jan. 1960. *Br J Radiol* 1960; **33:** 480–483.
8. Gowing NFC. III. Pathological changes in the bladder following irradiation. *Br J Radiol* 1960; **33:** 484–487.
9. Mallik BMK. Study of radiation necrosis of the urinary bladder following treatment of carcinoma of the cervix. *Am J Obst Gynec* 1962; **83:** 393–400.
10. Rubin P, Casarett GW. Clinical Radiation Pathology, Vol. 1. Philadelphia: W. B. Saunders Company, 1968.
11. Ram MD. Complications of radiotherapy for carcinoma of the bladder. *Proc Roy Soc Med* 1970; **63:** 93–95.
12. Rosen VJ. Radiation pathology of the genitourinary tract. In: Berdjis CC, ed. Pathology of Irradiation. Baltimore: The Williams and Wilkins Company, 1971: 592–596.
13. Maier J. Effects of radiations on kidney, bladder and prostate. In: Vaeth JM, ed. Frontiers of Radiation Therapy and Oncology, Vol. 6, Radiation Effect and Tolerance. Normal Tissue. Basic Concepts in Radiation Pathology. Proceedings of the Sixth Annual San Francisco Cancer Symposium, San Francisco, California. Basel: S. Karger, 1972: 196–227.
14. Loveless KJ. Effects of radiation upon cytology of benign and malignant bladder epithelia. *Acta Cytol* 1973; **17:** 355–360.
15. Duncan RE, Bennett DW, Evans AT, Aron BS, Schellhas HF. Radiation induced bladder tumors. *J Urol* 1977; **118:** 43–45.
16. Antonakopoulos GN, Hicks RM, Hamilton E, Berry RJ. Early and late morphological changes (including carcinoma of the urothelium) induced by irradiation of the rat urinary bladder. *Br J Cancer* 1982; **46:** 403–416.
17. Hutch JA. Anatomy and Physiology of the Bladder, Trigone and Urethra. London: Butterworths, New York: Meredith Corporation, 1972.
18. Schreiber H, Oehlert W, Kugler K. Regeneration und proliferationkinetik der normalen und strahlengeschädigten Urothels der Ratte. *Virchow's Arch B Cell Path* 1969; **4:** 30–34.
19. Stewart FA, Denekamp J, Hirst DG. Proliferation of the mouse bladder after irradiation. *Cell Tissue Kinet* 1980; **13:** 75–89.
20. Toner PG, Carr KE. Cell Structure. An Introduction to Biological Electron Microscopy. Edinburgh and London: Livingstone, 1968.
21. Koss LG. Tumors of the urinary bladder. Atlas of Tumor Pathology, Second Series, Fascicle 11. Washington DC: Armed Forces Institute of Pathology, 1975.
22. Casarett GW. Similarities and contrasts between radiation and time pathology. *Adv Gerontol Res* 1964; **1:** 109–163.
23. Robbins SL. Pathologic Basis of Disease. Philadelphia, London, Toronto: W.B. Saunders Company, 1974.
24. Hopewell JW. The late vascular effects of radiation. *Br J Radiol* 1977; **47:** 157–158.
25. Stearner SP, Devine RL, Christian EJB. Late changes in the irradiated microvasculature: an electron microscope study of the effects of fission neutrons. *Radiation Research* 1976; **65:** 351–370.
26. Michailov MCh, Elsäber E, Welscher UE. Immediate mechanical reactions of isolated human detrusor muscle on X-irradiation. *Strahlentherapie* 1979; **155:** 284–286.

JOURNAL OF PATHOLOGY, VOL. **143:** 117–125 (1984)

PATHWAYS OF CELLULAR EFFLUX AND PARTICULATE CLEARANCE AFTER CARBON INSTILLATION TO THE LUNG*

D. H. BOWDEN AND I. Y. R. ADAMSON

Pathology Department, University of Manitoba, Winnipeg, Canada

Received 27 January 1984
Accepted 13 February 1984

SUMMARY

The pulmonary response to the deposition of carbon particles was investigated to determine the routes of cellular efflux and the mechanisms of particulate clearance. At intervals to 6 months after the intratracheal instillation of 4 mg carbon, the lungs of mice were fixed *in situ* by perfusion without lavage. Within a few hours, migration of granulocytes into the bronchioles was observed; large numbers of PMNs were not seen in alveoli until 24 h. Associated with the PMN efflux there was transient oedema with no evidence of pulmonary cell necrosis. The number of free macrophages increased in response to the carbon and mononuclear cell migration into alveoli and bronchioles was also observed. The bronchiolar component of the cellular efflux indicates that PMNs and macrophages recovered from the lung by lavage are not entirely of alveolar origin. Whereas most particles, either free or in phagocytic cells, were cleared by the bronchial tree, some transepithelial passage of free particles to the interstitium was observed. Some carbon was found in hilar lymph nodes but overall lymphatic clearance was low.

KEY WORDS—Lung clearance, alveolar macrophages, bronchiolar clearance.

INTRODUCTION

Deposition of small particles in the lung results in a rapid exudate of polymorphonuclear cells (PMN) followed by an increase in free alveolar macrophages. In studies where this inflammatory response has been examined[1–3] or the cytokinetics of the macrophagic system determined,[4,5] the lungs have been lavaged to recover the free cells. Using this procedure it has not been possible to determine if the cellular efflux is totally alveolar or whether there is a transbronchiolar component to the inflammatory reaction. This question is addressed in the present morphologic study, in which lungs are fixed by perfusion to examine serially the routes of cellular migration to the air spaces after the administration of carbon particles. This method leaves undisturbed the free carbon and alveolar cells so that particulate localization, transport to the interstitium and lymph nodes, and sites of long term particle retention in the lung can be studied.

MATERIALS AND METHODS

Four milligrams of colloidal carbon (0·03 μm in diameter) in 0·1 ml sterile water was instilled by intratracheal injection into 60 Swiss Webster mice under mild pentobarbital anaesthesia. Groups of three animals were killed at hours 3 and 7, at days 1, 2, 3, 5, 7, 10, 14, 21 and 28 then at monthly intervals to 6 months.

At sacrifice the chest was opened prior to fixing the lungs by vascular perfusion. A small hole was cut in one side of the heart while 10 ml of 2 per cent buffered glutaraldehyde was injected slowly into the other side. This procedure flushed out the vasculature and filled the pulmonary vessels with fixative, leaving air spaces undisturbed. The lungs were tied off, removed and immersed in fixative for 1 h. Slices were then cut and fixed for a further

* This research was supported by the Medical Research Council of Canada.

Addressee for correspondence: Dr D. H. Bowden, Pathology Department, 770 Bannatyne Avenue, Winnipeg, Manitoba, Canada R3E 0W3.

0022–3417/84/060117–09$01.00

hour in glutaraldehyde. At least four random slices per animal were post-fixed in formalin, dehydrated and embedded in glycol methacrylate. Sections (1μm) were cut and stained by haematoxylin and eosin. Random pieces of the remaining lung were post fixed in osmic acid, dehydrated and embedded in Spurr plastic for electron microscopy.

Two hilar lymph nodes were also removed from each animal; these were fixed and embedded for electron microscopy.

RESULTS

Animals killed 3 h after the injection of carbon exhibit uniformly black lungs and, by light microscopy, the carbon is observed as a thin, black lining to the airways and air sacs (Fig. 1). No bronchial or alveolar cellular exudates are observed at this time, but a few polymorphonuclear granulocytes (PMN) are seen in perivascular and peribronchiolar spaces. At 7 h there are very few PMNs within the alveoli whereas many are seen in the peribronchial interstitium and some granulocytes are observed between bronchiolar epithelial cells (Figs 2, 3). In some areas the surface of the bronchial epithelium is covered by a mixture of PMNs and free carbon particles (Fig. 4). By 24 h the bronchial-derived cells are supplemented by a PMN response in the alveoli. These cells are seen in capillary walls and free in the alveolar lumen (Fig. 5). The PMN response, maximal between 2 and 3 days, is accompanied by focal intraalveolar oedema (Fig. 6). The accumulated fluid disappears from the lungs by 5 days. No ultrastructural evidence of cell necrosis is seen in endothelial or epithelial cells in the lung at any stage of the study.

Phagocytosis of carbon is accomplished by PMNs and by free alveolar macrophages which increase in number by 24 h. As previously shown, the macrophages are derived from blood monocytes and from a population of interstitial cells.[4,5]

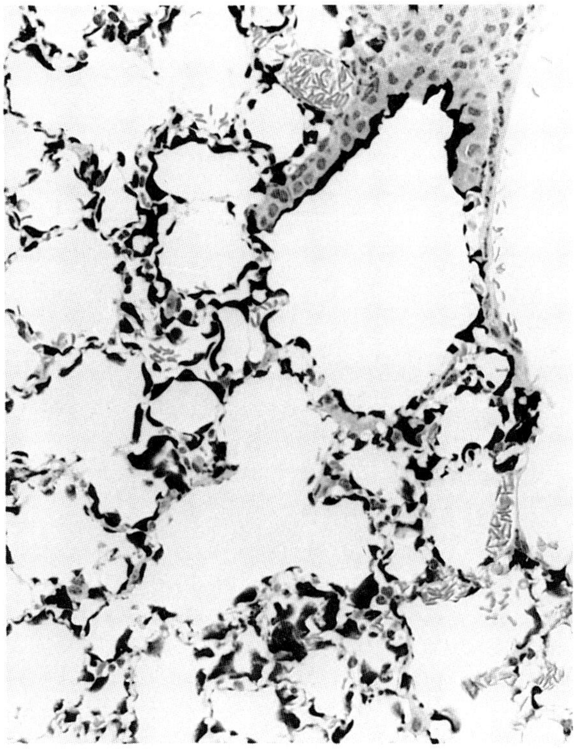

Fig. 1—Three hours after carbon deposition, the distribution of particles is uniform over the epithelial surface of the lung. Haematoxylin and eosin (H & E) stain, ×270

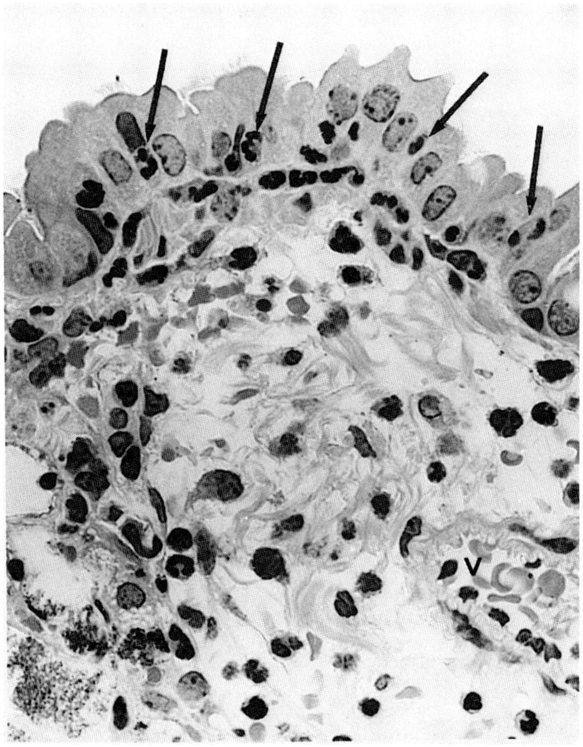

Fig. 2—Seven hours after carbon deposition, PMNs are seen around a large vessel (V), and between bronchiolar epithelial cells (arrows). H & E, ×810

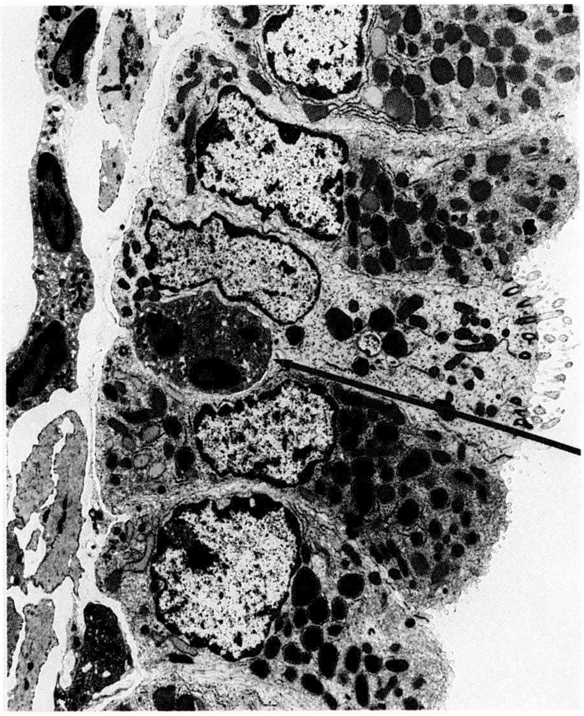

Fig. 3—PMN (arrow) is seen between bronchiolar epithelial cells. EM, ×4410

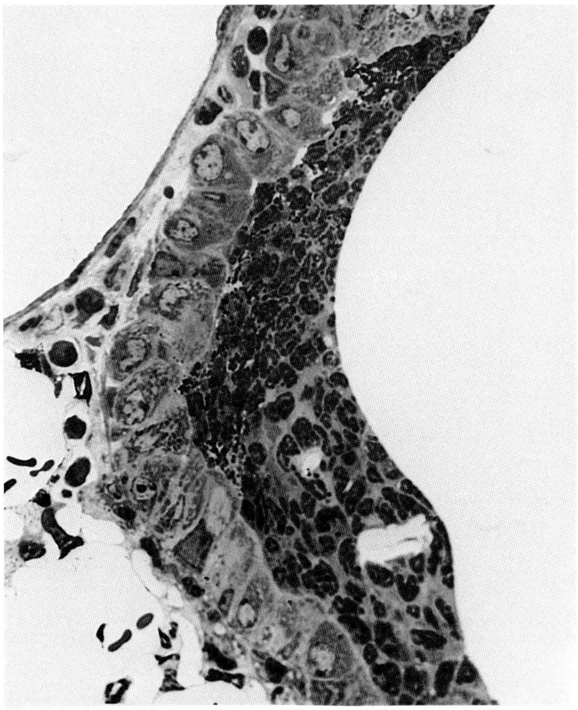

Fig. 4—Mixture of PMNs and carbon particles covers the bronchiolar surface, 7 h after carbon deposition. H & E, ×765

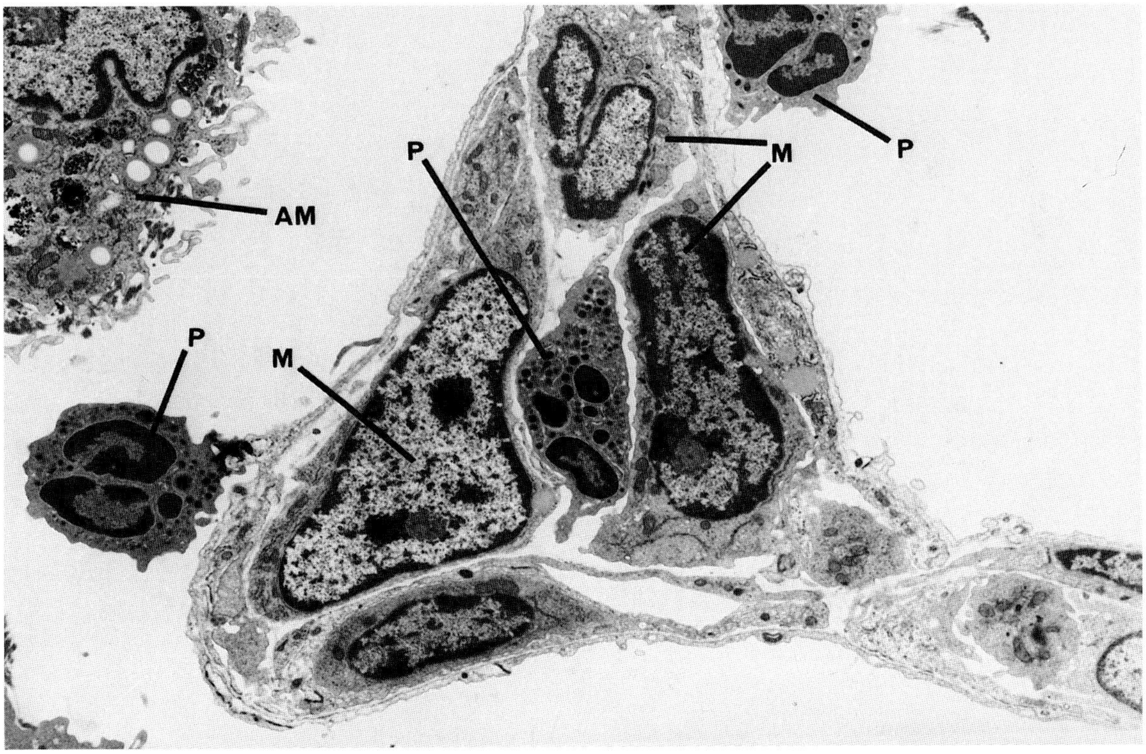

Fig. 5—One day after carbon deposition, PMNs (P) are seen in the alveolar interstitium and free in the alveoli; several mononuclear cells (M) in the alveolar wall and an alveolar macrophage (AM) with carbon are also shown. EM, ×5400

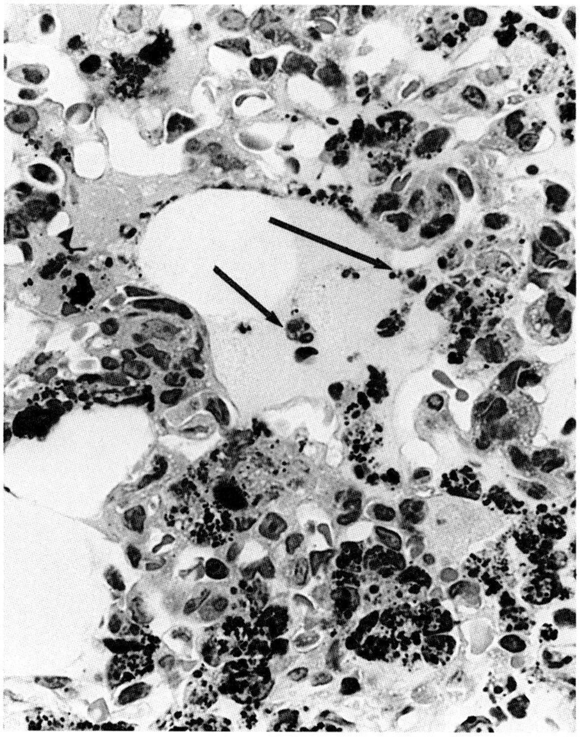

Fig. 6—Two days after carbon deposition, some alveoli contain oedema fluid and PMNs (arrows). H & E, ×720

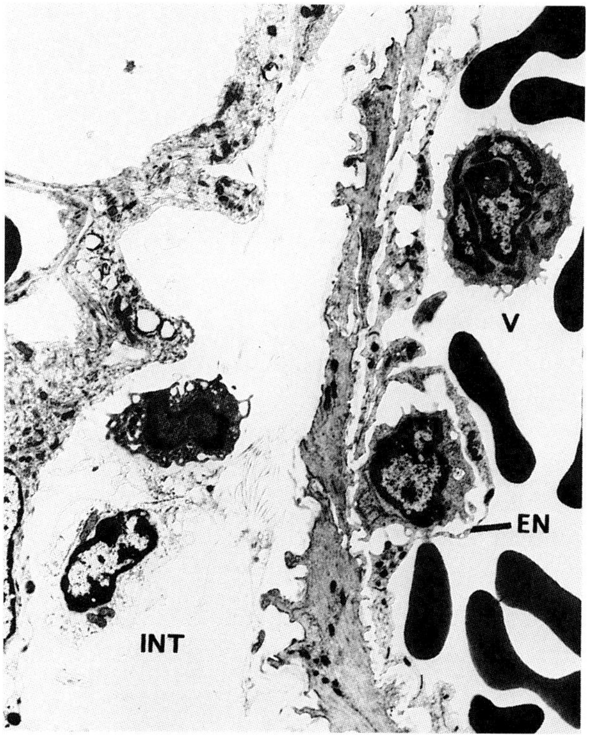

Fig. 8—Mononuclear cells in vascular lumen (V), beneath the endothelium (EN) and in the interstitium (INT). EM, ×4410

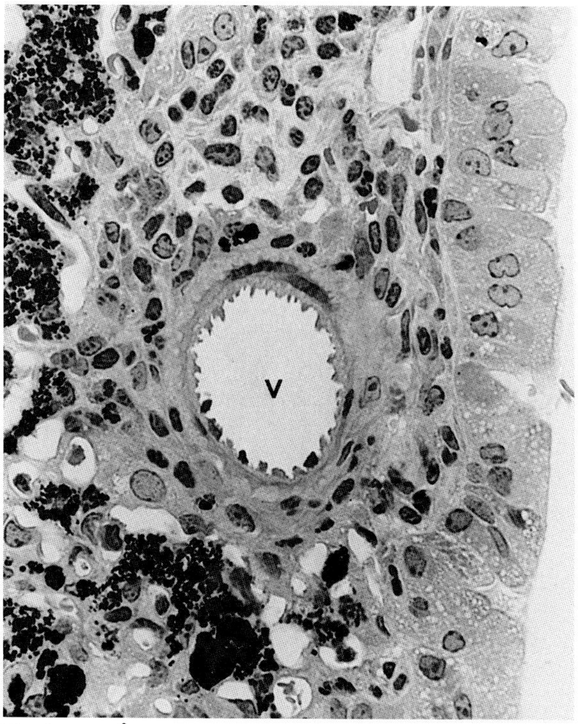

Fig. 7—Two days after carbon deposition, there is an increase in mononuclear cells in the interstitium surrounding a blood vessel (V). H & E, ×720

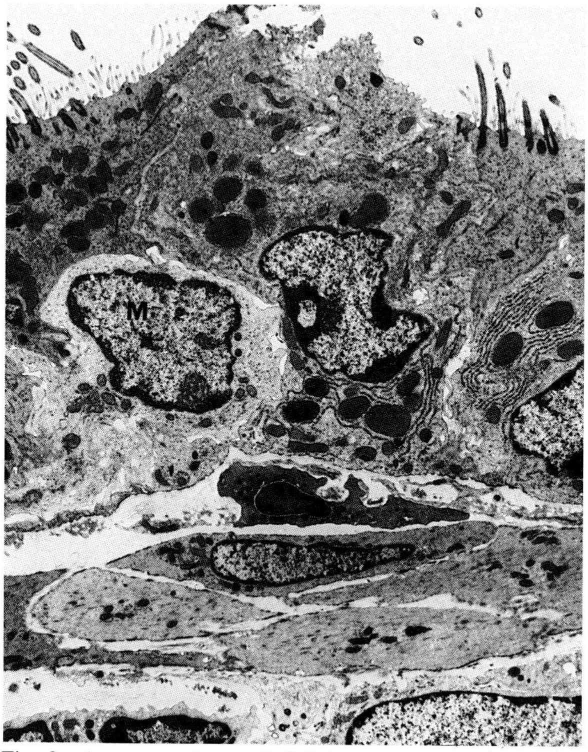

Fig. 9—A mononuclear cell (M) is seen apparently passing between bronchiolar epithelial cells. EM, ×4950

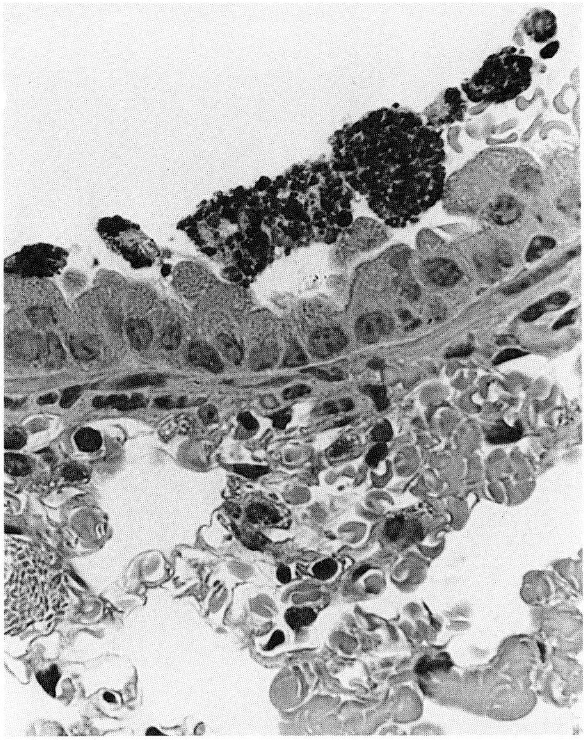

Fig. 10—Five days after carbon deposition, many carbon-laden macrophages are seen on the bronchial surface. H & E, ×765

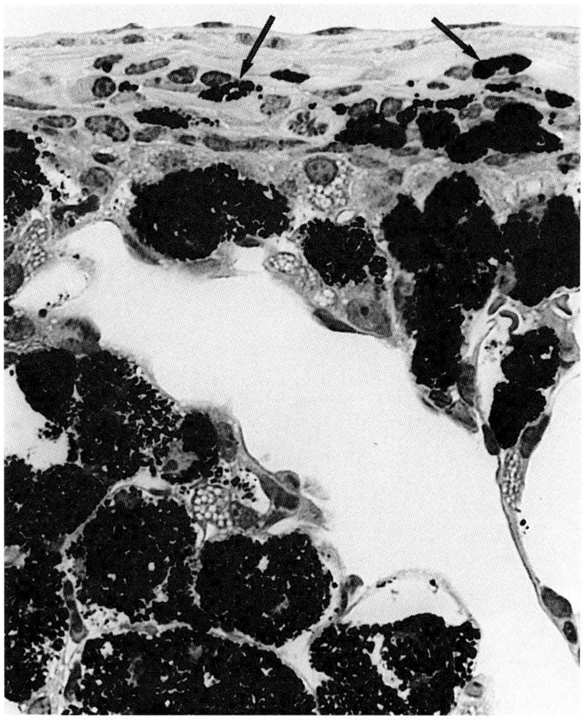

Fig. 12—Six weeks after carbon deposition, many large carbon-laden macrophages are seen in peribronchial alveoli. Smaller amounts of carbon are also seen in perivascular interstitial cells (arrows). H & E, ×810

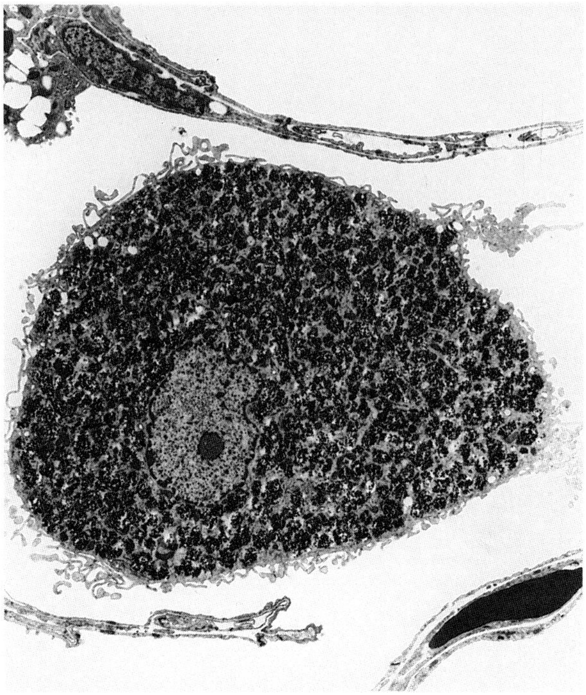

Fig. 11—Six weeks after carbon deposition, an alveolus is almost filled by a 40 μm diameter macrophage loaded with carbon. EM, ×4410

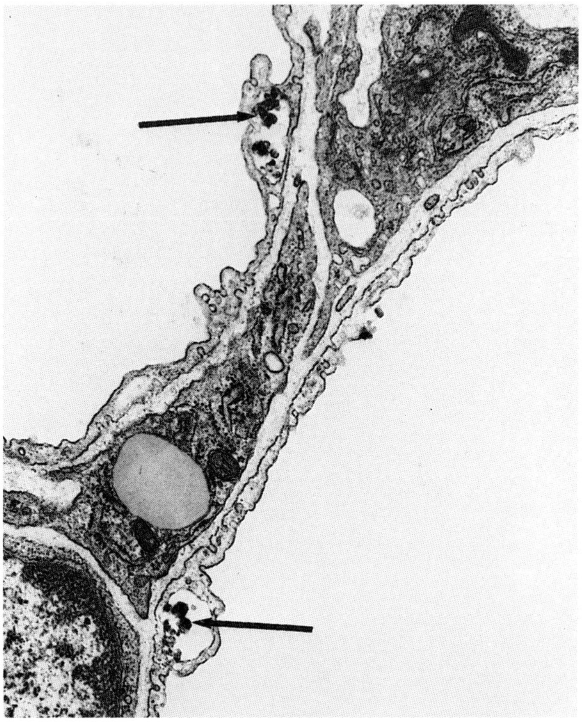

Fig. 13—Carbon particles (arrows) are seen in the cytoplasm of type 1 epithelial cells at 1 day. EM, ×22 500

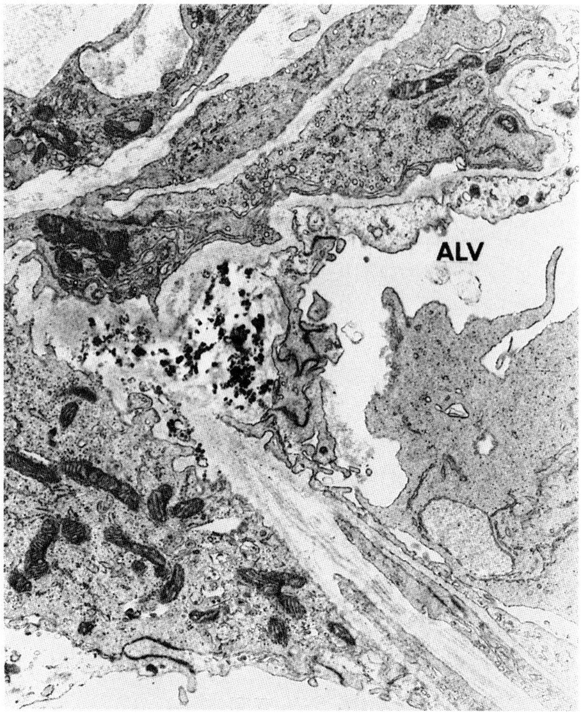

Fig. 14—Free carbon particles are seen in the interstitium at 1 day. ALV—alveolus. EM, ×12 600

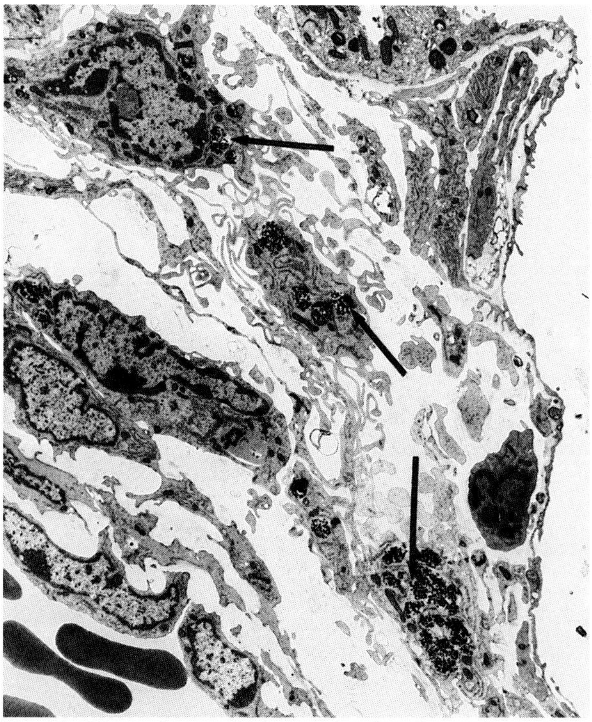

Fig. 15—Macrophages with ingested carbon (arrows) are shown in the perivascular interstitium at 3 days. EM, ×4410

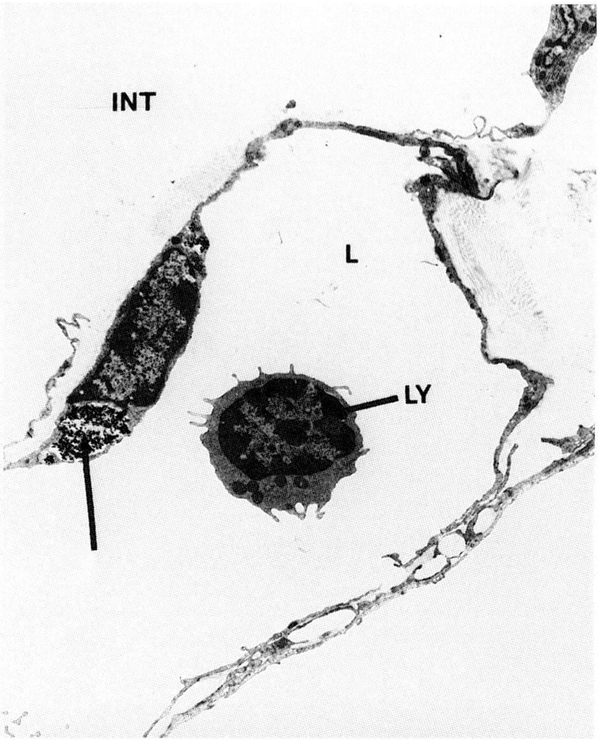

Fig. 16—One day after carbon deposition, particles (arrows) are seen in the cytoplasm of an endothelial cell lining a lymphatic (L) in the bronchial wall. INT—interstitium; LY—lymphocyte. EM, ×4410

At 1 day, blood vessels are packed with monocytes and, from 2–3 days, an increase in mononuclear interstitial cells is observed in alveolar walls (Fig. 5) and in peribronchial and perivascular areas (Fig. 7). Mononuclear cells are frequently seen, presumably in transit, crossing the vascular endothelium (Fig. 8) and bronchiolar epithelium (Fig. 9). From 3 days onward, the number of PMNs decreases as particulate clearance from the alveoli is predominantly accomplished by macrophages (Fig. 10).

Whereas the majority of macrophages are cleared via the bronchial tree, some heavily laden cells, often larger than 40 μm diameter, appear to linger for many weeks or even months in the air sacs (Fig. 11). The majority of these cells are clustered in alveoli adjacent to blood vessels and bronchioles (Fig. 12). Re-entry of these cells into the interstitium has not been seen.

Phagocytosis and bronchial clearance are not the only routes for the removal of carbon from the lung. Free particles are seen within the cytoplasm

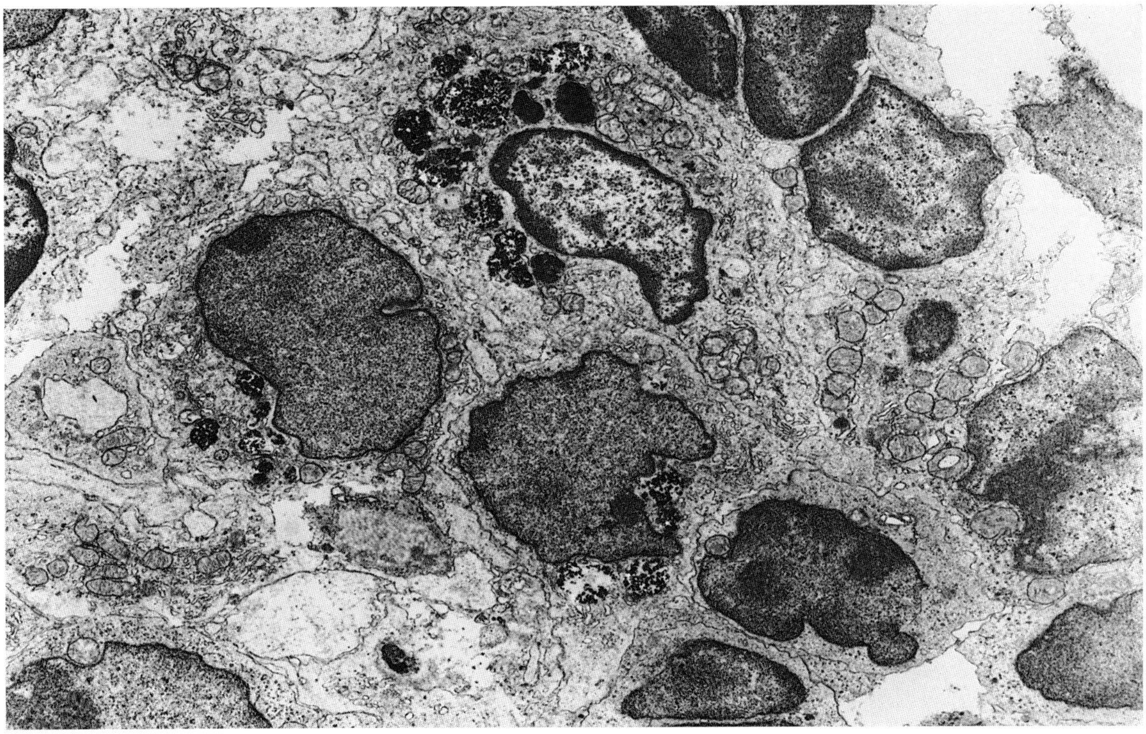

Fig. 17—Two days after carbon deposition, a few carbon particles are seen in macrophages of a hilar lymph node. EM, × 6300

of type 1 epithelial cells at 24 h (Fig. 13) then free within the interstitial tissue (Fig. 14). Subsequently, interstitial carbon is phagocytosed by macrophages located predominantly in peribronchial and perivascular connective tissue (Figs 12 and 15) where some particle-laden cells are found up to 6 months.

Some of the carbon that reaches the pulmonary interstitium is cleared by the lymphatics. A few free carbon particles are seen within the cytoplasm of bronchial lymphatic endothelial cells within 24 h of the instillation (Fig. 16). Thereafter carbon is found by electron microscopy in macrophages of the hilar lymph node at 2 days and by light microscopy after several weeks (Figs 17, 18). Although the hilar lymph nodes appear grey on gross examination by 4 weeks, the amount of carbon seen in sections suggests that the lymphatic system is not the major clearance route for inhaled particles.

At 6 months the lungs appear free of carbon by gross examination; by microscopy focal accumulations of carbon are limited to peribronchial areas and lymph nodes. No evidence of fibrosis or of alveolar dilatation or destruction is observed.

DISCUSSION

Administration of particles by the intratracheal route is a convenient method of studying serial cellular responses in the lung since a known dose can be administered at one time. The distribution of carbon is uniform over the whole lung and particles are deposited in both bronchiolar and alveolar regions. Deposition and clearance of particles injected intratracheally is generally similar to that seen following inhalation of a carbon suspension[6] and the pattern of sequential recruitment of cells and clearance corresponds to that described for the handling of bacteria instilled into the trachea.[7] In previous studies using bronchoalveolar lavage, we have shown that the magnitude of the cellular response to carbon is dose related[8] but, as Brain[1] has suggested, the system may have a saturation point.

The initial cellular response to carbon instillation is granulocytic; large numbers of PMNs and free particles are observed on the bronchial surface at a time when very few PMNs are seen in the alveoli. It is usually assumed that PMNs seen on the bronchial surface or obtained by bron-

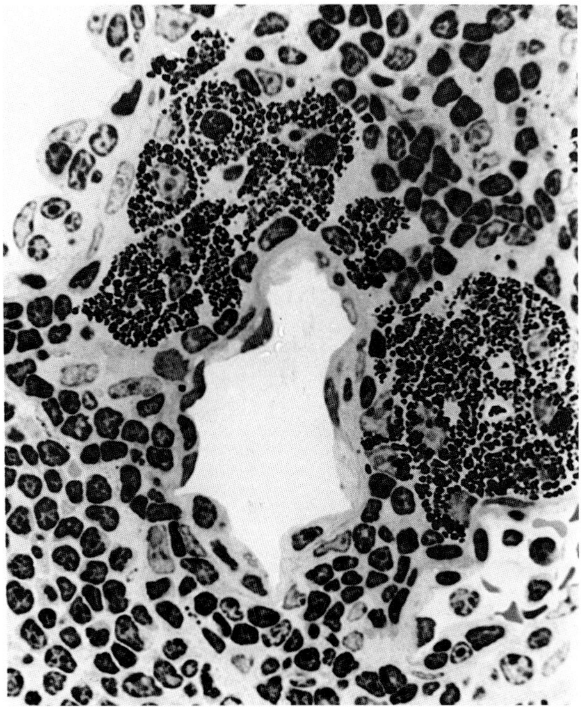

Fig. 18—Eight weeks after carbon deposition, some carbon-laden macrophages are found in a hilar lymph node. Toluidine blue, ×765

choalveolar lavage are alveolar in origin. However, the present observations made on cellular distribution *in situ* suggest that the initial efflux of PMNs occurs directly into the bronchioles. Cells are seen marginating in larger vessels, within the perivascular and peribronchiolar interstitium and passing between the bronchiolar epithelial cells, several hours before PMNs cross the alveolar walls.

The peak of the PMN response, as measured by bronchoalveolar lavage, occurs between 1 and 2 days, then the number of PMNs falls rapidly.[4] In the present experiment in which the inflammatory exudate is undisturbed, the PMN response at 2 and 3 days is accompanied by focal intraalveolar oedema; the oedema and granulocytes disappear by 5 days. The temporal relationship between the presence of PMNs and oedema is the usual inflammatory response associated with the release of toxic products from the neutrophils.[9,10] Some recent studies have indicated that PMN-derived products, such as oxygen free radicals, may destroy alveolar lining cells;[9,11] however, in this study, no evidence of endothelial or epithelial necrosis was found. Furthermore, cytokinetic studies following the instillation of carbon showed no change in DNA synthesis by endothelial or epithelial cells[4] as would be expected if cellular regeneration following injury was underway. Therefore, in spite of a massive PMN outpouring, changes to cells in the alveolar wall are minimal and are confined to increased vascular permeability resulting in transient, reversible oedema.

Although the initial particle clearance involves phagocytosis by PMNs and mucociliary transport, over the longer term carbon elimination requires an adaptive increase in the number of macrophages.[4,8] It has previously been shown that the majority of these new cells arise from monocytes crossing the blood-air barrier to reach the alveoli, with a smaller contribution from dividing cells in the pulmonary interstitium.[4,5] The number of pulmonary macrophages recovered by bronchoalveolar lavage increases with the number of particles administered until a saturation point is reached.[1,8] The PMN and macrophagic responses appear to be triggered by chemotactic factors released during macrophage–particle interactions.[2,12,13] It is generally assumed that the macrophages recovered by lavage are all of alveolar origin, however, we observed many mononuclear interstitial cells in perivascular and peribronchial locations and occasionally macrophage-like cells were seen apparently passing between bronchiolar epithelial cells. This suggests that some mononuclear cells, responding to a chemotactic stimulus generated in the bronchiolar lumen, migrate directly to that site.

At the conclusion of the study there was no evidence of fibrotic or destructive lung disease and most of the carbon had been cleared from the lung. However, a few very large macrophages were seen in peribronchiolar alveoli suggesting that these cells are long-lived and perhaps they may be too large, or too heavy or immobile to pass into the bronchiolar openings. Particle-laden macrophages are also seen in the interstitium at 6 months. This serial study has confirmed that free particles cross the type 1 epithelial cell prior to phagocytosis by interstitial macrophages.[6,14,15] These cells are probably long-lived though some may be cleared by the lymphatics or migrate into the alveoli. This latter route may operate in response to a further chemotactic stimulus in the alveolus and the clearance of pigmented cells from lungs in lobar pneumonia may be explained on this basis.[16]

Direct clearance of particulates from the lung by

the lymphatic system is another pathway of elimination.[17] A few carbon particles that reach the interstitium have been observed in the endothelial cells of bronchial lymphatic channels. Particles may be then transported to the hilar lymph nodes directly prior to phagocytosis by macrophages, or carbon-laden interstitial macrophages may migrate into the lymphatics.[15] The relative importance of these routes has been estimated in a quantitative study of titanium dioxide clearance which showed that, after 25 days, about 45 per cent of deposited particles were eliminated by the tracheo-bronchial route while only 0·7 per cent was removed by the lymphatics at low levels of exposure and not more than 4 per cent at high exposure levels.[18] The present study supports the conclusion that particulate clearance by the lymphatic route is relatively small.

REFERENCES

1. Brain JD. The effects of increased particles on the number of alveolar macrophages. In: Walton WH, ed. Inhaled Particles, Vol. III. Old Woking, England: Unwin Brothers, 1971: 209.
2. Kazmierowski JA, Gallin JI, Reynolds HY. Mechanism for the inflammatory response in primate lungs: demonstration and partial characterization of an alveolar macrophage-derived chemotactic factor with preferential activity for polymorphonuclear leukocytes. *J Clin Invest* 1977; **59:** 273.
3. Gross P, deTreville RTP, Tolker EB, Kaschak M, Babyak MA. The pulmonary macrophage response to irritants: an attempt at quantitation. *Arch Environ Health* 1969; **18:** 174.
4. Bowden DH, Adamson IYR. Adaptive responses of the pulmonary macrophagic system to carbon. I. Kinetic studies. *Lab Invest* 1978; **38:** 422.
5. Bowden DH, Adamson IYR. Role of monocytes and interstitial cells in the generation of alveolar macrophages. I. Kinetic studies of normal mice. *Lab Invest* 1980; **42:** 511.
6. Heppleston AG, Young AE. Uptake of inert particulate matter by alveolar cells: an ultrastructural study. *J Pathol* 1973; **111:** 159.
7. Lipscomb MF, Onofrio JM, Nash EJ, Pierce AK, Toews GB. A morphologic study of the role of phagocytes in the clearance of *Staphylococcus aureus* from the lung. *J Reticuloendothel Soc* 1983; **33:** 429.
8. Adamson IYR, Bowden DH. Dose response of the pulmonary macrophagic system to various particulates and its relationship to transepithelial passage of free particles. *Exp Lung Res* 1981; **2:** 165.
9. Tate RM, Repine JE. Neutrophils and the adult respiratory distress syndrome. *Am Rev Resp Dis* 1983; **128:** 552.
10. Flick MR, Perel G, Staub NC. Leukocytes are required for increased lung microvascular permeability after microembolism in sheep. *Circ Res* 1981; **48:** 344.
11. Johnson KJ, Fantone JC, Kaplan J, Ward PA. *In vivo* damage of rat lungs by oxygen metabolites. *J Clin Invest* 1981; **67:** 983.
12. Dauber JH, Daniele RP. Secretion of chemotaxins by guinea pig lung macrophages. I. Spectrum of inflammatory cell responses. *Exp Lung Res* 1980; **1:** 25.
13. Adamson IYR, Bowden DH. Chemotactic and mitogenic components of the alveolar macrophage response to particles and neutrophil chemoattractant. *Am J Pathol* 1982; **109:** 71.
14. Brody AR, Hill LH. Interstitial accumulation of inhaled chrysotile asbestos fibers and consequent formation of microcalcifications. *Am J Pathol* 1982; **109:** 107.
15. Adamson IYR, Bowden DH. Adaptive responses of the pulmonary macrophagic system to carbon. II. Morphologic studies. *Lab Invest* 1978; **38:** 430.
16. Gross P, Brown JHO. The mobility of pneumoconiotic deposits. *Am J Clin Pathol* 1952; **22:** 821.
17. Leak LV. Lymphatic removal of fluids and particles in the mammalian lung. *Environ Hlth Perspec* 1980; **35:** 55.
18. Ferin J, Feldstein ML. Pulmonary clearance and hilar lymph node content in rats after particle exposure. *Environ Res* 1978; **16:** 342.

JOURNAL OF PATHOLOGY, VOL. **143:** 127–137 (1984)

SEQUENTIAL AND DOSE-DEPENDENT ALTERATIONS IN RAT BRONCHIOLAR EPITHELIUM DURING *O,O,S*-TRIMETHYL PHOSPHOROTHIOATE INDUCED DELAYED TOXICITY

JAY GANDY, T. ROY FUKUTO AND TOSHIKO IMAMURA

Division of Toxicology and Physiology, Department of Entomology, University of California, Riverside, CA 92521, U.S.A.

Received 8 September 1983
Accepted 8 October 1983

SUMMARY

The sequential and dose-dependent effects of *O,O,S*-trimethyl phosphorothioate (OOS-Me) on rat lung bronchiolar epithelium were investigated using scanning electron microscopy. At 12 h after oral treatment (20 mg/kg), there was a small increase in debris in the bronchioles and, by 24 h, there was much debris as well as phagocytic cells in the bronchioles. After 3 days, there was a decrease in the number of bronchiolar Clara cells as determined by the loss of their characteristic apical bulges. Concomitantly, there was a significant increase in lactate dehydrogenase activity in bronchopulmonary lavage fluid. By day 7, the Clara cells appeared to be reforming and, by day 14, the morphology of bronchiolar epithelium had returned to normal. Dose-dependent studies revealed a threshold dose level of OOS-Me between 10 and 20 mg/kg which produced the observed effects in Clara cells. Both sequential and dose-dependent effects of OOS-Me on Clara cells were correlated with changes in bronchopulmonary lavage lactate dehydrogenase activity.

KEY WORDS—Bronchiolar epithelium, Clara cells, trimethyl phosphorothioate toxicity, scanning EM.

INTRODUCTION

O,O,S-Trimethyl phosphorothioate (OOS-Me), an impurity found in many commonly used organophosphorus insecticides, such as malathion, fenitrothion and phenthoate, causes a delayed toxicity in rats.[1–4] When OOS-Me is administered at low doses, rats display anorexia, laboured breathing and red staining around the nose, mouth and eyes. An oral dose of 20 mg/kg causes an approximate 30 per cent weight loss 3 days after treatment but, after this time, OOS-Me-treated rats begin gaining weight at an even greater rate than controls.[5] No typical cholinergic signs of toxicity are produced by OOS-Me.

The specific mechanisms of the delayed toxicity are unknown; however, morphological studies have indicated that OOS-Me causes lung abnormalities in rats.[6,7] We have recently reported that the morphology of lung bronchiolar epithelium is altered after an oral dose of 20 mg/kg OOS. The treatment produced a decrease in the number and an increase in the size of nonciliated bronchiolar (Clara) cells.[8] The morphological changes were correlated with an increase in bronchopulmonary lavage fluid lactate dehydrogenase (LDH) levels. This paper provides the results of a more detailed study of the dose-response and time course effects of OOS-Me on bronchiolar epithelium of rat lungs.

Addressee for correspondence: Dr Toshiko Imamura, Division of Toxicology and Physiology, Department of Entomology, University of California, Riverside, CA 92521, U.S.A.

0022–3417/84/060127–11$01.10

MATERIALS AND METHODS

Animals

Male Sprague–Dawley rats were used which had been bred in our animal facility, housed in cages at 25°C, and maintained under an alternating 12 h light/dark cycle. Food and water were available *ad libitum*. Animals were fasted 16 h prior to oral treatment with either OOS-Me or corn oil as the vehicle control.

Chemicals and treatment

Crude OOS-Me was synthesized and purified according to the methods of Umetsu *et al.*[1] and determined to be more than 99·9 per cent pure by TLC and GLC. Glutaraldehyde and osmium tetroxide were purchased from Ted Pella, Inc. (Tustin, CA).

OOS-Me was dissolved in corn oil (10 mg/ml) and administered orally. For dose–response experiments, groups of rats were treated with 10 mg/kg ($n = 3$), 20 mg/kg ($n = 4$), or 40 mg/kg ($n = 3$). These animals were killed 3 days after treatment and the lungs were prepared for scanning electron microscopy (SEM). For time-course experiments, groups of rats were each treated with 20 mg/kg OOS-Me and killed at 12 h ($n = 3$), 24 h ($n = 3$), 3 days ($n = 4$), 7 days ($n = 3$) or 14 days ($n = 2$) after dosage, and prepared for SEM. Control animals ($n = 6$) received corn oil alone at 2 ml/kg. Separate groups of rats treated at these dose levels and time courses were used for enzyme assays.

Electron microscopy

The lungs from each animal were prepared for scanning electron microscopy using the modified techniques of Andrews.[9] Each animal was anaesthetized with an i.p. injection of pentobarbital; the trachea was cannulated, and the animal killed by aortic transection. The thorax was opened, and the lungs perfused through the pulmonary artery with 0·9 per cent NaCl in order to wash out the blood. The lungs were perfused with fixative (2·0 per cent glutaraldehyde in 0·1 M phosphate buffer, pH 7·2) through the pulmonary artery and filled with fixative by intratracheal injection. The trachea was ligated, and the lungs were excised and immersed in fixative. After 24 h, the lungs were sectioned with a razor blade into multiple cross sections varying in size from 2 × 2 mm to 4 × 3 mm, washed with 0·1 M phosphate buffer, pH 7·2, and post-fixed with osmium tetroxide. After thorough washing, the tissue was dehydrated in an ascending series of acetone solutions. After three changes of absolute acetone, the tissue was dried with liquid CO_2 in a Tousimis Samdri PVT-3 critical point dryer using three 5-min soaks in liquid CO_2 and four 2-min liquid CO_2 rinses to ensure adequate transition fluid/acetone exchange. After drying, the specimens were mounted on stubs with conductive silver paint, coated with gold–palladium and examined with a JEOL JEM 35 scanning electron microscope at an accelerating voltage of 15 kV.

From several specimens of each rat, five electron micrographs were taken at the same magnification. The micrographs were taken only when the entire frame of 4 × 5-in Polaroid film (59 × 76·7 μm surface area) was filled by epithelium from terminal bronchioles. On each of these micrographs the number of Clara cells was counted, and the maximum diameter of the apical bulge of 10 randomly selected cells was measured.

Enzyme preparation and assays

On the days of sacrifice, each animal was anaesthetized with 60 mg/kg sodium pentobarbital, i.p., and the trachea was cannulated with PE tubing. Isotonic NaCl (3 ml) (0·9 per cent) at room temperature was introduced gently into the cannula via a syringe and immediately withdrawn. This procedure was repeated once and the recovered lavage fluid volumes from the two washes were combined. The sample was stored in ice, then centrifuged at 600 *g* for 5 min at room temperature. The activity of LDH in the fluid was assayed by the spectrophotometric method of Bergmeyer and Bernt.[10] Protein was measured by the method of Sedmak and Grossberg.[11] Five to eight animals were tested per treatment.

Statistical analysis

All data were calculated as mean ± S.E. Values within groups were normally distributed and statistical comparisons between groups were done by one-way analysis of variance followed by Duncan's multiple range test. A p value of 0·05 or less was considered to be significant.[12]

RESULTS

Controls

The epithelium of terminal bronchioles was examined by SEM. In control rats, terminal bronchioles were characterized by the appearance of ciliated cells and nonciliated Clara cells (Fig. 1). The Clara cells were evenly distributed among the ciliated cells. Clara cells typically displayed an apical bulge which was surrounded at its base by a flat zone. The number of Clara cells per $76{\cdot}7 \times 59\ \mu m$ in terminal bronchioles of each animal ranged from 43·7 to 79·4, and the mean diameters of these cells ranged from 3·7 to 5·8 μm (Table I).

Time course effects

At 12 h after oral treatment with 20 mg/kg OOS-Me terminal bronchioles began to show only a few changes. The morphology of the bronchiolar epithelium was normal in appearance, except that there was an increase in debris on the surfaces of bronchioles (Fig. 2). The nature and origins of this debris are not known. Clara cells remained prominent throughout the terminal bronchioles and appeared unaffected except for the debris adhering to their surfaces. The number and mean diameter of Clara cells did not differ significantly from controls (Table I).

At 24 h after treatment, the amount of debris on the bronchiolar surfaces had greatly increased, being present in almost every terminal bronchiole examined (Fig. 3). Additionally, cells were present lying on the surface of bronchioles covered with microvilli which appeared to be macrophages. The number of Clara cells per unit area was decreased in one animal, while they remained similar to controls in the other two animals (Table I). The mean diameters of Clara cells did not change after 24 h (Table I).

After 3 days, the morphology of terminal bronchiolar epithelium had been significantly altered (Fig. 4). The number of Clara cells per $76{\cdot}7 \times 59\ \mu m$ area was decreased to a range of 7·6–27·0, while the mean diameters of these cells was increased to 7·0–7·1 μm (Table I). The appearance of the Clara cells was no longer characteristic. Rather than possess a distinct apical bulge, the non-ciliated cells had flat surfaces (Fig. 4, arrow); these probably represent Clara cells which had sloughed or withdrawn their apical bulge. In some areas it appeared that cilia were beginning to form on these surfaces that were once

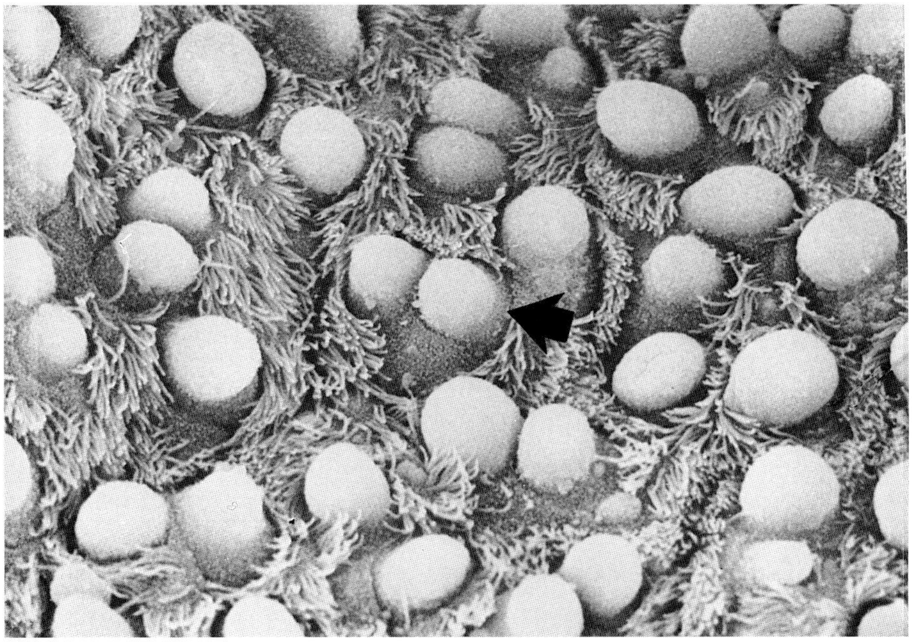

Fig. 1—Scanning electron micrograph of normal epithelium of rat lung terminal bronchioles from control animals showing Clara cells (arrow) and ciliated cells. $\times 1860$

Table I—Time course. The number of Clara cells per $76{\cdot}7 \times 59$ μm area of rat bronchiolar epithelium and mean diameter of Clara cells at varying times after oral treatment with corn oil or *O,O,S*-trimethyl phosphorothioate (OOS-Me)

Animals	Treatment	Cell number*	Mean diameter of Clara cells (μm)†‡
1	Control (corn oil)	62·4 ± 4·9	4·8 ± 0·1
2	(2·0 ml/kg)	43·7 ± 2·6	5·4 ± 0·3
3		54·6 ± 5·5	5·8 ± 0·1
4		62·4 ± 4·5	3·7 ± 0·1
5		79·4 ± 6·4	4·2 ± 0·1
6		66·6 ± 3·7	4·2 ± 0·2
7	OOS-Me	56·4 ± 6·2	5·2 ± 0·1
8	12 h	46·0 ± 5·8	5·4 ± 0·1
9	(20 mg/kg)	64·6 ± 5·3	5·2 ± 0·1
10	OOS-Me	52·0 ± 6·9	4·9 ± 0·1
11	24 h	29·6 ± 2·0	5·3 ± 0·2
12	(20 mg/kg)	40·6 ± 6·7	4·9 ± 0·1
13	OOS-Me	7·6 ± 2·4	7·0 ± 0·2
14	3 day	27·0 ± 5·0	7·1 ± 0·3
15	(20 mg/kg)	20·3 ± 3·7	7·0 ± 0·3
16		25·2 ± 5·2	7·1 ± 0·2
17	OOS-Me	51·1 ± 5·4	3·8 ± 0·1
18	7 day	40·1 ± 3·4	3·5 ± 0·1
19	(20 mg/kg)	46·6 ± 2·7	3·9 ± 0·2
20	OOS-Me	54·9 ± 3·4	3·9 ± 0·1
21	14 day	48·5 ± 3·0	3·8 ± 0·1
	(20 mg/kg)		

* Values are the mean ± S.E. for $n = 6$. Statistical comparisons between groups were done by one-way analysis of variance followed by Duncan's multiple range test. Groups not underscored by the same line are significantly different from one another, $p < 0{\cdot}05$.

5, 6, 9, 3, 4, 7, 20, 2, 10, 17, 21, 8, 1, 19, 12, 18, 11, 13, 15, 14, 16.

† Mean diameter (μm) of 10 cells per micrograph.

‡ Values of the mean ± S.E. for $n = 6$. Statistical comparison: see footnote *.

13, 15, 14, 16, 2, 1, 8, 11, 9, 7, 10, 12, 3, 5, 6, 20, 19, 21, 4, 17, 18.

nonciliated Clara cells. The debris in the bronchioles was no longer as evident.

At 7 days after treatment, Clara cells began showing recovery from the effects of OOS-Me. Apical bulges were again arising from most of the non-ciliated flat zones; however, there were still a few bare, flat surfaces without their apical projections, and many of the apical bulges that were present were smaller than those seen in controls (Fig. 5). Presumably this is because the Clara cells were still in the process of reforming their lost bulges. The number of Clara cells per unit area was comparable to control values.

By day 14 the bronchiolar epithelium had recovered from the morphological alterations caused by OOS-Me (Fig. 6). Well-formed Clara

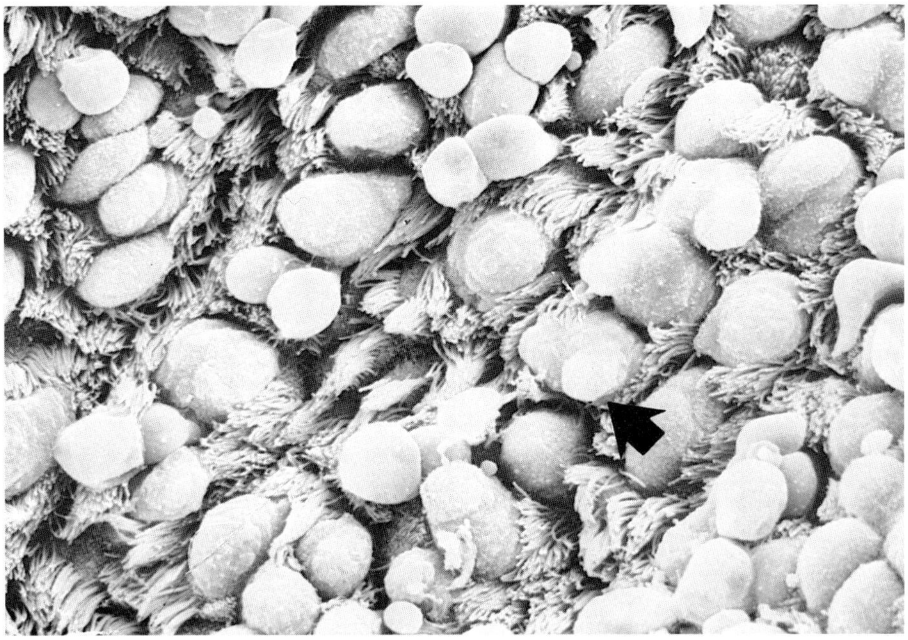

Fig. 2—Terminal bronchiole 12 h after oral treatment with OOS-Me (20 mg/kg). Little change was seen at this time, although some Clara cells appeared to have formed multiple projections of their apical bulges (arrows). ×1860

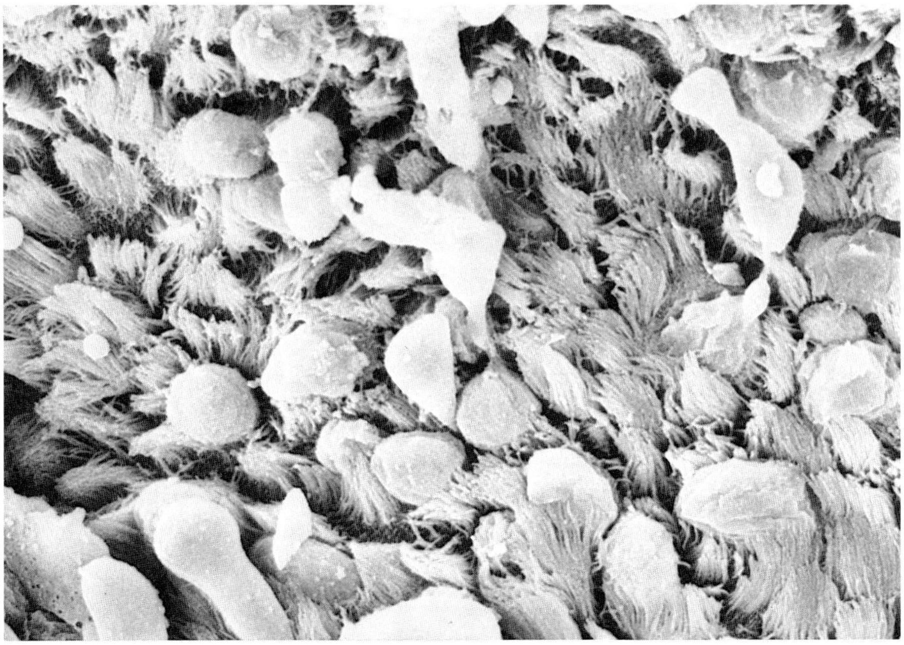

Fig. 3—Scanning electron micrograph of terminal bronchiole 24 h after oral treatment with OOS-Me (20 mg/kg) revealing an increase in debris found in the bronchiolar lining. ×1860

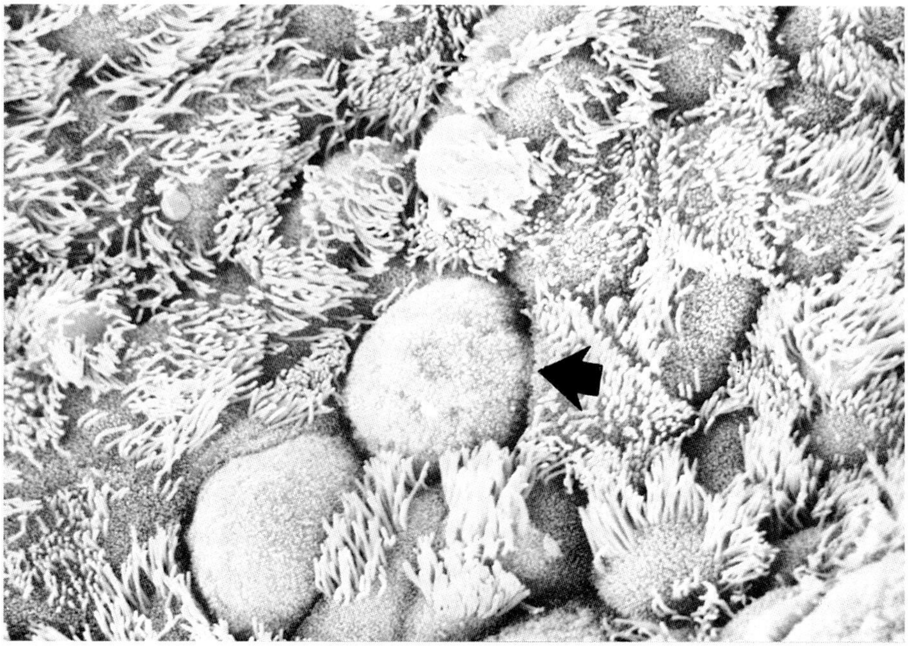

Fig. 4—Terminal bronchiolar epithelium 3 days after treatment with OOS-Me (20 mg/kg). Note the decrease in the number of Clara cell apical bulges and the appearance of flat, bare surfaces (arrow) and the apparent increase of cilia. ×1860

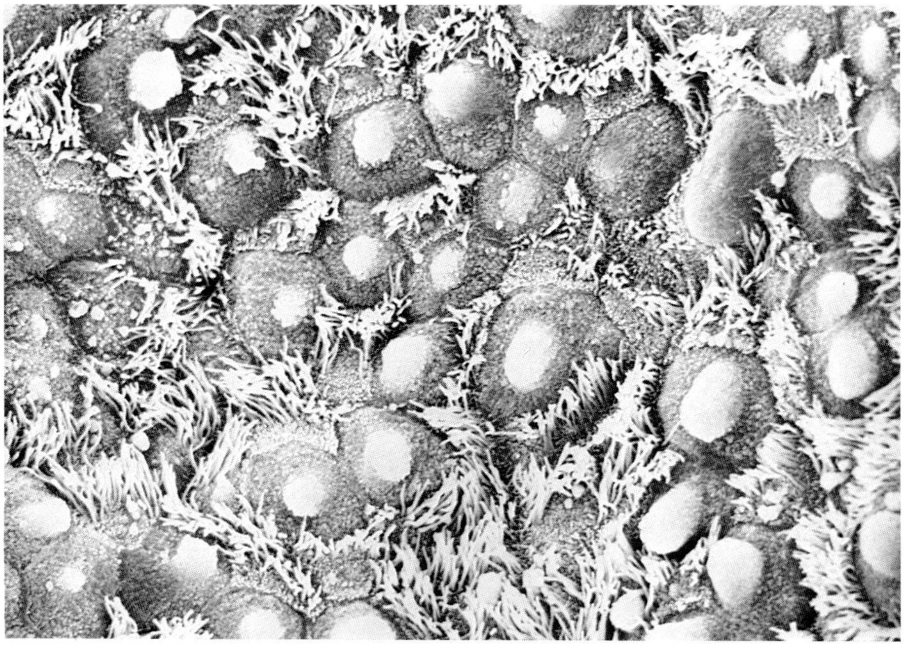

Fig. 5—Terminal bronchiole 7 days after oral treatment with OOS-Me (20 mg/kg). Clara cells appear to be reforming their apical bulges. ×1860

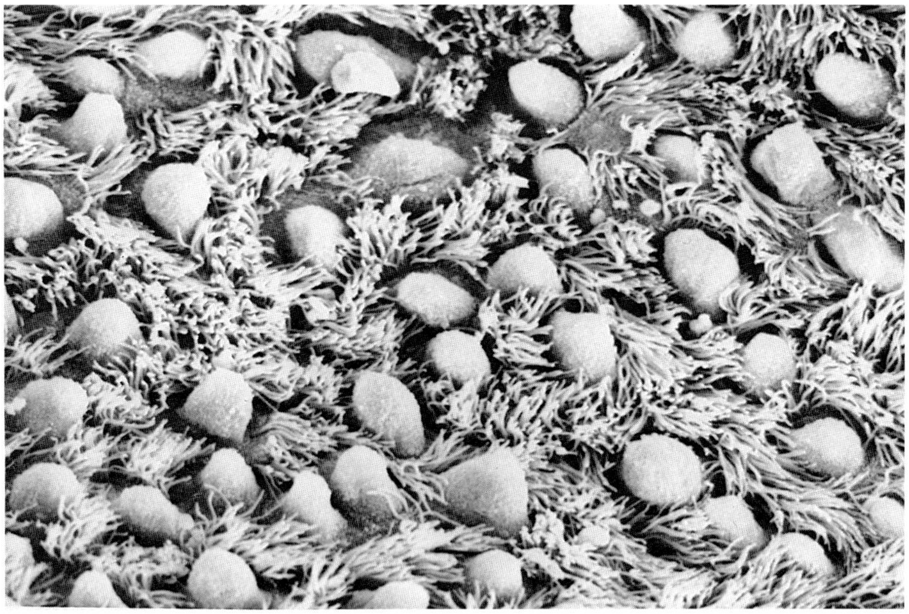

Fig. 6—Terminal bronchiolar epithelium 14 days after oral treatment with OOS-Me (20 mg/kg). The morphology of the bronchioles has returned to its normal appearance. The size and distribution of Clara cells are comparable to controls. ×1860

cells with their apical bulges were prominent throughout the terminal bronchioles. Both numbers of Clara cells per unit area and mean diameters of Clara cells were within the ranges seen in control animals.

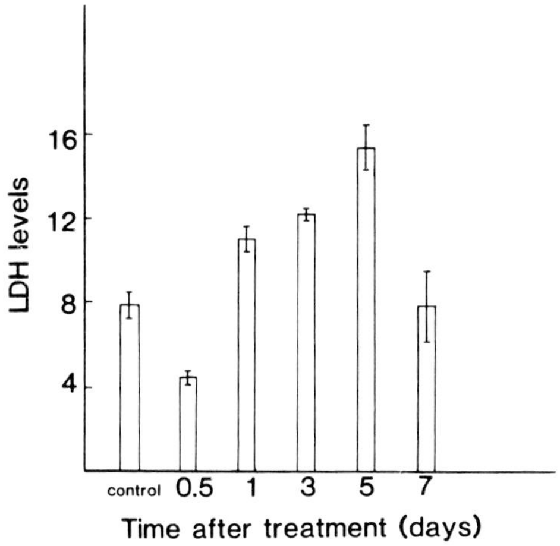

Fig. 7—Lactate dehydrogenase (LDH) activity (U/100 ml) of lung lavage fluid measured from groups of rats after the same OOS-Me (20 mg/kg) treatment intervals as those used for SEM study

Increased LDH activity in bronchopulmonary lavage fluid has been shown to be a marker for detecting lung injury resulting from pneumotoxic chemicals.[13, 14] It has previously been found that lung lavage fluid LDH is significantly increased 3 days after treatment with OOS-Me, 20 mg/kg.[8] Lung lavage fluid LDH activity was, therefore, measured from groups of rats after the same treatment intervals as those used for SEM study. After 12 h, mean LDH activity was lower than control values, but by 24 h the mean activity had increased by 29 per cent over controls (Fig. 7). By day 3, the mean LDH activity had increased by 36 per cent over that seen in control rats but, by day 7, the activity had returned to control levels. Additionally, a 5-day time-course group was examined, and its LDH activity was found to be higher than the 3-day group, reaching a maximum mean LDH value 45 per cent greater than control values (Fig. 7).

Dose–response relationship

Since the effects of OOS-Me are most prevalent 3 days after treatment, all dose–response animals were killed at this time. At a dose of 10 mg/kg, few changes were seen in terminal bronchioles (Fig. 8).

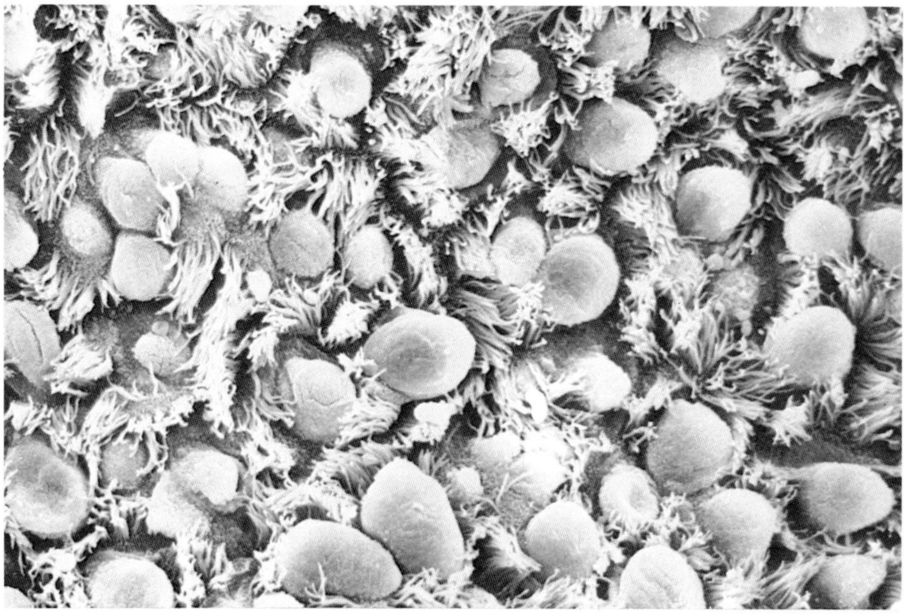

Fig. 8—Terminal bronchiolar epithelium after a 10 mg/kg oral dose of OOS-Me (3 days after treatment). No change can be seen in the number or size of Clara cells, although some Clara cells show small creases in their cell surfaces that were not seen in controls. ×1860

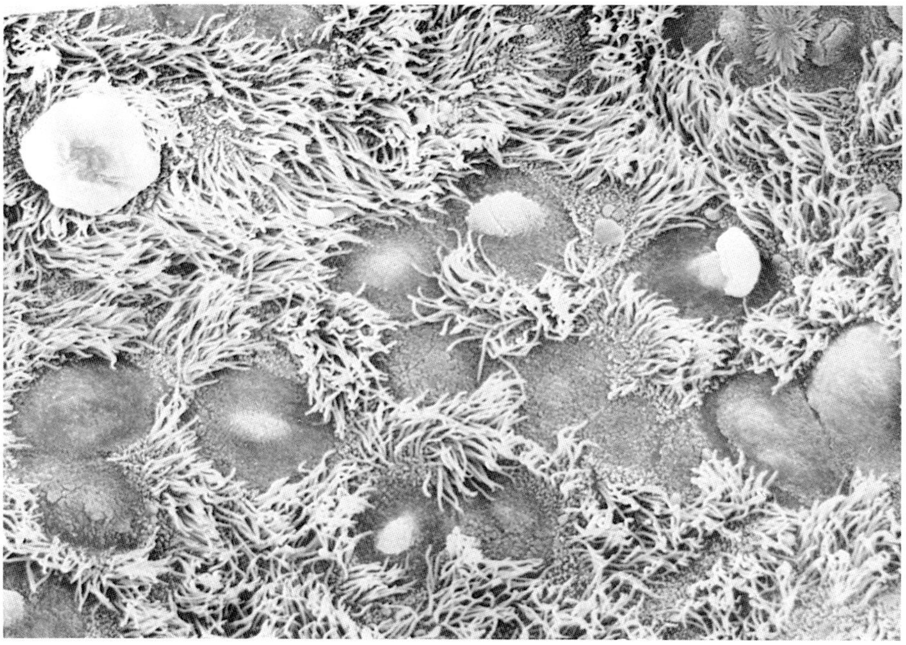

Fig. 9—Terminal bronchiolar epithelium after a 40 mg/kg oral dose of OOS-Me (3 days after treatment). Many non-ciliated Clara cells no longer possess their apical bulge, leaving a bare, flat area. ×1860

Table II—Dose–response. The number of Clara cells per $76 \cdot 7 \times 59$ μm area of rat bronchiolar epithelium and mean diameter of Clara cells 3 days after oral treatment with corn oil or varying doses of *O,O,S*-trimethyl phosphorothioate (OOS-Me)

Animals	Treatment	Cell number*	Mean diameter (μm)†‡
1	Control (corn oil)	62·4 ± 4·9	4·9 ± 0·1
2		43·7 ± 2·6	5·4 ± 0·3
3		54·6 ± 5·5	5·8 ± 0·1
4		62·4 ± 4·5	3·7 ± 0·1
5		79·4 ± 6·4	4·2 ± 0·1
6		66·6 ± 3·7	4·2 ± 0·2
7	OOS-Me 10 mg/kg	57·6 ± 2·0	4·4 ± 0·2
8		51·4 ± 7·8	4·3 ± 0·1
9		57·6 ± 3·9	4·9 ± 0·2
10	OOS-Me 20 mg/kg	7·6 ± 2·4	7·0 ± 0·2
11		27·0 ± 5·0	7·1 ± 0·3
12		20·2 ± 3·7	7·0 ± 0·3
13		25·2 ± 5·2	7·1 ± 0·2
14	OOS-Me 40 mg/kg	29·4 ± 9·1	5·3 ± 0·1
15		14·2 ± 0·6	5·0 ± 0·2
16		23·4 ± 5·4	4·9 ± 0·1

* Values are the mean ± S.E. for $n = 6$. Statistical comparisons between groups were done by one-way analysis of variance followed by Duncan's multiple range test. Groups not underscored by the same line are significantly different from one another, $p < 0 \cdot 05$.

5, 6, 3, 4, 7, 9, 2, 8, 1, 14, 10, 12, 16, 11, 15, 13.

† Mean diameter (μm) of 10 cells per micrograph.

‡ Values of the mean ± S.E. for $n = 6$. Statistical comparison: see footnote*.

10, 12, 11, 13, 2, 1, 14, 15, 9, 3, 16, 7, 5, 6, 8, 4.

The numbers and mean diameters of Clara cells were not different from those of control rats (Table II). Some Clara cells had small creases in their surfaces that were not seen in controls.

The effects of a 20 mg/kg dose of OOS-Me on day 3 are described above in the time-course section and can be seen in Fig. 4 and are summarized in Table II.

At 40 mg/kg, terminal bronchioles were effected in a similar manner as with the 20 mg/kg dose. Many of the non-ciliated cells no longer had distinct apical bulges, leaving a bare, flat area (Fig. 9). The numbers of Clara cells per unit area were less than the numbers seen in the control groups, although the reduction was no greater than the reduction seen with the 20 mg/kg dose. The mean diameters of the Clara cells were not increased

Table III—Mean LDH activity 3 days after oral treatment with varying doses of *O,O,S*-trimethyl phosphorothioate

Group No.	Dose	LDH (U/100 ml)*	n
1	Control	7·92 ± 0·67	5
2	10 mg/kg	7·37 ± 1·08	6
3	20 mg/kg	12·25 ± 1·02	5
4	40 mg/kg	9·46 ± 1·00	8

* Values are the mean ± S.E. Statistical comparisons between groups were done by one-way analysis of variance followed by Duncan's multiple range test. Groups not underscored by the same line are significantly different from one another, $p < 0 \cdot 05$.

3, 4, 1, 2.

with the 40 mg/kg dose as it was with the 20 mg/kg dose (Table II).

LDH activity was measured at the 10, 20 and 40 mg/kg dose levels. The activity did not change on day 3 after a 10 mg/kg treatment. The 20 mg/kg dose produced the greatest change (35 per cent increase), while 40 mg/kg produced an 18 per cent increase (Table III).

DISCUSSION

In a previous communication,[8] we described the initial findings that treatment with OOS-Me results in changes in the morphological appearance of terminal bronchiolar epithelium. In this present study, we have presented a thorough sequential and dose-dependent analysis of these alterations, which correlated with changes in bronchopulmonary LDH activity.

The earliest noticeable effects of OOS-Me to the bronchioles was the increased amount of debris 12 and 24 h after treatment. The origin of this debris is not known. It possibly results from the sloughing of Clara cell apical bulges. However, the greatest amounts of debris (24 h) were observed prior to the most pronounced reduction in the number of Clara cell apical bulges and, therefore, the debris could likely be due to a necrosis of another specific lung cell type. For example, Dinsdale *et al.*[7] found that *O,S,S*-trimethyl phosphorodithioate and *O,O,S*-triethyl phosphorothioate caused damage to type I pneumocytes within 24 h after treatment. We are currently investigating whether OOS-Me effects type I and type II alveolar cells. The small creases seen in the surfaces of some Clara cells following the 10 mg/kg dose could be due to the direct effects of OOS-Me (or one of its metabolites), or it could be due to an increased fragility of the cellular structure after treatment that causes the creases to occur when the tissue is fixed with glutaraldehyde.

The cells seen lying on the epithelial surfaces of the bronchioles at 12 and 24 h after OOS-Me (20 mg/kg) treatment appeared to be macrophages. No macrophages were observed in bronchioles of control animals, although one would expect to see them in small numbers. Therefore, the macrophages seen in treated animals most likely represent an increase in macrophage numbers. Macrophages migrate toward chemotactic factors produced as a result of tissue damage.[15] Therefore, the observed macrophages have possibly migrated into the bronchioles in response to the increase in debris, to aid in the removal of the debris.

The rise in mean bronchopulmonary LDH activity, an indication of tissue damage, seems to correlate well with the sequential morphological changes observed. However, we cannot explain the decrease in LDH activity seen 12 h after OOS-Me treatment. For the dose–response experiments, the increase in LDH levels exhibited a threshold level between 10 and 20 mg/kg. A threshold dose level for increasing LDH activity is consistent with the observed dose–response effects on bronchiolar morphology, since a 10 mg/kg dose did not result in significant changes of the Clara cells, while 20 and 40 mg/kg doses produced effects that were similar.

Clara cells are one of the loci of pulmonary mixed-function oxidase (MFO) activity. This makes them potential target cells for toxins that require MFO-mediated activation.[16,17] Available evidence suggests that OOS-Me must be metabolized to an active form(s) to produce toxic effects.[18,19] It is possible that Clara cells are a site of the conversion of parent compound into its toxic form(s), thereby making these cells susceptible to the toxic action of OOS-Me. Another possibility is that a metabolite(s) of OOS-Me which is activated in some other organ(s) selectively produces toxic effects on Clara cells.

Histochemical and ultrastructural characteristics of Clara cells indicate that they have a secretory function,[20–22] and it is believed that they contribute to the surfactant lining of the bronchioles.[23–25] It has been proposed that normally Clara cells release their secretory products by merocrine secretion but, after exposure to pulmonary toxicants such as naphthalene or NO_2, or as a result of chronic bronchitis, Clara cells respond by a decapitation secretion mechanism,[26,27] insuring adequate release of Clara cell surfactant necessary in preventing blockage of peripheral airways. It is possible that the changes we see in Clara cells may not be a direct toxic effect of OOS-Me but rather an indirect functional response to a damage produced elsewhere in the lung.

Our present studies provide additional evidence that the lung is a target organ for OOS-Me toxicity. At this time we cannot be certain whether the effects on Clara cells are due to a direct toxicity of OOS-Me or due to a toxic lesion produced to other cell types in the lung.

ACKNOWLEDGEMENTS

The authors wish to thank Ms Leslie Hasegawa for her excellent technical assistance, and Ms Linda McCloud for the care and breeding of the experimental animals. This work was supported in part by Public Health Service Grant ES 02225.

REFERENCES

1. Umetsu N, Grose FH, Allahyari R, Abu-El-Hajs S, Fukuto TR. Effects of impurities on the mammalian toxicity of technical malathion and acephate. *J Agric Food Chem* 1977; **25:** 946–953.
2. Aldridge WN, Miles JW, Mount DL, Verschoyle RD. The toxicological properties of impurities in malathion. *Arch Toxicol* 1979; **42:** 95–106.
3. Mallipudi NM, Umetsu N, Toia RF, Talcott RE, Fukuto TR. Toxicity of *O,O,S*-trimethyl and triethyl phosphorothioate to the rat. *J Agric Food Chem* 1979; **27:** 463–466.
4. Toia RF, March RB, Umetsu N, Mallipudi NM, Allahyari R, Fukuto TR. Identification and toxicological evaluation of impurities in technical malathion and fenthion. *J Agric Food Chem* 1980; **28:** 599–604.
5. Imamura T, Gray AJ, Umetsu N, Fukuto TR. Biochemical and physiological investigation into the delayed toxicity produced by *O,O,S*-trimethyl phosphorothioate in rats. *Pestic Biochem Physiol* 1983; **19:** 66–73.
6. Verschoyle RD, Aldridge WN, Cabral JRP. Toxicology of trimethyl- and triethyl phosphorothioates. In: Holmstedt B, Lauwerys R, Mercier M, Roberfroid M, eds. Mechanisms of Toxicity and Hazard Evaluation. Amsterdam: Elsevier/North Holland Biomedical Press, 1980: 631–634.
7. Dinsdale D, Verschoyle RD, Cabral JRP. Cellular responses to trialkylphorothioate-induced injury in rat lung. *Arch Toxicol* 1982; **51:** 79–89.
8. Imamura T, Gandy J, Fukuto TR, Talbot P. An impurity of malathion alters the morphology of rat lung bronchiolar epithelium. *Toxicol* 1983; **26:** 73–79.
9. Andrews PM. The respiratory system. In: Hodges GM, Hallowes RC, eds. Biomedical Research Applications of Scanning Electron Microscopy. London: Academic Press, 1979: 177–202.
10. Bergmeyer HU, Bernt E. Lactate dehydrogenase UV-assay with pyruvate and NADH. In: Bergmeyer HU, ed. Methods of Enzymatic Analysis. Vol 2. New York: 1974: 574–579.
11. Sedmak JJ, Grossberg SE. A rapid, sensitive and versatile assay for protein using Coomassie brilliant blue G250. *Anal Biochem* 1977; **79:** 544–552.
12. Steel RGD, Torrie JH. Principles and Procedures of Statistics. 2nd ed. New York, 1980.
13. Henderson RF, Damon EG, Henderson TR. Early damage indicator in the lung. I. Lactate dehydrogenase activity in the airways. *Toxicol Appl Pharmacol* 1978; **44:** 291–297.
14. Roth RA. Effect of pneumotoxicants on lactate dehydrogenase activity in airways of rats. *Toxicol Appl Pharmacol* 1981; **57:** 69–78.
15. Snyderman R, Stahl C. Chemotaxis of mononuclear leukocytes. In: Sorbit E, ed. Chemotaxis: Its Biology and Biochemistry. 1974: 284–295.
16. Boyd MR. Evidence for the Clara cell as a site of cytochrome P-450-dependent mixed-function oxidase activity in lung. *Nature* 1977; **269:** 713–715.
17. Boyd MR, Statham CN, Longo NS. The pulmonary Clara cell as a target for toxic chemicals requiring metabolic activation; studies with carbon tetrachloride. *J Pharmacol Exper Ther* 1980; **212:** 109–114.
18. Imamura T, Hasegawa L. Role of metabolic activation, covalent binding and glutathione depletion in pulmonary toxicity produced by an impurity of malathion. *Toxicol Appl Pharmacol* 1983; **32:** 3191–3195.
19. Verschoyle RD, Cabral JRP. Investigation of the acute toxicity of some trimethyl and triethyl phosphorothioates with particular reference to those causing lung damage. *Arch Toxicol* 1982; **51:** 221–231.
20. Azzopardi A, Thurlbeck WM. The histochemistry of the nonciliated bronchiolar epithelial cell. *Amer Rev Resp Dis* 1969; **99:** 516–525.
21. Niden AH, Yamada E. Some observations on the fine structure of the non-ciliated bronchiolar cells. In: Uyeda R, ed. Proceedings of the VI International Congress for Electron Microscopy, Vol 2. Tokyo: 1966: 599.
22. Petrik P. Fine structure identification of peroxisomes in mouse and rat bronchiolar and alveolar epithelium. *J Histochem* 1971; **19:** 339–348.
23. Gil J, Weibel ER. Extracellular lining of bronchioles after perfusion-fixation of rat lung for electron microscopy. *Anatomical Record* 1971; **169:** 185–199.
24. Niden AH. Bronchiolar and large alveolar cell in pulmonary phospholipid metabolism. *Science* 1967; **158:** 1323–1324.
25. Petrik P, Collet AJ. Quantitative electron microscopic autoradiography of *in vivo* incorporation of ^{3}H-choline, ^{3}H-leucine, ^{3}H-acetate, and ^{3}H-galactose in non-ciliated bronchiolar (Clara) cells of mice. *Am J Anatomy* 1974; **139:** 519–533.
26. Mahvi D, Bank H, Harley R. Morphology of a naphthalene-induced bronchiolar lesion. *Am J Pathol* 1977; **86:** 559–572.
27. Evans MJ, Johnson LV, Stephens RJ, Freeman G. Renewal of terminal bronchiolar epithelium in the rat following exposure to NO_2 or O_3. *Lab Investigation* 1976; **35:** 246–257.

BOOK REVIEWS

Acute Inflammation (Second Edition). J. V. HURLEY. Churchill-Livingstone, Edinburgh, 1983. No. of pages: 157. Price: £17. ISBN: 0443 02507.

Clarity of style gives an immediately favourable impression of this book. This derives from the way one is led with deceptively simple logic through complex and disputed topics, such as the nature of normal vascular permeability and the role of chemical mediators in increased permeability. This second edition, 10 years on, is somewhat longer than the first but with a larger page format and more illustrations of the same high quality. Very occasional typing errors are the only blemish.

Of course the criticism might be made that such a slim monograph is not as comprehensive as larger multiauthor texts on such topics as prostaglandin metabolism or the detailed enzymology of the various inflammatory cell types. But this book is the authoritative account of histological events, both structural and cellular, at light and electron microscopic level. It is largely based on results from investigative techniques applied at those levels. The final chapters on the terminations of acute inflammation, including an additional one on healing by scar formation, seem to lack the authority of the main part, and contain little more on chronic inflammation and healing than general pathology texts.

On a more sombre note, it is very obvious, on comparing the reference lists of the two editions, that the additional references from the last 10 years are taken largely from non-pathological journals. One suspects that the subject has lost much of its input from academic pathologists, and that the lead has now passed over to scientists in other disciplines, while so many histopathologists confine themselves to tumour immunohistochemistry.

W. D. THOMPSON
Glasgow

History of Staining (Third Edition). Edited by G. CLARK and F. H. KASTEN. Williams and Wilkins, Baltimore, 1983. No. of pages: 304. Price: £22.25. ISBN: 0683 017 055.

Twenty-four very readable chapters comprise this third edition of the *History of Staining*, a worthy successor to two previous editions by the hand of Dr H. J. Conn. In adding six new chapters the editors (Clark and Kasten) have substantially continued the policies laid down in the Preface to the Second Edition (1948). Here it was proposed that the whole history of staining should be covered, but "in a somewhat sketchy manner", avoiding precise technical details of the work of any particular individual.

The third edition represents a comprehensive and imposing catalogue of names in which it is difficult to find any serious omissions. It remains possible, however, to find a few surprising inclusions.

Three of the six new chapters range from brief to vanishingly brief but the other three, all from the pen of Dr F. H. Kasten, make ample amends and run to a total of 60 pages. Chapter 1 is a complete exposition of the life and works of Ralph Dougall Lillie (1896–1979), who did so much to sustain and improve the deliberations and publications of the Biological Stain Commission. Chapter 23 is a treatise on the 'Development of Fluorescence Microscopy' and Chapter 24 covers 'Protein and Nucleic Acid Histochemistry'. Together they form a splendid scholarly culmination to the work, which concludes with an extensive bibliography. Here, as in many other places, the technology of staining encroaches on the territory of histochemistry and cytochemistry. The *History of Staining* is an essential source book for adherents of these two specialties and also for those concerned with the principal biological disciplines, putting into perspective all the important techniques of the present day and, in the process, rescuing from oblivion so many whose efforts and skills deserve to be remembered.

A. G. E. PEARSE
Hammersmith Hospital, London

Biology and Pathology of the Vessel Wall (Proceedings of the Royal College of Pathologists Symposium). Edited by NEVILLE WOOLFE. Praeger, Eastbourne, 1983. No. of pages: 351. Price £17.50. ISBN: 003 0641 497.

A quarter of a century ago a visitor to any academic department of pathology was almost bound to meet someone engaged in research into atheromatous vascular disease and to find in the animal house a batch of rabbits quietly munching some form of cholesterol diet. The scene has changed as such departments are now more likely to be awash with monoclonal antibodies. Histopathologists, with a few notable exceptions, have largely abandoned vascular pathology and epidemiologists, biochemists, haematologists, pharmacologists and diverse experimentalists have filled the vacuum. In those far-off days, because of Duguid's resuscitation of Rokitansky's 'thrombogenic hypothesis', the major controversy concerned the relative contributions made to the disease complex by platelets and fibrin on the one hand and by lipid deposition, the kernel of the 'dietary or infiltration hypothesis', on the other. As judged by the published proceedings of the College symposium the argument still goes on but, inevitably, attempts are now being made to reconcile and synthesize the two theories. However, this book is not just about atheroma but ranges widely through structure, physiology, pharmacology and pathology of the vessel wall and includes contributions on the inflammatory response, hypertension, diabetes and other disorders.

The editor of the Proceedings, Professor Neville Woolf, is to be congratulated on declining to mourn the passing of the days "when the artery wall was regarded as a more or less passive site for the deposition of lipid derived from the plasma" and, by implication, that morphology tended to hog the scene. The book is well edited with remarkably few printing errors detectable, it is cheap by current prices and it has been produced soon after the Symposium. It is, therefore, commended to all those, whatever their discipline, who have an interest in blood vessels. How can one not?

W. B. Robertson
St George's Hospital Medical School, London

The Human Teratomas. Experimental and Clinical Biology. Edited by Ivan Damjanov, Barbara B. Knowles and Davor Salter. Humana Press, Clifton, New Jersey, 1983. No. of pages: 358. Price: £44.65. ISBN: 0896 030 407.

This book consists of 50 chapters by different authors which cover clinical, epidemiological and pathological aspects of human teratomas as well as their biology and aspects of experimental work in human and animal models.

Each chapter is subdivided by appropriate headings, most have an introductory section and many end with a general discussion or brief summary so that most may be read satisfactorily in isolation. With two exceptions, careful editing has produced pleasing continuity and avoidance of unnecessary repetition.

A historical review, which includes the theories of origin of these tumours precedes well-referenced contributions on general and specific aspects of the pathology and biology of teratomas, their epidemiology and treatment. The last four chapters are concerned with laboratory work on human and mouse teratoma cell lines.

Some of the photomicrographs are of poor quality and two chapters are so full of abbreviations that they precipitate lexical hiccups.

Reference to experimental work throughout the book and detailed accounts of *in vitro* work with human and animal teratomas, with which most pathologists will be unfamiliar, make fascinating reading. The book shows the relevance of many aspects of teratoma behaviour to histological reporting and patient management. It also adds to our understanding of embryological development and its control. It would make a useful addition to the pathology department library.

J. W. Keeling
John Radcliffe Hospital, Oxford

Substance P (Volume 3). Petr Skrabanek and David Powell. Eden Press, Montreal, 1983. No. of pages: 290. ISBN: 0906 783 178.

This book is the second update of Drs Skrabanek and Powell's excellent 'megareview' of substance P which is now, as the authors point out, the third most active field in the life sciences.

This compact volume provides concise and yet detailed reports of every aspect of research into substance P which has been published between autumn 1979 and the end of 1981. The authors are to be commended for ploughing through such a mass of literature and breaking it down into such an easily digestible form. Their book is an invaluable source of information for those involved in a variety of fields, including biochemistry, neurophysiology, endocrinology and pathology.

Julia Polak
Royal Postgraduate Medical School, London

Catalogue of Chromosome Aberrations in Cancer. (Reprint from *Cytogenetics and Cell Genetics*, Vol. 36, Nos 1–2, 1983). Edited by F. Mitelman. S. Karger AG, Basel, 1983. No. of pages: 516. Soft cover. Price: Sfr. 132 (DM 158) (US $79.00). ISBN: 3 8055 3813 8.

This is not a book for leisure reading. As the title indicates it is a comprehensive catalogue of karyotypic changes in 3844 referenced cases of neoplasia, classified by chromosome number and histopathology. It has limited shelf life, scanty text and a high cost which suggest that, whilst of considerable value to those actively engaged in the molecular biology and cytogenetics of cancer, few hospitals or individuals will rate it as a high priority purchase.

I. D. Young
Leicester Royal Infirmary

Pathology Annual: Part 1. Volume 18, 1983. Series Editors: S. C. SOMMERS and P. P. ROSEN. Prentice-Hall International, Hemel Hempstead, 1983. No. of pages: 420. Price: £35.80. ISBN: 0838 577 318.

This issue includes three articles on lung neoplasms, two on Crohn's disease, two on thyroid tumours and one each on transitional cell cancer of the bladder, sebaceous neoplasms of salivary gland origin, phaeochromocytoma (with particular reference to the organ of Zuckerkandl), the diagnosis of viral infections by electron microscopic examination of tissue specimens, adenomas of large bowel, light microscopy and photomicrography, Creutzfeldt–Jakob disease and fine needle aspiration biopsy of the breast.

The writers of the review on lymphoreticular tumours of the lung discuss the distinction from similar non-neoplastic infiltrates. In another chapter, the categorization of a variety of lower respiratory tract tumours is considered in the light of recent electron microscopic, histochemical and immunological investigations. Attention is drawn to the heterogeneity of differentiation in lung tumours and the same point arises in the section devoted to pulmonary neuroendocrine cells and neoplasms.

Aspects of Crohn's disease discussed include the significance of mast cell infiltrates and the correlation of general pathological features with prediction of recrudescence.

The diagnosis and behaviour of follicular and papillary thyroid tumours are the subjects of two articles. The interesting observation that only 33 per cent follicular carcinomas were correctly identified by frozen section examination perhaps raises the question whether this investigation should be used for thyroid tumours.

Although not specified in the title, the section on adenomas refers to those of the large bowel. The statement that ". . . adenomas may be benign or malignant" seems ill chosen and "The presence of hyperplasia therefore enhances cell proliferation . . ." needs clarification.

Except for some of the low magnification photomicrographs, the illustrations are mostly good, but almost all of them are separated by a page or more from the relevant text. Typographical errors are few, e.g. "vascular vessel" in the legend to Fig. 17, p. 271. An irritating recurrent error of English usage is "comprised of" and there is the occasional "indeterminant" for indeterminate.

On the whole the articles are well-written and cover a variety of interesting and important topics, each with an extensive, up-to-date bibliography. The book can be highly recommended as a worthwhile addition to the pathologist's bookshelf.

P. V. BEST
University of Aberdeen

Arterial Pollution—An Integrated View on Atherosclerosis. Edited by H. PEETERS, G. A. GRESHAM and R. PAOLETTI. NATO ASI Series, Series A: Life Sciences, Vol. 58. Plenum Press, New York, London, 1983. No. of pages: 422. Price: $55.

This volume gives an account of a 2 week course on atherosclerosis, sponsored by NATO, held in 1981. The course was intended to broaden the view of the disease held by research workers who might be active in a relatively narrow field of study. It reviews, therefore, the natural history of atherosclerosis, animal models of the disease, physiopathology, epidemiology and risk factors, prevention, regression and therapy.

I am sure that the course served its purpose. The review of the development of atheroma in man is clear and, even if a little dated (some uncritical statements about neonatal coronary vessels are made), provides a clear account for the non-pathologist. The reviews of metabolic aspects, animal models and the cellular components of the lesion are also succinct and informative. This general section is followed by articles on ultrasound, myocardial lipids, the biochemistry of the infarcted heart, apolipoproteins and determinants of HDL levels, giving an idea of the diversity of research techniques applied to this disease.

Later sections succeed in putting epidemiology and risk factors in a useful framework for the generalist, although the sections on regression and therapy are not so well presented.

The volume will be most useful for non-pathologists who work on this disease. Pathologists will find many data collected here which might otherwise need searching for.

C. L. BERRY
The London Hospital

Multiple Choice Questions in Pathology. I. L. BROWN. Arnold, London, 1983. Price: £1.95. No.of pages: 62. ISBN: 071314436X.

This booklet is based very firmly on the current edition of Muir's *Text Book of Pathology,* and this is emphasized by the fact that it carries the same pictorial cover. It contains 150 selected questions derived from all sections of the parent book. Inevitably, these are insufficient to cover each section comprehensively but the selected questions are well chosen from the important topics. The book is aimed at both students and staff, and students who tackle it conscientiously will certainly revise significant subjects and will reveal their major gaps—as indeed will staff. I proved this myself by going through the complete set. My final score must remain classified information but the series clearly revealed gaps that I had long suppressed from consciousness—in the details of modern immunology and of the coagulation cascades.

As predicted by Professor Anderson in his preface, I would like to disagree with some of the answers and explanatory comments so helpfully provided on the pages facing the questions, but only on points of detail. There seems to be one error, however—to me Sheehan's syndrome does not really match up with 'post-mortem necrosis'.

I don't really like MCQs as, like this one, they show me up, but they are with us to stay and this is a more benign and educatively helpful set than some. At a cost of £1.95 it should be affordable by all and it can certainly be recommended.

G. B. Scott
University of Aberdeen

New Frontiers in Mammary Pathology Vol. 2. Edited by K. H. Hollmann and J. M. Verley. Plenum Press, New York, 1981. No. of pages: 328. Price: £55. ISBN: 0306 406 551.

The second volume in this series comprises the proceedings of the Symposium of the International Society Against Breast Cancer held in December 1981. The majority of papers are from invited speakers with a small number of free papers included.

The emphasis is on the development of breast neoplasia with several chapters devoted to risk factors, precancerous and *in situ* neoplastic lesions. There is an extensive tabulated reference list of potential risk factors which was up to date at the time of the symposium. The papers concerned with pre-cancerous and *in situ* lesions are predominantly histopathological and consider lobular neoplasia in some detail. Interesting questions are raised but little new information is presented. In one paper, immunohistochemical data are invoked with insufficient details about antibodies being given, a practice which should be discouraged.

Individual chapters are devoted to angiogenesis, genetic markers, cell markers and steroid binding and are clearly written. The former two provide fairly extensive experimental details and the latter manage to consider the area adequately in the space allotted.

The section relating to cytology and histological analysis of breast tumours consist of papers of varying standard, some being rather limited both in their content and the numbers considered.

Reflecting the interests of the editors, the section concerned with tumour immunity is well planned, with one paper giving a general overview and others being devoted to cellular immunity, immunomorphology and immunotherapy, all well referenced.

The quality of many of the papers is high, but the standard of some is poor, in regard to the material presented and the referencing. This volume may be of use to pathologists wanting a review of certain areas of interest in breast neoplasia, but will provide little that is new to those who are up to date.

Rosemary A. Walker
Leicester Royal Infirmary

Pre-Eclampsia. The Hypertensive Disease of Pregnancy. I. MacGillivray. W. B. Saunders, London, 1983. No. of pages: 392. Price: £19.50. ISBN: 07216 1195 8.

Pre-eclampsia remains the enigma of obstetrics. There is no universally acceptable clinical definition and the diagnosis depends on recognition of disputed symptoms and signs. It is a disease which almost certainly begins in the first trimester yet becomes clinically manifest in the latter half of pregnancy. Professor MacGillivray has attempted to provide a broad outline within the confines of a reasonable sized textbook. The majority of the text is devoted to epidemiology and clinical aspects and, as such, is clearly aimed at obstetricians. Much laboratory data are included covering biochemistry, endocrinology, haematology and immunology. I found this section comprehensive and readable. Much of the factual information inevitably relates to the effects of the disease rather than its cause. The final chapters consider the morbid anatomy and aetiology. There are inequalities in the former, thus coverage of the lesions in maternal organs is adequate but the discussion of placental pathology is disappointing. Some of the illustrations chosen are curious, e.g. Figs. 11.10, 11.13; others are meaningless, Fig. 11.15, as the duration of pregnancy is not stated. The chapter on aetiology provides a concise view of current hypotheses. The references are carefully chosen and up-to-date.

This book will find its way into few pathology departments, but is recommended to those providing laboratory services in maternity hospitals and to those contemplating research into pre-eclampsia.

D. I. Rushton
The Birmingham Maternity Hospital

JOURNAL OF PATHOLOGY, VOL. **143:** 143 (1984)

ANNOUNCEMENT

THE BRITISH SOCIETY FOR DERMATOPATHOLOGY

are holding a 1-day symposium on

MONOCLONAL ANTIBODIES IN DERMATOPATHOLOGY

This will take place at Keele University on Wednesday 19 September 1984 immediately prior to the winter meeting of the British Society of Investigative Dermatology. Guest speakers include Dr Kirk Ruiter from Leiden and Dr Julia Polak from London.

Further details from: Dr Robin Russell Jones, Secretary, British Society for Dermatopathology, St John's Hospital for Diseases of the Skin, Lisle Street, Leicester Square, London WC2H 7BJ, U.K.

PUBLISHING AGREEMENT

1. It is our custom to request authors to vest the worldwide copyright of their papers in John Wiley & Sons Limited for the full term of copyright and we would be grateful if you would confirm your acceptance of these terms by signing and returning the agreement below. We will not withhold permission for any reasonable request from you to publish any part of this paper in connection with any other work by you, provided the usual acknowledgements are given regarding copyright notice and reference to the original publication.
2. If it is appropriate, the author's employer may sign this agreement, and in any event the employer may reserve the right to use the paper internally or for promotional purposes only, by so indicating on this agreement. It is understood that proprietary rights other than copyright (including patent rights) are reserved.
3. If the author is a U.S. Government employee and this work was done in that capacity the assignment applies only to the extent allowable by U.S. law. If at least one co-author is *not* a government employee, said author should sign the agreement.
4. If the author is an employee of the British Government then HMSO will grant a non-exclusive licence to publish this paper in the Journal in any form or media provided British crown copyright and user rights (including patent rights) are reserved.
5. The author warrants that the manuscript is the author's original work, and has not been published before. (If excerpts from copyrighted works are included, the author will obtain written permission from the copyright owners and show credit to the sources in the manuscript.) The author also warrants that the article contains no libellous or unlawful statements, and does not infringe on the rights of others.
6. If the work was prepared jointly the author agrees to inform co-authors of the terms of the agreement, and to sign on their behalf.

With the qualifications listed above I assign to John Wiley & Sons Limited, the copyright of my paper entitled ______________________________

____

for publication in ______________________________

______________________________ Signed

______________________________ Date

If the paper is rejected this assignment is null and void.

JOURNAL OF PATHOLOGY, VOL. **143**: 145–146 (1984)

EDITORIAL
THE DIAGNOSIS OF MALIGNANT MESOTHELIOMA

It is 24 years since Wagner *et al.* first recognized the association between malignant mesothelioma (MM) of the pleura and exposure to asbestos, particularly crocidolite.[1] During this period pathologists have become increasingly aware of this tumour and have become better able to recognize it and differentiate it from metastatic or pulmonary adenocarcinoma. In 1960 many pathologists, notably Willis,[2] doubted the existence of MM, while others had already recognized it as a primary tumour.[3] Wagner diagnosed many of his original cases on biopsy material alone, but most pathologists continued to consider that definitive diagnosis depended on the exclusion of an extra pleural primary at necropsy. Although diagnostic accuracy was improved by the demonstration (in some cases) of hyaluronidase sensitive mucopolysaccharides in tumour cells,[4] it was improved more by pathologists' familiarity with the highly characteristic histological appearances of MM.[5] The pendulum has now swung to such an extent that some cytopathologists are prepared to make a firm diagnosis of MM on cytological material alone.[6,7] This has been encouraged as a way of avoiding the risks of thoracotomy and open biopsy.[8] The disadvantage of cytology alone is that, because hyperplastic mesothelial cells can closely mimic MM, false positives can occur even with the most experienced observers.[7]

With the implications both of the financial compensation now available to patients with MM previously exposed to asbestos and of the increasing use of surgical treatment for MM (pleurectomy and pleuropneumonectomy), there is considerable pressure on pathologists and cytologists to provide early accurate diagnosis. The paper by Whittaker and Shilkin in this journal[9] gives valuable practical advice about making full use of information derived from pleural fluid analysis and Abram's needle biopsy. This may provide a definitive diagnosis in some cases but, more often, a presumptive one. There is an inherent fallacy in the concept that two probabilities make a certainty. A pleural fluid which contains morulae of atypical mesothelial cells lacking definite criteria of malignancy, and a biopsy showing invasive tumour but not of certain mesothelial origin, do not combine to give a definitive diagnosis of MM. Hyperplastic mesothelial cells can mimic MM, particularly in cirrhosis and pulmonary infarction, but also in the pleural reaction to metastatic carcinoma.[10]

From our own experience in Southampton, where we see more than 10 new cases of MM per year in surgical biopsy material, we would urge the greater use of thoracoscopy for diagnosis of this disease. This is a much simpler procedure than thoracotomy and provides a definite diagnosis in most cases (unpublished observations). Tracking of tumour through to the chest wall has not proved to be a major problem but can occur with any procedure, including aspiration of fluid.[8] Using the type of practical approach outlined by Whittaker and Shilkin, cases can be selected for a biopsy which will provide adequate material for histological diagnosis and confirmatory histochemical techniques.

AMANDA HERBERT
Southampton General Hospital

REFERENCES

1. Wagner JC, Sleggs CA and Marchand P. Diffuse pleural mesothelioma and asbestos exposure in the North West Cape Province. *Br J Industr Med* 1960; **17**: 260–271.
2. Willis RA. In: Pathology of Tumours. Vol. 53, 1st and 2nd edn. London: Butterworth, 1948.
3. McCaughey WTE. Primary tumours of the pleura. *J Pathol Bacteriol* 1958; **76**: 517–529.
4. Wagner JC, Munday DE and Harington JS. Histochemical demonstration of hyaluronic acid in pleural mesotheliomas. *J Pathol Bacteriol* 1962; **84**: 73–78.
5. McCaughey WTE. Criteria for the diagnosis of malignant mesothelial tumors. *Ann NY Acad Sci* 1965; **132**: 603.
6. Naylor B. The exfoliative cytology of diffuse malignant mesotheliomas. *J Pathol Bacteriol* 1963; **86**: 293.
7. Butler EB and Berry AV. Diffuse mesothelioma:

diagnostic criteria using exfoliative cytology. In: Biological Effects of Asbestos. Lyon: International Agency for Research on Cancer, 1973: 68.

8. Elmes PC and Simpson MJC. The clinical aspects of mesothelioma. *Am J Med* 1976, **45:** 427–449.
9. Whittaker D and Shilkin KM. Diagnosis of pleural malignant mesothelioma in life—a practical approach. *J Path* 1984; **143:** 147–175.
10. Herbert A and Gallagher PJ. Pleural biopsy in the diagnosis of malignant mesothelioma. *Thorax* 1982; **37:** 816–821.

JOURNAL OF PATHOLOGY, VOL. **143**: 147–175 (1984)

DIAGNOSIS OF PLEURAL MALIGNANT MESOTHELIOMA IN LIFE—A PRACTICAL APPROACH

DARREL WHITAKER*‡ AND KEITH B. SHILKIN†

**Cytology Unit, Combined Anatomical Pathology Services, and †Department of Histopathology, Sir Charles Gairdner Hospital, Nedlands 6009, Western Australia*

Received 30 December 1983
Accepted 29 February 1984

SUMMARY

This review documents a practical approach to the pathological diagnosis of pleural malignant mesothelioma based on the closed needle biopsy and effusion cytology, thus avoiding the need to resort to open surgery. Tissue diagnosis is often difficult, and the pathologist's opinion may be influenced by a consideration of three factors: the clinical setting; the adequacy and availability of specimens; and the criteria for assessment and interpretation of these. The level of confidence with which a tissue diagnosis of mesothelioma can be established using limited material depends on there being an appropriate clinical background including a history of asbestos exposure. Without this, the diagnosis should be a qualified or tentative one. For an adequate tissue sample to be obtained, the closed needle biopsy procedure is best performed by an experienced operator. All aspirated pleural effusions should be forwarded for cytological evaluation. In addition to conventional morphological studies, adequate samples permit ancillary tests to be carried out. A combined interpretive approach utilizing both histopathology and cytology is recommended in order to increase the accuracy of the diagnosis.

KEY WORDS—Mesothelioma, diagnosis, pleural biopsy, cytopathology.

INTRODUCTION

Many pleural malignant mesotheliomas are still diagnosed only at necropsy. In life, the diagnosis is often established only after open chest surgery which, unfortunately, is hazardous in this disease. To enable correct management of these patients there is a need for early diagnosis using minimal intervention. Further, in those exposed industrially to asbestos early diagnosis is of importance if they are to receive compensation during their lifetime.

This review examines the problems associated with making an early tissue diagnosis of malignant mesothelioma. Guided by our experience over the past 10 years we shall describe our present approach to this problem. Earlier reviewers, in addressing themselves to the many facets of this subject have invariably concluded that the early diagnosis of malignant mesothelioma is difficult, if not impossible, without resorting to open surgical biopsy[1–4] despite that procedure's well-recognized complication of neoplastic spread into the surgical wound and from there into the chest wall and nearby structures.[5,6]

With the increasing incidence of the disease there is a greater awareness of mesothelioma; there is also widespread sharing of data derived from national and international review panels and programmes of surveillance. In our view, significant improvements can now be made to increase the accuracy of diagnosis during life. This requires a new approach to the use of the closed needle pleural biopsy and the cytological assessment of pleural fluid. We will discuss firstly our use of these specimens and the various investigations that may contribute to the diagnosis of malignant mesothelioma. We will then consider in more

‡Author to whom correspondence should be addressed.

0022–3417/84/070147–29$02.90

detail the relative contribution of histopathology, cytology, and ancillary tests. Finally, we will examine an approach that correlates this information to provide the basis for an accurate diagnosis without the need to resort to open surgery.

GENERAL CONSIDERATIONS

Specimens

Two types of specimen are most frequently submitted to the laboratory when a diagnosis of mesothelioma is being considered: firstly, a core or fragment of pleural tissue obtained by closed needle biopsy and, secondly, pleural effusions. Both specimens are valuable and permit several forms of investigation, although the contribution to diagnosis from each may vary.

Although pleural malignant mesothelioma is a diffuse disease, a needle biopsy taken in the early stages of its development or by inexperienced operators may miss the lesion or may sample only thickened fibrous pleura not containing neoplasm. It is not uncommon for such blind biopsies to contain no recognizable mesothelial cells, and, in our own material, 15 per cent of our cases of mesothelioma fell into this category on the initial biopsy.[7] Obviously, such biopsies must be interpreted as being non-contributory rather than negative. Concerning fluids for cytological assessment, clinicians should be encouraged to forward adequate volumes, if not all of the effusion, to the laboratory for analysis and not to discard most of it, as is commonplace.

Investigations

There are many investigations which may be undertaken. We consider that several examinations should be performed routinely and that the pathologist's opinion is best based on an appraisal of all the information gained from both fluid and tissue samples. Such a combined approach to the diagnosis of malignant pleural disease is not new. Using cytology of effusions and histology of closed needle biopsies Salyer *et al.*[8] were able to increase their diagnostic accuracy of pleural malignancy from 56 per cent using biopsy alone, or 66 per cent using cytology alone, to 90 per cent when both methods were used. Kannerstein and his colleagues[9] were the first investigators to advocate this approach for mesothelioma; however, this combined method of study has found only partial acceptance.[6]

HISTOPATHOLOGY OF MESOTHELIOMA

The classical appearances of mesothelioma are now well recognized and several excellent and detailed descriptions are available.[1, 10–12] These illustrative accounts are based on the histological examination of abundant tissue, including necropsy material, this being necessary to gain a broad perspective of the variability of histological pattern. In this section we emphasize the histological problems associated with small closed needle biopsy samples.

Histological patterns

The epithelial pattern is characterized by papillary, tubular, acinar-like, or solid growth, which is composed of pavement-like cells in a stroma of variable cellularity and density (Figs 1–3). Slit-like spaces are often present. When forming papillae or tubules, the tumour cells are usually cuboidal, when lining the slit-like spaces they are frequently flattened. Although this type of histological pattern has some similarities to an adenocarcinoma, including papillary adenocarcinoma, the slit-like spaces and cuboidal nature of the cells are helpful distinguishing features, and the overall appearance is generally characteristic of mesothelioma. There is a wide variation, however, in appearance, and poorly-differentiated tumours remain a problem.

The sarcomatous pattern of mesothelioma is characterized by spindle-cell growth. Often this has a monotonous picture of well-aligned malignant spindle cells, but whorls or herring bone arrangements are not uncommon. Occasionally, the spindle-cell pattern has no particular arrangement.

Desmoplastic variants are recognized in which the degree of cellularity and pleomorphism can vary greatly. Epithelial-like cell structures are characteristically absent in this form of mesothelioma. Sometimes the cellularity is so sparse that distinction from a benign fibrous reaction is difficult.

Biphasic mesotheliomas are common and many

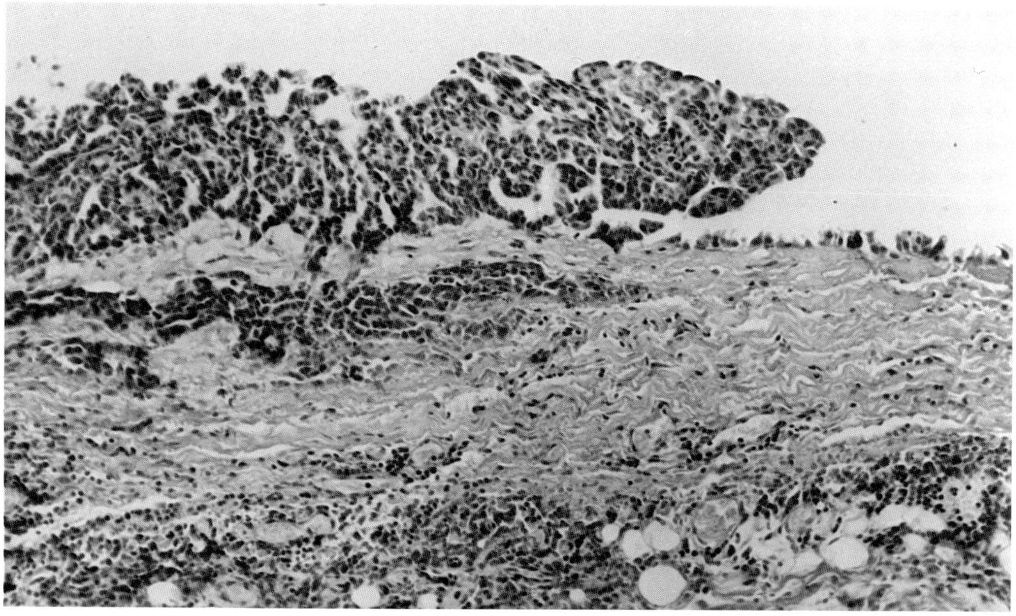

Fig. 1—Mesothelioma. Surface tubopapillary growth with tumour infiltrating into the serosa. Several collections of lymphocytes are also present. Pleural needle biopsy

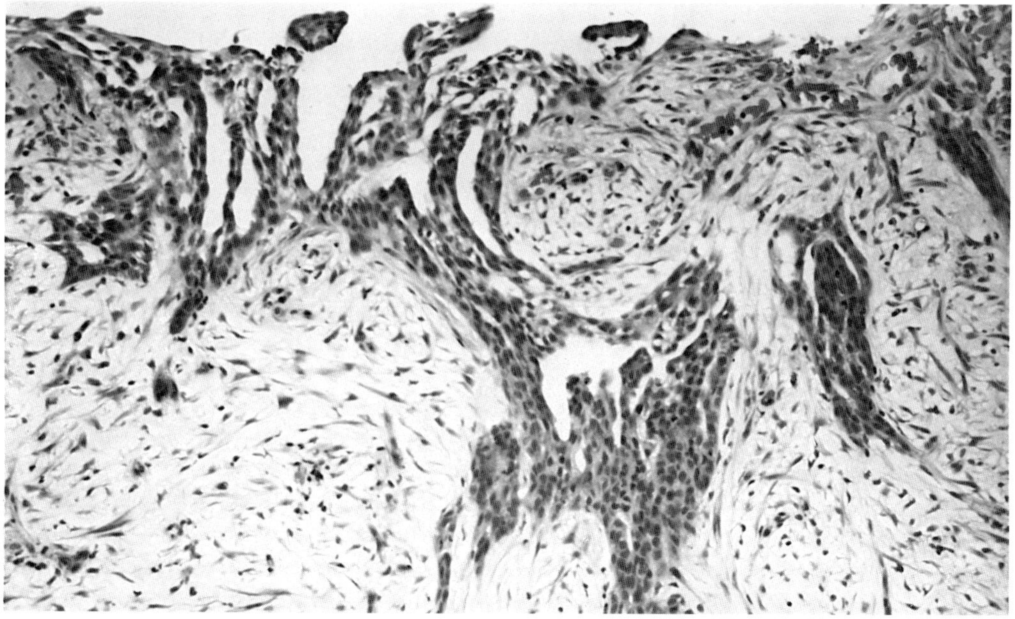

Fig. 2—Mesothelioma. Both surface papillary growth and tongues of infiltrating tumour are shown. Several small slit-like spaces are also seen. Pleural needle biopsy

pathologists believe that with sufficient sampling most malignant mesotheliomas can be so characterized. Foci of epithelial growth, usually either solid or tubo-papillary but which may be of any pattern, are found interspersed within sarcomatous growth. The proportion of each varies. This biphasic pattern, while not entirely pathognomic, is quite characteristic of mesothelioma.

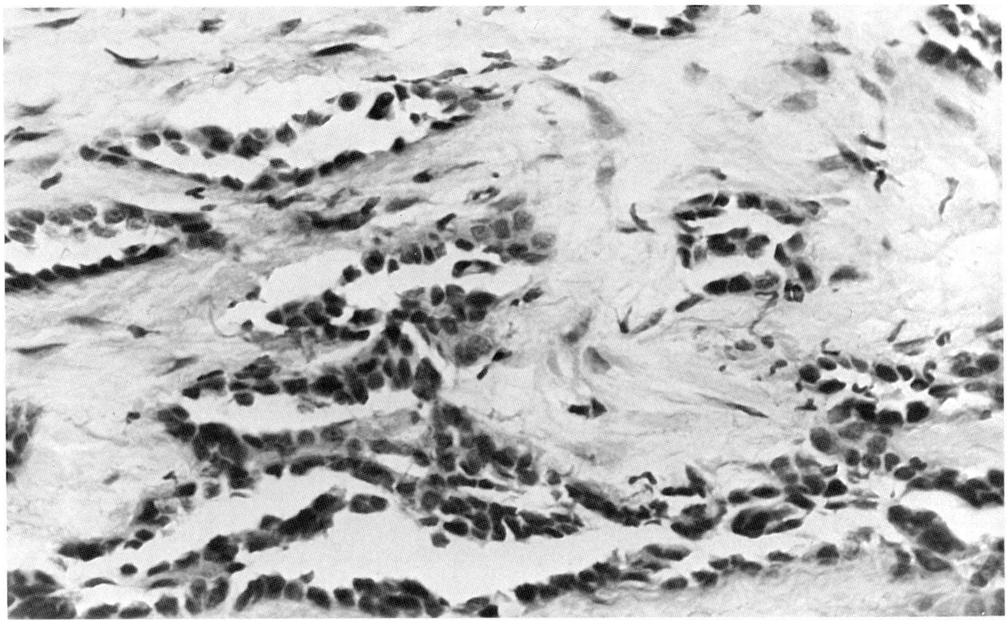

Fig. 3—Mesothelioma. Several neoplastic tubules with slit-like spaces are lined by cuboidal mesothelioma cells. Pleural needle biopsy

The role of closed pleural needle biopsy

While this technique is frequently used to diagnose metastatic malignant pleural disease, it is held to be of limited value in establishing a diagnosis of malignant mesothelioma.[1,4,9,13] Data on the accuracy of the technique are not easy to obtain, but a success rate of 60 per cent is claimed by Edge and Choudhury.[6] In our series 39 per cent of mesotheliomas were correctly diagnosed initially by closed needle biopsy.[7]

There are two inter-related problems associated with this technique: obtaining sufficient material; and the histological interpretation of small biopsy samples. While it is held that inadequacy of material is the most common difficulty, Herbert and Gallagher[14] found their interpretation to be more perplexing. Obtaining an adequate albeit small amount of tissue depends on the skill of the operator. The problem of interpretation can be divided into two distinct facets: firstly, to distinguish malignant mesothelioma from benign reactive mesothelial proliferation and, secondly, to distinguish malignant mesothelioma from metastatic pleural tumours.

It should be stressed that no absolute criteria exist for the definitive diagnosis of malignant mesothelioma on such small biopsies alone. What follows are guidelines enabling a tentative assessment to be made which, when considered with other data such as cytology of effusions and the clinical setting, may more clearly indicate the true nature of the disease and enable the pathologist to increase the confidence of his opinion.

Special histological features of closed needle biopsies

The cellular 'hallmarks' of malignancy, such as pleomorphism, nuclear enlargement, irregularity, hyperchromasia, and nucleolar prominence, are characteristically found in mesothelioma[14, 17–19] (Fig. 4). Mitotic activity is only a common feature in less well-differentiated types.[12] Mesothelial cell cytoplasm, benign or malignant, is abundant, optically dense, and usually intensely eosinophilic, but frequently has a slightly basophilic hue.[11,20] The cytoplasm is often finely vacuolated producing a bubbly[12, 13, 17] or even ground glass appearance,[2] the outer cytoplasm often being encircled by a ring of vacuoles and ending in a dense, homogenous rim (Figs 5, 6).

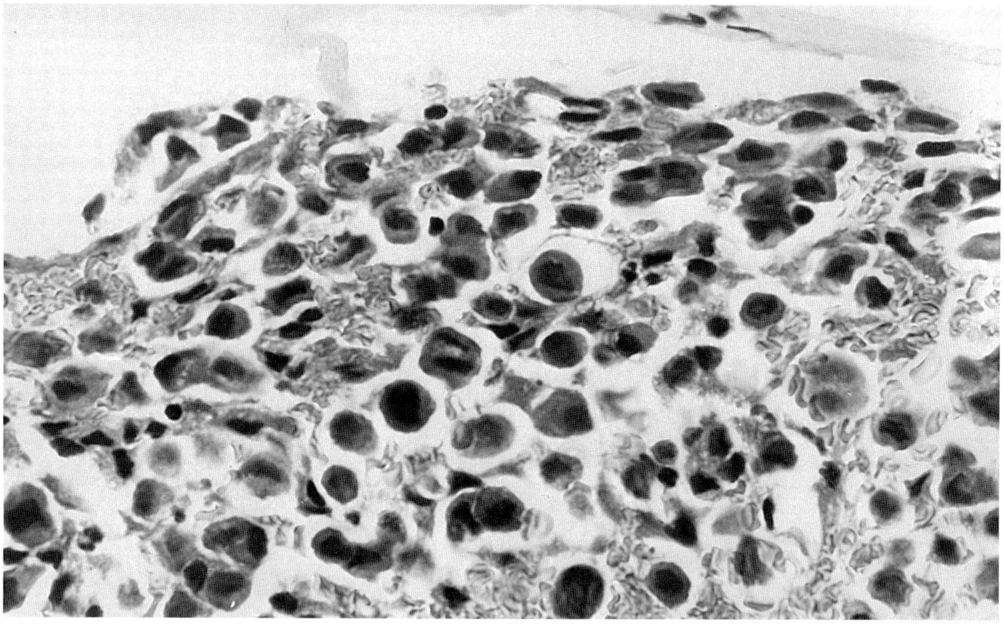

Fig. 4—Mesothelioma. Showing only single rounded malignant cells with no particular architectural arrangement. Pleural needle biopsy

Mesothelial cell shape is variable depending on the presence or absence of an effusion and location.[16] When mesothelial cells are situated on the serosal surface as a single layer, they are cuboidal, dome-shaped, or even peg-like, and produce an uneven, picket-fence arrangement. Kawai *et al.*[21] also describe infrequent columnar mesothelial cells. While elongated forms are

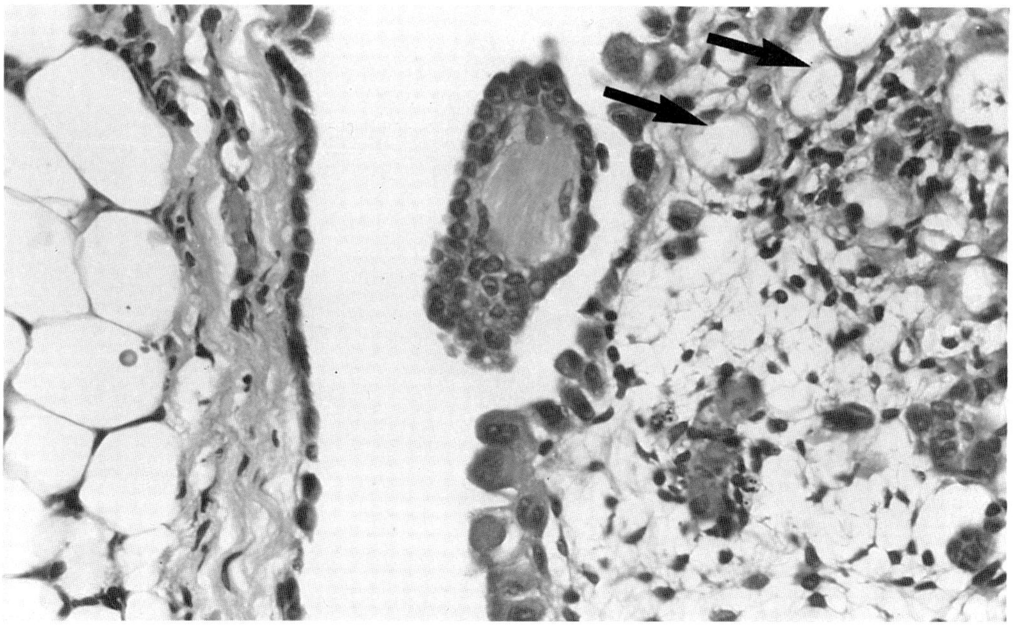

Fig. 5—Atypical proliferation. Enlarged atypical mesothelial cells, signet ring forms (arrows) and a papillary structure are present. Pleural tissue from thoracotomy

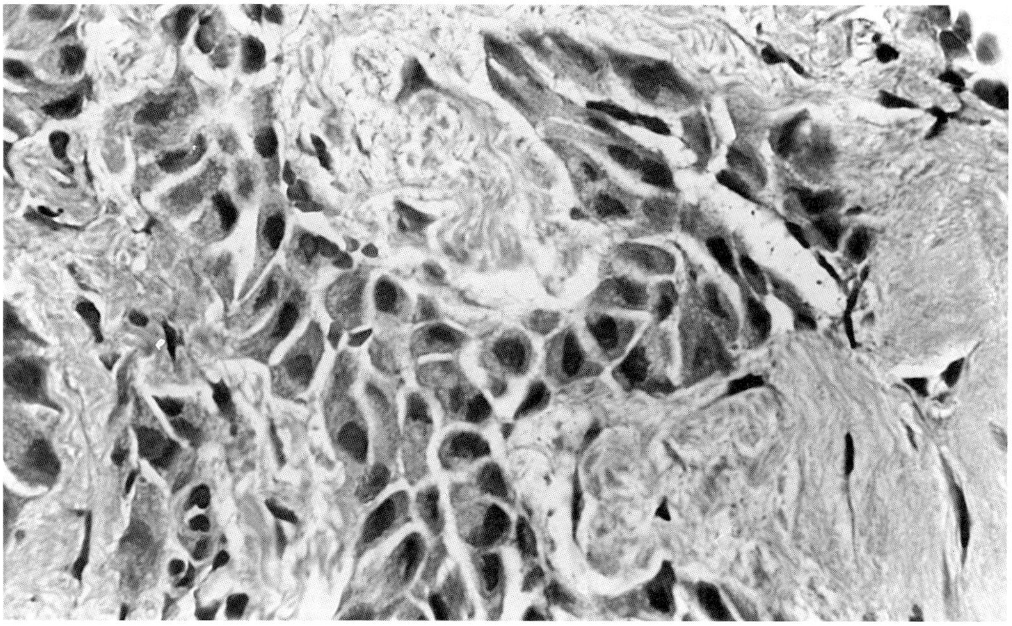

Fig. 6—Mesothelioma. Showing a collection of squamoid-like mesothelioma cells with finely vacuolated cytoplasm. Pleural needle biopsy

occasionally found, their nuclei are usually located in the central or luminal aspect of the cell (Fig. 7) and not at its base as is more typical of columnar cells. We believe that the cell shape is of considerable importance irrespective of the architectural arrangement: cuboidal cells favour mesothelioma, whereas columnar cells are more suggestive of adenocarcinoma. Shedding of

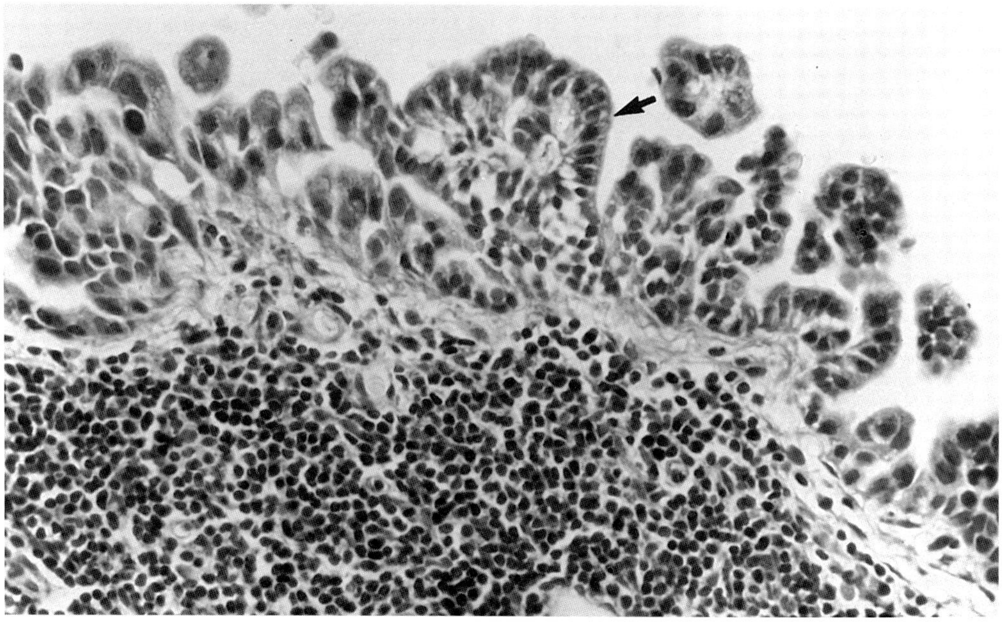

Fig. 7—Mesothelioma. Surface papillary formation with a spectrum of cell shapes. A few cells are elongated (arrow), and others are rounded or cuboidal. Note the dense lymphocytic infiltrate in the serosa. Pleural needle biopsy

mesothelial cells results in dissociated collections of round cells (Fig. 4). In more compact sheets, they form a mosaic of polygonal cells.

The identification of multilayering and irregular cell crowding is considered a prerequisite for the diagnosis of malignant mesothelioma.[17] The problem of false multilayering caused by tangential cutting of the flat surfaces of mesothelial cells was highlighted by Sheldon *et al.*[18] One can avoid this potential trap if the following points are remembered: in sections with tangential cuts, the mesothelial sheet will usually have peaks and troughs, resembling a mosaic with prominent inter-cellular bridges (Fig. 8); in such false multilayering the nuclei are regular and round; on the other hand, collections of mesothelioma cells show nuclear atypia and have an irregular configuration (Figs 3, 6).

Papillary growth is a particularly common feature in the epithelial form of malignant mesothelioma (Figs 7, 9). While longstanding serous effusion of any aetiology can result in mesothelial papillary formation, its recognition in needle biopsies of the pleura other than in mesothelioma is rare.[14]

Mesothelial invasion into the subserosa and adjacent tissues is perhaps the strongest evidence for a malignant process. It should be noted that, in rare instances, tubular and acinar-like structures composed of benign mesothelial cells can be seen trapped in the subserosa in reactive pleurisy[9,22] (Fig. 10). These commonly appear as rounded discrete structures, whereas true invasion is characterized by foci of tumour cells having irregular, elongated, penetrating outlines (Fig. 11).

When adequate tissue is available for examination, most malignant mesotheliomas of the pleura can be characterized as biphasic;[11] however, it is unusual to find both these elements in small needle biopsies. Although sarcomatous mesothelioma can be diagnosed by this method, it is far more common to find only the epithelial-like growth on the serosal surface constituting most of the material in a needle biopsy. This is almost certainly due to preferential epithelial differentiation in the proximity of an effusion.[23]

Problems in differential diagnosis in closed needle biopsies

In this section we wish to highlight five main problems in differential diagnosis.

Reactive mesothelial proliferation.
Metastatic malignancy, particularly adenocarcinoma.

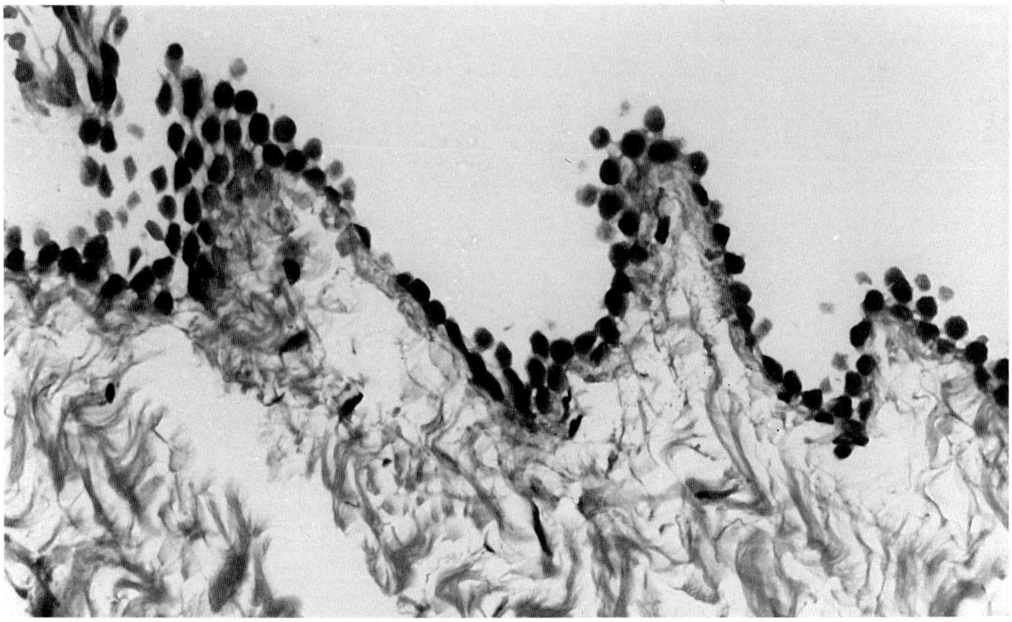

Fig. 8—Apparent hyperplasia due to tangential cutting. Note the peak and trough arrangement and mesothelial cell stacks showing intercellular 'bridges'. Pleural needle biopsy

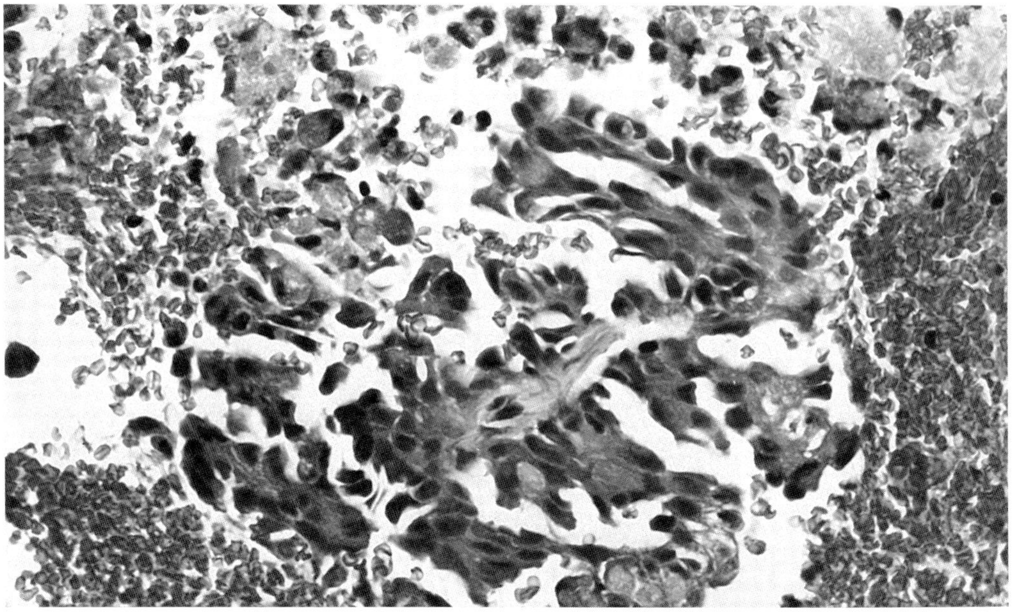

Fig. 9—Mesothelioma. A fibrovascular papillary structure is composed of mesothelial cells showing nuclear atypia. Pleural needle biopsy

Anaplastic and unusual forms of mesothelioma.
Reactive fibrosis.
Lymphocytic infiltration.

Reactive mesothelial proliferation—Without doubt, the greatest problem in the differential diagnosis of mesothelioma in small biopsies lies in distinguishing malignant from reactive prolifera-

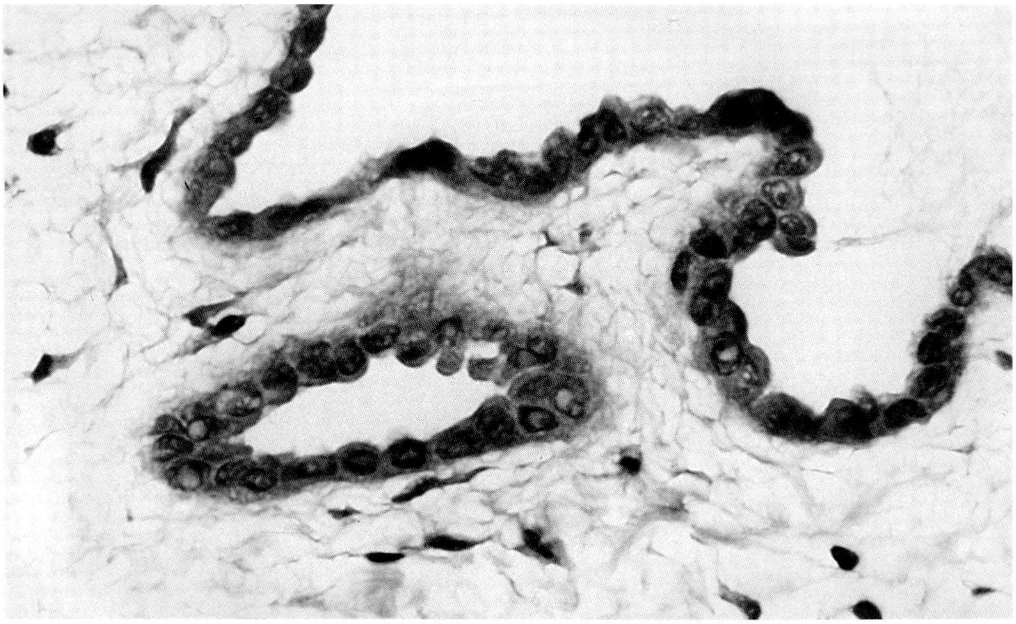

Fig. 10—Benign reaction. There is a single layer of cuboidal mesothelial cells with a pseudo-gland structure possibly representing entrapped benign mesothelium. Pleural needle biopsy

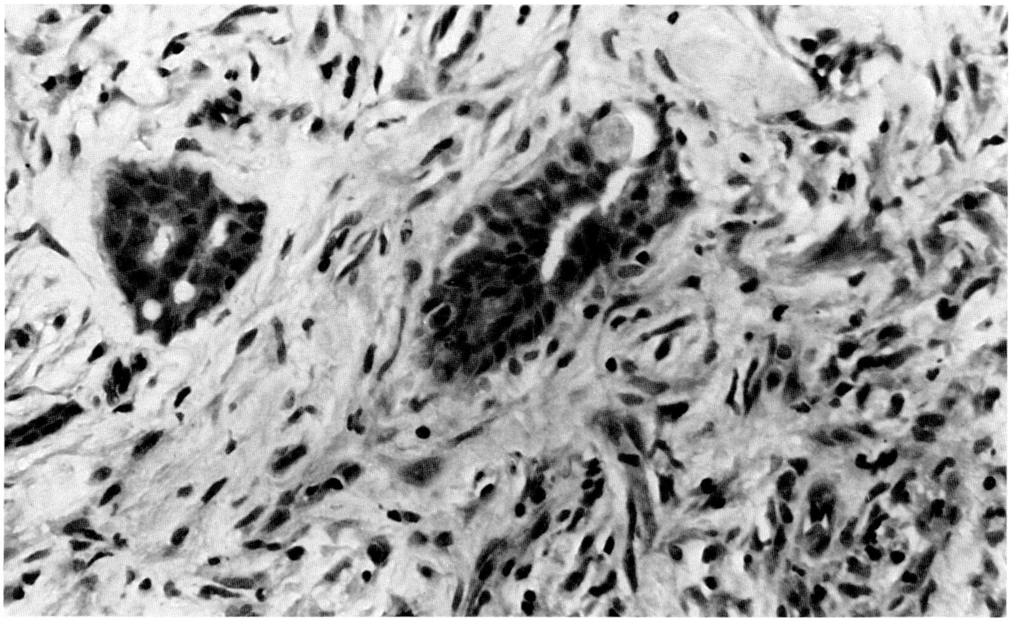

Fig. 11—Mesothelioma. Two pseudo-acini of mesothelioma. Compare the irregular shape of this malignant infiltrate with the benign rounded structure in Fig. 10. Pleural needle biopsy

tions of mesothelial cells. The latter usually appears as mesothelial hyperplasia with multilayering and is commonly seen as a consequence of long-standing effusions. It is frequently present in needle biopsies taken during and after pleurisy from any cause. Mesothelial hyperplasia is most commonly located superficially, appearing as compact stacks of cells or focal collections of shed, separated cells lying amongst fibrin (Fig. 12). Occasionally, it is also possible to identify better

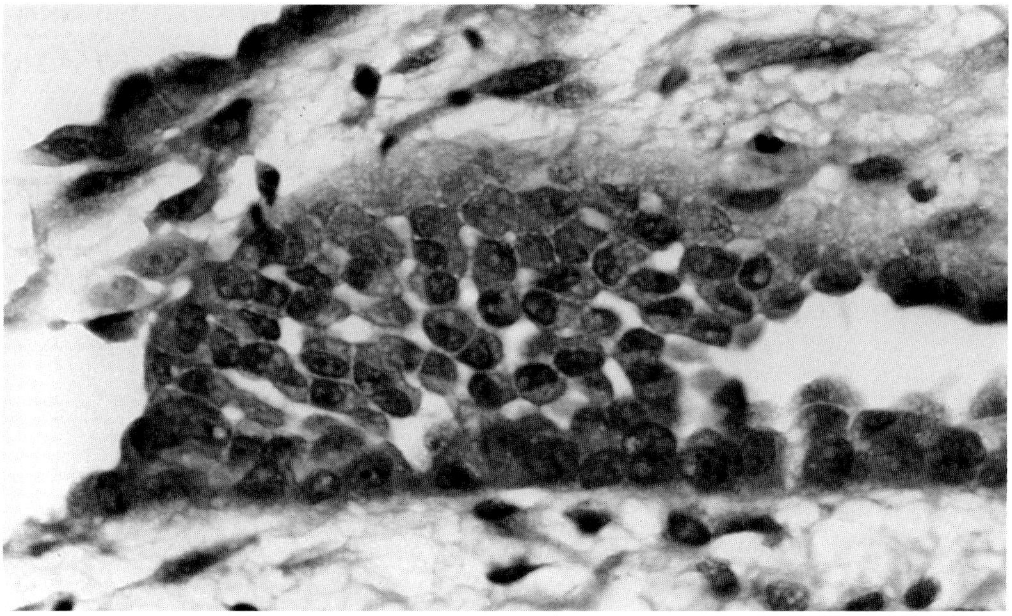

Fig. 12—Benign reaction. This demonstrates a collection of rounded and polygonal mesothelial cells within a tubular structure. Pleural needle biopsy

defined mesothelial structures, including papillary, acinar, and tubular arrangements. Such patterns cause the greatest interpretive problems.

Benign papillary formations are a well-recognized differential diagnostic problem in the pericardium[24,25] and in hernial sacs,[26] yet they occur less frequently in the pleura.[14] Herbert and Gallagher[14] studied the histopathology of mesothelial proliferation and mesothelioma in small needle biopsies and found that mesothelial papillae were a strong indication of malignant mesothelioma. We concur with their findings. In our retrospective studies, at least two cases initially reported as unusual atypical mesothelial proliferation with papillae were subsequently proven to be mesotheliomas. One additional case suspected (but as yet unproven) of being a mesothelioma had several well-developed surface mesothelial papillary structures but no evidence of invasion (Fig. 13). Nevertheless, such structures are not pathognomic of mesothelioma and we have seen two cases which featured well-developed mesothelial papillae in sections of benign pleural tissue obtained at thoracotomy. One such example was from a 20-year-old female who had an apical pleurectomy for recurrent spontaneous pneumothorax (Fig. 14).

Nuclear size was considered to be an important discriminator between reactive proliferations and mesothelioma by Kwee *et al.*[27] These authors measured the nuclear areas of benign and malignant mesothelial cells morphometrically; nuclear areas below 30 μm^2 were found only in the reactive mesothelium.

Metastatic malignancy, particularly adenocarcinoma—The histological distinction between the more common metastatic malignancies and malignant mesothelioma of the serous cavities can be difficult. This diagnostic problem, however, is greater in the peritoneum, especially in females, than in the pleura.[10] In the pleura, papillary adenocarcinomas may be confused with the epithelial form of mesothelioma,[10,28] whereas metastatic spindle-cell tumours may be indistinguishable from the sarcomatous variety of mesothelioma. Nevertheless, only a few malignant cells, devoid of any architectural arrangement, may be present in a needle biopsy. In this instance, the distinction lies in the recognition of mesothelial cell characteristics (previously described). To compound the problem it is possible in pleural metastatic carcinoma for cells to be distributed as a monolayer on the serosal membrane thus mimicking mesothelioma (Fig. 15). In cases of difficulty, ancillary tests, such as histochemistry and im-

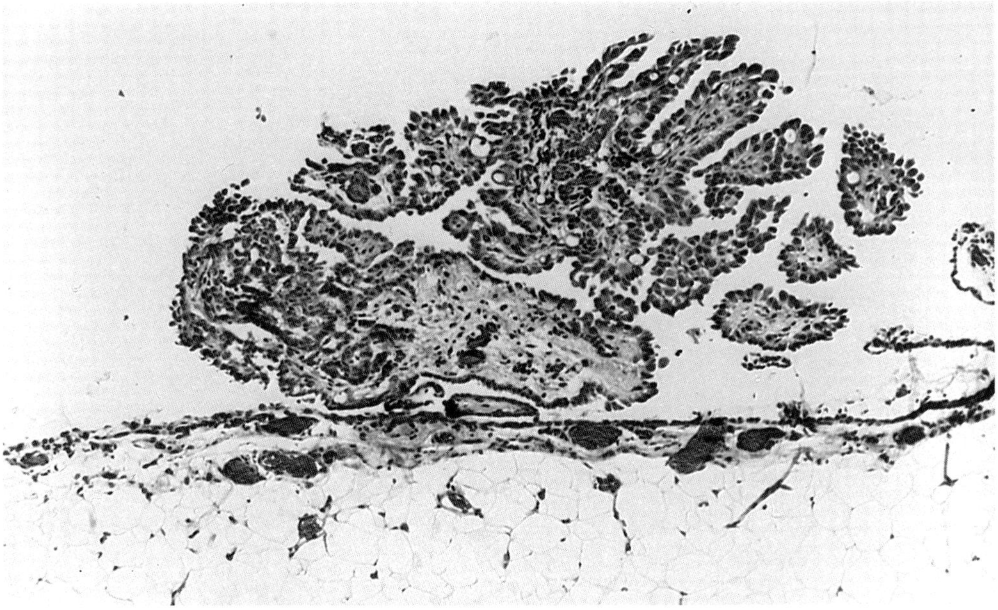

Fig. 13—Atypical proliferation. A focal atypical cellular proliferation of mesothelium protrudes from the parietal serosa. Pleural tissue from thoracotomy

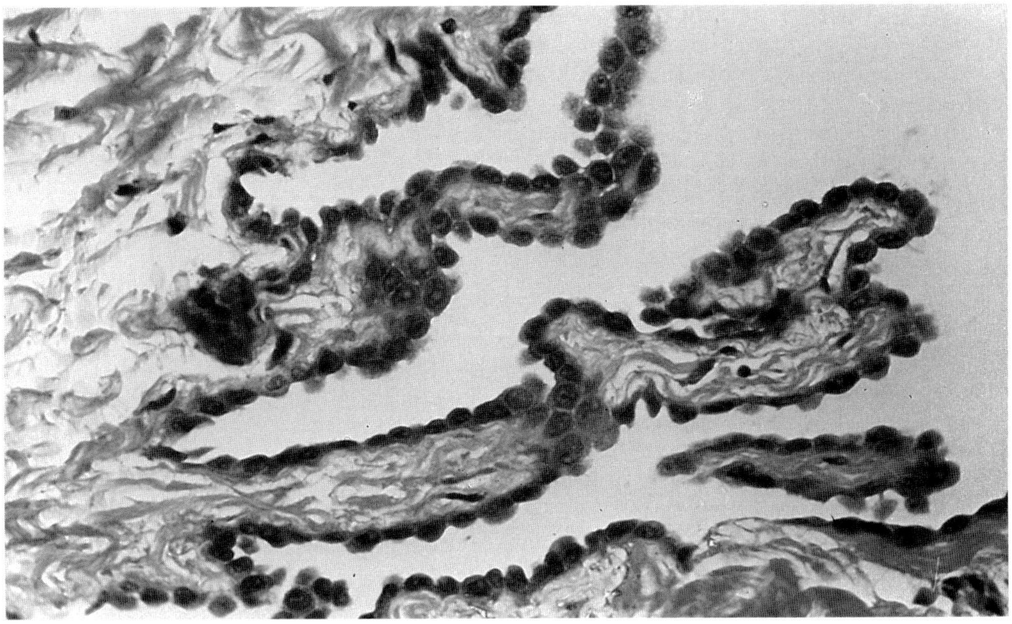

Fig. 14—Benign papillary formation. Multiple simple papillary structures protrude from the serosal surface. Pleural tissue from thoracotomy

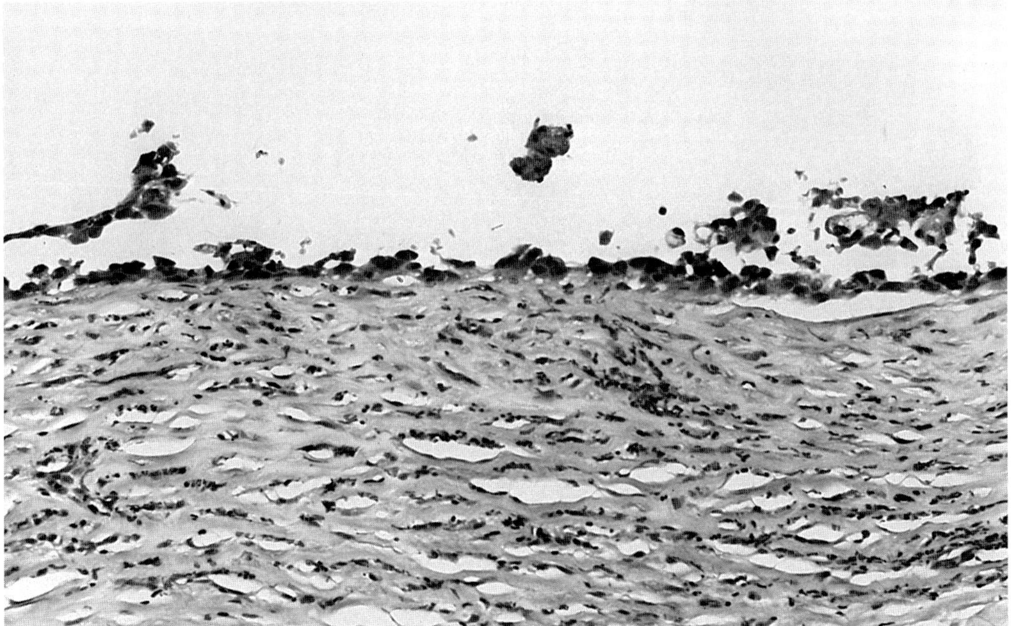

Fig. 15—Metastatic carcinoma. Note the monolayer distribution of tumour cells mimicking early mesothelioma. Pleural needle biopsy

munohistochemistry, are useful in distinguishing mesothelioma from metastatic carcinoma especially adenocarcinoma, and this is discussed later.

Anaplastic and unusual forms of mesothelioma—The great diversity of appearances found in mesothelioma is well recognized. Kannerstein *et al.*[1] have described these variations in terms of 'vertical differentiation' or degree of anaplasia, and 'horizontal differentiation' or cell type. The problem of tumour typing is greater when only small samples are available from needle biopsy specimens in that they may not be wholly representative. Unless clinically suspected, anaplastic or poorly differentiated varieties will rarely be classified correctly in the first instance. The less common forms of mesothelioma include desmoplastic tumours,[29,30] adenomatoid-like or microcystic-like,[1,12] and 'adeno-squamous'[31] tumours. Awareness of these histological patterns will be helpful when mesothelioma is being considered by the pathologist. Additionally, there is a need to be aware of the entity of benign pleural fibroma[16] whenever there is a pleural mass and the biopsy contains poorly cellular fibrous tissue.

Reactive fibroblasts—Because malignant mesothelioma can present as a spindle-cell or biphasic neoplasm, the interpretation of plump, spindle cells in the subserosal connective tissue warrants careful evaluation. The finding of abnormal fibroblastic-like growth, with such features as nuclear hyperchromasia and irregularity, is suggestive of mesothelioma[14,30] (Fig. 16).

Lymphocytes—The presence of numerous inflammatory cells, particularly a dense lymphocytic infiltration, can make the histological interpretation of a pleural needle biopsy difficult. Mesothelial proliferation within such a biopsy should probably be viewed as benign in the absence of other strong evidence of a malignant process;[22] however, focal accumulations of lymphocytes are not uncommon in malignant mesothelioma[1,2,17] and may be found in needle biopsies (Figs 1, 6). Leigh and Webster[32] found some form of lymphocytic infiltration in 30 per cent of their mesotheliomas and believed they indicated longer survival.

CYTOPATHOLOGY OF MESOTHELIOMA

The value of cytology in the diagnosis of malignant mesothelioma is controversial, some investigators claiming good results[27,33–38] others[2,14,39–41] finding it of little value. Kannerstein *et al.*[1] stress that a 'high level of competence

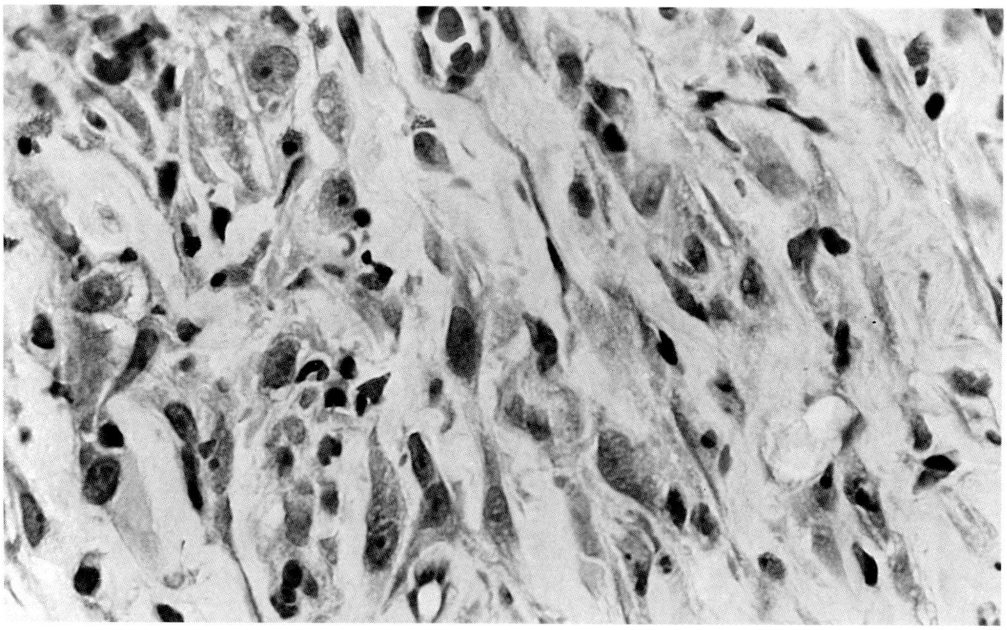

Fig. 16—Mesothelioma. Malignant spindle cells are seen within the stroma. Pleural needle biopsy

and experience are necessary in the application of the cytologic modality'. We believe that, with experience, it is possible in many cases to make a confident diagnosis of malignant mesothelioma through the cytological study of effusions. Further, as we discuss and emphasize here, cytology has an important role when used in conjunction with closed needle biopsy of tissues. At the outset it should be stated that we completely agree with Tao[37] that the cytology of effusions has little or no value in the diagnosis of benign pleural tumours.

Application

Effusions are common in mesotheliomas and these offer the possibility of a good sample in most cases. In a recent paper Chahinian *et al.*[41] reported that 95 per cent of their cases had a serous effusion; our figure was closer to 75 per cent.[7] Regrettably, effusions are sometimes discarded and not sent for cytodiagnosis. Physicians' awareness of the value of cytology in the diagnosis of mesothelioma can prevent the loss of such samples, and this, together with increasing accuracy in cytodiagnosis, leads to increasing acceptance and use of fluid for cytological evaluation. Before 1975, 72 per cent of mesotheliomatous pleural effusions were sent to our laboratory, whereas presently the figure is 92 per cent.

Accuracy

To enhance the success of cytodiagnosis two aspects require particular attention: laboratory technique and interpretation. While considerable interest has been directed to cyto-morphology, less attention has been paid to technique. Butler and Berry[35] were the first to advocate the use of smears and cell blocks as well as ancillary techniques. When the cell-block method[14,20] is used solely, limited information usually results. Gupta and Frost[40] also recently stressed the need for the collection of good samples, the use of several techniques, and the need for clinical information as well as the application of definitive diagnostic criteria. We also use this approach[36] and with increasing experience accuracy is enhanced and overall performance also increases. Before 1975 we correctly diagnosed malignant mesothelioma through the cytology of effusions on 25 per cent of occasions; the present sensitivity of this test in our department is 62 per cent. This success rate may be partially explained by a high awareness of the possibility of mesothelioma provided by information concerning asbestos exposure on the consultation request forms and our special interest in the cytology of mesothelioma. This combination of special interest in the cytodiagnosis of mesothelioma and a cohort in which advice concerning asbestos exposure was available, previously resulted in the detection of 20 out of 26 cases (77 per cent).[6]

Descriptive cytology

The cytological diagnosis of malignant mesothelioma is a two-phase process and is based on recognizing cells with malignant characteristics, and that these cells are mesothelial in nature.[9,35,36] Normally, the cytological diagnosis of malignancy is based on nuclear criteria, such as pleomorphism, irregularity of nuclear membrane, chromatin distribution, and nuclear and nucleolar shape; however, in some cases of mesothelioma the effusion is so overwhelmingly cellular, possessing numerous large aggregates of atypical mesothelial cells, that mesothelioma may be suspected in the absence of overt malignant nuclei.

Characteristic cytological features (epithelial and biphasic varieties) include the following.

Cell aggregates.
Characteristic cytoplasm with cell enlargement.
Specialized cell borders.
Multinucleation.
Cell-to-cell apposition.
Uniform cell population.

Cell aggregates—Without doubt, the finding of numerous cell aggregates of varying size is the most distinctive feature of mesothelioma[37,42–44] (Figs 17, 18). These structures are composed of 5–200 or more cells and are frequently rounded with a knobbly edge; they can, however, be elongated or even frond-like and represent broken off papillary fragments floating in the effusion. In sections of cell blocks made from such effusions, the structure of the aggregates is more clearly seen. While many are hollow and consist of a ring of cells with centrally placed nuclei,[35] others have a collagenous core, confirming their true papillary nature (Figs 18, 19). Once malignancy has been established, the presence of aggregates with collagen cores has diagnostic significance. While

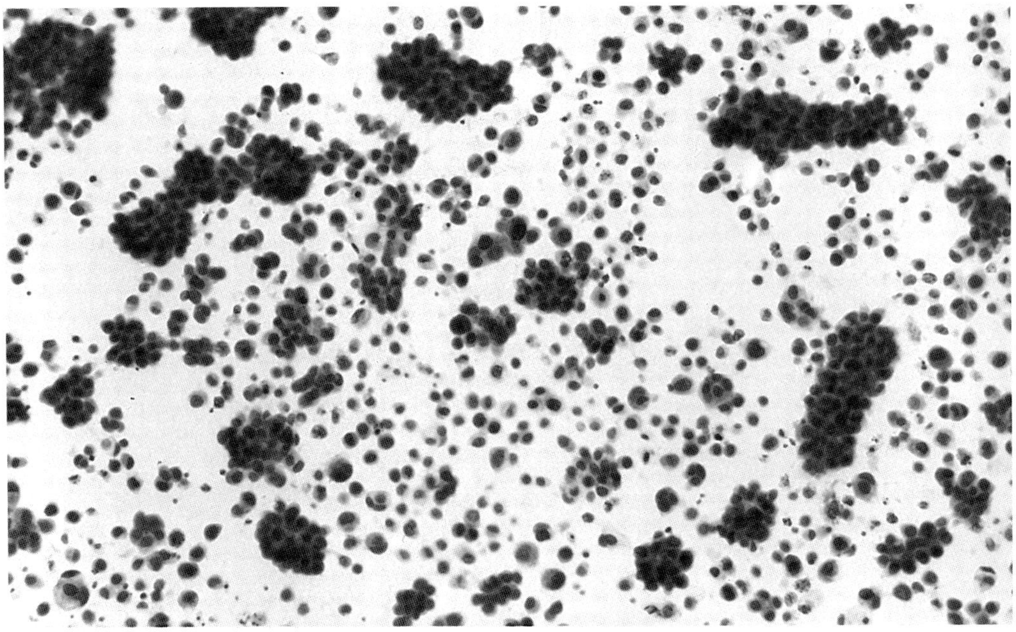

Fig. 17—Mesothelioma. Numerous cell clusters and many free mesothelioma cells are seen. Effusion smear. Papanicolaou stain

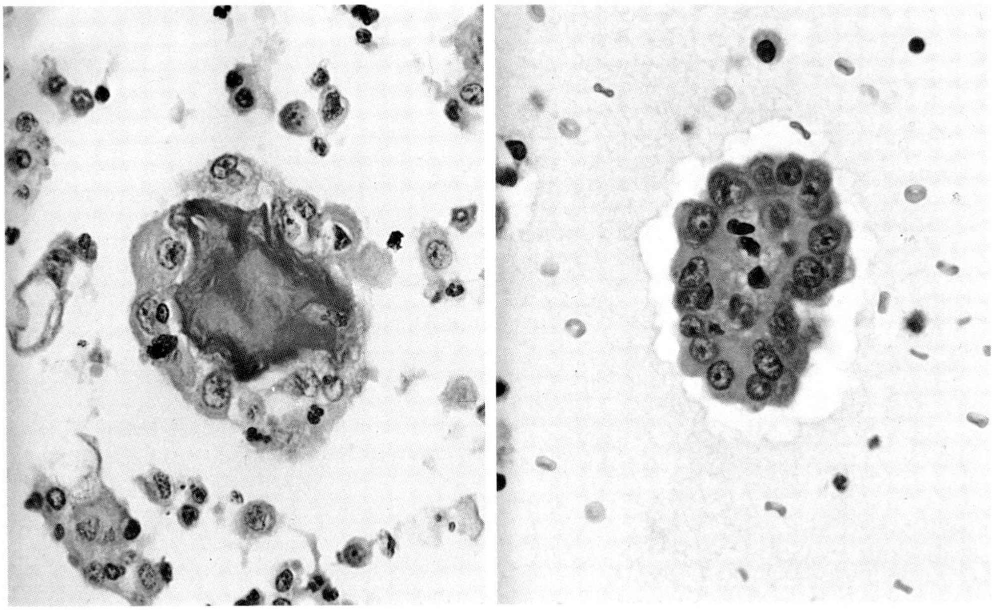

(a) (b)

Fig. 18—(a) Mesothelioma. A papillary cluster showing a collagen core. Cell block. (b) Mesothelioma. Showing a solid cluster of cuboidal cells. Cell block

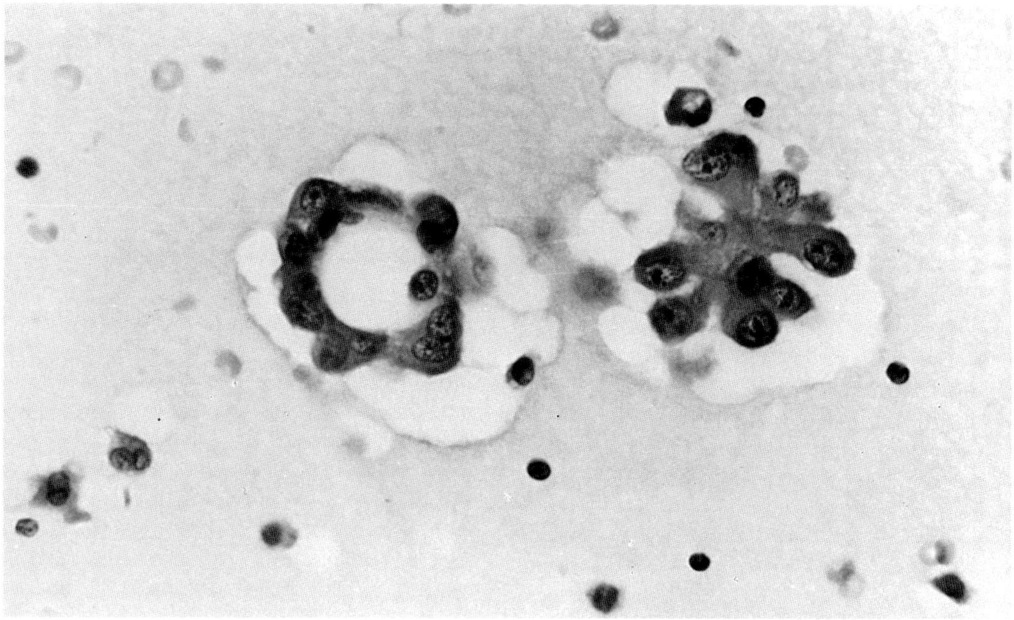

Fig. 19—Mesothelioma. Two small clusters of cuboidal mesothelioma cells, one with pseudo-acinar structure the other with a characteristically papillary arrangement. Effusion smear. Papanicolaou stain

they are common in mesothelioma, true papillary aggregates are uncommon in metastatic adenocarcinoma.[43] We have found abundant mesothelial aggregates of varying size together with large numbers of free malignant mesothelial cells to be the most characteristic picture of mesothelioma.

Characteristic cytoplasm—Mesothelial cytoplasm of benign or malignant cells has a characteristic, optically dense appearance demonstrating unusual tinctorial properties when stained by the Papanicolaou technique, the edge of the cell being green, whereas the central, thicker portion close to the nucleus is often red or orange. There may be peripheral vacuolation,[44] and commonly, there is cellular enlargement[42] to 20–25 μm,[40] the normal size range being 10–20 μm[38] (Figs 20–22).

Cell periphery—A brush-like border is frequently seen in mesothelial cells[38] representing the fine microvillous edge of the cytoplasm. Peripheral, cytoplasmic blebbing is also seen and, while these may have no value in discriminating between mesothelioma and metastatic malignant cells,[27] they are more common in malignant mesothelial cells than in benign and thus have some diagnostic value (Fig. 23).

Multinucleation—Multinucleated forms in various stages of evolution (including cell-in-cell or cell engulfment forms) are common.[34,36,37,44] This cell-in-cell feature is rarely seen in benign mesothelial cells[45] and should prompt a serious consideration of mesothelioma (Figs 20–22). Although binucleate forms of benign mesothelial cell are common, many large mutinucleate cells with 'malignant' nuclei are one of the cytological hallmarks of the epithelial form of mesothelioma.

Cell-to-cell apposition—This feature is accepted by most cytopathologists as being a characteristic of mesothelial cells both benign and/or malignant. Where two or more mesothelial cells are attached to one another, their common borders are flatly apposed but often show a 'window' or gap between the two cells (Fig. 21). They are joined only at the terminal edges of the cells, the remaining points of contact being cell junctions. This 'window' effect has been attributed to the prominent microvillous border of mesothelial cells.[46]

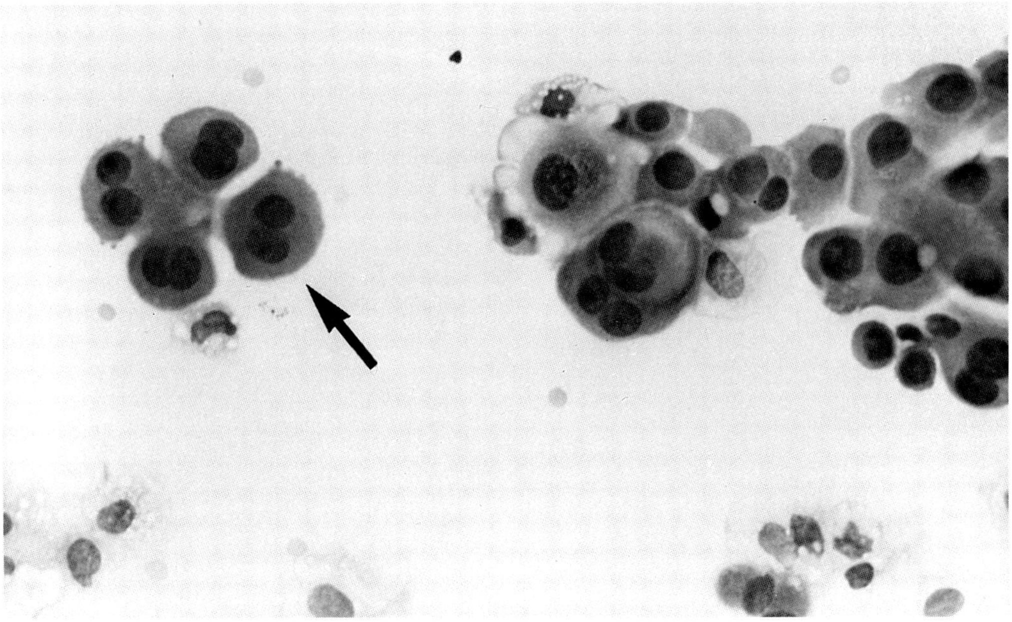

Fig. 20—Mesothelioma. A small cluster of four cells (arrow) and a group of mesothelioma cells showing cell engulfment and close cell to cell apposition. Cytoplasmic blebbing is also evident. The arrangement of cells arrowed is often seen in mesothelioma. Effusion smear. Papanicolaou stain

Uniform cell population—A diagnostic feature of metastatic carcinoma in a serous effusion is the presence of two cell types, reactive mesothelial cells and metastatic malignant cells. Characteristically, this feature is lacking in mesotheliomatous effusions; however, there is frequently a mixture of mesothelial cell types, some normal, some reactive, and some malignant. This observation

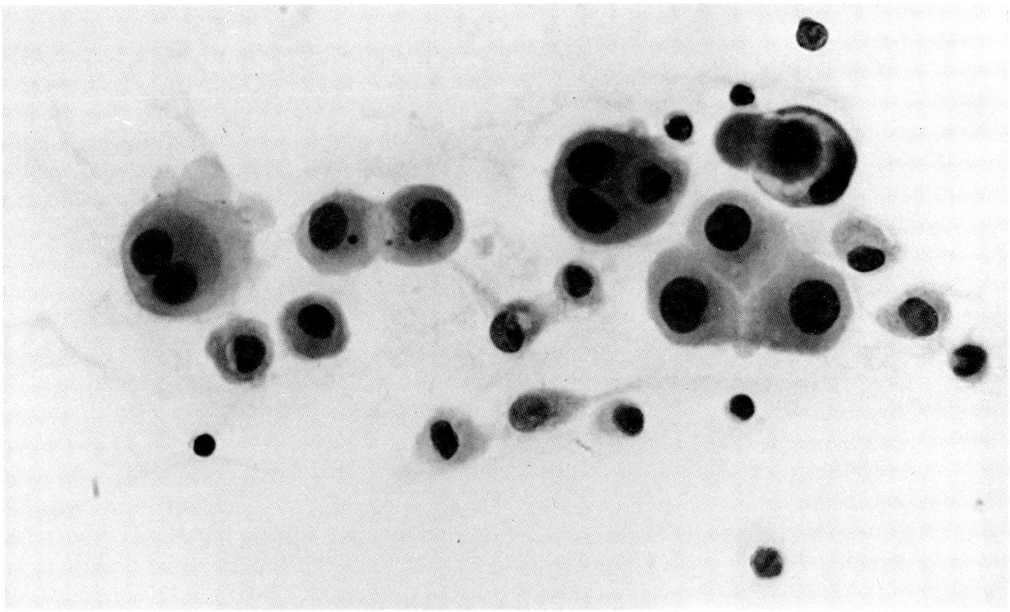

Fig. 21—Mesothelioma. Malignant cells have dense cytoplasm, prominent intercellular borders, blebbing and cell engulfment. Effusion smear. Papanicolaou stain

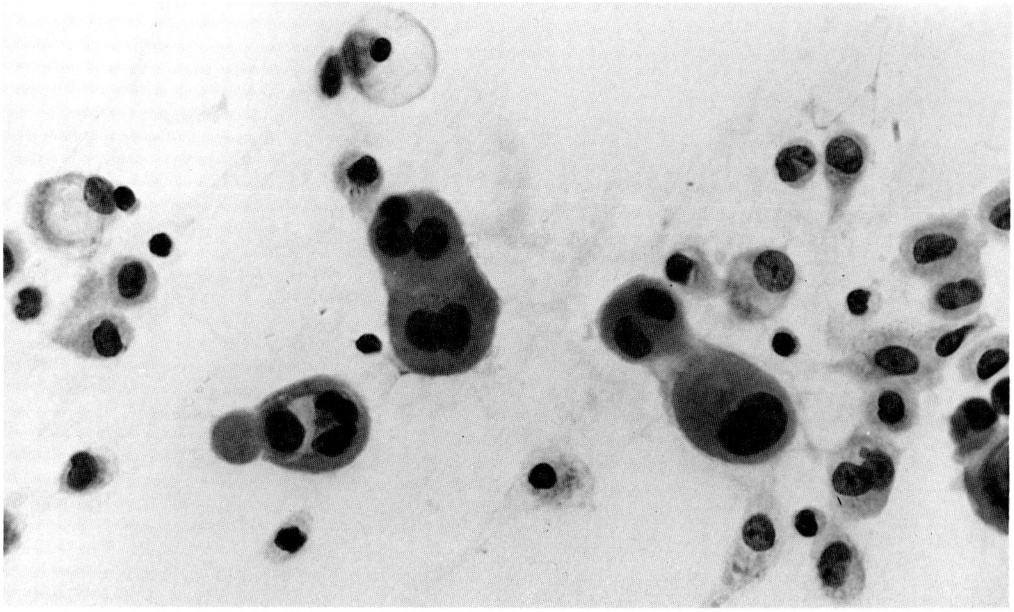

Fig. 22—Mesothelioma. The malignant cells show dense cytoplasm and multinucleation. Effusion smear. MGG stain

has been explained as exfoliation from serosal surfaces both involved and uninvolved by mesothelioma.[36]

Problems in cytological differential diagnosis

The following major points are to be covered here.

Metastatic adenocarcinoma.
Cellular aggregates in a reactive process.
Atypical mesothelial cells.
Well-differentiated mesothelioma.
Sarcomatous mesothelioma.
Undifferentiated and unusual forms of mesothelioma.
Mesothelioma presenting in unusual sites.
Lack of mesothelial cells.

Metastatic adenocarcinoma—Without doubt the most common problem is to distinguish malignant mesothelioma from metastatic adenocarcinoma. When two separate cell populations, benign mesothelial cells and malignant cells lacking mesothelial characteristics, can be identified, the recognition of metastatic malignancy can be easy.[20,35,38] In the absence of this contrasting picture and especially when the malignant cells appear only in aggregates, the distinction between malignant mesothelial and malignant non-mesothelial cells is sometimes not obvious. Papillary adenocarcinomas in general may shed cell clusters that mimic mesothelioma. In particular, well-differentiated adenocarcinomas of the lung, bronchiolar–alveolar carcinoma, and papillary carcinoma of the thyroid, are specific examples where problems arise due to the similarity of presentation of papillary aggregates. All of these tumours including mesothelioma can contain psammoma bodies in smears; however, intranuclear invagination, which is characteristic of papillary thyroid cancer cells and can be found in adenocarcinoma and bronchiolar–alveolar carcinoma of the lung,[47] is very uncommon in mesothelioma.

The configuration of cell aggregates has some differential diagnostic significance. In smears, the shape of aggregates from mesothelioma is quite variable there being elongated and frond-like structures as well as rounded ones. In contrast, most aggregates from adenocarcinomas have a rounded construction.

The value of the cell block method in distinguishing mesothelioma from adenocarcinoma is now well established.[35,43,45] With this technique not only can the columnar morphology with basal

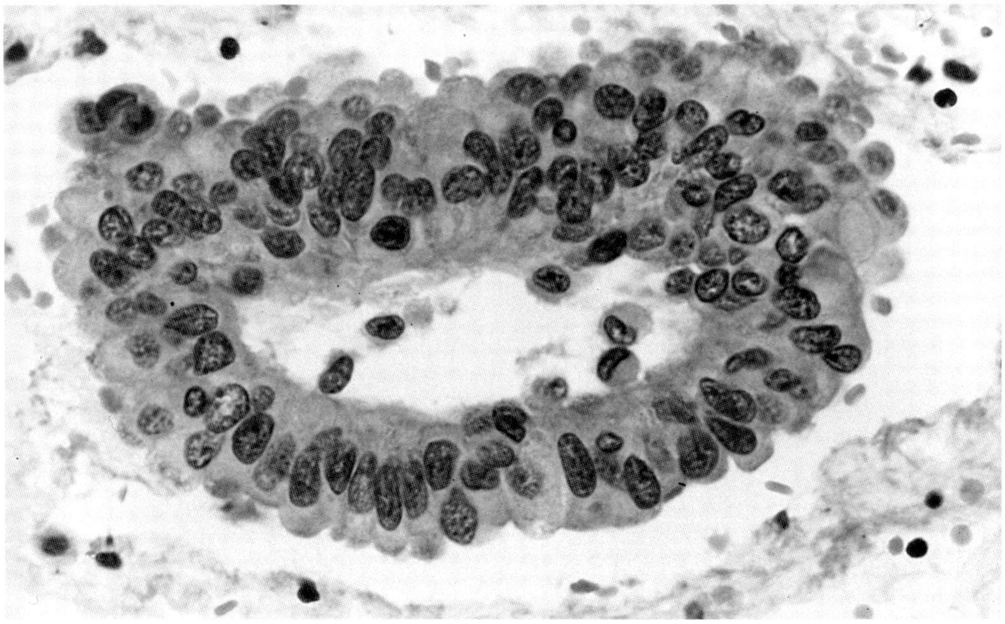

Fig. 23—Adenocarcinoma. A group of columnar adenocarcinoma cells in an acinus is shown. Cell block

nuclei be identified in adenocarcinoma cells (Fig. 23), but the cuboidal or elongated cells of mesothelioma are shown to have centrally or luminally situated nuclei (Fig. 18). In addition, in sections of papillary-like aggregates from adenocarcinomas there is rarely a collagenous central core[43] whereas this stromal structure may often be seen in mesothelioma.

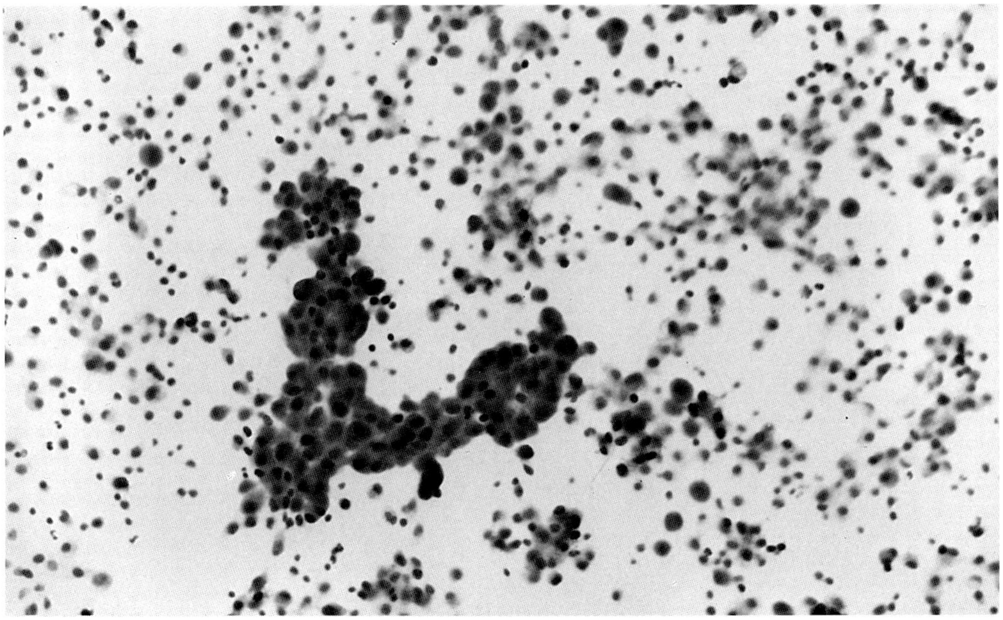

Fig. 24—Benign reaction. An aggregate of benign mesothelial cells in a flat sheet arrangement is present, from an effusion resulting from a pulmonary infarction. Effusion smear. Papanicolaou stain

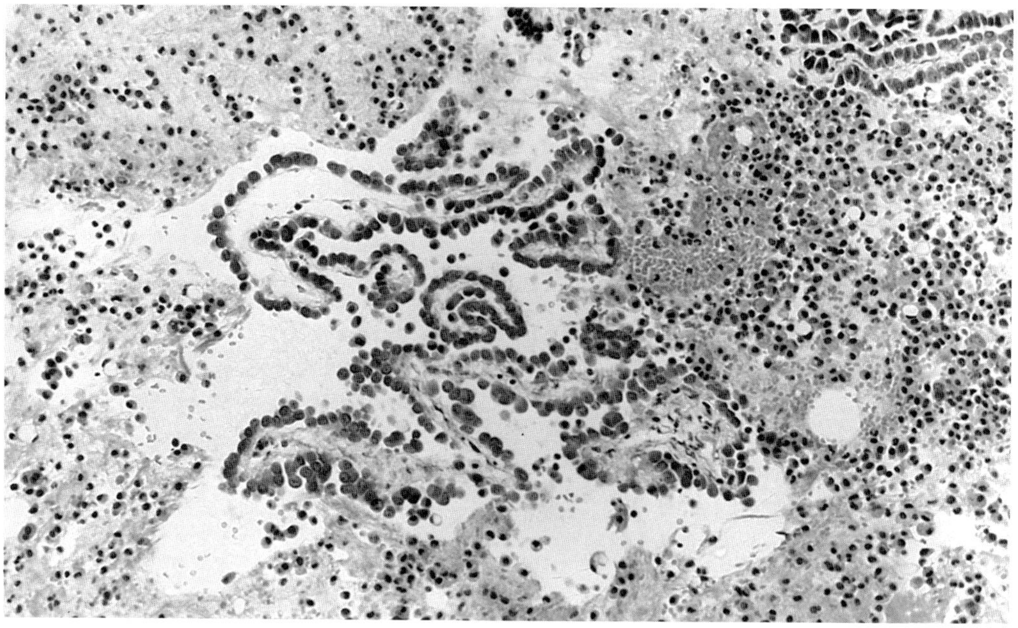

Fig. 25—Benign mesothelial reaction. This cluster of benign mesothelial papillae is from an effusion following chest trauma. Cell block

Cellular aggregates in a reactive process—Mesothelial papillae may form as a consequence of any longstanding, benign serous effusion; however, such structures are more common and abundant in pericardial[24,25] or peritoneal[48] than pleural effusions. Clusters of mesothelial cells are recognized and are commonly found in pleural effusions after pulmonary infarction. We have found them occasionally after pneumonia and chest trauma (Fig. 24). Generally speaking, the aggregates seen in reactive mesothelium are fewer, smaller, and less complex than those seen in mesothelioma.[38] It is our impression that benign aggregates are also flatter and rarely form three-dimensional structures. Sometimes large or numerous papillary fragments (Fig. 25) can be identified, and, in these circumstances, careful reference to the clinical presentation should prompt a cautious approach to their interpretation. Nevertheless, even in a patient with a suspected history of pulmonary embolism, the finding of aggregates of mesothelial cells in a smear should lead to a consideration of malignancy in the mind of the pathologist. In one such case, a female aged 29 years, who had samples of fluid repeatedly sent for cytology, it was only on the third sample that the possibility of malignant mesothelioma was canvassed with her clinician. Subsequently, mesothelioma was proven, and it emerged that the patient had spent her childhood as a resident of an asbestos mining town and had frequent contact with asbestos.

Atypical mesothelial cells—Under certain conditions including chest trauma,[49] radiation,[38] and chemotherapy,[50] an effusion may develop in which atypical mesothelial cells may be found. These cells may have sufficiently abnormal nuclei to mimic mesothelioma.[51] We have seen such atypical mesothelial cells in pleural effusion during cyclophosphamide therapy and also in recurrent effusion after pneumonia. The usual cytological picture is of a moderate number of single cells or small flat sheets of mesothelial cells showing such nuclear atypia as pleomorphism and enlarged, irregular nucleoli (Fig. 26). Caution must be exercised in the interpretation of even highly atypical cells in squamoid-like sheets and it is our experience that these are invariably benign.

We have also observed cases of apparently benign asbestos pleurisy containing both small mesothelial aggregates and atypical mesothelial cells. Clearly, such cases warrant close clinical follow-up, as at least one of Gaensler's and Kaplan's cases[52] eventually developed mesothelioma.

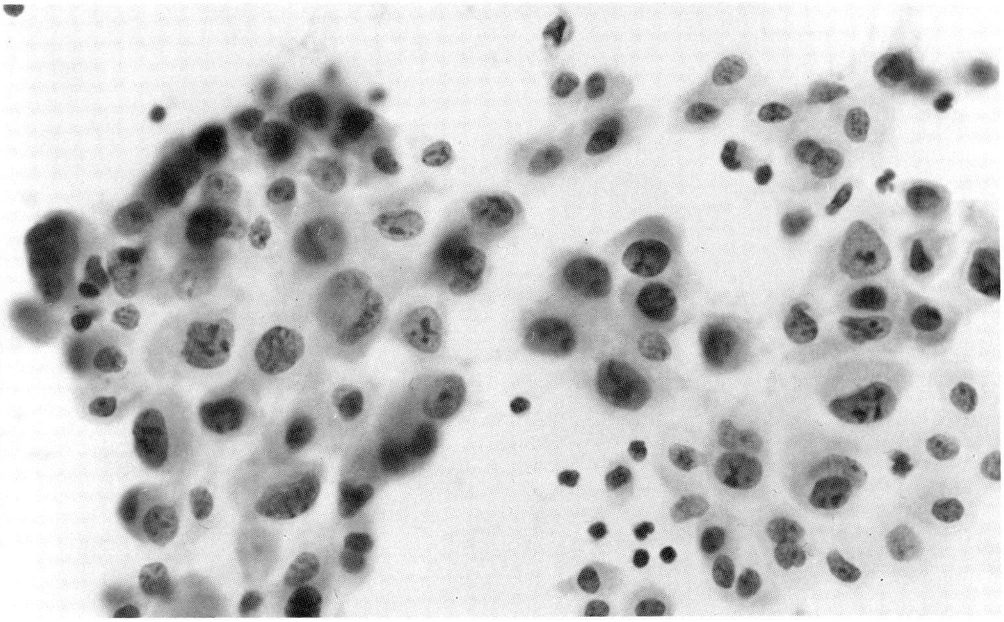

Fig. 26—Benign reaction. Flat sheet of highly atypical mesothelial cells showing nuclear enlargement, irregularity, and prominent multiple nucleoli was from a patient on cyclophosphamide treatment. Effusion smear. Papanicolaou stain

Well-differentiated mesothelioma—Occasionally, a mesothelioma may be so well-differentiated that the exfoliated cells in the effusion closely resemble benign reactive mesothelial cells and so provide a cytologically perplexing problem.[1] Even when mesothelioma is strongly suspected because of the clinical evidence or the cytological finding of numerous cell aggregates, a definite cytological diagnosis of mesothelioma cannot be made unless the cells possess obviously malignant nuclei; however, the identification of the mesothelial nature of the process when considered with the histological findings of the closed needle biopsy will often contribute to a definitive diagnosis.

Sarcomatous mesothelioma—This form of mesothelioma frequently presents clinically without a pleural effusion. When fluid is available, malignant spindle cells can only sometimes be identified and, occasionally, small sheets of new growth may be found.[36,38] Such spindle cells appearing in a pleural effusion should always lead to a consideration of the possibility of mesothelioma.

Undifferentiated and unusual forms of mesothelioma—Definitive diagnosis, on cytological grounds alone, of such tumours is often impossible.[9,35,37] Poorly-differentiated malignant cells in pleural effusion often defy classification, perhaps with the exception of small cell carcinoma of the lung. Rarely, mesothelioma can present with an unusual pattern. We have seen a case of signet-ring-like mesothelioma not dissimilar to that reported by Boon *et al.*[53] and discussed by Spriggs and Grunze.[54] A small cell variant of mesothelioma has also been described.[48]

Mesothelioma presenting in unusual sites—With the advent of fine needle aspiration cytology, mesothelioma can sometimes be diagnosed from lymph node or chest wall aspirates.[46,47] We have also identified four cases of metastatic mesothelioma in sputum samples. In one case this was concurrent with the effusion, and in the other three the positive sputum developed a few weeks after the onset of the pleural effusion. A finding of malignant cells in sputum would generally not prompt a diagnosis of mesothelioma as this occurrence is alleged to be rare.

Lack of mesothelial cells—During a review of cytology slides from known mesotheliomas previously reported by us as negative, a few showing numerous lymphocytes but no mesothelial cells held our attention. It is well recognized that the common cytological picture in tuberculous pleurisy is characterized by plentiful lymphocytes and lack of mesothelial cells.[45,55] Bearing this in mind, at least two of the above cases were initially thought to be due to tuberculosis, but this proved not to be so. Thus, the absence of recognizable mesothelial cells in an effusion from a case suspected of being mesothelioma should lead to examination of any remaining fluid, a diligent search for spindle cells, and, if necessary, a request for a further fluid if the effusion re-accumulates.

In summary, we believe that the cytological evaluation of pleural effusions is a valuable diagnostic test. Its usefulness increases with experience and cytology alone may often provide the definitive diagnosis. When used together with biopsied tissue it can, at the very least, enhance the chances of an accurate diagnosis.

ANCILLARY TESTS

General role

The definitive diagnosis of malignant mesothelioma during life is based on an accumulation of evidence. Laboratory tests of an ancillary nature may be used whenever it is necessary for added support. The possible range of tests is constantly changing and increasing and presently includes electron microscopy, measurements of serous effusion levels of hyaluronic acid, histochemical stains for glycogen and mucins, immunochemical reactions, morphometry, and cytogenetic analysis. Obviously the availability of specialized facilities will affect the choice of tests and the relative importance they might have in contributing to a diagnosis. At the present time no single test provides a unique marker for malignant mesothelioma. In general two broad types of ancillary test are applied in attempting to arrive at a diagnosis. Firstly, there are those which discriminate between mesothelial cells, either benign or malignant, on the one hand, and metastatic malignancy on the other. Such tests aim to identify histogenetic markers and include ultrastructure, hyaluronic acid assay, epithelial mucin, and immunoperoxidase techniques employing carcinoembryonic antigen (CEA) and keratin antisera. The second type of test aims to distinguish benign and malignant cells, may include epithelial membrane antigen (EMA) and Cal antisera, morphometry, and cytogenetic analysis.

Ultrastructure of mesothelioma

Both scanning electron microscopy (SEM) and transmission electron microscopy (TEM) have been used in the differential diagnosis of malignant mesothelioma. Most ultrastructural descriptions are based on examination of the tissue obtained at thoracotomy or autopsy.[12,56–58] The technique has also been advocated for assessing closed pleural needle biopsies[21,59] and the cell content of serous effusions.[13,53,59,60,62,63]

While SEM of serous effusions may distinguish between any variety of mesothelial cell and metastatic malignant cells[64,65] it does not discriminate between single benign and malignant mesothelial cells.[59,62] The finding by light microscopy of numerous cell aggregates demonstrated to be mesothelial by SEM may aid in the diagnosis of mesothelioma. The value of SEM assessment of tissue samples is unproven in its application to the diagnosis of mesothelioma.[67]

The TEM appearances of the various forms of mesothelioma are now well-documented.[13,57,59,66,68] Using the limited material available from closed needle biopsies and effusions it may only be possible to characterize with confidence the better differentiated epithelial forms. In the context of attempting to arrive at a diagnosis on minimal material we have found TEM of the cell deposits from serous effusion to be the single most rewarding ultrastructural exercise. This approach is not new, having been advocated by Murad[61] and Legrand and Pariente[60] and it is now finding more support.[13,43,59,63] Mesotheliomas characteristically have recurrent accumulations of fluid and, when present, there is usually ample fresh cellular material either from the initial or subsequent samples. Part of the cell sediment can be fixed in glutaraldehyde to be processed further only if required, depending on the outcome of the primary histological and cytological assessment.

While recognizing the usefulness of TEM in distinguishing between malignant mesothelial or metastatic cells in serous effusions we, like others,[13,69] remained unconvinced of its value in distinguishing between benign and malignant mesothelial cells and believe that the malignant nature of the process needs to be ascertained by

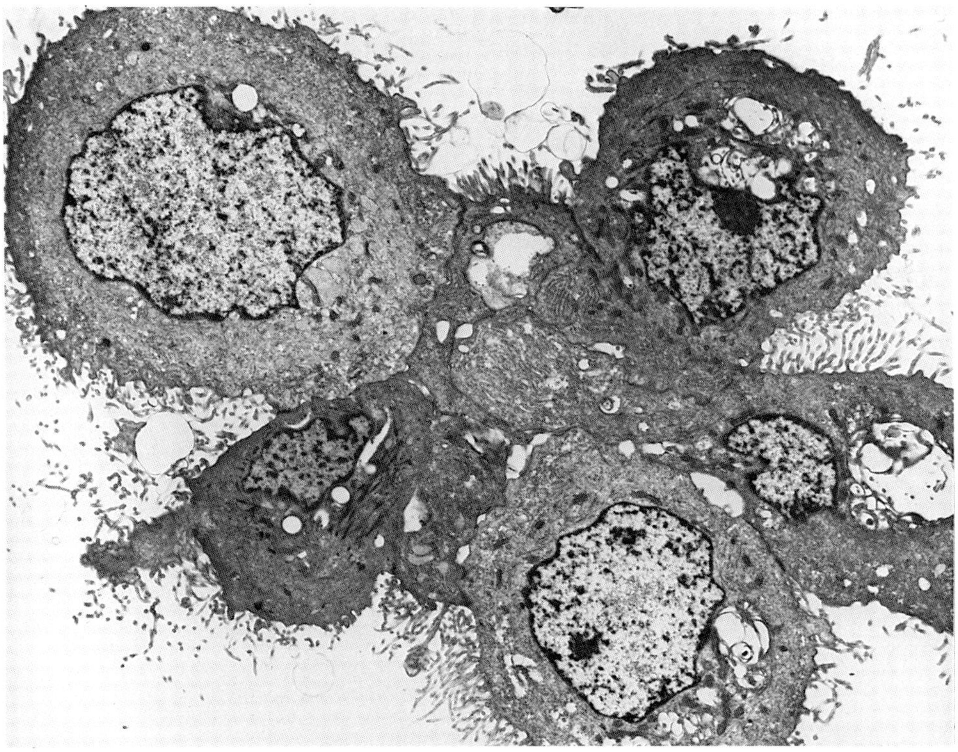

Fig. 27—Mesothelioma. A cluster of mesothelioma cells showing abundant long thin microvilli. Effusion smear. Electron micrograph ×4000

other means. The characteristic ultrastructural features of mesothelioma cells are numerous long, thin microvilli and abundant intermediate filaments, often with a terminal filamentous webb.[13,68] Provided the malignant nature of the cells is ascertained before ultrastructural examination is performed, the mesothelial origin of the cells and cell aggregates can frequently be confirmed by this technique (Fig. 27).

Hyaluronic acid

The demonstration of the glycosaminoglycan, hyaluronic acid, has long been a mainstay of supplementary aids in the differential diagnosis of malignant mesothelioma. Mesodermally-derived tissues, including the mesothelium, and their neoplasms may produce large quantitites of this acid mucopolysaccharide. Traditionally, tests for hyaluronic acid have involved some form of biochemical analysis of the effusion and its histochemical demonstration by the dye alcian blue.

Tissue hyaluronic acid—The successful demonstration of hyaluronic acid in tissue depends on the method of fixation[70] the degree of tumour differentiation[71] and the identification of the reaction product within the epithelial-like cells.[15] Recently Kwee *et al.*[19] found hyaluronic acid in 49 per cent of their mesotheliomas. Nevertheless, this test is often difficult to interpret because stromal connective tissue is also heavily stained with alcian blue and this may overwhelm any intracytoplasmic positivity, inhibiting its value as a definitive diagnostic discriminator.[72] In general we have replaced this test in our laboratory by immunocytochemical tests.

Hyaluronic acid levels in serous effusions—As early as 1908, Miller and Wynn[73] commented on the viscosity of mesotheliomatous effusions and a test for hyaluronic acid was introduced in 1963.[74] Since then very high levels have been demonstrated,[75,76] greater than 212 mg/l being considered by some to be diagnostic of malignant mesothelioma.[77] We have measured hyaluronic acid levels in ten cases of human mesothelioma, six of benign effusion, and five of metastastic malignant effusion, using the method of Rowley *et al.*[78] Six of the cases of mesothelioma contained more than 200 mg of hyaluronic acid per litre, the highest being 3130 mg/l, but none of the other cases contained more than 90 mg/l. This biochemical test may, therefore, have a useful ancillary role in the differential diagnosis of malignant mesothelioma.

Cytochemistry

Mesotheliomatous cells characteristically contain abundant glycogen and Fisher and Hellstrom[79] described its fine, granular distribution. Wagner *et al.*[80] also observed much glycogen and demonstrated the lack of epithelial mucin in mesotheliomas. They advocated the use of the PAS stain, both with and without diastase digestion, to demonstrate glycogen and/or mucin in alternate histological sections as a differential diagnostic test to distinguish between mesothelioma and adenocarcinoma.

Although this method has great value, it is not without some problems of interpretation. When found in adenocarcinoma cells as a single large inclusion, the mucin is readily identifiable, but when it occurs as rounded globules of generally small size, its mucinous nature may not be recognized. Intracellular glycogen, because of its fine, even, granular distribution is usually readily distinguished as it is removed by diastase; however, all PAS-positive–diastase-resistant material is not mucin and, occasionally, diastase-resistant protein or lipoprotein droplets can be found within cells and they may be difficult, if not impossible, to identify. Notwithstanding these hazards it remains a very useful test,[1,19] particularly as it is easy to perform. Some laboratories may prefer to use mucicarmine or some other stain for epithelial mucin.

Immunocytochemistry

This relatively new area of investigation is rapidly establishing itself as a significant adjunct to the conventional morphological studies in identification and histogenetic typing of neoplasms. Demonstration of cell and tissue antigens by these methods can be exacting and, despite standardization of technique and reagents, results may vary from centre to centre giving rise to a variable degree of confidence in the accuracy and value of such investigations. Nevertheless, with perseverance, critical evaluation and careful interpretation, the place of immunocytochemistry in relation to a given problem can be stabilized. Five markers have been utilized with mesothelioma. Two, CEA and keratin, are histogenetic markers; the other three, EMA, Cal, and α-1-antichymotrypsin, are potential markers for malignancy. It should, therefore, be emphasized that CEA and keratin antibody tests do not distinguish between benign and malignant mesothelial cells. A specific antimesothelial-cell serum has also been developed and used by one group of investigators who found that only benign and malignant mesothelial tissue reacted positively.[81]

CEA—We have found the CEA test, initially advocated by Wang *et al.*[82] to be valuable in distinguishing between mesothelial tissues, which are invariably negative, and adenocarcinoma which is frequently CEA-positive. Occasionally, a focal weak positive reaction is described in mesothelioma,[83,84] but a strong deposition of reaction product located on the glycocalyx is never seen in mesothelioma.[85] The technique has greatest diagnostic value when used in conjunction with conventional mucin stains, enabling most mesotheliomas to be clearly distinguished from adenocarcinomas.[19,85]

Keratin—Native mesothelial cells,[86] reactive mesothelium, and mesothelioma contain many intermediate filaments of keratin or pre-keratin type.[83,84,87] When tested in a peroxidase–antiperoxidase system these keratin filaments were commonly found in mesothelioma but were lacking[83,84] or had a different distribution[87] in adenocarcinoma; however, there is some evidence that the demonstration of keratin in adenocarcinoma is subject to the particular antibody used and the method of fixation employed.[88]

EMA—EMA is an antigen directed against malignant epithelial cells and has been found by To *et al.*[89] to be valuable in discriminating between benign mesothelial cells and malignant epithelial cells, including carcinoma and mesothelioma, in serous effusions. They stress the need for stringent control of the technique and the reagents to obtain optimum results. We have also found this antigen to be helpful. In smears and in cell blocks, reactive mesothelial cells are negative or stain only weakly, whereas all cases of adenocarcinoma and mesothelioma studied were strongly positive.

Cal—The Cal antigen as developed by Ashall *et al.*[90] also seeks to distinguish benign from malignant tissue[91] or benign from malignant cells in effusions.[92] This antigen reacts positively with mesothelioma cells, whereas reactive mesothelial cells are claimed to be negative.[90] This antibody is presently under evaluation as a diagnostic test in several laboratories including our own, however some reports question its value in the differential diagnosis of mesothelioma in biopsy tissue[96] or effusion cells.[97]

α-1-Antichymotrypsin—Herbert and Gallagher[93] found this enzyme assists in the discrimination between reactive and malignant mesothelial cells in sections of tissue and cell block, but we have no experience with it.

Of all the available immunocytochemical investigations we attach greatest reliance to the results of the CEA test.

Other ancillary tests

There are at least two other ancillary tests which are claimed to have value in distinguishing between benign and malignant mesothelial cells. These are cytogenetics and morphometry. We have had no personal experience with these. Spriggs and Boddington[45] advocated cytogenetic analysis of cells from effusions in diagnosing mesothelioma, and Mark[94] found three common chromosomal abnormalities in malignant mesothelioma which were thought to be marker patterns: monosomy 13, monosomy 22, and one characterized by the deletion of part of the long arm of chromosome 13 ($13q^-$). Recently, Watts *et al.*[95] reported good results with this form of investigation using short term culture of effusion cells including mesotheliomas.

Kwee *et al.*[27] advocated quantitative assessment of mesothelial cells based on the measurement of nuclear and cytoplasmic size in discriminating between benign and malignant mesothelial cells. Both mean nuclear and cytoplasmic areas were found to be significantly higher in mesothelioma than in reactive benign mesothelial cells.

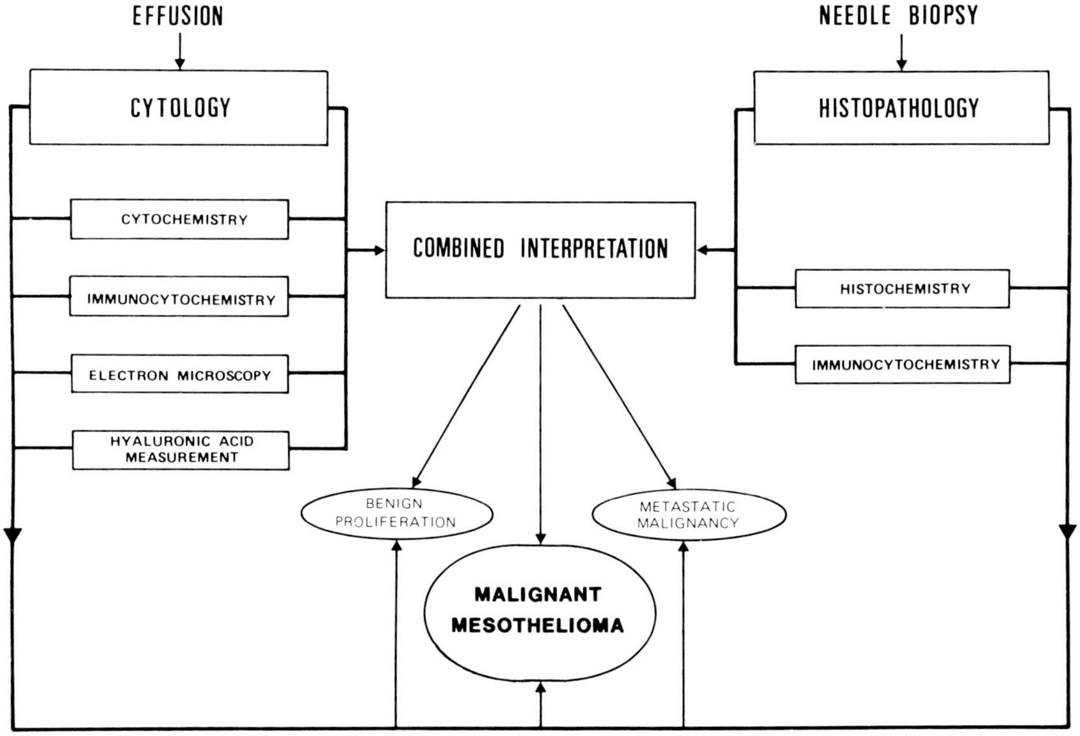

Fig. 28—Possible pathways of approach to the tissue diagnosis of malignant mesothelioma in life

PRACTICAL APPLICATION

In this section we wish to deal with the practical aspects of the approach to diagnosis when only small amounts of material are available.

Combined histological–cytological approach

The single most important factor in favour of the diagnosis of mesothelioma is an appropriate clinical presentation including a history of asbestos exposure, recurrent pleural effusion, chest pain, and pleural thickening. Against such a background a confident diagnosis of malignant mesothelioma based on needle biopsy and/or effusion can sometimes be made with relative ease. Commonly, some ancillary tests will be used to enhance the routine morphological findings. When the clinical presentation is not classical, however, the problems for the pathologist are greatest, and the ability to make a definitive tissue diagnosis with any degree of confidence is generally much reduced.

While the pathological diagnosis of malignant mesothelioma may be established by cytology alone or, in the absence of an effusion, solely by biopsy, there is a significant number of cases in which it will be rewarding to consider the cytological and histological findings together, particularly as it is common practice for the closed needle biopsy to be obtained at the same time as the effusion is drained. Such a combined approach creates the opportunity of raising the level of confidence of the morphological diagnosis. Although the contribution of each element in this combined approach may vary from case to case, in every instance something of additional value is gained, and this method is a routine practice in our

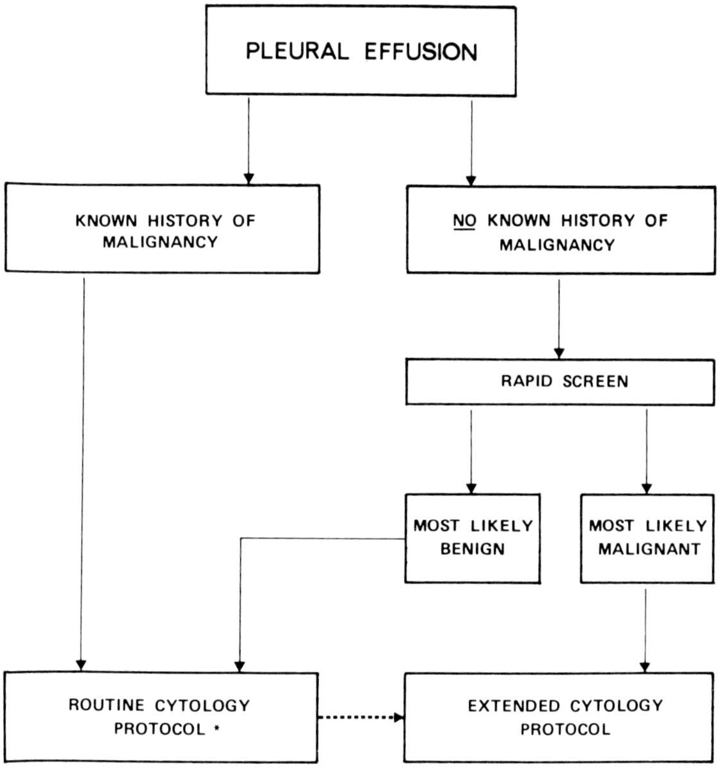

* NOTE. THE ROUTINE PROTOCOL INCLUDES DIRECT SMEAR AND CYTOCENTRIFUGE PREPARATIONS STAINED WITH PAPANICOLAOU AND MGG STAINS AND CELL BLOCK SECTIONS STAINED BY H&E AND PAS& DIASTASE

Fig. 29—Pleural effusion protocol

laboratory. There are at least three specific situations in which histopathology and cytology can complement each other and result in a more confident diagnosis.

(i) Histopathology=mesothelial; cytology=malignant. A biopsy may show what is considered to be an atypical surface proliferation of mesothelial cells. Alone, this would be insufficient for the diagnosis of malignant mesothelioma; however, when the cytology yields a population of malignant cells whose cytoplasmic characteristics are not typically mesothelial, both modalities may be assessed together to yield the diagnosis of malignant mesothelioma.

(ii) Histopathology = malignant; cytology = mesothelial. Biopsy tissue may occasionally show an invasive tumour, but the mesothelial nature of the process remains unclear. Taken together with cytology when there are atypical cells whose cytoplasmic features are characteristic of mesothelial cells, the diagnosis may be made.

(iii) Histopathology = suspicious of mesothelioma; cytology = suspicious of mesothelioma. Where both samples are suggestive of mesothelioma, but when each alone is inadequate for a definitive diagnosis, a greater degree of confidence in the diagnosis of mesothelioma may be achieved if they are assessed together.

In a series of 70 cases of confirmed mesothelioma which we have recently analysed,[7] 39 per cent were correctly diagnosed by the initial needle biopsy and 50 per cent were correctly diagnosed on cytological morphology alone; however, when using the combined approach, the number of cases in which the diagnosis could be made rose to 80 per cent.

Practical guide

As a result of our evolving experience with the use of histopathology, cytology, and ancillary investigations, we have developed a protocol for

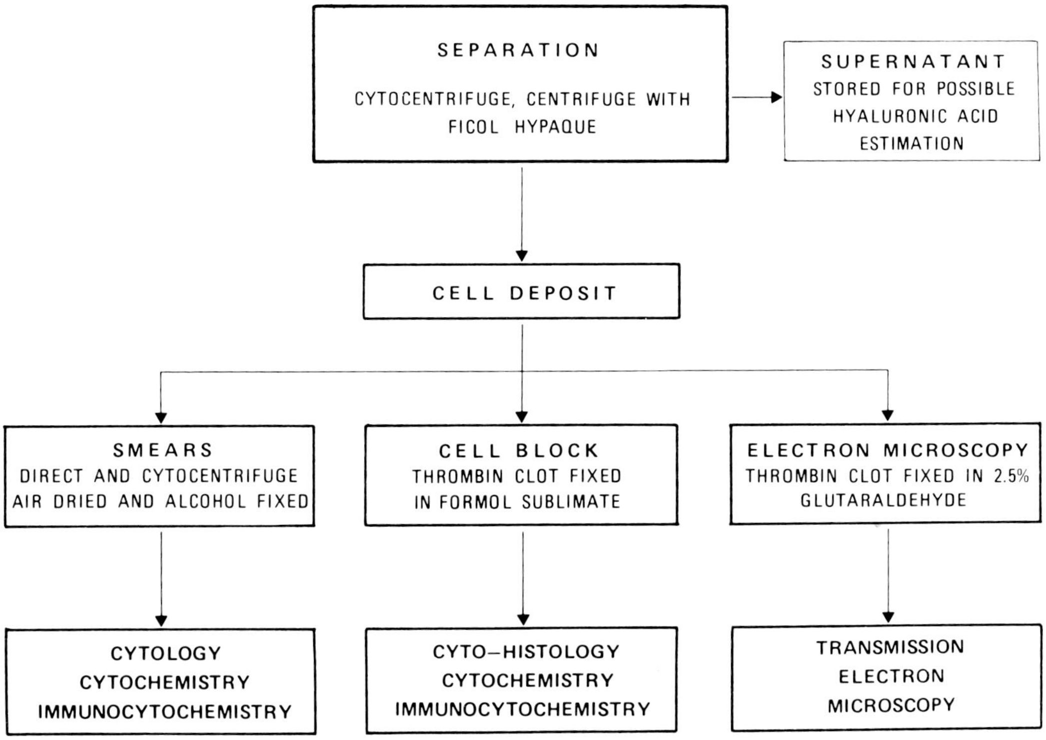

Fig. 30—Extended cytology protocol

the processing of specimens. The outline of the protocol is shown in Figs 28–30. We recognize that modalities, such as cytogenetics and morphometry, and other developments may well have a place in such a scheme. As we update and analyse our experience, modifications may be made, but, at present, it provides a convenient and valuable guide to the problems we have set out here. With the increasing impetus to establish a tissue diagnosis during life, without open surgery, there is a need to develop criteria based on limited biopsy material and pleural fluid. With extensive use of asbestos and the long latency before the clinical presentation of asbestos-associated disease, pathologists will be faced with this diagnostic problem for many years to come.

REFERENCES

1. Kannerstein M, Churg J, McCaughey WT. Asbestos and mesothelioma: A review. *Pathol Ann* 1978; **13** (part 1): 81–129.
2. Griffiths MH, Riddell RJ, Xipell JM. Malignant mesothelioma: a review of 35 cases with diagnosis and prognosis. *Pathology* 1980; **12:** 591–603.
3. Brenner J, Sordillo PP, Magill GB, Golbey RB. Malignant mesothelioma of the pleura: review of 123 patients. *Cancer* 1982; **49:** 2431–2435.
4. Churg A, Golden J. Current problems in pathology of asbestos-related disease. *Pathol Ann* 1982; **17** (part 2): 33–66.
5. Elmes PC, Simpson MJC. The clinical aspects of mesothelioma. *Quart J Med* 1976; **45:** 427–449.
6. Edge JR, Choudhury SL. Malignant mesothelioma of the pleura in Barrow-in-Furness. *Thorax* 1978; **33:** 26–30.
7. Shilkin KB, Whitaker D. Malignant mesothelioma in Western Australia: pathologic aspects. *Med J Aust* (in press).
8. Salyer WR, Eggleston JC, Erozan YS. Efficacy of pleural needle biopsy and pleural fluid cytopathology in the diagnosis of malignant neoplasm involving the pleura. *Chest* 1975; **67:** 536–539.
9. Kannerstein M, McCaughey WT, Churg J, Selikoff IJ. A critique of the criteria for the diagnosis of diffuse malignant mesothelioma. *Mt Sinai J Med* 1977; **44:** 485–494.
10. McCaughey WTE. Primary tumours of the pleura. *J. Pathol Bacteriol* 1958; **76:** 517–529.
11. Whitwell F, Rawcliffe M. Diffuse malignant pleural mesothelioma and asbestos exposure. *Thorax* 1971; **26:** 6–22.
12. Enzinger FM, Weiss SW. Soft Tissue Tumors. St Louis: Mosby, 1983: 550–579.
13. Suzuki Y. Pathology of human malignant mesothelioma. *Semin Oncol* 1980; **8:** 268–282.
14. Herbert A, Gallagher PJ. Pleural biopsy in the diagnosis of malignant mesothelioma. *Thorax* 1982; **37:** 816–821.
15. Henderson DW. Asbestos related pleuropulmonary diseases: asbestosis, mesothelioma and lung cancer. *Pathology* 1982; **14:** 239–243.
16. Whitaker D, Papadimitriou JM, Walters MN-I. The mesothelium and its reactions: a review. *CRC Crit Rev Toxicol* 1982; **10:** 81–144.
17. Klima M, Gyorkey F. Benign pleural lesion and malignant mesothelioma. *Virch Arch (Pathol Anat)* 1977; **376:** 181–193.
18. Sheldon CD, Herbert A, Gallagher PJ. Reactive mesothelial proliferation: a necropsy study. *Thorax* 1981; **36:** 901–905.
19. Kwee WS, Veldhuizen RW, Golding RP, *et al.* Histologic distinction between malignant mesothelioma, benign pleural lesion and carcinoma metastasis. *Virch Arch (Pathol Anat)* 1982; **397:** 287–299.
20. Carter D. Histologic classification and differential diagnosis of mesothelioma. *Yale J Biol Med* 1981; **54:** 173–180.
21. Kawai T, Suzuki M, Kageyama K. Reactive mesothelial cell and mesothelioma of the pleura. *Virch Arch (Pathol Anat)* 1981; **393:** 251–263.
22. Hourihane DO'B. A biopsy series of mesotheliomata and attempts to identify asbestos within some of the tumors. *Ann NY Acad Sci* 1965; **132:** 647–673.
23. Whitaker D, Shilkin KB, Walters MN-I. The cytologic and tissue culture characteristics of asbestos-induced mesothelioma in rats. *Acta Cytol* 1984, **28:** 185–189.
24. Becker SN, Pepin DW, Rosenthal DL. Mesothelial papilloma: a case of mistaken identity in a pericardial effusion. *Acta Cytol* 1979; **20:** 266–268.
25. Spriggs AI, Jerome DW. Benign mesothelial proliferation with collagen formation in pericardial fluid. *Acta Cytol* 1979; **23:** 428–430.
26. Rosai J, Dehner LP. Nodular mesothelial hyperplasia in hernia sacs: a benign reactive condition simulating a neoplastic process. *Cancer* 1975; **35:** 165–175.
27. Kwee WS, Veldhuizen RW, Alons CL, Morawetz F, Boon ME. Quantitative and qualitative differences between benign and malignant mesothelial cells in pleural fluid. *Acta Cytol* 1982; **26:** 401–406.
28. Harwood TR, Gracey DR, Yokoo H. Pseudomesotheliomatous carcinoma of the lung. A variant of peripheral lung cancer. *Am J Clin Pathol* 1976; **65:** 159–167.
29. Kannerstein M, Churg J. Desmoplastic diffuse malignant mesothelioma. In: Fenoglio CM, Wolff, eds. Progress in Surgical Pathology. Vol 2. New York: Masson, 1980: 19–29.
30. Cantin R, Al-Jabi M, McCaughey WTE. Desmoplastic diffuse mesothelioma. *Am J Surg Pathol* 1982; **6:** 215–222.
31. Kwee WS, Veldhuizen RW, Golding RP, Donner

R. Primary 'adenosquamous' mesothelioma of the pleura. *Virch Arch (Pathol Anat)* 1981; **393:** 353–357.
32. Leigh RA, Webster I. Lymphocytic infiltration of pleural mesothelioma and its significance for survival. *S Afr Med J* 1982; **61:** 1007–1009.
33. Klempman S. The exfoliative cytology of diffuse pleural mesothelioma. *Cancer* 1962; **15:** 691–704.
34. Roberts, GH, Campbell GM. Exfoliative cytology of diffuse mesothelioma. *J Clin Pathol* 1972; **25:** 577–582.
35. Butler EB, Berry AV. Diffuse mesotheliomas. Diagnostic criteria using exfoliative cytology. In: Bogovski P, Gilson JC, Timbrell V, Wagner JC, eds. Biological Effects of Asbestos. Lyon: International Agency for Research on Cancer, 1973: 68–73.
36. Whitaker D, Shilkin KB. The cytology of malignant mesothelioma in Western Australia. *Acta Cytol* 1978; **22:** 67–70.
37. Tao LC. The cytopathology of mesothelioma. *Acta Cytol* 1979; **23:** 209–213.
38. Koss LG. Diagnostic Cytology and its Histopathologic Bases. 3rd edn. Philadelphia: Lippincott, 1979.
39. McCaughey WTE. Criteria for diagnosis of diffuse mesothelial tumors. *Ann NY Acad Sci* 1965; **132:** 603–613.
40. Gupta K, Frost K. Cytologic changes associated with asbestos exposure. *Sem Oncol* 1981; **8:** 283–289.
41. Chahinian AP, Pajak TF, Holland JF, Norton L, Ambinder RM, Mandell EM. Diffuse malignant mesothelioma. Prospective evaluation of 69 patients. *Ann Intern Med* 1982; **96:** 746–755.
42. Naylor B. The exfoliative cytology of diffuse malignant mesothelioma. *J Pathol Bacteriol* 1963; **86:** 293–298.
43. Whitaker D. Cell aggregates in malignant mesothelioma. *Acta Cytol* 1977; **21:** 236–239.
44. Boon ME, Kwee WS, Alons CL, Morawetz F, Veldhuizen RW. Discrimination between primary pleural and primary peritoneal mesotheliomas by morphometry and analysis of vacuolization pattern of the exfoliated mesothelial cells. *Acta Cytol* 1982; **26:** 103–108.
45. Spriggs AI, Boddington MM. The Cytology of Effusions. 2nd edn. London: Heinemann, 1968.
46. Bonfiglio T. Cytopathologic interpretation of transthoracic fine-needle biopsies. In: Johnston WW, ed. Masson Monographs in Diagnostic Cytopathology. Vol 4. New York: Masson, 1983: 131, 181.
47. Orell SR, Sterrett GF, Walters MN-I, Whitaker D. Manual and Atlas of Fine Needle Aspiration Cytology. Edinburgh: Churchill Livingstone, 1984.
48. Ashton PR. Diagnostic cytology seminar. *Acta Cytol* 1982; **26:** 851–882.
49. Naib ZN. Exfoliative Cytopathology. 2nd edn. Boston: Little Brown, 1976: 301.
50. Von Haam E. Cytology of transudates and exudates. In: Wied GL, ed. Monographs in Clinical Cytology. Vol 5. Basel: Karger, 1977: 93–99.
51. Hughes HE, Dodds TC. Handbook of Diagnostic cytology. Edinburgh: Livingstone, 1968: 159.
52. Gaensler EA, Kaplan AI. Asbestos pleural effusion. *Ann Inter Med* 1971; **74:** 178–191.
53. Boon ME, Posthuma HS, Ruiter DJ, v Andel JG. Secreting peritoneal mesothelioma. *Virch Arch (Pathol Anat)* 1981; **392:** 33–44.
54. Spriggs AI, Grunze H. An unusual cytologic presentation of mesothelioma in serous effusions. *Acta Cytol* 1983; **27:** 288–292.
55. Winkelmann M, Pfitzer P. Blind pleural biopsy in combination with cytology of pleural effusions. *Acta Cytol* 1981; **25:** 373–376.
56. Kay S, Silverberg SG. Ultrastructural studies of a malignant fibrous mesothelioma of the pleura. *Arch Pathol* 1971; **92:** 449–455.
57. Wang NS. Electron microscopy in the diagnosis of pleural mesotheliomas. *Cancer* 1973; **31:** 1046–1054.
58. Pritchett PS, Murad TM. Electron microscopic studies of mesothelioma. *Ala J Med Sci* 1978; **15:** 178–189.
59. Stoebner P, Brambilla E. Ultrastructural diagnosis of pleural tumors. *Path Res Pract* 1982; **173:** 402–416.
60. Legrand M, Pariente R. Ultrastructural study of pleural fluid in mesothelioma. *Thorax* 1974; **29:** 164–171.
61. Murad TM. Electron microscopic studies of cells in pleural and peritoneal effusions. *Acta Cytol* 1973; **17:** 401–409.
62. Butler EB, Johnson JF. The use of electron microscopy in the diagnosis of diffuse mesotheliomas using human pleural effusions. In: Wagner JC, ed. Biological Effects of Mineral Fibres. Lyon: IARC Sci Publ 1980; **30:** 409–418.
63. Warhol MJ, Hickey WF, Corson JM. Malignant mesothelioma. Ultrastructural distinction from adenocarcinoma. *Am J Surg Pathol* 1982; **6:** 307–314.
64. Gondos B, Lai CE, King EB. Distinction between atypical mesothelial cells and malignant cells by scanning electron microscopy. *Acta Cytol* 1979; **23:** 321–326.
65. Domagala W, Woyke S. Transmission and scanning electron microscopic studies of cells in effusions. *Acta Cytol* 1975; **19:** 214–224.
66. Davis JM. Ultrastructure of human mesotheliomas. *J Natl Cancer Inst* 1974; **52:** 1715–1725.
67. Dionne GP, Wang NS. A scanning electron microscopic study of diffuse mesothelioma and some lung carcinomas. *Cancer* 1977; **40:** 707–715.
68. Henderson DW, Papadimitriou JM. Ultrastructural

appearances of tumours: A Diagnostic Atlas. Edinburgh: Churchill Livingstone, 1981: 109–115.

69. Seymour AE, Henderson HW. Electron microscopy in surgical pathology: a selective review. *Pathology* 1981; **13:** 111–135.
70. Wagner JC, Munday DE, Harington JS. Histochemical demonstration of hyaluronic acid in pleural mesotheliomas. *J Pathol Bacteriol* 1962; **84:** 73–78.
71. Jagueux M, Pieron R, Cosset JM. Current data on malignant mesothelioma. Histochemical characterization of hyaluronic acid. *J Fr Med Chir Thorac (Paris)* 1972; **26:** 5–24.
72. Kannerstein M, Churg J, Magner D. Histochemistry in the diagnosis of malignant mesothelioma. *Ann Clin Lab Sci* 1973; **3:** 207–211.
73. Miller J, Wynn WH. A malignant tumour arising from the endothelium of the peritoneum, and producing a mucoid ascitic fluid. *J Pathol Bacteriol* 1908; **12:** 267–278.
74. Harington JS, Wagner JC, Smith M. The detection of hyaluronic acid in pleural fluids of cases with diffuse pleural mesotheliomas. *Br J Exp Pathol* 1963; **44:** 81–83.
75. Boersma A, Degand P, Biserte G. Hyaluronic acid analysis and the diagnosis of pleural mesothelioma. *Bull Physiopathol Respir (Nancy)* 1980; **16:** 41–45.
76. Waxler B, Eisenstein R, Barrifora H. Electrophoresis of tissue glycosaminoglycans as an aid in the diagnosis of mesotheliomas. *Cancer* 1979; **44:** 221–227.
77. Matzel W. Differential diagnosis of pleural diseases. *Zeitschrift Gur die Gesamte Inneae Medizin* 1979; **34:** 50–52.
78. Rowley G, Antonas KN, Hilbert J. Quantitation of hyaluronic acid in equine synovia. *Am J Vet Res* 1982; **43:** 1096–1099.
79. Fisher ER, Hellstrom R. The periodic acid–Schiff reaction as an aid in the identification of mesothelioma. *Cancer* 1960; **13:** 837–841.
80. Wagner JC, Munday DE, Harington JS. Histochemical demonstration of hyaluronic acid in pleural mesotheliomas. *J Pathol Bacteriol* 1962; **84:** 73–78.
81. Singh G, Whiteside TL, Dekker A. Immunodiagnosis of mesothelioma. Use of antimesothelial cell serum in an indirect immunofluorescence assay. *Cancer* 1979; **43:** 2288–2296.
82. Wang NS, Huang SN, Gold P. Absence of carcinoembryonic antigen-like material in mesothelioma: an immunohistochemical differentiation from other lung cancers. *Cancer* 1979; **44:** 937–943.
83. Corson JM, Pinkus GS. Mesothelioma: profile of keratin proteins and carcinoembryonic antigen. *Am J Pathol* 1982; **108:** 80–88.
84. Said JW, Nash G, Tepper G, Banks-Schlegel S. Keratin proteins and carcinoembryonic antigen in lung carcinoma. *Hum Pathol* 1983; **14:** 70–76.
85. Whitaker D, Sterrett GF, Shilkin KB. Detection of tissue CEA-like substance as aid in the differential diagnosis of malignant mesothelioma. *Pathology* 1982; **14:** 255–258.
86. Whitaker D. The mesothelium of the rat and its response to injury. PhD thesis. Perth: University of Western Australia, 1983.
87. Kahn HJ, Hanna W, Yeger H, Baumal R. Immunohistochemical localization of prekeratin filaments in benign and malignant cells in effusions. *Am J Pathol* 1982; **109:** 206–214.
88. Ramaekers F, Puts J, Moesker O, Kant A, Jap P, Vooijs P. Demonstration of keratin in human adenocarcinomas. *Am J Pathol* 1983; **111:** 213–223.
89. To A, Dearnaley DP, Ormerod MJ, Canti G, Coleman DV. Indirect immunoalkaline phosphatase staining of cytologic smears of serous effusions for tumour marker studies. *Acta Cytol* 1983; **27:** 109–113.
90. Ashall F, Bramwell ME, Harris H. A new marker for human cancer cells: 1. The ca antigen and the cal antibody. *Lancet* 1982; **ii:** 1–6.
91. McGee JO'D, Woods JC, Ashall F, Bramwell ME, Harris H. A new marker for human cancer cells 2. Immunohistochemical detection of the ca antigen in human tissues with the cal antibody. *Lancet* 1982; **ii:** 7–10.
92. Woods JC, Spriggs AI, Harris H, McGee JO'D. A new marker for human cancer cells 3. Immunocytochemical detection of malignant cells in serous fluids with the cal antibody. *Lancet* 1982; **ii:** 511–513.
93. Herbert A, Gallagher PJ. Interpretation of pleural biopsy specimens and aspirates with the immunoperoxidase technique. *Thorax* 1982; **37:** 822–827.
94. Mark J. Three chromosomal abnormalities observed in cells of two malignant mesotheliomas studied by banding technique. *Acta Cytol* 1978; **22:** 398–401.
95. Watts KC, Boyo-Ekwueme H, To A, Posnansky M, Coleman DV. Chromosome studies on cells cultured from serous effusions: use in routine cytologic practice. *Acta Cytol* 1983; **27:** 38–44.
96. Burnett RA, Deery ARS, Adamson MR, Liddle C, Thomas M, Roberts GH. Evaluation of Ca 1 antibody in pleural biopsy tissue. *Lancet* 1983; **i:** 1158.
97. Pallesen G, Jepsen FL, Hastrup J, Ipsen A, Hvidberg N. Experience with the Oxford tumour marker (Ca 1) in serous effusions. *Lancet* 1983; **i:** 1326.

JOURNAL OF PATHOLOGY, VOL **143**: 177–182 (1984)

HYPERTENSION, CEREBRAL VASCULAR CHANGES AND STROKE IN GHANA. 1—MICROANEURYSM FORMATION AND STROKE

J. T. ANIM AND A. D. KOFI

Department of Pathology, University of Ghana Medical School, Accra, Ghana

Received 7 July 1983
Accepted 28 November 1983

SUMMARY

A modification of the post-mortem arteriographic technique of Ross Russell[1] was used to study the brains of 284 consecutive autopsy cases dying from non-traumatic causes; and made up of 159 hypertensives and 125 normotensives. Microaneurysms were demonstrated in 30·8 per cent of the hypertensives compared with 9·6 per cent normotensives. Haemorrhagic stroke was the cause of death in 37·6 per cent of the hypertensives, the majority of which were in younger age groups compared with hypertensive strokes in whites. The much lower incidence of microaneurysms in the brain of black hypertensives (even those with haemorrhagic strokes) compared with that found by workers among white hypertensives further emphasized the different nature of hypertension in blacks. It is suggested that, in the absence of significant structural differences in the cerebral vasculature between blacks and whites, the high incidence of haemorrhagic strokes occurring in the relatively younger subjects in Ghana may be due to the direct effect of high blood pressures on small intracerebral vessels and that microaneurysm formation may not be as important as in the much older white subjects dying of haemorrhagic strokes.

KEY WORDS—Hypertension, cerebral haemorrhage, microaneurysms.

INTRODUCTION

It is well accepted now that hypertension among blacks is a different disease from hypertension in whites,[2,3] both from the point of view of natural history and from its complications which may ultimately bring about the demise of the patient.[4–7] Whereas coronary disease with or without myocardial infarction is the commonest cardiovascular complication of hypertension among whites,[8,9] in blacks, stroke or cerebrovascular accident (CVA) and hypertensive cardiac failure are the most common.[10–12]

Many clinical investigators in Africa have stated that thrombotic and embolic stokes are commoner than haemorrhagic strokes.[6,10,13–17] However, post mortem findings, especially in West Africa, have shown a different pattern from that documented by clinical investigators. Edington[18] working in Ghana has shown a high incidence of haemorrhagic strokes compared with thrombo-embolic strokes and this has been confirmed by Laing[19] and Anim.[20]

0022–3417/84/070177–06$01.00

This much higher incidence of haemorrhagic strokes among blacks raises the following questions regarding the cause of the haemorrhage: (a) Is it due to rapidly evolving changes in the cerebral blood vessel walls due to the direct effect of persistently high pressures, since most of the cases are either undetected or poorly controlled hypertensives? (b) Or, is it due to accelerated formation of microaneurysms or even larger aneurysms which ultimately rupture to cause haemorrhage? (c) Or, is it due to an inherent defect in the cerebral vasculature which, like hypertension in blacks is both racial and genetic and presumably predisposes the vessels to rupture?

This study was carried out in an attempt to answer some of the above questions.

MATERIALS AND METHODS

Consecutive post mortem cases were included in the study. These were both hypertensives and normotensives over the age of 20 years. Since the study was carried out in the Korle Bu Hospital Mortuary (which caters for both hospital and medico-legal cases), only fresh corpses were included in the study to ensure that fresh brains were taken for study. All traumatic deaths were excluded. A a modification of the post mortem arteriographic technique of Ross Russell[1] was; employed, using a Harvard infusion pump to inject contrast medium (micropaque without gelatin) simultaneously into the two cannulated intenal carotid stumps at the base of the brain.[21]

After injection, the brains were fixed in 10 per cent formalin for a perod of 3 weeks after which 1 cm thick coronal slices were made using a long brain knife. The slices were exposed to X-rays (30 kV, 4·5 mA, 25 s exposure) in a Softex machine using fine grain Industrex Kodak films which were, subsequently, processed and examined for microaneurysms using a hand lens. Blocks were selected, dehydrated and cleared in methyl salicylate for examination under a dissecting microscope to confirm the presence of microaneurysms. Suitable blocks were further processed for histology using routine haematoxylin and eosin, Van Gieson, Mallory's trichrome stain and PTAH.

Table I—Cases studied Accra (1983)

Total number of cases	310
Hypertensives	181
Normotensives	129
Injected cases	297
Cases rejected	13
Cases examined for microaneurysms	284
Hypertensives	159
Known	94
Unknown	65
Normotensives	125

RESULTS

The number of cases studied was 310, out of which 297 were injected. Of the injected cases 13 were rejected on account of poor injection of poor fixation leaving a total of 294 cases which were studied for microaneurysms (Table I). The 284 cases were made up of 159 hypertensives and 125 normotensives. Before autopsy 94 hypertensives were known hypertensives, but 65 were unknown which were declared hypertensive after autopsy on the basis of heart weight of 360 g or more for males and 300 g or more for females. These heart weights were taken in conjunction with granular kidneys as evidence of pre-existent hypertension.

Microaneurysms

The age distribution of microaneurysms in both hypertensives and normotensives is shown in Table II and Fig. 1. Microaneurysms are commoner in hypertensives (30·8 per cent) than normotensives (9·6 per cent) and occurred in the usual areas of the brain as described by Ross Russell[1] and Cole and Yates,[22] viz., the basal ganglia, internal and external capsules, and thalamus. Fewer microaneurysms were found in the cerebral cortex, cerebellum and brain stem. They were multiple in all cases but fewer in the younger age groups increasing in number with age. The age distribu-

Table II—Age distribution of microaneurysms in hypertensives and normotensives

	Hypertensives			Controls (normotensives)		
Age group	Number	Micro-aneurysms	%	Number	Micro-aneurysms	%
20–29	13	0	0	23	0	0
30–39	24	1	4·2	27	0	0
40–49	29	5	20	25	0	0
50–59	49	17	34·7	21	1	4·8
60–69	24	13	54·2	13	3	23·1
70–79	16	10	62·5	11	4	36·4
80–89	3	2	67	3	2	67
90–99	1	1	100	2	2	100
Total	159	49	30·8	125	12	9·6

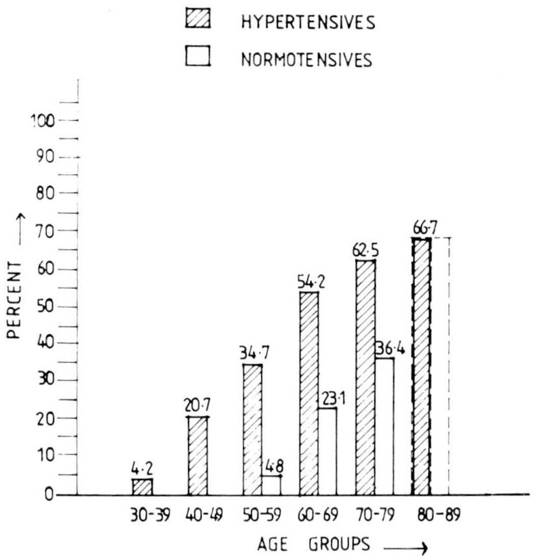

Fig. 1—Age distribution of microaneurysms in hypertensives and normotensives

tion in normotensives shows that formation of microaneurysms is also age-dependent.

Cerebral haemorrhage

Of all the complications of hypertension, cerebral haemorrhage is the most common cause of death as shown in Table III. There were 68 deaths from cerebral haemorrhage, 64 of which were massive as defined by Russell[23] while the remaining four were small but multiple. Fifty-six of these haemorrhagic brains (all massive) were injected out of which 25 showed microaneurysms in the usual sites (44·6 per cent). This percentage is higher than the percentage of microaneurysms in all hypertensives. The remaining hypertensives without

Table III—Causes of death in hypertensives studied

Disease	Number	%
Cerebral haemorrhage	68	37·6
Cerebral infarction		40·9
(atherothrombotic)	6	3·3
Hypertensive cardiac failure	70	38·7
Myocardial infarction	2	1·1
Other	35	19·3
Total	181	100

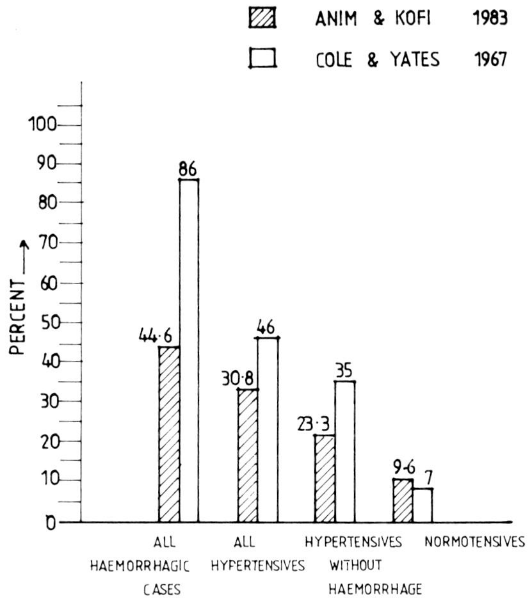

Fig. 2—Percentage of microaneurysms in various categories of cases

haemorrhage showed only 23·3 per cent microaneurysms (Fig. 2).

Infarcts

There were only six deaths from thromboembolic CVA, all hypertensives. Table IV and Fig. 3 show the age distribution of these infarcts indicating that they occur in older subjects than cerebral haemorrhage. Four of the six cases of brain infarction had microaneurysms and they were in the seventh and eighth decades (67 per cent).

Table IV—Age distribution of infarcts in hypertensives

	All hypertensives		
Age group	Number	Infarct	%
20–29	13	0	0
30–39	26	0	0
40–49	37	0	0
50–59	54	2	3·7
60–69	30	2	6·7
70–79	17	2	11·8
80–89	3	0	0
90–99	1	0	0
Total	181	6	2·8

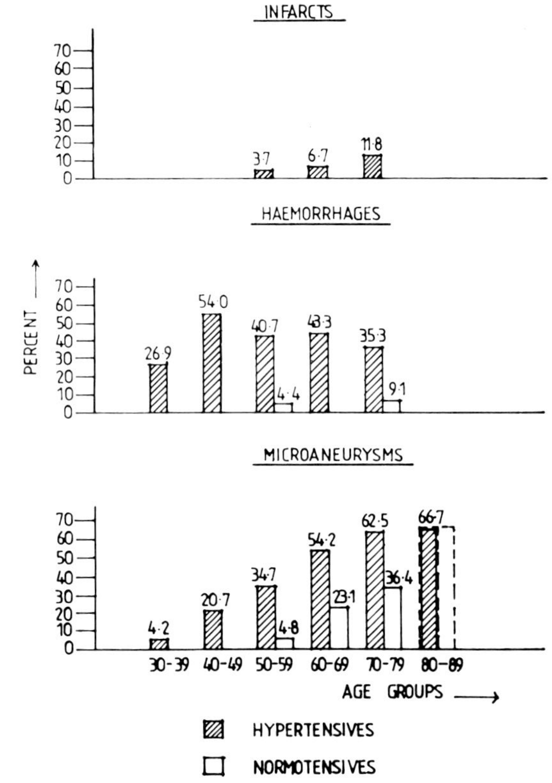

Fig. 3—Age distribution of infarcts and haemorrhages compared to microaneurysms

DISCUSSION

This study further confirms earlier findings,[18–20] that CVA is the most common cause of death in hypertensives in Ghana (Table V) and that haemorrhagic strokes are more common than infarcts. The pattern is different among hypertensive whites who show higher mortality from myocardial infarction and coronary artery disease in general. Stroke when it occurs in white hypertensives seems to be commonly the infarctive type, haemorrhagic stroke being less common.[24–26]

The sites of haemorrhage in the haemorrhagic strokes are similar to those described both among whites and negroes[27,28] (Table VI), but with slightly higher incidence of haemorrhage into the pons as, found by Freytag[28] in negroes when compared with whites.

The much higher incidence of haemorrhages appears to occur in younger age groups in this study than among whites, as stated by Cole and Yates[22] and Ross Russell.[1] Table VII shows that over 70 per cent of hypertensives in this study are below 60 years and about 80 per cent of the unknown hypertensives are below 60 years. Figure 3 is a composite chart comparing the age incidence of cerebral infarcts and haemorrhages with microaneurysm formation and shows that, while the few cases of cerebral infarction occur in the older age groups, cerebral haemorrhage is more common in the younger age groups. Coincidentally,

Table VI—Sites of haemorrhage (comparison of various studies)

Site of haemorrhage	Dinsdale[27] (in whites)	Freytag[28] (in negroes)	Anim and Kofi[21]
Intracerebral	83·9%	72%	70·6%
Cerebellar	10·1%	12%	13.·2
Pontine	6·0%	16%	11·8%
Sub-arachnoid	—	—	4·4%

Table V—Type of CVA (comparison of various studies)

Type of CVA	Adams and Cohen[24] (U.S.) Autopsy 329/1400	Zimmermann[33] (U.S.) Autopsy 182/4240	Edington[18] (Ghana) Autopsy 73 cases	Anim[20] Autopsy 1179/10 720
Haemorrhagic strokes	21%	47%	90·4%	88·8%
Infarct (atherothrombotic and embolic strokes)	73%	46%	9·6%	11·2%

Table VII—Age distribution of all cases studied

Age groups	All hypert.	Known hypert.	Unknown hypert.	Controls	Total
20–29	13	1	12	23	36
30–39	26	14	12	27	53
40–49	37	22	15	25	62
50–59	54	36	18	23	77
60–69	30	22	8	15	45
70–79	17	13	4	11	28
80–89	3	1	2	3	6
90–99	1	—	1	2	3
Total	181	109	72	129	310

these are the age groups in which most unknown or undiagnosed and, therefore, uncontrolled hypertensives occur. As shown in Fig. 3, microaneurysms are commoner among the older age groups and, in this study, the incidence of microaneurysms among cerebral infarcts (although the numbers are small) is higher presumably because the subjects were much older. Although the incidence of microaneurysms among the cerebral haemorrhages is higher than in all the hypertensives studied (including cerebral haemorrhages), it is lower than those found by Cole and Yates.[22] However, their hypertensives are much older and their cerebral haemorrhages also occur in older subjects who are more likely to have microaneurysms.

Microaneurysm formation although it appears to be increased in hypertensives is also age dependent.[1,22] In the much younger hypertensives in Ghana, although hypertension is associated with the formation of microaneurysms, the overall incidence of 30·8 per cent is lower than that found by these same workers and is lower than expected in view of the much higher incidence of cerebral haemorrhage.

It is well accepted that blood pressures are much higher on the average in blacks than in whites.[2,3,29] In this study, of the 78 cases in whom the value of blood pressure was stated, only 16 showed some measure of control, with diastolic pressure of 100 mmHg or less and systolic pressure between 120 and 170 mmHg. The remaining 62 were not controlled and showed average diastolic pressure of 120 mmHg, occasionally reaching 180 mmHg, and average systolic pressure of 200 mmHg, occasionally reaching 280 mmHg. This means, therefore, that even among the known hypertensives blood pressure is poorly controlled.

Since a large proportion of haemorrhages occur in younger hypertensives or, if known, poorly controlled and in whom microaneurysm formation is only just beginning, the haemorrhage is more likely to be due to direct effect of the persistently raised blood pressures on the arteriolar wall resulting in damage to the wall. Histological studies so far carried out have shown no new lesions in the smaller vessels or the brain apart from those described earlier by other workers,[7,30,31]—i.e. changes such as adventitial fibrosis in larger intracerebral vessels, medial fibrosis in smaller vessels with hyalinosis and sometimes fibrinoid necrosis in addition to the formation of microaneurysms.

Treatment of hypertension has been shown to reduce the incidence of cerebral haemorrhage.[32] Adequate treatment of hypertensives in Ghana, therefore, is likely to reduce the incidence of haemorrhagic strokes considerably since, as found by Kannel[9] in the Framingham study, the incidence of stroke is directly related to high blood pressure while coronary heart disease is less dependent on it. Whether by adequately treating hypertensives the pattern of causes of death in Ghanaian hypertensives will change such that coronary heart disease becomes more important is debatable because there are other factors that must be taken into account.

ACKNOWLEDGEMENTS

This study was funded by the Wellcome Trust and we wish to record our sincere gratitude to the Board of Trustees for making it possible. We also express our appreciation to Professor C. C. Bird of the Department of Pathology, University of Leeds, for considerable material assistance as well as helpful suggestions and criticisms; and Mr R. I. Banks of the same department for help in procuring much needed items of equipment and material. We also thank Professor J. O. M. Pobee of the Department of Medicine, University of Ghana Medical School, for helpful suggestion on this manuscript and Professor E. C. Christina for permission to carry out the project in the department. Finally, our sincere thanks go to Mr S. W. Briandt of the Medical Illustrations Unit, University of Ghana Medical School for preparing the illustrations and Miss Sophia Mackenzie for secretarial assistance.

REFERENCES

1. Ross Russell WR. Observations on intracerebral aneurysms. *Brain* 1963; **86:** 425.
2. Ajkinkugbe OO, Akinkugbe FM, Ayeni O, Solomon H, French K. Biracial study of arterial pressures in the first and second decades of life. *British Med J* 1977; **1:** 1132.
3. Boyle E. Biological pattens in hypertension by race, sex, body weight and skin colour. *J Amer Med Ass* 1970; **213:** 1637.
4. Moriyama I, Krueger DE, Stamler J. Cardiovascular disease in the United States. Vital and Health Statistics Monographs, American Public Health Association. Cambridge, Massachusetts: Harvard University Press.
5. McDonough JR, Hames CG, Stulb MS. *et al.* Coronary heart disease among negroes and whites in Evans County, Georgia. *J Chronic Diseases* 1965; **18:** 443.
6. Dada TO, Johnson FA, Araba AB Cerebrovascular accidents in Nigerians: a review of 205 cases. *W Afr Med J* 1969; **18:** 95.
7. Kuller L, Reisler DM. An explanation for variations in distribution of stroke and arteriosclerosic heart disease among populations and racial groups. *Amer J Epidemiol* 1971; **93:** 1.
8. Kannel WB, Wolv PA, Verter J, McNamara PM. Epidemiological assessment of the role of blood pressure in stroke: the Framingham study. *J Amer Med Ass* 1970; **24:** 301.
9. Kannel WB. The Framingham study. *Brit Med J* 1976; **2:** 1255.
10. Haddock DRW. Cerebrovascular accidents in Ghana. *Trans Roy Soc Trop Med Hyg* 1970; **64:** 300.
11. Williams AO, Resch JA, Loewenson RB. Cerebral atherosclerosis—a comparative autopsy study between Nigerian Negroes and American Negroes and Caucasians. *Neurology (Minneap)* 1969; **19:** 205.
12. Williams AO, Loewenson RB, Lippert MS, Resch J. Cerebral atherosclerosis and its relationship to selected diseases in Nigerians: a pathological study. *Stroke* 1975; **6:** 395.
13. Haddock DRW. Neurological disorders in Tanzania. *J Trop Med Hyg* 1965; **68:** 161.
14. Hutton PW. Neurological disease in Uganda. *E Afr Med J* 1956; **33:** 209.
15. Shaper AG, Shaper L. Analysis of medical admissions to Mulago Hospital, 1957. *E Afr Med J* 1958; **35:** 647.
16. Ojiambo HP. Neurological diseases at Kenyatta National Hospital, Nairobi. *E Afr Med J* 1966; **43:** 366.
17. Kaushik SC. In: Lambo TA. ed. The pattern of neurological disease in Ibadan. First Pan-African Psychiatric Conference, Abeokuta, Nigeria, Ibadan: Government Printer, 1961: 1978.
18. Edington GM. Cardiovascular disease as a cause of death in the Gold Coast. *Trans Roy Soc Trop Med Hyg* 1954; **48:** 419.
19. Laing WN. Sudden, unexpected and unexplained deaths in Accra. *Ghana Med J* 1968; **7:** 1.
20. Anim JT. Mortality from stroke and other complications of hypertension in Accra: a study of post-mortems in Korle Bu Teaching Hospital—1972–1981. *West Afr J Med* in press.
21. Anim JT, Kofi AD. Postmortem angiographic study of cerebral vasculature in the Ghanaian adult population—methodology. *Ghana Med J* in press.
22. Cole FM, Yates PO. The occurrence and significance of intracerebral microaneurysms. *J Path Bact* 1967; **93:** 393.
23. Russell DS. The pathology of spontaneous intraranical haemorrhage. *Pròc R Soc Med* 1954; **47:** 689.
24. Adams RD, Cohen ME. Vascular disease of the brain. *Bull New Eng Med Center* 1947; **9:** 180.
25. Groch SN, McDevitt E, Wright IS. Long-term study of cerebral vascular disease. *Ann Int Med* 1961; **55:** 358.
26. Brain, R. Cerebral vascular disorders. *Ann Int Med* 1954; **41:** 675.
27. Dinsdale HB. Spontaneous haemorrhage in the posterior fossa: a study of primary cerebellar and pontine haemorrhages with observations on their pathogenesis. *Arch Neurol (Chicago)* 1964; **10:** 200.
28. Freytag E. Fatal hypertensive intracerebral haematomas: a survey of the pathological anatomy of 393 cases. *J Neurol Neurosurg Psychiat* 1968; **31:** 616.
29. Pobee JOM, Dodu SRA, Larbi EB, Belcher DW, Wurapa FK. Blood pressure distribution in a rural Ghanaian population. *Trans Roy Soc Trop Med Hyg* 1977; **71:** 66.
30. Ross RWR. How does blood pressure cause stroke? *Lancet* 1975; **ii:** 1283.
31. Baker AB, Iannone A. Cerebrovascular disease III. The intracerebral arterioles. *Neurology* 1959; **9:** 441.
32. Smirk H, Hodge JV. Causes of death in treated hypertensive patients. *Brit Med J* 1963; **2:** 1221.
33. Zimmermann HM. Cerebral apoplexy: mechanism and differential diagnosis. *New York J Med* 1949; **49:** 2153.
34. Clawson BJ. In: Bell ET, ed. The Heart in Essential Hypertension. Minneapolis: University of Minnesota Press, 1951; 239.

JOURNAL OF PATHOLOGY, VOL. **143**: 183–186 (1984)

AGE RELATED DETECTION OF TISSUE AMYLOID P IN THE SKIN

A. M. KHAN AND F. WALKER

Department of Pathology, University of Leicester, Leicester, England

Received 19 December 1983
Accepted 25 January 1984

SUMMARY

The presence of tissue amyloid P component in normal skin from fetuses and children was studied using direct, fluorescent, immunohistochemical techniques on frozen sections. Tissue amyloid P is not detected in fetuses or in children up to the age of 2 years but from the age of 4 years upwards it is readily detected and invariably present. Though the function of human amyloid P is unknown its role appears to be age or maturity related.

KEY WORDS—Amyloid P component, skin, fetus, children.

INTRODUCTION

Tissue amyloid P component (TAP) is a pentameric glycoprotein which was originally isolated from all types of amyloid deposits.[1] Subsequently, it has been demonstrated that TAP is not peculiar to amyloid deposits but is a constituent of normal connective tissues.[2–6] The tissues investigated in all of these studies were from adults.

A component apparently identical to TAP is present in the blood and is known as serum amyloid P (SAP). Umbilical cord blood contains very low levels of SAP[7] but these increase rapidly to reach the lower part of the adult range during the first few weeks of extra-uterine life.[8] There have been no comparable studies of TAP in childhood. It was, therefore, decided to investigate the presence of TAP in tissue from a young age group. The localization of TAP in adult skin is well documented[4,9] so this organ was selected for study in fetuses and children.

MATERIALS AND METHODS

In order to obtain an adequate number and appropriate age range of normal skin specimens the site selected for study was the prepuce. Fifty-two specimens, ranging in age from 27 weeks *in utero* to 15 years, were obtained from post mortems on stillbirths and neonates and from surgical circumcisions. (Table I).

The tissues were snap frozen in liquid nitrogen. Sections of approximately 8 μm thickness were cut on a cryostat and air dried at room temperature for 30 min. TAP was demonstrated using direct immunofluorescence as previously described.[4] Briefly FITC conjugated goat anti-human AP (Atlantic Antibodies, Nonesuch Road, Scarborough, U.S.A., Batch No. PCO FITC-012-1 Cat. No. 053-04), previously shown to react with and be absorbed by amyloid deposits was applied to the sections at a dilution of 1:20 PBS, pH 7·2, for 30 min.

With each specimen an unstained section was examined to detect levels of elastic fibre autofluorescence. Adult skin was used as a positive control. For negative controls inappropriate antiserum, namely FITC conjugated goat anti-human immunoglobulin, was applied to the specimen.

Parallel sections were stained with haematoxylin and eosin, and with orcein.

RESULTS

No specific anti-TAP fluorescence is detected in any of the specimens from fetuses or from children

Addressee for correspondence: Dr A. M. Khan, Department of Pathology, Clinical Sciences Building, Leicester Royal Infirmary, P.O. Box 65, Leicester LE2 7LX, England.

0022–3417/84/070183–04$01.00

Table I—Age and number of specimens

Age	27–40 weeks	0–1 yr	1–2 yr	2–3 yr	4 yr and upwards
No.	11	10	5	5	21

up to 2 years in age (Fig. 1). In specimens from children aged 4 years and upwards specific anti-TAP fluorescence is invariably and readily detected (Fig. 2). By the age of 5 years the intensity of the fluorescence is comparable to that of adult control specimens. The distribution in the child is the same as that in the adult and corresponds with orcein staining fibres, i.e. elastic fibres.

Anti-TAP fluorescence is equivocal or barely detected in specimens from 3 year-old children.

DISCUSSION

These results clearly show that the presence of TAP in human skin is age dependent. It is undetectable until the third year then increases to approximate to adult proportions by the fifth year. Presumably this also occurs in other organs.

This time scale differs markedly from that of SAP which rises from low or undetectable levels at birth[7] to adult levels in the first few weeks of extra-uterine life.[8] While the techniques used to detect SAP—immunoassay—and TAP—direct immunofluorescence—differ, their sensitivities are not dissimilar. It is, therefore, concluded that the time differential of about 4 years between SAP and TAP reaching detectable levels in serum and tissue is a true biological phenomenon and not just a manifestation of a technical difference.

In addition as present evidence indicates that TAP and SAP are either identical or very similar, we suggest that the body's AP component exists in two pools. One of these, SAP, circulates in the serum, reaches adult levels in a few weeks and remains remarkably constant though the component only has a half-life of the order of hours.[10] The other pool, TAP, is fixed in the connective tissues

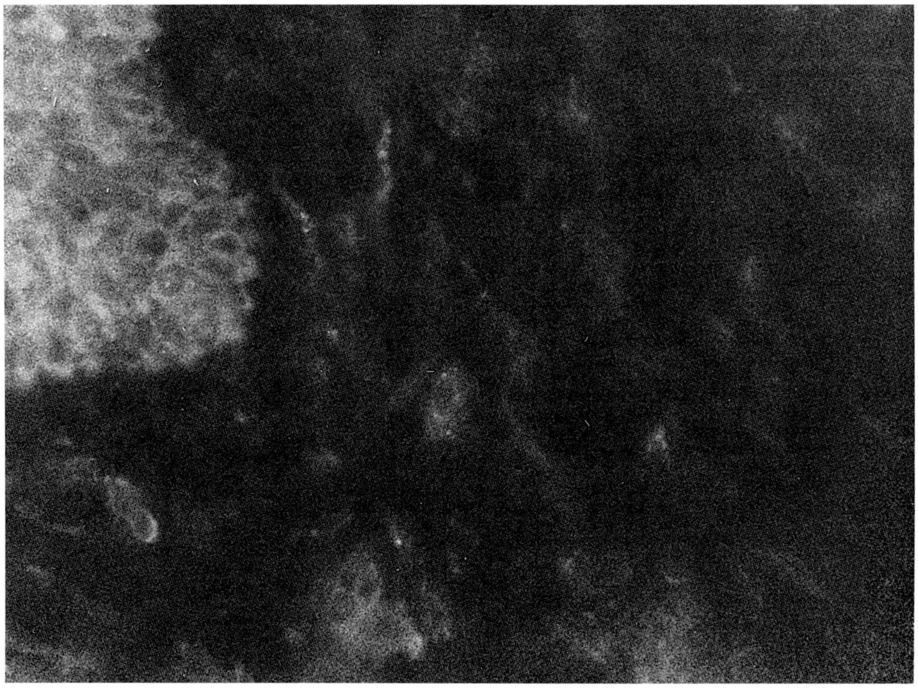

Fig. 1—Two-year old skin, epidermis top left for orientation, showing absence of specific staining with FITC conjugated anti-amyloid P-component. (×450)

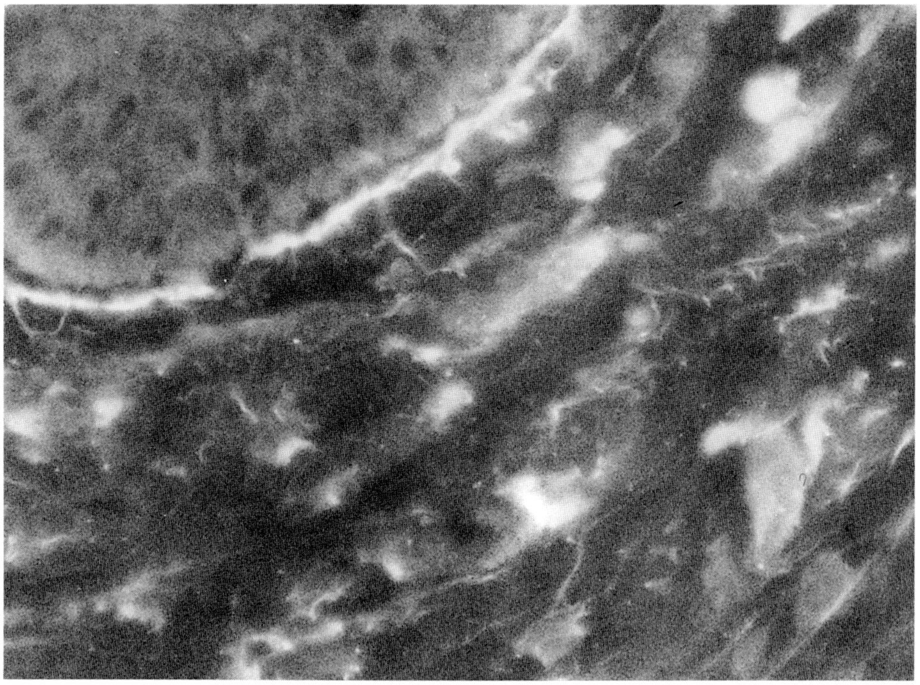

Fig. 2—Four-year old skin, epidermis top left for orientation, showing abundant specific staining with FITC conjugated anti-amyloid P-component. (×450)

and takes several years to reach adult proportions. At present there is no direct information relating to the normal tissue levels or to the biological half-life of TAP. Both warrant investigation.

The microfibrils of elastic tissue appear first in elastogenesis and their diameter increases with fetal and childhood maturation to reach adult size by the age of 8 years[11,12] suggesting that maturation of elastic fibre continues for several years after birth.[11] The central amorphous material i.e. elastin, is laid down at a later stage. Amyloid P appears to be associated very closely with the microfibril component of the elastic fibre but the nature of this relationship is, as yet, undefined.[3]

The function of human AP is unknown but our TAP observations and the SAP results of other investigators do show that in the young its role is age related. Possibly, more precisely, its role may be maturity related for though TAP is not detectable in the term fetus it is readily detectable in the term placenta (unpublished observations).

SAP and C-reactive protein are closely related[13,14] and in the mouse, but not in man, SAP acts as an acute-phase reactant.[15] Speculatively, AP may be regarded in man as a chronic phase reactant: chronic in this context including both age effects on the whole organism and maturity effects on individual organs. In either case it would be of interest to quantify TAP in different organs—particularly in the aged.

ACKNOWLEDGEMENTS

The technical and clerical assistance of Mr M. J. L. Rae, Mr P. Sanderson and Mrs G. L. Holmes is gratefully acknowledged. This paper was presented in part at the 147th Meeting of the Pathological Society of Great Britain and Ireland, at Edinburgh in July 1983.

REFERENCES

1. Cathcart ES, Comerford FR, Cohen AS. Immunologic studies on a protein extracted from human secondary amyloid. *New England Journal of Medicine* 1965; **273:** 143–146.

2. Schneider HM, Loos M. Amyloid P component—a special type of collagen? *Virchows Archiv B (Cell Pathology)* 1978; **29:** 225–228.
3. Breathnach SM, Melrose Suzan M, Bhogal B, De Beer FC, Dyck RF, Tennent Glenys, Black MM, Pepys MB. Amyloid P component is located on elastic fibre microfibrils in normal human tissue. *Nature* 1981; **293:** 652–654.
4. Hamon MD, Walker F. The distribution of amyloid P component in normal human skin. *Virchows Archiv B (Cell Pathology)* 1982; **40:** 411–415.
5. Clayton SJ, Walker F. The distribution of amyloid P component in normal human cervix. *Virchows Archiv B (Cell Pathology)* 1983; **43:** 63–66.
6. Kendall CH, Walker F. Amyloid P component in human thyroid. *Virchows Archiv B (Cell Pathology)* 1984; **45:** 75–78.
7. Cathcart ES, Wollheim FA, Cohen AS. Immunoassay of P-component in amyloidotic sera. *Proceedings of the Society for Experimental Biology and Medicine* 1967; **125:** 1123–1125.
8. Pepys MB, Baltz ML, De Beer FC, Dyck RF, Holford S, Breathnach SM, Black MM, Tribe CR, Evans DJ, Feinstein A. Biology of serum amyloid P component. *Annals of New York Academy of Sciences* 1982; **389:** 286–298.
9. Breathnach SM, Bhogal B, Dyck RF, De Beer FC, Black MM, Pepys MB. Immunohistochemical demonstration of amyloid P component in skin of normal subjects and patients with cutaneous amyloidosis. *British Journal of Dermatology* 1981; **105:** 115–124.
10. Skinner M, Sipe JD, Yood RA, Shirahama T, Cohen AS. Characterization of P-component (AP) isolated from amyloidotic tissue: half-life studies of human and murine AP. *Annals of New York Academy of Sciences* 1982; **389:** 190–198.
11. Tsuji T, Hamada T. Age-related changes in human dermal elastic fibres. *British Journal of Dermatology* 1981; **105:** 57–63.
12. Cleary EG, Fanning JC, Prosser I. Possible roles of microfibrils in elastogenesis. *Connective Tissue Research* 1981; **8:** 161–166.
13. Oliveira EB, Gotschlich EC, Liu T-H. Primary structure of human C-reactive protein. *Proceedings of the National Academy of Sciences, U.S.A.* 1977; **74:** 3148–3151.
14. Oliveira EB, Gotschlich EC, Liu T-H. Primary structure of human C-reactive protein. *Journal of Biological Chemistry* 1979; **254:** 489–496.
15. Pepys MB, Baltz M, Gomer K, Davies AJS, Doenhoff, M. Serum amyloid P-component is an acute-phase reactant in the mouse. *Nature* 1979; **278:** 259–261.

JOURNAL OF PATHOLOGY, VOL. **143**: 187–191 (1984)

THE ROUTINE HISTOLOGICAL INVESTIGATION OF AXILLARY LYMPH NODES FOR METASTATIC BREAST CANCER

F. HARTVEIT

Department of Pathology, The Gade Institute, The University, Bergen, Norway

Received 6 January 1984
Accepted 1 February 1984

SUMMARY

A simple method of preparing axillary nodes from breast cancer patients for routine histology is presented. It is based on appreciation of nodal anatomy and the pathophysiology of tumour growth in them. Current methods assume that the latter is a random process, but this is not so. It has long been known that tumour cells enter via the afferent lymphatics. They may also exit by the efferent. It has not been generally realized that these vessels enter/leave the node *in the same plane of section,* or that a section in this plane, a hilar section, is theoretically the one of choice for the identification of tumour cells in the node. It is shown here that use of *hilar sections alone* allows the identification of tumour-free and tumour-bearing nodes, as well as the tumour status of the efferent vessels, with considerable certainty. The use of random sections, in contrast, carries a high risk of false negative reporting.

KEY WORDS—Breast cancer, lymph nodes, metastatic spread.

INTRODUCTION

The prognosis in breast cancer patients with and without tumour spread to the axillary nodes differs radically. It is therefore the duty of the pathologist to give a reliable report on nodal status.

It has been claimed that serial sectioning is necessary to achieve this end,[1] as nodes reported as negative on routine examination have been shown by this means to contain tumour in up to 30 per cent of cases. This procedure is beyond the means of most investigators but, even so, it is hard to accept a false negative level as high as this. To get round this difficulty mathematical models have been developed that describe, for example, the optimal method of sectioning a node to find a randomly placed metastasis using a minimum of cuts.[2] The method gives high accuracy in small nodes, but this drops rapidly as nodal size increases.

In this study the problem is approached from a different angle. The anatomy of the axillary node is shown to determine the location of metastases, giving a firm basis for the proposed system of sectioning.

MATERIAL AND METHODS

The axillary dissection specimens from 267 women were studied. All these patients had been treated by modified radical mastectomy with axillary node dissection for infiltrating breast carcinoma.

After fixation in formalin for 48 h the lymph nodes in the axillary dissection specimens were easily palpated. If less time is used for fixation even large nodes may be missed. The nodes were dissected free by blunt dissection. The efferent

Addressee for correspondence: Professor F. Hartveit, Dept. of Pathology, 5016 Haukeland Hospital, Bergen, Norway.

0022–3417/84/070187–05$01.00

vessels are readily identified in the process as they are stronger than the surrounding tissue. They leave the node at its hilum which is usually on its concave border. The afferent vessels break easily and are difficult to identify with the naked eye.

The majority of the nodes in the axillae are kidney-shaped. When placed on a flat surface the hilum with its vessels will lie at one side. As shown in Fig. 1 the nodes were bisected through the hilum and the node's longest axis; the cut was made parallel to the surface on which the node was lying. Both parts were prepared for paraffin embedding, the cut surface down. They were embedded together in one block, or in two if their size made this necessary. If these pieces were thicker than 1–2 mm further cuts were made parallel to the first; the cut surface of the additional tissue was prepared for sectioning. In this way two surfaces were made available for hilar sections, while the additional tissue from the periphery was also sectioned in larger nodes. In some very large nodes the surface area was too great to cut in one block. These were divided. A total of 2447 nodes were prepared in this way. From 5 to 7 min were needed for this procedure per axilla.

In 167 cases the axillary specimens were cleared in cedar wood oil after the palpable nodes had been removed. A further 893 nodes were recovered from these cleared specimens. The majority were embedded in one block; 22 nodes from 15 cases were embedded in two blocks. More than two blocks were not required.

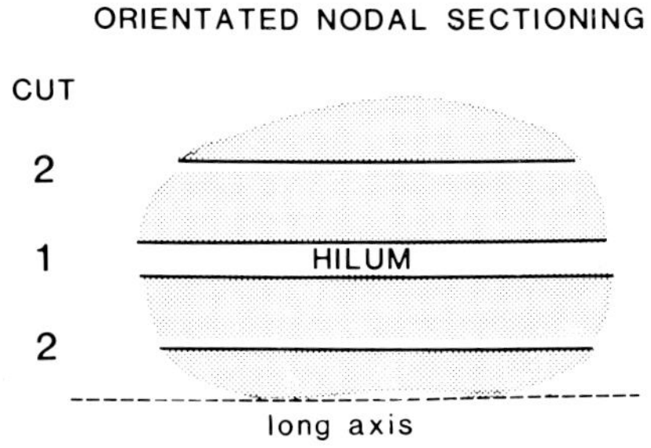

Fig. 1—Diagram of an axillary node lying on a flat surface showing the planes of section used in this study. The first cut (1) goes through the hilum and the longest axis of the node. Secondary cuts (2) are made parallel to the first at 1–2 mm intervals as required. The dark surfaces are those sectioned.

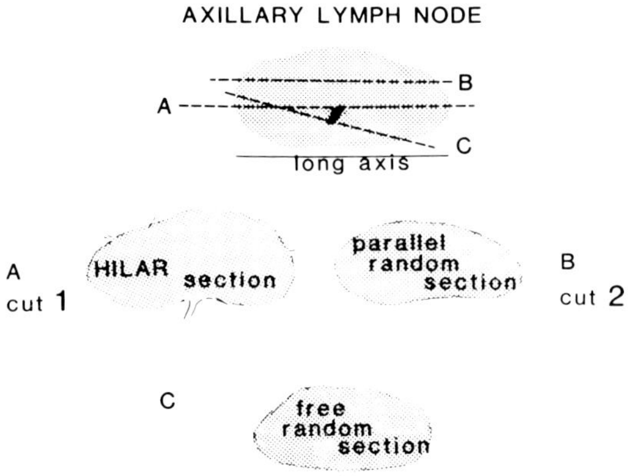

Fig. 2—Terminology used to describe the lymph node sections, see also Fig. 1.

The axillary specimens had been orientated in the majority of cases at operation; the apex was marked with a suture. After fixation the specimen was divided into three levels—upper, middle and lower[3]—and the nodes identified accordingly. One histological section was examined per block and stained with haematoxylin and eosin. The presence/absence of tumour cells in the efferent nodal vessels (efferent vascular invasion = EVI) was recorded from the hilar sections,[4] (see Fig. 2).

RESULTS

The *number of blocks* taken using this system of investigation is related to the tumour status of the nodes and the axilla in Table I. The use of multiple parallel blocks, though usual in tumour-bearing nodes, was not confined to them. The greatest difference in the number of nodes requiring three or more blocks was between the tumour positive, and negative nodes from positive axillae. This difference is statistically significant ($\chi^2 = 5{\cdot}4$, $p < 0{\cdot}025$), as is that between nodes from a negative axilla and the positive nodes ($\chi^2 = 4{\cdot}8$, $p < 0{\cdot}05$). The overall difference between the positive and negative axillae is not.

A total of 517 (14 per cent) of all the nodes were tumour-bearing; 50 per cent of these positive nodes were embedded in one block, compared with 75–80 per cent of the negative. (Divided sections were needed in 6 per cent of the nodes, 4·7 per cent of the negative and 7·5 per cent of the positive.)

Table I—The number of nodes investigated and their tumour status related to the number of blocks taken for histology

Tumour status axilla	Nodes	No. of cases	No. of blocks/node 1	2	3 or more (%)	Total no. of nodes
Negative	Negative	150	1381	331	122 (6·6)	1834
Positive	Positive	117	259	173	85 (16·4)	517
	Negative		772	167	50 (5·1)	989
	All	117	1031	340	135 (9·0)	1504
Total		267	2412	671	257 (7·7)	3340

Table II—The number of nodes from which multiple parallel blocks were taken related to their level in the axillary specimen

Tumour status axilla	Nodes	No. of nodes in axillary specimen with three or more blocks: Upper	Middle	Lower	Total no. of orientated nodes
Negative	Negative	36	62	17	115
Positive	Positive	15	52	9	76
	Negative	21	16	11	48
	All	36	68	20	124
Total		72	130	37	239

A mean of 12·2 ± 6·0 nodes was recovered from node-negative cases, 12·9 ± 5·6 from node-positive.

The level in the axilla at which nodes requiring multiple blocks were found is shown in Table II. Well over half were in the middle axillary area, in both node-negative and node-positive cases. They were more evenly distributed in node-negative from a positive axilla; while they were most prominent in the middle area in positive nodes. Thus, the distribution of nodal size gives little indication of nodal tumour status.

Of nodes requiring multiple blocks 53 per cent needed three blocks, 42 per cent four blocks, 2·8 per cent five blocks, the remainder six or seven. There was little difference in the incidence of these very large nodes, that often consisted mainly of fat, in positive/negative axillae.

Tumour distribution

When tumour was found it was present in one of the hilar sections in all 517 nodes, and in 87 per cent of all sections, from these nodes. It was usually present in both hilar sections but, in 13 of the 85 positive nodes with multiple blocks, one of the putative hilar sections was tumour negative. In eight the hilum was in a different section, and in four additional hilar areas were found in parallel lateral blocks. (Hilar distortion may be due to asymmetrical tumour growth or difficulty in defining the longer axis in a round node, as opposed to one that is kidney-shaped.)

When tumour was not found in the hilar section none was found in the others. Thus, tumour was not found in hilar sections from 2651 nodes, and not found when additional parallel blocks were also taken from a further 172 nodes.

When hilar sections were excluded the distribution of tumour in the remaining blocks showed that in nodes with tumour in the hilar section 101 of 122 parallel sections were tumour-bearing, in contrast to none of 257 in those without. This difference is statistically significant ($\chi^2 = 29$ (2*dl*) $p<0{\cdot}0005$).

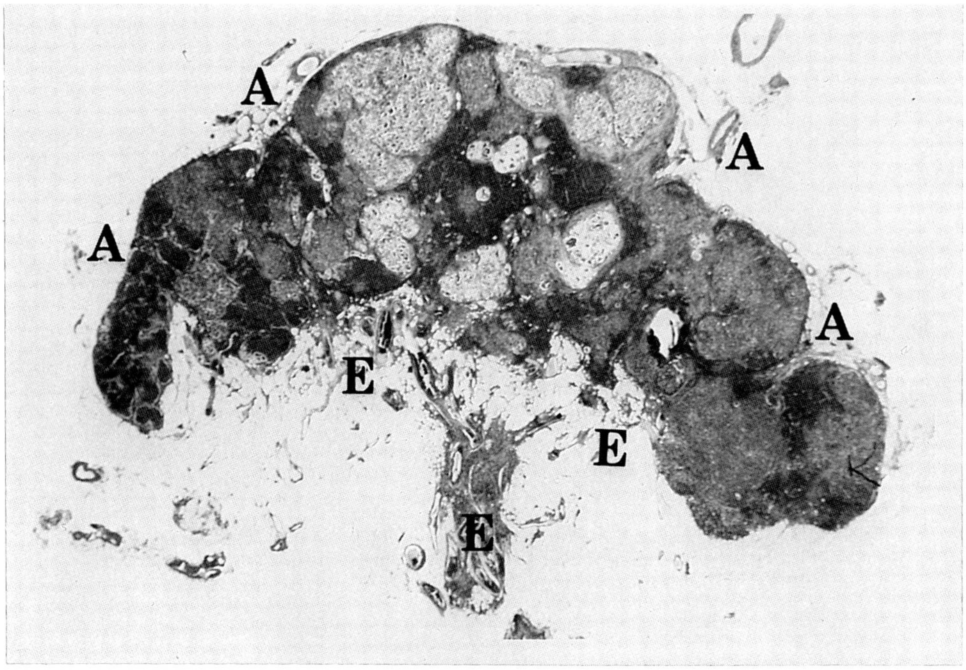

Fig. 3—A hilar section of an axillary node from a patient with breast carcinoma. Afferent lymphatic vessels (A) enter the afferent sinus along the convex border of the node; efferent vessels (E) leave from the concave hilar area. Both sets of vessels contain embolic tumour cells, and tumour growth is established in the node. Haematoxylin and eosin, ×7

Positive nodes with multiple sections

In 61 of these 85 nodes (72 per cent) *all the sections showed tumour,* and 38 of them were EVI positive. When such nodes were EVI negative (23) other EVI positive nodes were present in the axilla in all but two cases.

In 24 nodes (28 per cent) *some sections were tumour-negative.* Six of these nodes were EVI positive and two of them were the only EVI positive nodes in the axilla. The number of tumour-bearing nodes in these cases with negative blocks was 3·8 ± 4·1 (others 7·8 ± 5·3).

In six cases the multiply sectioned node that was EVI negative was the only tumour-bearing node in the axilla, the others were one of two or three. In four only small deposits were found in the hilar sections.

Figure 3 illustrates the principles involved in the identification of a hilar section.

DISCUSSION

It has long been accepted that tumour cells enter lymph nodes by the afferent lymphatics. They may then colonize the node and leave it via the efferent vessels.[4] In man the efferent vessels leave the nodes at the hilum, while the afferent vessels enter on the convex surface.[5] The present work points out that both these sets of vessels enter/leave the node *in the same plane of section.*

On this basis the hilar sections used in this series would theoretically be those of choice for finding tumour cells in the nodes. In practice this proved to be the case. Tumour, when demonstrated in the nodes, was consistently found in a hilar section. Conversely if it were not present in the hilar sections it was not found elsewhere. This indicates that the *distribution of tumour in the nodes is not a random process,* but one that follows a set pattern. Whatever detours the lymph flow may make within the node, the hilar plane would seem to be that of transport in and out. Since tumour cells arrive with the afferent lymph and, as tumour growth is first established in the cortex,[6] it is logical that when present it should be found in hilar sections. This does not exclude that tumour cells may enter the nodes and pass through them without establishing growth. Such cells are unlikely to be found in transit. If slicing of the specimen is used in preference to palpation, orientation of the nodes is not possible, as they will have been cut at random in the process. The method of cutting the nodes described here for the identification of metastases differs from that recommended for the examination of lymphoid tissue, in which cutting through the greatest nodal width is recommended.[7] Sections from such blocks would neatly avoid most of the afferent vessels. The method described here is a variant of three level sectioning',[8] but has the advantage inherent in prior nodal orientation.

The assumption that metastatic growth occurs *at random* in the nodes must thus be abandoned, as should their random sectioning.

The observation that the afferent and efferent vessels are to be found in the same plane of section allows us to use the 'section of choice', which is the hilar section, when looking for tumour cells in these nodes. As a bonus such sections offer the opportunity of recording the status of the efferent vessels; the presence of tumour cells in them denotes poor prognosis,[9] irrespective of the number of tumour-bearing nodes identified.

Clearing of the axillary specimen is not necessary to identify cases with such EVI positive nodes,[10] but multiple sectioning of large nodes may be advisable in rare cases. Such a node, if it contains tumour, may be the only EVI positive node in the axilla, and if EVI negative, the only tumour-bearing node. In general, as the nodes are basically bilaterally symmetrical, the first cut through the node will include the hilar area and give the information needed. If, however, the node was distorted, by tumour or previous scarring, the hilum may have been missed in the first cut. If this happens, and the other nodes in the axilla are either tumour-free or EVI negative, the examination of further cuts from the large node is indicated.

This method of routine histological investigation of the axillary nodes in breast carcinoma adds reliability to the pathologist's report, at the cost of attention to detail, but little extra time or laboratory work. It may be that previous lack of trust in the information given, due to fear of high false negative reporting, has been responsible for the conservative approach to nodal sampling that is common today. If this trend continues valuable prognostic data will be lost, and with it the patient's chance to receive appropriate therapy.

ACKNOWLEDGEMENTS

My thanks are due to the many surgeons who provided the material on which the present study was based, and to the Norwegian Cancer Society that financed the laboratory and clerical work.

REFERENCES

1. Saphir O, Amromin GD. Obscure axillary lymph node metastases in carcinoma of breast. *Cancer* 1948; **1:** 238.
2. Wilkinson EJ, Hause L. Probability in lymph node sectioning. *Cancer* 1974; **33:** 1269.
3. Hartveit F, Tangen M, Halvorsen JF. The axillary nodes and tumour size in breast cancer. *Breast Cancer Research and Treatment* 1982; **2:** 105.
4. Hartveit F. Tumour cells and the axillary nodes in breast cancer. *Invest Cell Path* 1979; **2:** 123.
5. Clark WE, Le Gros. The Tissues of the Body, 2nd edn. Oxford: Clarendon Press, 1945: 232.
6. Hartveit F, Mæhle BO, Halvorsen JF, Tangen M. On the progressive nature of tumour growth in the axillary nodes in breast cancer. *Oncology* 1983; **40:** 309.
7. Wright DH, Isaacson PG. Biopsy Pathology of the Lymphoreticular System. London: Chapman and Hall, 1983; 311.
8. Pickren JW. Significance of occult metastases. A study of breast cancer. *Cancer* 1961; **14:** 1266.
9. Mæhle BO, Skjærven R, Hartveit F. Efferent vascular invasion and the mean nuclear area of axillary nodal tumour cells in breast cancer. *Diagnostic Histopathol* 1982; **5:** 297.
10. Hartveit F, Samsonsen G, Tangen M, Halvorsen JF. Routine histological investigation of the axillary nodes in breast cancer. *Clin Oncology* 1982; **8:** 121.

JOURNAL OF PATHOLOGY, VOL. **143**: 193–197 (1984)

DEGRADATION OF BASEMENT MEMBRANE COLLAGENS BY METALLOPROTEASES RELEASED BY HUMAN, MURINE AND AMPHIBIAN TUMOURS

S. E. SHIELDS, D. J. OGILVIE, R. G. MCKINNELL*† AND D. TARIN‡

Nuffield Department of Pathology, (University of Oxford), John Radcliffe Hospital, Oxford OX3 9DU, U.K.

Received 4 July 1983
Accepted 4 October 1983

SUMMARY

In this investigation it has been found that naturally-occurring (i.e. indigenous, not transplanted) tumours of diverse organs in a spectrum of vertebrates from frogs to man can secrete enzymes which degrade basement membrane collagens (types IV and V). The enzymes are inhibited by chelating agents (EDTA) but not by other protease antagonists and are, therefore, specific metalloproteases. Individual tumours do not necessarily secrete collagenases active against all collagen types (I, IV and V) and release of these different enzymes does not, therefore, appear to be coordinated. These biochemical findings support those reported for serially transplanted tumour cell lines and provide a plausible mechanism for the destruction of basement membranes and stromal collagen fibres observed morphologically in tumour spread.

KEY WORDS—Tumour invasion, basement membrane, collagenases.

INTRODUCTION

Morphological investigations on invading primary tumours and metastatic deposits show that there is extensive destruction of adjacent basement membranes and interstitial collagen.[1,2] It is inferred from such observations that in the vicinity of disseminating neoplasms there is release of proteases which digest elements of the connective tissue and allow disorganized expansion of the tumour. Biochemical evidence confirming the release of specific proteases capable of digesting type I and type III (fibrous) collagens by various tumours has been provided by several investigators[3–8] and a correlation of enhanced collagenase secretion with metastatic colonization potential[9] has also been shown. However, type IV and type V collagen, which are major components of basement membranes throughout the body and are structurally and genetically distinct types of collagen, have been reported to be resistant to cleavage by purified collagenases capable of splitting interstitial collagens (I, II and III).[10,11] These investigations were conducted with enzymes derived both from normal and from neoplastic tissues. Despite this, histopathological and electron microscopical observations[2] have repeatedly shown that tumour cells traverse and demolish epithelial basement membranes, and those surrounding blood vessels, during invasion and metastasis. Liotta *et al.*[11] first reported the secretion, by cells of a *transplantable* murine tumour, of a metalloprotease specifically active against type IV collagen and recently Barsky *et al.*[12] described immunocytochemical localization of type IV collagenase in invading breast carcinoma cells. We now extend these findings by reporting the *secretion* of metalloproteases capable of cleaving type IV and type V collagen by a variety of *naturally-occurring* (indigenous) invasive tumours in man and other animals.

---

* Royal Society Guest Research Fellow.
† Permanent address: Department of Genetics and Cell Biology, University of Minnesota, Saint Paul, Minnesota 55108-1095, U.S.A.
‡ Addressee for reprints.

0022–3417/84/070193–05$01.00

MATERIALS AND METHODS

The samples studied consisted of supernatants obtained from explant cultures of five spontaneous murine mammary tumours, three human breast carcinomas, one human endometrial carcinoma and two spontaneous frog renal tumours (Lucké adenocarcinomas). The explants consisted of minced fragments (approx. 1 mm diameter) derived from a known weight of viable histologically confirmed tumour tissue (usually 200 mg/culture flask). These were cultured in insulin and amino acid supplemented, serum-free, Minimum Essential Medium (mammalian tissue) or Wolf–Quimby medium (amphibian tissue) for 2 weeks after a 2–3 day period of initiation on medium containing 10 per cent newborn calf serum. The culture supernatants were harvested at intervals of 3–4 days, centrifuged and stabilized with one-twentieth volume of 1 M Tris–HCl buffer pH 7·4 containing 100 mM $CaCl_2$ and 0·02 per cent (w/v) sodium azide, prior to storage at −20°C. The samples, *which were not concentrated,* were tested for collagenolytic activity by incubation with purified collagen type IV and type V. These substrates were extracted from pepsin-digested human placentae by the method of Bailey *et al.*[13] modified by incorporation of a heat gelation step[14] to remove residual type I collagen. Excess EDTA was added to reaction mixtures, after 18 h incubation at 25°C, to arrest collagenolytic activity (see Fig. 1 for details) and digestion products were displayed by polyacrylamide gel electrophoresis (PAGE) afer reduction with 2-mercaptoethanol and heat denaturation by boiling in the presence of 4 per cent sodium dodecyl sulphate (SDS).

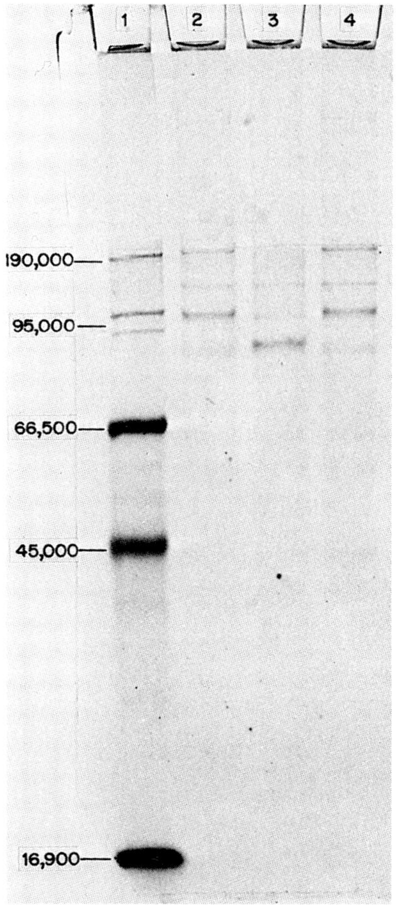

Fig. 1—Polyacrylamide slab gel electrophorogram demonstrating digestion of type IV collagen by a metalloprotease secreted by a human endometrial carcinoma in culture (day 14 supernatant). Track 2: type IV collagen substrate alone. Track 3: type IV collagen plus trypsin-activated culture supernatant. Track 4: type IV collagen plus trypsin-activated culture supernatant plus EDTA. Track 1: molecular weight markers; rat-tail type I collagen β chains, 190 000; rat-tail type I collagen α chains, 95 000; bovine serum albumin, 66 500; ovalbumin, 45 000; myoglobin, 16 900. Digestion of the 120 K and 100 K components by the supernatant accompanied by appearance of an 85 K band representing cleavage product is seen (track 3). The collagenolysis is totally inhibited by EDTA (track 4).

The total volume of the reaction mixture in each of the above assays was 50 μl containing 8 mM $CaCl_2$, 30 mM Tris–HCl pH 7·5, 20 μl of type IV collagen solution and 10 μl of culture supernatant. In wells not containing 80 mM EDTA compensation was made for final assay volume by addition of distilled water. See text for mode of trypsin activation of supernatants. Incubations were conducted at 25°C for 18 h. Before electrophoresis, the samples were diluted 1 : 1 with a reduction-solubilization cocktail for PAGE containing 2-mercaptoethanol and SDS, boiled for 3 min and applied on polyacrylamide gels (5 per cent stacking gel; 7·5 per cent resolving gel). All concentrations given are final concentrations in the reaction mixture

RESULTS

Disappearance or diminution in the intensity of the specific bands representing type IV and type V collagen, together with the appearance of new bands representing characteristic cleavage products obtained by scission of the molecules at specific sites was observed (Figs 1–3). This constitutes qualitative evidence for the presence of collagenolytic metalloproteases in the supernatant. Confirmation is provided by inhibition of enzyme activity in the presence of EDTA in the reaction mixture during digestion[15] and by absence of inhibition by serine protease inhibitors (Soybean Trypsin Inhibitor—SBTI; Phenyl Methyl

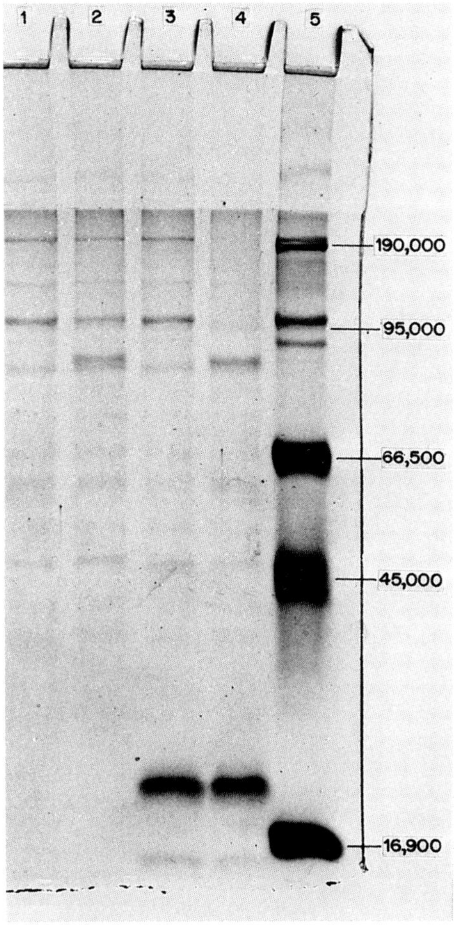

Fig. 2—Polyacrylamide slab gel electrophorogram demonstrating digestion of type IV collagen by a metalloprotease secreted by a frog Lucké renal adenocarcinoma in culture (day 11 supernatant). Track 1: type IV collagen substrate plus culture supernatant plus EDTA. Track 2: type IV collagen plus culture supernatant (no EDTA). Track 3: type IV collagen plus trypsin-activated culture supernatant plus EDTA. Track 4: type IV collagen plus trypsin-activated culture supernatant (no EDTA present). Track 5: contains molecular weight markers (as in Fig. 1). The 120 K and 100 K components of the type IV collagen are cleaved by the supernatant and this activity is completely inhibited by EDTA. Note the 85 K reaction product associated with cleavage of the substrate. The activated culture supernatant (track 4) cleaves more effectively than the unactivated supernatant (track 2). The quantitative composition of the reaction mixture and the mode of preparation of samples for electrophoresis were as described in Fig. 1

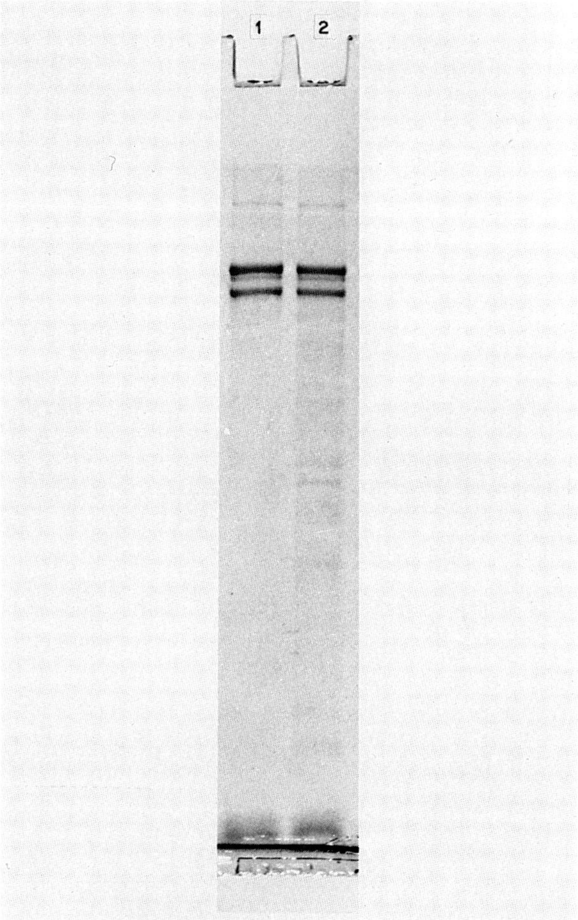

Fig. 3—Polyacrylamide slab gel electrophorogram demonstrating digestion of type V collagen by a metalloprotease secreted by a mouse mammary carcinoma in culture (day 10 supernatant). Track 1: type V collagen substrate plus trypsin-activated culture supernatant plus EDTA. Track 2: type V collagen substrate plus trypsin-activated culture supernatant (no EDTA). The substrate is partially cleaved and digestion products can be seen in track 2; these are missing in the EDTA-containing sample. Type V collagen (20 ml) was incubated with 10 μl of a trypsin-activated supernatant from a cultured mouse mammary tumour. The assay conditions and mode of preparation of samples for electrophoresis were as described in Fig. 1

Sulphonyl Fluoride—PMSF). We have also corroborated the specificity of action of the metalloprotease in these supernatants by tests with other non-specific proteases such as trypsin which attack the pepsin extracted collagen fragments but produce different reaction products and are inhibited by PMSF but not by EDTA.

In this investigation it was found that metalloprotease activity capable of digesting type IV collagen was present in tumour supernatants harvested from all the human, murine and frog tumours tested (see Figs 1, 2) and weak collagenase activity capable of digesting type V collagen was found in several murine mammary as well as one of the human mammary tumours (Fig. 3). It should be clarified, however, that this does not necessarily mean that all tumours in these vertebrates secrete these proteases. The supernatants selected for testing were chosen because they also had significant activity against type I collagen. It was found that murine and human supernatants required prior activation by light trypsin digestion (10 min exposure to 50 μg/ml trypsin at 25°C arrested by addition of 10-fold excess SBTI) to demonstrate cleavage of the collagen (IV) substrate. One amphibian supernatant was used only after trypsin activation but the other was tested for collagenolytic activity before and after trypsin activation. This was the only supernatant which showed some collagenolytic activity against type IV collagen without prior trypsin activation, though it was less marked than that shown after trypsin activation.

DISCUSSION

From this information it is clear that some naturally-occurring tumours are capable of releasing specific metalloprotease activity against type IV and type V collagen *in vitro*. Whether they do so *in vivo* and, if so, under what conditions remains unknown. This supports the reports of Liotta and colleagues[11, 16, 17] who showed collagenase capable of cleaving type IV and V in serially-transplanted cell lines of a murine fibrosarcoma and a reticulum cell sarcoma. The capability of cleaving basement membrane collagens is, therefore, a property possessed by many separate individual 'wild' type tumours of diverse organs in a spectrum of vertebrates ranging from the frog to man. These observations are, at this stage, qualitative but equivalent amounts of substrate protein were applied to each of the tracks on these polyacrylamide gels and it is already evident that the amounts of type IV and type V collagenase activity secreted varies from tumour to tumour and that the activity against one substrate is not necessarily matched by activity against the other. Fully quantitative studies on these differences and their possible relationship to invasive and metastatic behaviour in spontaneous neoplasms, together with investigation of which cells produce the enzymes, are currently in progress in our laboratory. The recent brief report by Barsky *et al.*[12] indicates that type IV collagenase can be detected immunocytochemically within the invading tumour cells.

We have not yet purified from our tumour supernatants the enzymes responsible for cleaving these collagenous proteins and, therefore, cannot state with certainty that two separate enzymes with different specificities are present. Further studies are in progress in this laboratory to investigate this issue but, meanwhile, the observation that the levels of activities against type IV and type V substrates vary independently indicates that separate specific enzymes are secreted by these tumours. This conclusion is supported by earlier work on enzymes derived from normal[10] and malignant tissues.[11] These studies demonstrated that the enzymes which cleaved the interstitial collagens and each of the basement membrane collagens are separate specific entities. Mainardi *et al.*[18] have reported that elastase, secreted by granulocytes, cleaves type IV collagen, but histological studies on all of these tumour types show remarkably few of these cells.

Our finding that most of the supernatants required trypsin activation to reveal collagenase activity showed that the culture conditions favour accumulation of latent enzyme but we cannot at this stage comment on whether it is originally secreted in active or latent form. There is considerable controversy[19] as to whether latent type I collagenase is a pro-enzyme or an enzyme–inhibitor complex and information on whether latent type IV and type V collagenases fall into either of these categories is currently not available.

This demonstration, in various types of tumours, of proteolytic activity capable of lysing major structural components of basement membranes correlates well with the electron microscopical observation of basement membrane destruction in tumours in various species. The release of the enzyme activity by tumours in such widely different vertebrates and the individual variation in degree of substrate cleavage between different tumours both suggest that elaboration of these specific proteases may be an important general mechanism in tumour invasion and metastasis.

ACKNOWLEDGEMENTS

This work was supported by a grant from the Cancer Research Campaign and a Royal Society Guest Research Fellowship awarded to Dr D. Tarin to invite Professor R. G. McKinnell to work in Oxford. The help of these organizations is gratefully acknowledged. We also wish to thank

Professor A. J. Bailey for advice on the preparation of collagen types IV and V, Professor A. C. Turnbull for help with obtaining human placentae, Mr E. G. Lee and Mr A. C. Vass for supplies of human tumour tissue, Professor G. W. Nace for amphibian tumours and Mrs P. Messer and Mrs B. Carter for help in preparation of the manuscript.

REFERENCES

1. Tarin D. Sequential electron microscopical study of experimental mouse skin carcinogenesis. *Int J Cancer* 1967; **2:** 195.
2. Tarin D. Cellular interactions in neoplasia. In Weiss L. ed. Fundamental Aspects of Metastasis. Amsterdam: North-Holland, 1976: 151.
3. Dresden MH, Heilman A, Schmidt JD. Collagenolytic enzymes in human neoplasms. *Cancer Res* 1972; **32:** 993.
4. Yamanishi Y, Dabbous MK, Hashimoto K. Effect of collagenolytic activity in basal cell epithelioma of the skin on reconstituted collagen and physical properties and kinetics of the crude enzyme. *Cancer Res* 1972; **32:** 2551.
5. Hashimoto K, Yamanishi Y, Maeyens E, Dabbous MK, Kanzaki T. Collagenolytic activities of squamous-cell carcinoma of skin. *Cancer Res* 1973; **33:** 2790.
6. Abramson M, Schilling RW, Huang C-C, Salome RG. Collagenase activity in epidermoid carcinoma of the oral cavity and larynx. *Ann Otol Rhinol Laryngol* 1975: **84:** 158.
7. Dabbous MK, Roberts AN, Brinkley B. Collagenase and neutral protease activities in cultures of rabbit VX-2 carcinoma. *Cancer Res* 1977; **37:** 3537.
8. Kuettner KE, Soble L, Croxen RL, Marczynska B, Hiti J, Harper E. Tumor cell collagenase and its inhibition by a cartilage-derived protease inhibitor. *Science* 1977; **196:** 653.
9. Tarin D, Hoyt BJ, Evans DJ. Correlation of collagenase secretion with metastatic colonization potential in naturally occurring murine mammary tumours. *Br J Cancer* 1982; **46:** 266.
10. Woolley DE, Glanville RW, Roberts DR, Evanson JM. Purification, characterization and inhibition of human skin collagenase. *Biochem J* 1978; **169:** 265.
11. Liotta LA, Abe S, Robey PG, Martin GR. Preferential digestion of basement membrane collagen by an enzyme derived from a metastatic murine tumor. *Proc Natl Acad Sci* 1979; **76:** 2268.
12. Barsky SH, Togo S, Garbisa S, Liotta LA. Type IV collagenase immunoreactivity in invasive breast carcinoma. *Lancet* 1983; **i:** 296.
13. Bailey AJ, Sims TJ, Duance VC, Light ND. Partial characterization of a second basement membrane collagen in human placenta. *FEBS Letters* 1979; **99:** 361.
14. Trelstad RL, Lawley KR. Isolation and initial characterization of human basement membrane collagens. *Biochem Biophys Res Comm* 1977; **76:** 376.
15. Gross J. An essay on biological degradation of collagen. In: Hay ED. ed. Cell Biology of Extracellular Matrix. New York: Plenum Press, 1981: 217.
16. Liotta LA, Tryggvason K, Garbisa S, Robey PG, Abe S. Partial purification and characterization of a neutral protease which cleaves type IV collagen. *Biochem* 1981; **20:** 100.
17. Liotta LA, Lanzer WL, Garbisa S. Identification of a type of V collagenolytic enzyme. *Biochem Biophys Res Comm* 1981; **98:** 84.
18. Mainardi CL, Dixit SN, Kang AH. Degradation of type IV (basement membrane) collagen by a proteinase isolated from human polymorphonuclear leukocyte granules. *J Biol Chem* 1980; **255:** 5435.
19. Harris EDJr, Vater CA. Methodology of collagenase research: substrate preparation, enzyme activation and purification. In: Woolley DE, Evanson JM. eds. Collagenase in Normal and Pathological Connective Tissues. Chichester: John Wiley, 1980: 37.

JOURNAL OF PATHOLOGY, VOL. **143:** 199–204 (1984)

IMMUNOLOCALIZATION OF PREALBUMIN AS A MARKER FOR CARCINOID TUMOURS

I. D. MILLER,* W. A. REID,†‡, CHRISTINE N. LIDDLE† AND C. H. W. HORNE*§

**Department of Pathology, University Medical Buildings, Foresterhill, Aberdeen AB9 2ZD, Scotland and †University Department of Pathology, Royal Infirmary, Glasgow G4 0SF, Scotland*

Received 17 February 1984
Accepted 27 February 1984

SUMMARY

Using a PAP immunoperoxidase technique, we have demonstrated the plasma protein prealbumin in 92 (87 per cent) out of a series of 106 carcinoid tumours from various sites. The frequency of detection was greater than with the conventional stains; 83 (78 per cent) of the cases were positive for one or more of these stains. The Grimelius technique was by far the most effective of the conventional stains; it was positive in 81 (76 per cent) cases. We were unable to detect prealbumin in a variety of carcinomas. Although prealbumin identification did not appear to have any advantage over the routine stains in midgut-derived carcinoids, it was much more effective in the diagnosis of bronchial (foregut) and rectal (hindgut) carcinoids. We believe that prealbumin staining offers a cheap, reliable and valuable method for the detection of carcinoid tumours in routine histopathology.

KEY WORDS—Prealbumin, carcinoid tumours, immunoperoxidase, histochemical stains.

INTRODUCTION

Carcinoid tumours are uncommon tumours of the diffuse neuroendocrine (APUD) cell system. The derivation of this system in the embryo is controversial and initially a common neural crest origin was suggested.[1] Carcinoid tumours occur in the appendix, oesophagus, stomach, duodenum, jejunum, ileum, colon, rectum, ovary, biliary tract and bronchi.[2] These tumours are, on the whole, easily recognized by their typical light-microscopic picture: solid nests, trabecular or ribbon-like, tubular, acinar or rosette-like cellular patterns are seen. In the routine laboratory confirmation of the diagnosis generally depends on the results of the conventional silver impregnation techniques (argyrophil or argentaffin). Electron microscopy can also reveal the characteristic neurosecretory granules. More recently, since these tumours are known to have the potential to produce a variety of proteins including peptide hormones, 5-hydroxytryptamine and neurone-specific enolase, immunocytochemistry can be performed as an aid to diagnosis.

Prealbumin, also known as thyroxine-binding prealbumin or vitamin A-transporting protein, is a major plasma protein of low molecular weight (54980).[3] It has been detected in human fetal cord blood from as early as 11·5 weeks gestation[4] and in adults, the generally accepted mean serum level is about 25 mg/100 ml.[5] In normal human tissue it is detectable by immunocytochemical techniques, in the α cells of the Islets of Langerhans and in single cells in the mucosa of the gastrointestinal tract, mainly stomach and colon.[6] There is a significant degree of homology between prealbumin and the polypeptide hormones glucagon, secretin and vasoactive intestinal peptide and it has been suggested that there may be an evolutionary link between them.[7] The distribution of prealbumin staining matches that of APUD cells and prelimin-

‡Present address: Department of Pathology, University of Leeds, Leeds LS2 9JT, England.

§Addressee for correspondence: Professor C. H. W. Horne, Department of Pathology, Royal Victoria Infirmary, Queen Victoria Road, Newcastle-upon-Tyne NE1 4LP, England.

0022–3417/84/070199–06$01.00

ary work has shown that it is detectable in carcinoid tumours.[8]

In the present study, a large series of carcinoid tumours from various sites were examined for prealbumin immunoreactivity and for comparison, the tumours were also stained using conventional histochemical methods.

MATERIALS AND METHODS

Tissues

Formalin-fixed paraffin-embedded tissue was obtained from the routine surgical files of Aberdeen Royal Infirmary, Raigmore Hospital, Inverness, Glasgow Royal, Victoria and Western Infirmaries and Withington Hospital, West Didsbury, Manchester. Sections were cut to a thickness of 5 μm.

Criteria for selection of cases

The 111 carcinoids in the series were originally diagnosed primarily on the basis of histological appearance. Our criteria for considering them as carcinoids were that they satisfied at least two of the following conditions:

(a) histological appearance suggestive of a carcinoid;
(b) one or more conventional stain positive (diazo, Grimelius, Bodian, Fontana);
(c) electron microscopy positive for neurosecretory granules in cases which were negative for all our tests and positive for prealbumin only.

Five cases were excluded from the series as they failed to satisfy our criteria.

Immunocytochemical staining

Trypsinized sections were stained by the PAP immunoperoxidase technique modified from the method of Sternberger *et al.*[9] All staining employed commercially obtained antisera to prealbumin (Dakopatts, Seward), at a dilution of 1:200. Specificity of the antisera was shown by complete abolition of positive staining after blocking the antisera with purified prealbumin (Seward).

Histochemical staining

The stains employed were the Grimelius silver nitrate technique and the Bodian silver protargol technique for argyrophil cells. The alkaline diazo method and the Masson–Fontana technique were used for argentaffin cells.

Ultrastructural studies

The sections were processed, then layered with Epon–Araldite and after hardening, the embedded tissue was prised off the slide. A selected area containing tumour cells was excised and then attached to a block of Epon–Araldite and sectioned for electron microscopy.[10]

RESULTS

Prealbumin was detectable in all appendix carcinoids and in all but one of the small bowel tumours (see Table I). The peroxidase staining for prealbumin tended to be marked, particularly around the periphery of the tumour clumps (Fig. 1) and electron microscopy confirmed that the reaction product was in relation to the endocrine secretory granules, the average size of which was

Table I—Frequency and percentage of prealbumin and conventional staining in carcinoid tumours

Site of tumour	Total cases	Prealbumin positive	Positive conventional stains: Diazo	Grimelius	Fontana	Bodian
Appendix	22	22 (100%)	19 (86%)	21 (95%)	17 (77%)	21 (95%)
Small bowel	36	35 (97%)	26 (72%)	35 (97%)	21 (58%)	32 (88%)
Colon	7	4 (57%)	0	4 (57%)	0	2 (29%)
Stomach	5	2 (40%)	0	3 (60%)	0	1 (20%)
Bronchus	29	23 (79%)	1 (3%)	16 (55%)	0	7 (24%)
Rectum	5	4 (80%)	0	0	0	0
Metastases	2	2	1	2	2	2
Total	106	92 (87%)	47 (44%)	81 (76%)	40 (38%)	65 (61%)

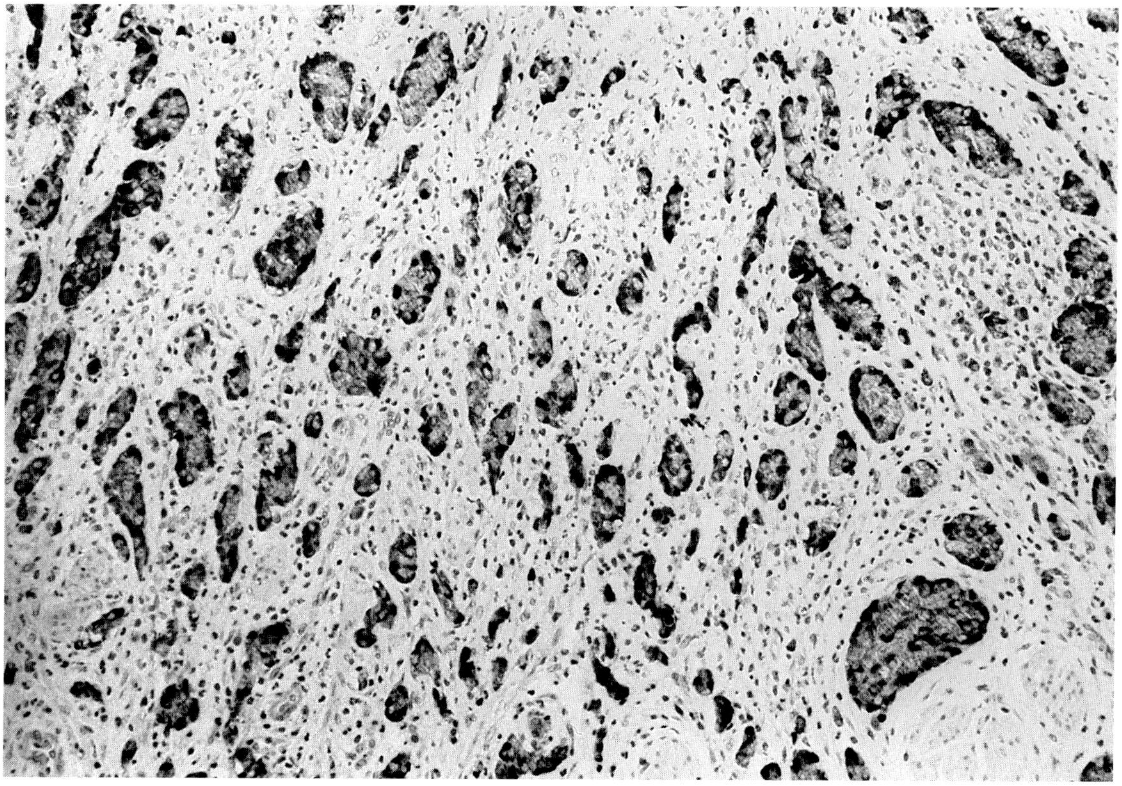

Fig. 1—Carcinoid tumour of appendix. Note the strong staining for prealbumin particularly around the periphery of the tumour cell nests. Immunoperoxidase (PAP)

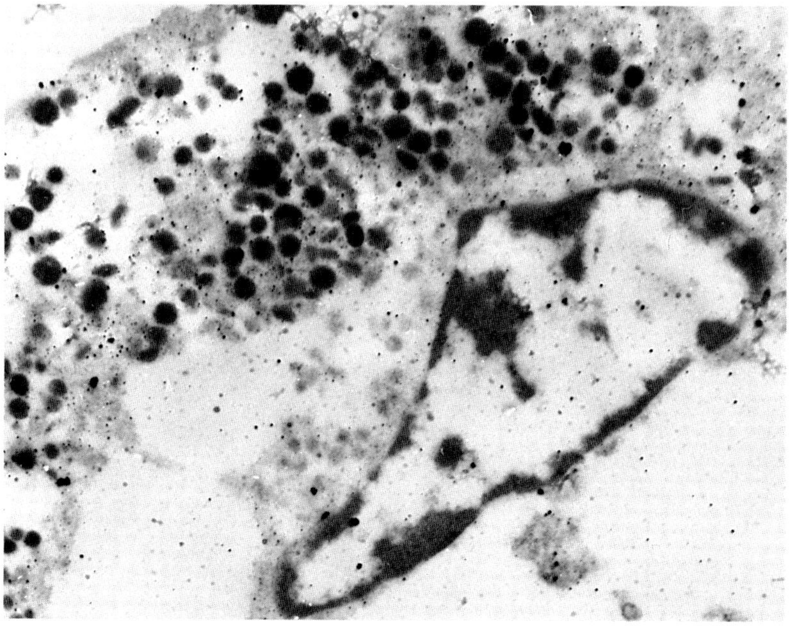

Fig. 2—Carcinoid tumour of appendix. The prealbumin/reaction product is associated with the neurosecretory granules Immunoperoxidase (PAP), E.M.×14744

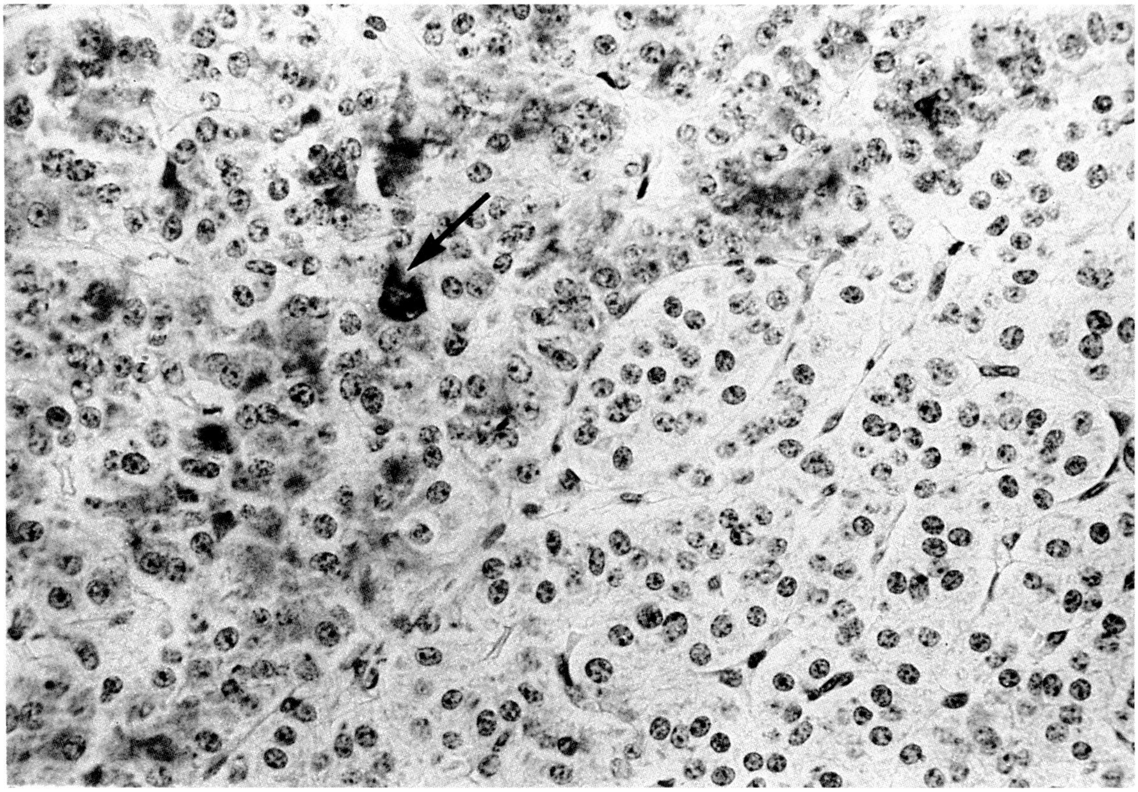

Fig. 3—Bronchial carcinoid. Note the patchy staining for prealbumin with strong staining in occasional cells (arrowed). Immunoperoxidase (PAP)

0·25 μm (Fig. 2). In some cases, particularly bronchial carcinoids, the peroxidase staining appeared to be focal but was marked in individual cells (Fig. 3).

The incidence of positive staining using conventional methods appeared to be similar to that of prealbumin, in carcinoids arising in appendix, small bowel, colon and stomach. As with prealbumin, the staining was most marked at the periphery of the tumour nests. However, in bronchial and rectal carcinoids, the number of cases positive for the conventional stains was considerably less than those positive for prealbumin.

Overall 87 per cent of the tumours in the series were positive for prealbumin, compared with 78 per cent for one or more of the routine stains. Twelve cases (11 per cent) which were negative with all the histochemical stains, were positive for prealbumin (lung (6), rectum (4), colon (1) and stomach (1)). In contrast, three cases (2·8 per cent) were positive only with the conventional stains (lung (2), caecum (1)). Eleven cases were negative for prealbumin and all the conventional stains.

All 29 control tumours examined (adenocarcinomas of lung and bowel, oat cell and squamous carcinomas of lung, malignant melanomas) were negative for prealbumin.

DISCUSSION

Prealbumin is one of many proteins which have been demonstrated in carcinoid tumours. Gould *et al.*[11] examined 22 cases of lung carcinoids and all but one showed immunoreactivity for at least one hormone. In 19 cases more than one hormone was detectable. The hormones included 5-hydroxytryptamine (16), bombesin (14), vasoactive intestinal peptide (13), leu-enkephalin (11), somatostatin (8) and calcitonin (2). He also noted that the distribution of these products tended to be notably heterogeneous. Wilander *et al.*[12] found gastrin and substance P immunoreactivity in a series of 16 gastroduodenal endocrine tumours. Few studies have attempted to evaluate these products as a specific marker for carcinoids or other apudomas. However, a study on a series of 90 apudomas showed that neurone-specific enolase, which is a neuronal form of the glycolytic enzyme enolase previously found to be present in APUD cells and neurones, stained all such tumours; it was not found in non-endocrine tumours.[13] It was also detectable in benign and malignant melanocytic lesions.[14] Neurone-specific enolase stained oat cell carcinomas; that observation would limit its use as a specific marker for bronchial carcinoids, whereas by contrast prealbumin was not detectable in oat cell carcinomas. A recent innovation was the use of monoclonal antibodies to 5-hydroxytryptamine to localize carcinoids,[15] but the disadvantage with this technique is that few foregut and hindgut carcinoids will stain, as most of these tumours show no signs of containing or secreting 5-hydroxytryptamine.[16]

Much reliance is often placed on the results of silver impregnation and diazo techniques in the diagnosis of carcinoid tumours, but the results of previous studies on their value have been somewhat variable. Marks[2] found that more than half of foregut and hindgut derived tumours in a large series were non-reactive. Soga and Tazawa[17] showed that foregut carcinoids were either argyrophil or non-reactive and hindgut carcinoids non-reactive. The great majority of midgut tumours were argentaffin positive. In total, 32 out of 62 carcinoids were non-reactive. In contrast, Blondal *et al.*[18] looked at 46 lung carcinoids and all were Grimelius positive. However, they observed that the argyrophil reaction often varied within each case and in some cases non-reactive areas were seen. Wilander *et al.*[19] found that the Grimelius technique stained all 45 gastrointestinal carcinoids irrespective of location, although rectal carcinoids sometimes needed re-impregnation. In our series the Grimelius silver nitrate technique was by far the most effective of the stains, although only 76 per cent were positive.

The results of our study demonstrate that the immunolocalization of prealbumin in carcinoid tumours seems to be a more useful marker for such tumours than are the conventional stains. Prealbumin staining is particularly valuable in the diagnosis of bronchial and rectal carcinoids; the frequency of positive silver and diazo staining is much less. It is not specific to carcinoids as it also stains islet cell tumours and in an unpublished study we have been able to detect prealbumin in 13 out of 20 (65 per cent) islet cell tumours. However, we have not been able to detect it in phaeochromocytomas (2) medullary carcinomas (3) or in any non-APUD tumours.

Although carcinoid tumours can be diagnosed ultrastructurally, this facility is not universally available. Furthermore, it is fairly expensive and time-consuming. Prealbumin localization by the PAP technique, on the other hand, is cheap and reliable and can be performed in any routine laboratory. In our experience prealbumin would be the first choice as a special stain for these tumours.

REFERENCES

1. Pearse AGE, Polak JM. Neural crest origin of the endocrine polypeptide (APUD) cells of the gastrointestinal tract and pancreas. *Gut* 1971; **12:** 783–788.
2. Marks C. Carcinoid tumours: a clinicopathological study. Boston: G. K. Hall and Co., 1979.
3. Kanda Y, Goodman DS, Canfield RE, Morgan FJ. The amino acid sequence of human plasma prealbumin. *J Biol Chem* 1974; **249:** 6795–6805.
4. Rossi T, Hirvonen T, Toivanen P. The concentration of prealbumin in human and infant sera. *Scand J Clin Lab Invest* 1970; **26:** 35–36.
5. Hutchinson DR, Halliwell RP, Smith MG, Parke DV. Serum prealbumin as an index of liver function in human hepatobiliary disease. *Clin Chim Acta* 1981; **114:** 69–74.
6. Liddle CN, Reid WA, Kennedy JS, Miller ID, Horne CHW. Immunolocalisation of prealbumin: distribution in normal tissue. *J Pathol,* in press.
7. Jörnvall H, Carlström A, Pettersson T, Jacobsson B, Persson M, Mutt V. Structural homologies between prealbumin, gastrointestinal prohormones and other proteins. *Nature* 1981; **291:** 261–263.
8. Reid WA, Miller ID, Liddle CN, Horne CHW. Prealbumin as a marker for carcinoid tumours. *Protides of the Biological Fluids* 1984; **31:** 379–382.
9. Sternberger LA, Hardy PHJR, Cuculis YJ, Meyer GH. The unlabelled antibody enzyme method of immunohistochemistry. Preparation and properties of soluble antigen–antibody complex (horseradish peroxidase) and its use in identification of spirochetes. *J Histochem Cytochem* 1970; **18:** 315–333.
10. Hashida Y. Electron microscopic demonstration of viral particles in sudden infant death syndrome. *Ultrastruct Pathol* 1980; **1:** 7–10.
11. Gould VE, Linnoila RI, Memoli VA, Warren WH. Neuroendocrine cells and neuroendocrine neoplasms of the lung. In: Sommers SC, Rosen PP, eds. Pathology Annual, Part I, Vol 18. Norwalk, Connecticut: Appleton-Century-Crofts, 1983: 287–330.
12. Wilander E, Grimelius L, Lundquist G, Skoog V. Polypeptide hormones in argentaffin and argyrophil

gastroduodenal endocrine tumours. *Am J Pathol* 1979; **96:** 519–530.

13. Tapia FJ, Polak JM, Barbosa AJA, Bloom SR, Marangos PJ, Dermody C, Pearse AGE. Neurone-specific enolase is produced by neuroendocrine tumours. *Lancet* 1981; **ii:** 808–811.
14. Royds JA, Parsons MA, Rennie IG, Timperley WR, Taylor CB. Enolase isoenzymes in benign and malignant melanocytic lesions. *Diagn Histopathol* 1982; **5:** 175–181.
15. Cuello AC, Wells C, Chaplin AJ, Milstein C. Serotonin immunoreactivity in carcinoid tumours demonstrated by a monoclonal antibody. *Lancet* 1982; **i:** 771–773.
16. Wilander E, Lundquist M. Accuracy in histological diagnosis of carcinoid tumours. *Lancet* 1982; **i:** 1471–1472.
17. Soga J, Tazawa K. Pathologic analysis of carcinoids. *Cancer* 1971; **28:** 990–998.
18. Blondal T, Grimelius L, Nou E, Wilander E, Aberg T. Argyrophil carcinoid tumours of the lung. *Chest* 1980; **78:** 840–844.
19. Wilander E, Portela-Gomes G, Grimelius L, Westermark P. Argentaffin and argyrophil reactions of human gastrointestinal carcinoids. *Gastroenterology* 1977; **73:** 733–736.

JOURNAL OF PATHOLOGY, VOL. **143:** 205–209 1984)

USEFULNESS OF ENZYME- AND IMMUNOHISTOCHEMISTRY IN THE DIAGNOSIS OF JUVENILE XANTHOGRANULOMA

C. DE WOLF-PEETERS†, F. FACCHETTI, H. DEGREEF*, J. J. VAN DEN OORD, A. VANNESTE AND V. J. DESMET

*Department of Pathology and *Department of Dermatology, A.Z. St.-Rafael, University of Leuven, Belgium*

Received 6 February 1984
Accepted 28 February 1984

SUMMARY

Skin biopsies from two children with juvenile xanthogranuloma were studied. Enzyme- and immunohistochemistry was used to establish the mononuclear phagocytic nature of the proliferating dermal elements. The usefulness of both techniques in the diagnosis and the differential diagnosis of this disease is suggested.

KEY WORDS—Juvenile xanthogranuloma, enzyme-histochemistry, immunohistochemistry, diagnostic histopathology.

INTRODUCTION

Juvenile xanthogranuloma is a benign, normolipaemic self-healing histiocytosis which develops almost always in the first year of life. The disease is characterized by an eruption of single or multiple papules or nodules which spontaneously disappear without scarring.[1]

Extracutaneous lesions can occur but are rare.[2] Establishment of the diagnosis can be difficult clinically as well as morphologically.[3–5]

The search for Birbeck granules by electron microscopy may be helpful[6] and even mandatory[5,7] to differentiate juvenile xanthogranuloma from histiocytosis X. The aim of this study is a further phenotyping of the proliferating histiocytes in juvenile xanthogranuloma with the help of enzyme- and immunohistochemistry.

CASE REPORTS

Case 1

A 4 month old boy presented with convulsions and skin lesions which developed 1 month before admission. These lesions corresponded to macular, slightly elevated, sharply delineated, ivory-yellowish to brownish stained plaques localized on the face (Fig. 1), xanthoma-like papules on the chin and the thumb and a few papules on the extremities. A first biopsy was taken from the knee. During the following 2 months all skin lesions developed a more clearcut xanthomatous aspect. A second biopsy was performed from a lesion on the chin.

The child was seen for the third time at the age of 14 months when almost the entire face was covered with heavily infiltrated xanthomatous plaques. The lesions on the thumb and the extremities had increased in number and size. A third biopsy was taken. No further clinical and biochemical abnormalities were found except for a 13–15 translocation on cytogenetic investigation. Clinically a diagnosis of juvenile xanthogranuloma of the macronodular type was proposed.

Case 2

A 1 year old girl presented with eight orange-yellowish stained, pea-sized, firm papules on her face (Fig. 2), scalp and knee. The lesions had been present for some months. No further clinical or

† Addressee for correspondence: C. De Wolf-Peeters, A.Z. St.-Rafael, Department of Pathology, Minderbroedersstraat 12, 3000 Leuven, Belgium.

0022–3417/84/070205–05$01.00

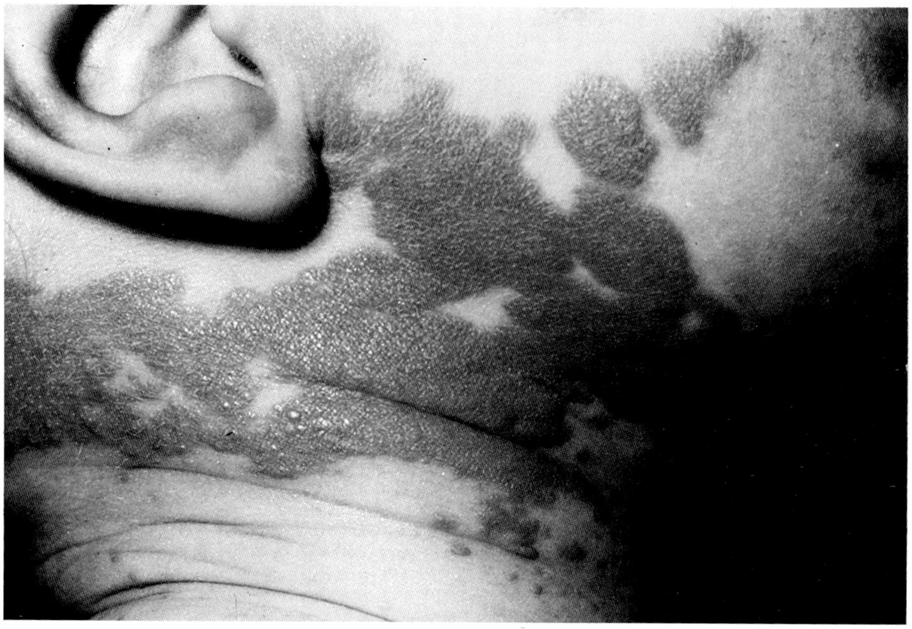

Fig. 1—Skin lesion of case 1. It shows macular, slightly elevated, clearly dilineated plaques on the face and side of the neck

biochemical anomalies were noted. A skin biopsy was taken from a lesion on the face.

The clinical presentation of the child suggested the micronodular variant of juvenile xanthogranuloma.

MATERIAL AND METHODS

Material from all skin biopsies was fixed in Bouin's fixative and paraffin-embedded. Fresh frozen tissue from the third biopsy of case 1 and

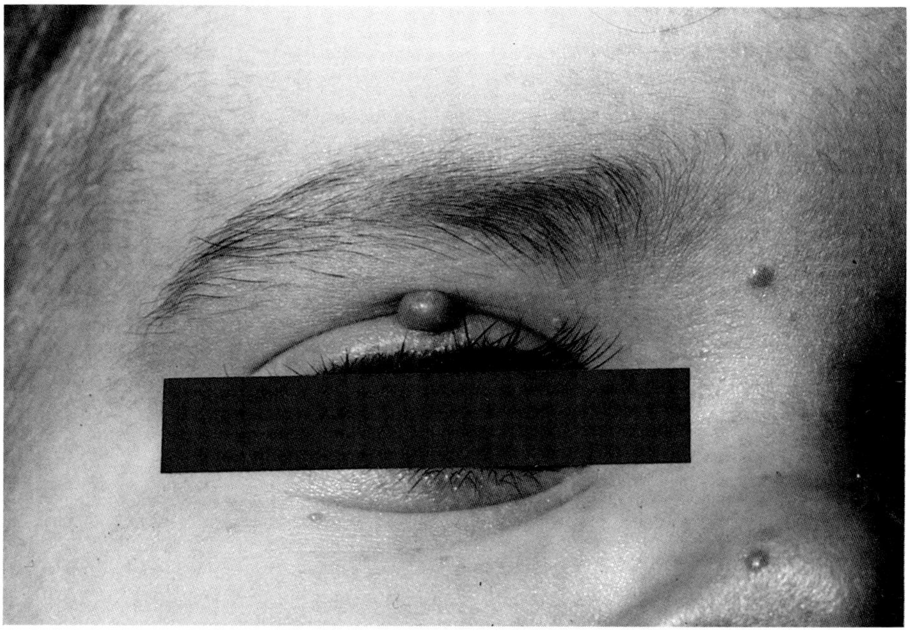

Fig. 2—Skin lesions of case 2. Various pea-sized papules are present on the face

from the biopsy of case 2 was available for immuno- and enzyme-histochemistry. Immunohistochemistry was performed using an indirect immunoperoxidase method.[8] Monoclonal antibodies directed to B lymphocytes (BA1, Hybritech Europe SA), T lymphocytes subsets, monocytes and the common framework of the HLA-Dr antigen (OKT4, OKT6, OKT8, OKM1 and OKIa1; Ortho-Pharmaceuticals, Ravitan, N.Y.) were applied. Serial sections were used for the demonstration of α-naphthyl acetate esterase and acid phosphatase.[9]

RESULTS

The first two biopsies from case 1 are characterized by an increased cellularity in the dermis without any epidermotropism (Fig. 3). Oval-shaped to elongated histiocytic elements are evenly distributed in the pars reticularis of the dermis. In the pars papillaris, small aggregates of similar histiocytic cells are found. The nuclei of these cells vary from round to deeply indented and small nucleoli are present. The cytoplasm of these cells is well delineated, abundant and rather eosinophilic. No foamy and no multinucleated cells are present. Lymphocytes, eosinophils and mast cells are admixed.

In the third biopsy the infiltrate is more dense and extends into the subcutaneous fatty tissue. Some mononuclear cells with a microvesicular or foamy cytoplasm as well as a few multinucleated cells of the Touton-type can be recognized. The skin biopsy from case 2 shows a diffuse dermal infiltrate, similar to the third biopsy of case 1, composed of mononuclear and some rare multinucleated cells.

The immunohistochemical results are similar in both cases. OKT6 + dendritic Langerhans cells are present in the epidermis. Only a few of them are found in the pars papillaris of the dermis mainly surrounding the adnexial structures (Fig. 4a). The histiocytic elements in the dermal infiltrate are OKIa1 +, OKM1 + as well as OKT4 + but OKT6 −. Some OKT8 + and OKT4 + lymphocytes can be recognized. No BA1 + cells are visualised.

Enzyme histochemistry reveals a strong positivity for acid phosphatase in the dermal infiltrate (Fig. 4b) while α-naphthyl acetate esterase is demonstrable only in the mononuclear cells lacking a foamy cytoplasm.

On electron microscopy the histiocytic elements

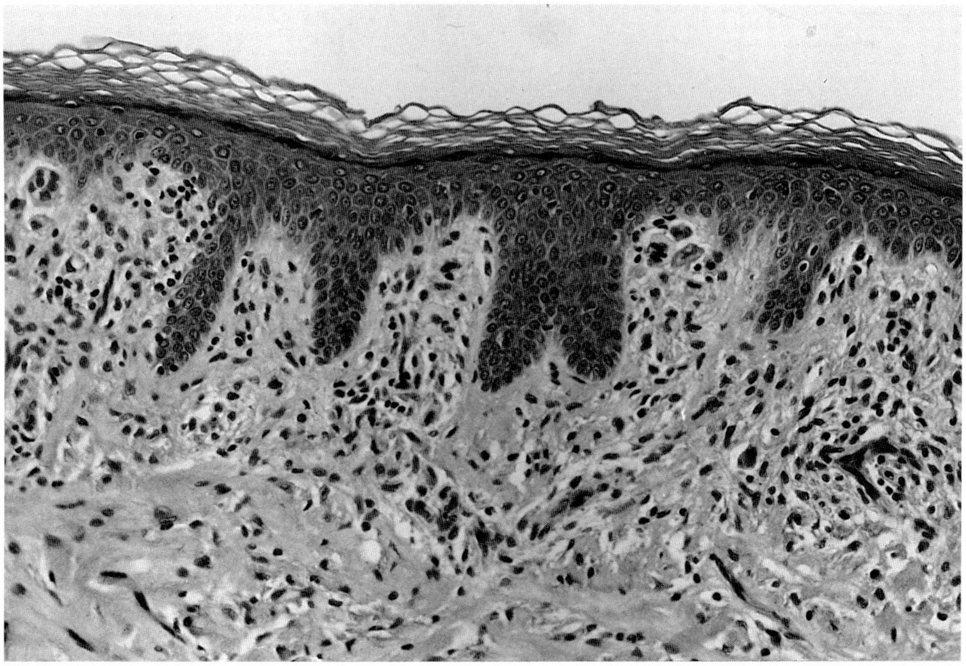

Fig. 3—Paraffin section from the second biopsy of case 1. Small aggregates of proliferating histiocytes admixed with some lymphocytes are found in the pars papillaris of the dermis

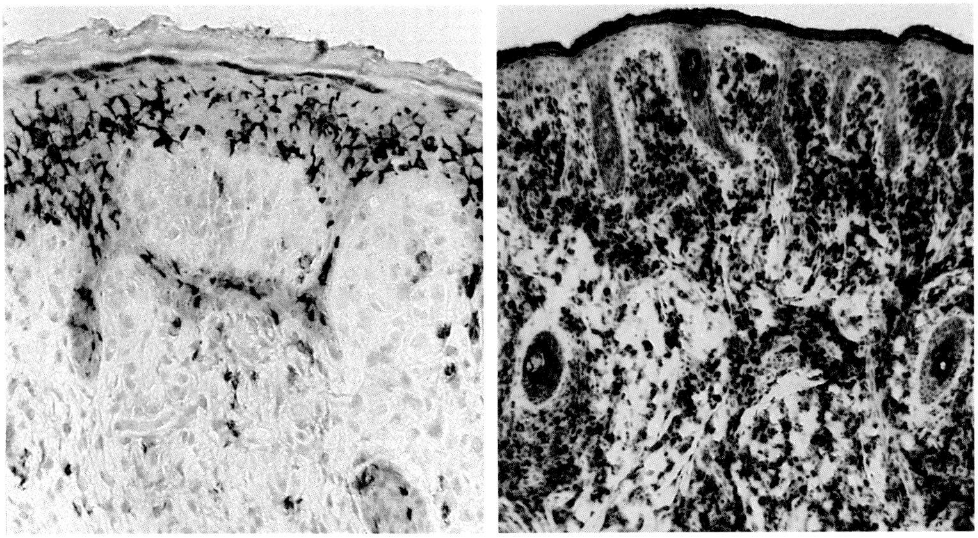

(a) (b)

Fig. 4—Serial frozen sections from the biopsy of case 2. (a) Stained with monoclonal antibody OKT6. Numerous dendritic OKT6 positive cells are seen in the epidermis. The dermal proliferating histiocytes are negative. (b) Stained for acid phosphatase. Most cells of the dermal infiltrate stain for acid phosphatase while epidermal Langerhans cells remain negative

of the dermal infiltrate are characterized by the presence of a variable number of lipid droplets and lipid vacuoles. Birbeck granules are not found in the dermal proliferating cells.

DISCUSSION

The clinical aspect of the skin lesions in both patients suggests a diagnosis of juvenile xanthogranuloma, presenting the macronodular type in case 1 and the micronodular variant in case 2. Juvenile xanthogranuloma with concomitant convulsions, as in case 1, has been previously reported.[5]

Fully-developed lesions of juvenile xanthogranuloma are characteristic on morphology: they correspond to a proliferation of histiocytic elements intermingled with a variable number of xanthomatous cells and Touton-like giant cells.[1,2] The morphological as well as the clinical diagnosis can, however, be problematical.[3–5]

The clinical aspect of the skin lesions in the two cases studied suggests a diagnosis of juvenile xanthogranuloma. The skin biopsies in both cases are less characteristic. Only the presence of some multinucleated giant cells and some foamy cells in the dermal infiltrate would suggest the histiocytic nature of the lesion. The positive results obtained for acid phosphatase and α-naphthyl acetate esterase staining as well as for OKM1 and OKIa1 immunostaining, establish the histiocytic nature of the proliferating cells.

Dermal histiocytic proliferations, characterized clinically by xanthomatous, reddish-brown papular lesions in childhood, can correspond to self-healing diseases as juvenile xanthogranuloma or to progressive disorders as histiocytosis X.[3]

The non-xanthomatous elements in juvenile xanthogranuloma are very similar to histiocytosis X cells. The presence of small aggregates of such elements in the dermal papillae as found in the first biopsy of case 1 further suggests a diagnosis of histiocytosis X. However, epidermotropism of the dermal infiltrate is lacking in all biopsies we received from both cases under study. On electron microscopy, Birbeck granules are lacking in the proliferating histiocytes in our cases. Based on the presence of Birbeck granules, histiocytosis X cells have been identified as proliferating Langerhans cells.[10] Both cell types react with monoclonal antibody OKT6[11] and do not present acid phosphatase activity.[12]

In the present biopsies the epidermal Langerhans cells are OKT6+, acid phosphatase and α-naphthyl acetate esterase negative. The proliferating dermal histiocytes are OKT6− and acid phosphatase and α-naphthyl acetate esterase positive. From these data we can conclude that the proliferating histiocytes in the cases under study do not correspond to histiocytosis X cells or Langerhans cells. On the contrary, they demonstrate characteristics of mononuclear phagocytes which transform into foamy cells and multinucleated giant cells in the fully developed lesions of juvenile xanthogranuloma. The proliferating histiocytes in the cases we studied are OKT4+. This monoclonal antibody is known to recognize T helper cells as well as monocytic–phagocytic cells.[13]

From this study we can conclude that juvenile xanthogranuloma is a proliferation of phagocytic histiocytes. Fully developed lesions can be recognized by the presence of foamy cells and multinucleated giant cells.

Problematical cases can be diagnosed and differentiated from histiocytosis X with the help of enzyme- and immunohistochemistry.

Finally our findings further support the difference in the proliferating histiocytes in juvenile xanthogranuloma and histiocytosis X as previously suggested on electron microscopy.[6]

ACKNOWLEDGEMENTS

The authors are grateful to E. Van Dessel for technical assistance, to A. Van den Panhuyzen for typing the manuscript and to M. Rooseleers for preparing the photographs.

REFERENCES

1. Helwig EB, Hackney VC. Juvenile xanthogranuloma (nevoxanthoendothelioma). *Am J Pathol* 1954; **30:** 625–626.
2. Webster SB, Reister HC, Harman LE. Juvenile xanthogranuloma with extracutaneous lesions. *Arch Dermatol* 1966; **93:** 71–76.
3. Altman J, Winkelmann RK. Xanthomatous cutaneous lesions of histiocytosis X. *Arch Dermatol* 1963; **87:** 164–170.
4. De Villez RL, Limmer BL. Juvenile xanthogranuloma and urticaria pigmentosa. *Arch Dermatol* 1975; **111:** 365–366.
5. Wolff HH, Vigl E, Braun-Falco O. Juveniles Xanthogranulom und Organmanifestationen. *Hautarzt* 1975; **26:** 268–272.
6. Gonzalez-Crussi F, Campbell RJ. Juvenile xanthogranuloma ultrastructural study. *Arch Pathol* 1970; **89:** 65–72.
7. Wolff HH, Braun-Falco O. Zur Diagnostik und Therapie des Morbus Hand-Shuller-Christian. *Hautarzt* 1972; **23:** 163–169.
8. Mason DY, Naiem M, Abdulaziz E, Nash JRG, Gatter KC, Stein H. Immunohistochemical applications of monoclonal antibodies. In: McMichael AJ, Fabre JW, eds. Monoclonal Antibodies in Clinical Medicine. London: Academic Press, 1982: 585–635.
9. Barka T, Anderson PJ. Histochemistry: Theory, Practice and Bibliography. New York: Hoeber Medical Division, Harper and Row, 1965: 239–242; 261–264.
10. Nezelof C, Basset F, Rousseau MF. Histiocytosis X: histogenetic arguments for a Langerhans cell origin. *Biomedicine* 1973; **18:** 365–371.
11. Murphy GF, Bhan AK, Sato S, Mihm MC, Harrist TJ. A new immunologic marker for human Langerhans cells. *New Engl J Med* 1981; **304:** 791–792.
12. Thomas JA, Janossy G, Chilosi M, Pritchard J, Pincott JR. Combined immunological and histochemical analysis of the skin and lymph node lesions in histiocytosis X. *J Clin Pathol* 1982; **35:** 327–337.
13. Wood GS, Warner NL, Warnke RA. Anti-Leu 3/T4 antibodies react with cells of monocyte/macrophage and Langerhans lineage. *J Immunol* 1983; **131:** 212–216.

JOURNAL OF PATHOLOGY, VOL. **143**: 211–218 (1984)

THE EFFECTS OF LONG-TERM ADMINISTRATION OF METHYLTESTOSTERONE ON THE DEVELOPMENT OF LIVER LESIONS IN BALB/c MICE

WILLIAM TAYLOR AND STANLEY SNOWBALL

Department of Physiological Sciences, The Medical School, The University, Newcastle-upon-Tyne NE1 7RU, U.K.

AND

MILENA LESNA

Department of Pathology, Royal Victoria Hospital, Shelley Road, Bournemouth BH1 4JG, U.K.

Received 23 February 1984
Accepted 16 March 1984

SUMMARY

Male and female BALB/c mice were treated orally with 5 mg/kg body weight of methyltestosterone for 10 months. Age-matched control animals received no steroid treatment. The livers of all animals were examined by standard histopathological methods. Hepatocellular dysplasia was found in livers of all treated mice, but not in control animals. The extent and severity of this dysplasia showed a sex difference. Most of the male mice (55/78) developed severe dysplasia and in 23/78 the dysplasia was only moderate; the corresponding numbers for female mice were: mild, 15/71; moderate, 48/71 and severe dysplasia, 8/71. Microscopic hepatocytic nodules were found in 6/78 males and 7/71 females. Hepatocellular carcinoma was seen in one male mouse. These findings indicate that methyltestosterone appears to act as a weak total hepatocarcinogen under the experimental conditions used.

KEY WORDS—Anabolic androgens, liver, dysplasia, carcinogenesis, mice.

INTRODUCTION

During the past decade there has been increasing concern about a possible association between the development of various types of liver tumours, including hepatocellular carcinoma, and the use of oral contraceptives by women, and also the treatment of adults and children of both sexes with anabolic-androgenic steroids. This concern is reflected in the many reviews on the subject which have appeared in recent years.[1–6] In the United Kingdom the Committee on the Safety of Drugs[7] reported that although various oral contraceptive steroids produced liver-cell tumours in rats, the tumour incidence was so low in the experimental animals that those steroidal preparations did not present a hazard to women. In human subjects it is considered that there is strong evidence for a causal relationship between treatment with anabolic androgens and development of liver tumours.[1,5,6] However, there have been no previous reports of successful attempts to induce liver tumours in experimental animals by administration of anabolic androgens alone to experimental animals in an attempt to assess the hepatocarcinogenic potential of this class of steroids (cf. Paradinas *et al.*[4]).

There are claims that steroids with a 17 α-alkyl substituent are more hepatotoxic and potentially carcinogenic than steroids lacking this substituent.[6] Therefore, the purpose of the present work was to observe the effect of oral treatment

Addressee for correspondence: Dr W. Taylor, Department of Physiological Sciences, The Medical School, The University, Newcastle-upon-Tyne NE1 7RU, U.K.

0022–3417/84/070211–08$01.00

with methyltestosterone (MeT) on liver structure in BALB/c mice. MeT was chosen as it has a 17 α-methyl substituent and is normally given to patients by the oral route. The animals were killed after only 10 months of treatment to lessen the possibility of development of spontaneous hepatic neoplasms.[8] The conditions of the experiment therefore approximated in dose (5 mg/kg body weight) and time to those used in human therapeutics.

Livers were studied by standard histopathological methods, and marked effects on hepatocytic morphology were observed in the treated animals but not in the controls.

A preliminary account of part of this work has been published elsewhere.[9]

MATERIALS AND METHODS

Animals and treatment

Male and female BALB/c mice, certified as free from pathogens and hepatitis virus(es) were obtained from a dealer registered with the Medical Research Council, U.K. The mice were 8–10 weeks old when received and were adapted to a schedule of 12 h artificial light and 12 h darkness for 2 weeks before use. Food was supplied *ad libitum* during the hours of darkness only, but there was no restriction on access to water. The diet was Rodent Standard Maintenance Diet 1 from Special Diet Services Ltd., Witham, Essex, U.K. The powdered MeT was mixed with diet calculated to provide a dose of 4·5–5·5 mg/kg body weight per day. This amount corresponds to that given to human subjects being treated orally with MeT. Control animals received diet only.

In the first experiment, 50 animals of each sex were assigned to treatment and control groups housed in sub-groups of five in standard mouse cages (experiment a). In the second experiment (experiment b) there were 40 animals in each group. In both experiments the treated animals were about 10 per cent heavier than control animals after 2–3 weeks of treatment, and this weight difference was maintained throughout the course of the experiments.

In experiment a, five animals of each sex from treatment and control groups were killed after 16 weeks, and a further seven females after 20 weeks. Two treated male and one female died between weeks 24–28 but could not be autopsied as death occurred overnight. In experiment b, five animals from each group were killed after 20 weeks, and three treated female mice died from unknown causes between weeks 29–34. The livers of all treated animals showed hepatocytic hyperplasia, whereas the livers of the control animals were normal.

After 10 months all remaining animals were killed by dislocation of the cervical vertebrae. The gall bladders were removed and the contents, pooled in batches of five, were stored frozen until analysed for bile acids and cholesterol, as previously described.[10] The livers were rapidly removed, cut into small pieces and placed in 10 per cent formol saline buffered at pH 7·4.

Table I—Lesions in livers of male and female BALB/c mice after oral treatment with methyltestosterone (5 mg/kg) for 10 months (two experimental groups, a and b)

		Male		Female		Total of two experiments	
						Male	Female
Experimental group		a	b	a	b		
Number of animals		43	35	39	32	78	71
Type of lesion	Extent of lesions						
Hepatocellular dysplasia	+	0	0	11	4	0	15
	++	23	0	20	28	23	48
	+++	20	35	6	2	55	8
Hepatocytic nodules		2	4	3	4	6	7
Hepatocellular carcinoma		0	1	0	0	1	0

The lesions are classified according to the system of Blackburn *et al.*[11] The degree of dysplasia has been graded from mild (+) to severe (+++), the latter with or without more demarcated areas of abnormal hepatocytes.

Histology

Multiple sections through all lobes of the livers were stained with haematoxylin and eosin, and some sections were stained for glycogen.

Histopathological assessment of liver lesions

The criteria for abnormality were based on the scheme proposed by the Workshop on Classification of Specific Hepatocellular Lesions in Rats as modified by Blackburn *et al.*[11] to include hepatocellular dysplasia and foci of cellular alterations (intermediate lesions), and the neoplastic lesions of nodules and hepatocellular carcinoma.

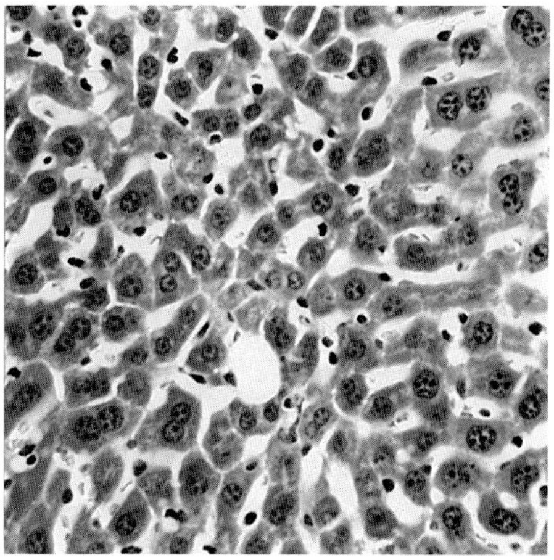

Fig. 2—Moderate dysplasia showing disturbance of cellular arrangement in centrizonal liver plates. There is a high proportion of binucleated hepatocytes and enlarged hyperchromatic nuclei. H & E, ×140

RESULTS

The effect of oral administration of 5 mg/kg of MeT for 10 months on the livers of male and female BALB/c mice is summarized in Table I. Dysplasia was considered to be a preneoplastic condition according to the criteria of Anthony, Vogel and Barker.[12] The degree of dysplasia was based on the extent and distribution of the lesion: thus, mild dysplasia (+) was confined to midzonal areas (Fig. 1), whereas in the severe form (+++) all of the zones were affected, occasionally interspersed with zones of smaller uniform hepatocytes. Moderate dysplasia (++) was ascribed to sections in which the extent of the lesions was neither obviously mild nor severe (Fig. 2). The nuclei of dysplastic hepatocytes displayed enlargement and hyperchromatism, lobulation or multinucleated forms. Coarse patterns of nuclear chromatin (Fig. 3) and occasional intranuclear eosinophilic inclusions were present, usually in the largest nuclei (not shown). In more severe forms of dysplasia the pattern of liver plates was disturbed by irregular arrangement of dysplastic hepatocytes, and in several cases of more severe dysplasia ill-defined foci of pale hepatocytes with small hyperchromatic nuclei had formed (Figs 4, 5).

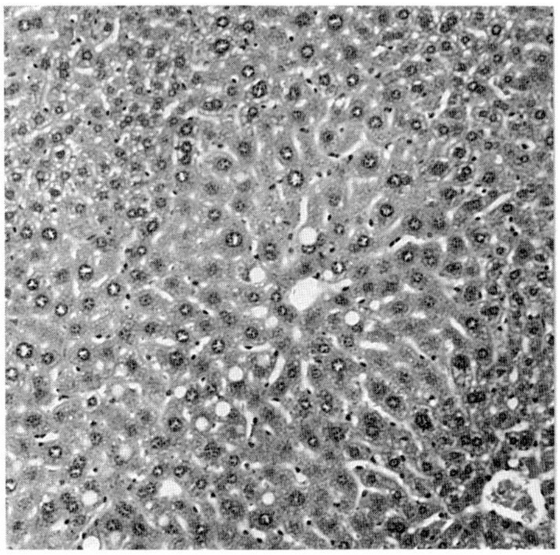

Fig. 1—Mild dysplasia in male mouse liver. Centrizonal and midzonal hepatocytes are enlarged due to an increase in the amount of cytoplasm and size of nucleus. Darker periportal hepatocytes are of normal size. Haematoxylin and eosin, ×80

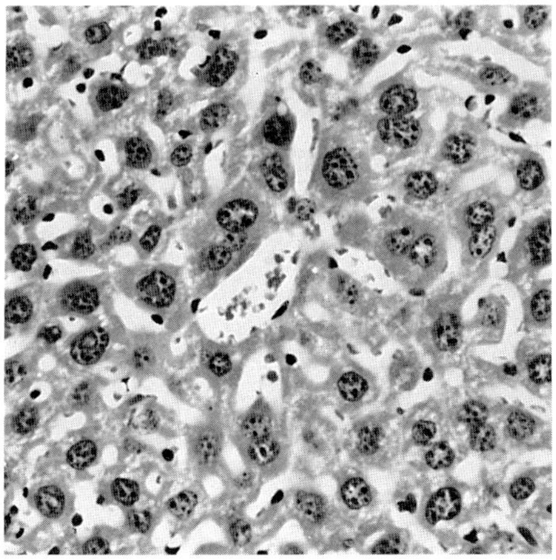

Fig. 3—Severe dysplasia. Irregular, hyperchromatic, enlarged nuclei of hepatocytes around the efferent venule; coarse pattern of chromatin. Alignment of hepatocytes is severely deranged. H & E, ×200

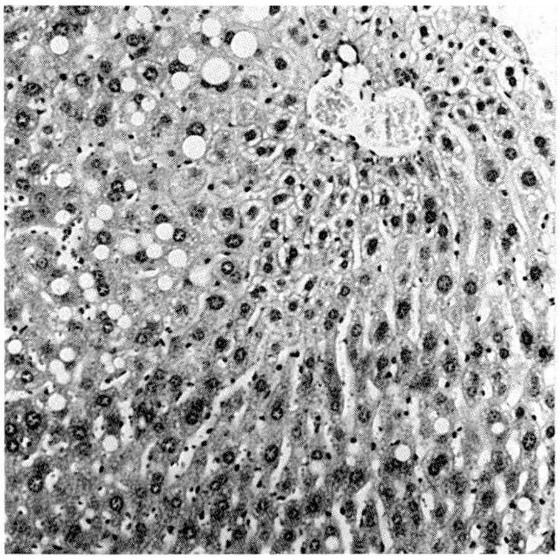

Fig. 4—Severe dysplasia with a more localized area of pale hepatocytes close to the edge of the liver (upper right). The large cytoplasmic vacuoles to the left of that zone are due to steatosis. H & E, ×80

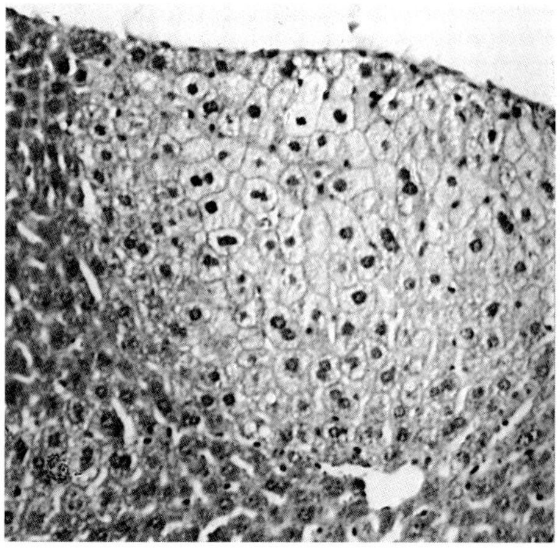

Fig. 6—A subcapsular clear-cell hepatocytic nodule typical of the kind found in both male and female mice. Note absence of compression of adjacent hepatocytes. H & E, ×80

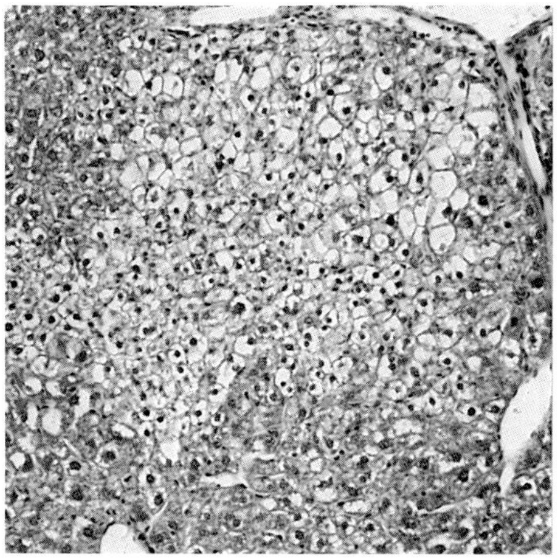

Fig. 5—A poorly demarcated nodule of clear hepatocytes with hyperchromatic nuclei. Severe dysplasia was also present in other regions of the same liver (not shown). H & E, ×50

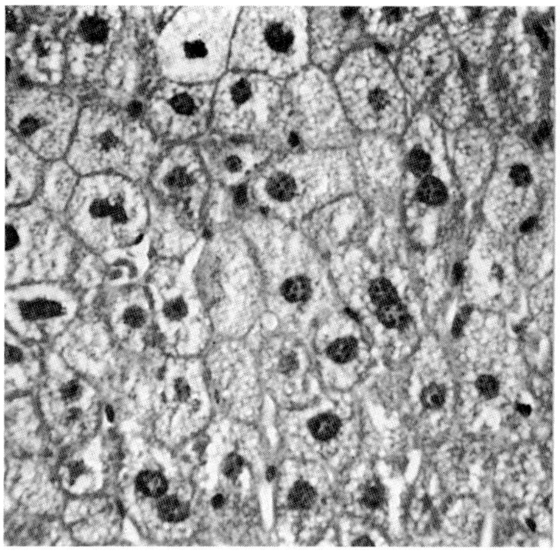

Fig. 7—Higher magnification of the nodule shown in Fig. 6 showing cellular enlargement, granular but pale cytoplasm and small hyperchromatic nuclei. Binucleated cells are also present. Excess glycogen was present in these cells (not shown). H & E, ×300

In both experiments a and b there appeared to be a sex difference in the severity of the induced lesions (Table I). All male mice showed at least a moderate degree of dysplasia, and 55/78 male mice developed severe dysplasia, whereas only 8/71 female mice showed dysplasia of this severity.

In addition to the above described changes, several well-demarcated hepatocytic nodules, microscopic in size, were found in six male and seven female mice. The majority of these lesions were of the clear-cell type (Figs 6, 7) and contained excess glycogen (not shown). Two nodules were composed of basophilic hepatocytes (Fig. 8) and showed numerous dilated sinusoids.

One large tumour in a male mouse liver in experiment b, tentatively described as 'hepatocellular carcinoma' (Figs 9, 10), bulged on the surface of the liver and occupied most of one lobe. It displayed histological features consistent with this type of neoplasm but it had not metastasized and, therefore, it cannot be dogmatically classified as hepatocellular carcinoma.

None of the control animals showed any liver lesions comparable to those found in treated mice,

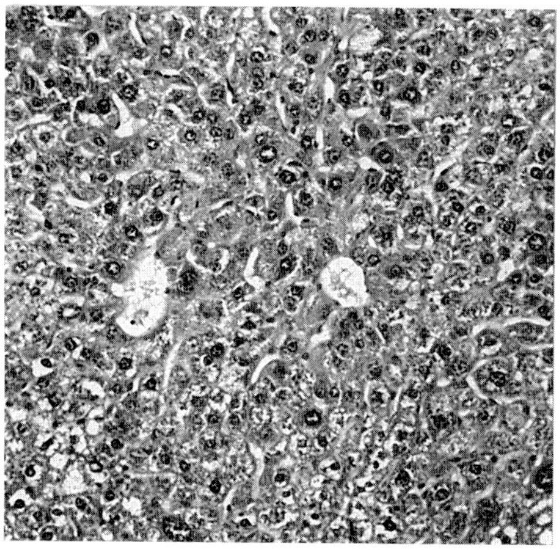

Fig. 8—A basophilic hepatocytic nodule/adenoma with dilated sinusoids forming cleft-like spaces. The lesion was not encapsulated and not associated with bile duct proliferation. H & E, × 100

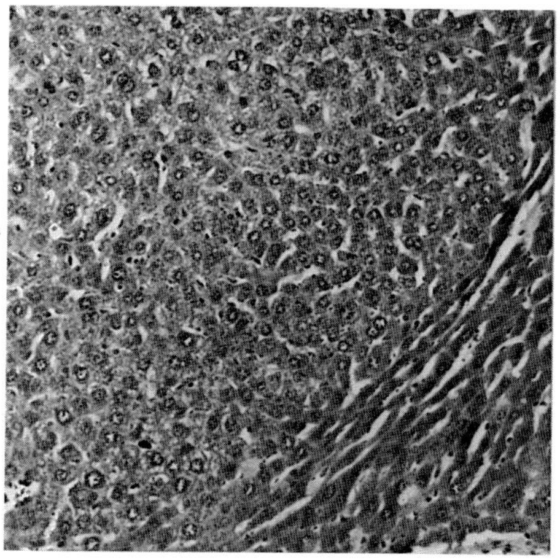

Fig. 9—The large tumour, found in a male mouse, projecting above the surface of one lobe and largely replacing it. Note absence of capsule and bile ducts, and the compact pattern with compression of adjacent liver parenchyma. H & E, × 80

and there was no sign of hepatocytic dysplasia or hyperplasia.

No changes were observed in the amount of total or individual bile acids nor in the amounts of cholesterol in the pooled gall bladder bile samples. The results (Table II) were remarkably similar to those found in bile of BALB/c mice treated with anabolic androgens for 10–12 weeks.[10]

DISCUSSION

When BALB/c mice were treated with 5 mg/kg of MeT for 10 months the major effect was the development of hepatocytic dysplasia in all animals. The lesion appeared to be more severe in male than in female mice (Table I). However, under the conditions used, the dysplasia progressed to apparent neoplasia in only 6/78 male and 7/71 female mice. Thus, there was no sex difference in the incidence of the microscopic hepatocytic nodules, and a lesion with the morphological characteristics of hepatocellular carcinoma was found in the liver of only one male mouse (Figs 9, 10). No such lesions were found in the untreated animals, the livers of which showed no distinctive features and were essentially normal.

Therefore, it can be stated with some certainty that the lesions in the livers of the treated mice were due to the action of MeT. This view is supported by the work of Sheldon.[8] In an extensive study of 2376 untreated female BALB/c mice, he

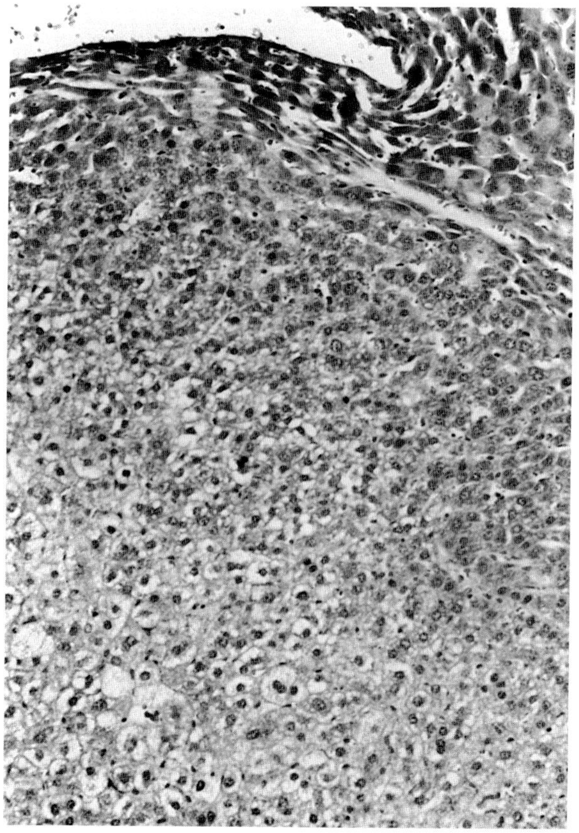

Fig. 10—Projecting part of the neoplasm shown in Fig. 9 showing compression of subcapsular hepatocytes and, centrally, a clear-cell pattern. Although metastases were not found, this tumour is considered to be hepatocellular carcinoma. H & E, × 100

Table II—Bile acids and cholesterol in pooled gall bladder bile of male and female BALB/c mice after treatment with methyltestosterone (5 mg/kg) for 10 months, and in control animals

	Male				Female			
	Control		Treated		Control		Treated	
Cholanoic acid	(mg/ml)	(% of total)	(mg/ml)	(% of total)	(mg/ml)	(% of total)	(mg/ml)	(% of total)
5α-3α,7α,12α	2·0, 0·04	3·0	2·4, 0·09	3·6	2·6, 0·10	3·8	2·3, 0·07	3·4
5β-3α,6β,7α	2·4, 0·07	3·6	2·1, 0·10	3·2	2·6, 0·12	3·8	2·0, 0·09	3·0
5β-3α,7α,12α	39·2, 0·34	59·8	40·0, 0·19	60·1	41·4, 0·27	60·7	40·9, 0·43	61·2
5β-3α,12α	4·9, 0·10	7·5	4·6, 0·21	6·9	5·1, 0·19	7·5	4·6, 0·23	6·9
5β-3α,6β	1·4, 0·12	2·1	1·2, 0·13	1·8	1·1, 0·20	1·6	1·4, 0·15	2·1
5β-3α,6β,7β	12·6, 0·23	19·2	13·0, 0·43	19·5	12·7, 0·32	18·6	12·4, 0·27	18·6
5β-3α,6α	3·1, 0·11	4·7	3·2, 0·23	4·8	2·7, 0·43	4·0	3·2, 0·21	4·8
Total bile acids	65·6		66·5		68·2		66·8	
Cholesterol (mg/ml)	3·6, 0·11		3·2, 0·20		3·6, 0·29		3·4, 0·12	
Number of observations	16		14		15		14	

Results for experimental groups a and b have been combined and show concentrations of total and individual bile acids and cholesterol (mg/ml) (mean, standard error), and individual bile acids as a percentage of total bile acids. The bile acids are designated as hydroxylated derivatives of 5α- or 5β-cholanoic acids.

found no hepatocytic lesions in 195 and 159 killed at 9 and 12 months. Only 45 animals from the 2376 developed spontaneous primary hepatocellular neoplastic lesions, including adenoma and hepatocellular carcinoma, all but two of which appeared when the animals were 17 months old. The validity of using mice for testing the hepatocarcinogenicity of various agents, but not anabolic androgens, has been discussed by Frith and Ward.[13] However, we consider that the development of the lesions in MeT-treated mice cannot be attributed to a non-specific toxic effect of that steroid. Only hepatocytic lesions were seen, whereas non-specific toxic agents tend to cause biliary and related lesions not seen in the present experiments. Furthermore, anabolic androgens, including endogenous male sex hormones, have a hyperplastic effect on the liver, which is now considered to be a target organ for steroidal gestagens.[14]

It is of interest that male mice seemed to be more affected by the steroid treatment than were female animals (Table I), since men are more prone than women to develop hepatic dysfunction and neoplasms after anabolic steroid treatment.[1,6] It is well known that males of many species are more susceptible than are females to the hepatotoxic and tumourigenic effects of a wide range of drugs, xenobiotics and carcinogens.[15] The reason for this sex difference is not fully understood, but the information expressing this difference must be imprinted in the liver early in life, since the long-term exposure of the mice to a relatively large dose of MeT would suppress normal gonadal function early in the course of treatment.

Cameron *et al.*[16] found that deoxy- and lithocholic acids are promoters of tumourigenesis in female rats, and that the former bile acid is a more active promoter than phenobarbital. Those authors, therefore, suggested that the hepatocarcinogenic effect of some cholestatic steroids might be secondary to an increased production of deoxycholic acid. Our findings do not support this view, since no differences in the amounts or types of bile acids were found between treated and control animals (Table II). It is generally assumed that endogenous and exogenous steroid sex hormones act mainly, if not exclusively, as promoters of tumourigenesis in organs of the digestive tract and liver[15] and there is much experimental evidence in support of this view.[14,17–19] Some authors have suggested that steroidal gestagens can act as weak hepatocarcinogens, i.e. both as initiators and promoters.[19,20] Our results tend to support this latter view.

The occurrence of spontaneous putative neoplastic cell populations has been demonstrated in livers of aged rats, and these lesions appear to have the same characteristics as those produced in rat liver by classical initiating and promoting agents.[21] In the present work the apparent sex difference in the development of hepatocytic dysplasia was not reflected in the numbers of neoplastic nodules found in the livers of the treated mice (Table I). Therefore, it is tempting to suggest that the nodules, and the one hepatocellular carcinoma, found in these mice might have been caused by promotion by MeT of cell populations which had been spontaneously initiated during the course of the experiment. Any spontaneous foci of initiated cells which might have developed in the livers of the control animals would not have progressed to neoplasia because of the absence of MeT from the diet.

As far as we are aware, this is the first report of the development of the preneoplastic lesion dysplasia and of neoplastic nodules, including one hepatocellular carcinoma, in the livers of animals treated with an anabolic steroid without prior treatment of the animals with a known initiator of hepatocarcinogenesis. The work provides evidence that there is a causative relationship between treatment with anabolic-androgenic steroids and neoplastic lesions of the liver, as some authors have advocated.[1,5] However, the experiments do not clearly show whether MeT acts as a promoter or an initiator, and were not designed for this purpose. Under the experimental conditions used, the anabolic steroid might have been acting as a weak complete carcinogen. Further work with larger doses of MeT and other anabolic androgens with and without a 17 α-alkyl substituent, with and without prior initiation with an agent such as diethylnitrosamine is required to establish the mechanism(s) by which anabolic androgens exert their tumourigenic effect in the liver.

ACKNOWLEDGEMENTS

This work was partially financed by grants from the Smith, Kline and French Foundation (WT) and the Dorset Area Health Authority (ML). S. Snowball was a Luccock Research Student of this Medical School; present address: Hepatology Department, Catholic University of Leuven, 3000 Leuven, Belgium.

We express our gratitude to the Department of Medical Photography and to the staff of the Histopathology Department (Boscombe Royal Victoria Hospital) for the preparation of the photographs and slides, respectively.

REFERENCES

1. Evans DJ. Liver tumors elicited by specific factors. In: Remmer H, Bolt HM, Bannasch P, Popper H, eds. Primary Liver Tumors. Lancaster: 1978: 213–216.
2. Goldfarb S. Sex hormones and hepatic neoplasia. *Cancer Res* 1976; **36:** 2584.
3. Ishak KG. Hepatic neoplasms associated with contraceptive and anabolic steroids. In: Lingeman CH, ed. Carcinogenic Hormones. Berlin: 1979: 73–128.
4. Paradinas FJ, Bull TB, Westaby D, Murray-Lyon IM. Hyperplasia and prolapse of hepatocytes into hepatic veins during long-term methyltestosterone therapy: possible relationships of these changes to the development of peliosis hepatis and liver tumours. *Histopathology* 1977; **1:** 225.
5. Popper H, Thomas LB. Environmental liver tumors. *Kurume Med J* 1979; **26:** 189.
6. Sherlock Sheila. Hepatic effects of sex steroids. In: Farber E, Fisher MM, eds. Toxic Injury of the Liver. New York: 1980: 597–627.
7. Committee of Safety of Medicines. Carcinogenicity Tests of Oral Contraceptives. London: H.M.S.O. 1972.
8. Sheldon WG. Spontaneous lesions in control BALB/c mice. *J Environ Path Toxicol* 1979; **3:** 155.
9. Taylor W, Lesna Milena. Preneoplastic and neoplastic lesions of BALB/c mice treated orally with methyltestosterone. Proc. 2nd. Internat. Congr., Hormones and Cancer, Monte Carlo. *J Steroid Biochem* 1983; **19** (Suppl.): 46S.
10. Dickson CM, Lesna Milena, Taylor W. The effects of anabolic androgens on gall-bladder bile acids and cholesterol in mice. *J Steroid Biochem* 1979; **11:** 1557.
11. Blackburn GR, Andrews JP, Custer RB, Sorof S. Early events during liver carcinogenesis involving two carcinogen: protein complexes. *Cancer Res* 1981; **41:** 4039.
12. Anthony PP, Vogel CL, Barker LF. Liver cell dysplasia: a premalignant condition. *J Clin Path* 1973; **26:** 217.
13. Frith CH, Ward JM. A morphological classification of proliferative and neoplastic lesions in mice. *J Environ Path Toxicol* 1980; **3:** 329.
14. Reuber MD. The importance of the testes in the induction of hyperplastic nodules, carcinomas and cirrhosis of the liver in rats ingesting *N*-2-fluorenyldiacetamide. *Eur J Cancer* 1976; **12:** 137.
15. Yamamoto RS, Weisburger EK. The role of

hormones on digestive and urinary tract carcinogenesis. *Rec Progr Horm Res* 1977; **33:** 617.

16. Cameron RG, Imaida K, Tsoda H, Ito N. Promotive effects of steroids and bile acids on hepatocarcinogenesis initiated by diethylnitrosamine. *Cancer Res* 1982; **42:** 4039.
17. Firminger HI, Reuber MD. Influence of adrenocortical, androgenic and anabolic hormones on the development of carcinoma and cirrhosis of the liver in A X C rats fed *N*-2-difluorenyldiacetamide. *J Natl Cancer Inst* 1961; **27:** 559.
18. Taper HS. The effect of estradiol-17-phenylpropionate and estradiol benzoate on *N*-nitrosomorpholine induced liver carcinogenesis in ovariectomised female rats. *Cancer* 1978; **42:** 461.
19. Yager JD, Yager R. Oral contraceptive steroids as promoters of hepatocarcinogenesis. *Cancer Res* 1980; **40:** 3680.
20. Yager JD. Oral contraceptive steroids as promoters or complete carcinogens for liver in female Sprague-Dawley rats. *Environ Health Perspectives* 1983; **50:** 109.
21. Schulte-Hermann R, Schuppler J, Ohde G, Bursch W, Timmermann-Trosiener I. Phenobarbital and other liver promoters. In: Nicolini C, ed. Chemical Carcinogenesis. New York: 1982: 231–260.

BOOK REVIEWS

Principles and Practice of Surgical Pathology. Edited by STEVEN G. SILVERBERG. Two vols. Total no. of pages: 1656. Price £124.50. John Wiley, New York, 1983. ISBN: 0471 05221 3.

This attractively produced two volume book is likely to secure a following among junior pathologists. In concept it is excellent and a welcome innovation is the arrangement of chapters in a sequence corresponding to the SNOMED classification of disease.

The chapters on infectious, autoimmune and iatrogenic diseases and metastatic tumours are useful. There is much to commend prefacing the discussion of the pathology of each organ or system by a resume of the normal anatomy, histology and physiology together with an outline of the clinical presentation of the commoner diseases. The addition of guidance on the handling of surgical specimens should also be useful. In the event, many of these sections prove to be discursive, uncritical and unhelpful. Some of the practical advice is needlessly repetitive: more stringent editing in this area would have shortened the book and enhanced its value considerably. It is unfortunate that there is insufficient detail in the descriptions of the diseased organs and their histology to act as a counterpoise to the turgid introduction of most chapters. The quality of reproduction of a number of the photomicrographs further militates against its use as a bench manual.

Multiple authors lead to variation in style and only occasionally does American syntax obtrude painfully. Inevitably, there is variation in the quality of the 52 chapters but there are a few grossly misleading statements, e.g. epitheliosis being synonymous with lobular carcinoma of breast. Muddled thinking is more frequent, e.g. the use of 'reticulum cell' in the chapter on lymph nodes, the discussion of epithelial proliferations in the breast and the discussion of glomerular disease. Is it really worthwhile saying ". . . data suggest that lobular and ductal hyperplasia represent precursors of carcinoma: thus the differential diagnosis in this case is a delicate one, and the judgement of a pathologist who is highly experienced in this domain is essential"? Surely some advice could be given. The differentiation of condyloma accuminatum and verrucous carcinoma receives similar unhelpful treatment. In spite of these criticisms there is much that is good also and we found chapters on skin, soft tissue tumours, bone, major salivary glands, the oesophagus, non-neoplastic lesions of the intestine, medical diseases of the liver, uterus and ovary particularly useful. The book is well supplied with references (9857 in number) though it is most unfortunate that very few of them are later than 1979, a manifestation of the problem associated with assembly of a multi-author text.

We conclude that this is a book which a junior pathologist in his early years and with ample time on his hands would find useful. There are undoubtedly more concise and no less reliable sources of information already available.

M. I. J. ANDREWS
R. BUCHANAN
J. BURSTON
St Mary's Hospital, Portsmouth

Review of Pathophysiology. C. E. KAUFMAN and S. PAPPER. Quarto Little Brown, Toronto, 1983. No. of pages: 555. Price: $26.25. ISBN: 0 316 48339 7.

The word 'pathophysiology' is a ridiculous contradiction which is slipping into general use with alarming speed. The preface describes the contents as 'alterations in normal body function that result from disease processes'. If pathology is the science of disease, what then is left?

It is easy to see why the volume has this title. Of the 48 distinguished authors only one lists pathology as his prime speciality; most are Professors of Medicine at well-known American medical schools, especially Oklahoma. The message for the readers of the *Journal of Pathology* is that our field, particularly the area encompassed in Florey's well-known textbook of general pathology, is being taken over by clinicians. This is not a new situation, for in Edinburgh a certain clinician, Professor James Syme, successfully lobbied the University Senate to abolish the Chair of Pathology. It took a major row to reinstate the Chair to the position it stands today.

Review of Pathophysiology is well laid out. It starts, appropriately, with a most interesting chapter on ageing. For example, we are told that by the fifth decade of life the number of skin cells is halved. The author describes the changes as 'associated with, or as the result of, the ageing process'. He thereby avoids the discussion on whether we are in fact time-programmed. A comment on progeria might be relevant. If a pathologist had been writing this chapter—rather than a clinician—I think he would have included a discussion on the remarkable multi-system change that occurs in elastic tissue.

We then move through chapters on cardiac arrhythmias, volume and pressure overload to atherosclerosis. This is regarded as synonymous with 'hardening of the arteries'. I think most pathologists would make a distinction here. Further, the two conditions are regarded as being associated with 'gradual and uneven narrowing of medium and large size arteries'. Standard pathology teaching is for a fusiform dilation of large arteries as part of the 'hardening' process.

The reviewer is bound to pay particular attention to areas of his own interest. The chapter on cancer of the breast is excellent and I was glad to see that Dr Slease emphasized the terminal duct origin of many cancers. My only criticism is that he does not emphasize the recent pathology contributions to this field, namely that breast cancer does not grow in the normal breast. In future, screening philosophy may be directed towards detecting the woman at risk rather than the woman with early cancer.

I will value my copy of this book as a reference source of disease mechanisms. It will be invaluable for teaching medical students and for preparing postgraduate lectures. It will also be a reference source for those studying for membership examinations. Further editions could be improved by including normal values at the end instead of blank pages for notes.

H. W. Simpson
University of Glasgow

Microanalysis and Quantification, Vol. 11: Methods and Achievements in Experimental Pathology. Series Editors: G. Jasmin and L. Proschek (Montreal). Karger, Basel, 1984. No. of pages: 189. Price: $69.50. ISBN: 3 8055 3717 4.

A wide range of quantitative methodology—image analysis, stereology, flow cytofluorimetry and x-ray microanalysis—is covered in the seven chapters of this slim, but rather expensive volume. Special applications, such as the assessment of muscle biopsies and dysplastic nasal epithelium, are considered in great detail. I suspect, however, that the most useful sections will be those that give a more general introduction to the methods: the chapters on image analysis and x-ray microanalysis are particularly good.

Major problems in the quantitative analysis of tissues are sampling and the determination of adequate sample size; I was disappointed to find so little consideration of these aspects, particularly in the rather unsatisfactory chapter on histomorphometry.

The illustrations are clear and the text contains few typographical errors.

If you are specifically interested in image analysis or x-ray microanalysis you will not be disappointed by the accounts given in this book. But, for the general reader who wants an introduction to stereological methods, there are better texts. The editing could have been a little tighter to ensure a more uniform standard between chapters.

J. C. E. Underwood
University of Sheffield Medical School

ANNOUNCEMENT

THE FOUNDATION FOR ADVANCED EDUCATION IN THE SCIENCES, INC.

will present

NEW SOLUTIONS TO OLD PROBLEMS IN SURGICAL PATHOLOGY

15–17 October 1984

Washington, D.C. area

This 3-day programme will address difficult or evolving areas of surgical pathology and will focus on areas which often pose diagnostic difficulty. New techniques applicable to the general surgical pathology laboratory will be presented and clinico-pathologic correlations of morphologic diagnoses will be stressed. Participants will receive a syllabus containing lecture outline material and references. The programme is designed for pathologists at the senior resident and practitioner levels. Twenty-one hours AMA Category I credit.

For further information or application write to: Surgical Pathology, c/o FAES, National Institutes of Health, Building 10, Room B1-L-101, Bethesda, MD 20205, U.S.A.

PUBLISHING AGREEMENT

1. It is our custom to request authors to vest the worldwide copyright of their papers in John Wiley & Sons Limited for the full term of copyright and we would be grateful if you would confirm your acceptance of these terms by signing and returning the agreement below. We will not withhold permission for any reasonable request from you to publish any part of this paper in connection with any other work by you, provided the usual acknowledgements are given regarding copyright notice and reference to the original publication.
2. If it is appropriate, the author's employer may sign this agreement, and in any event the employer may reserve the right to use the paper internally or for promotional purposes only, by so indicating on this agreement. It is understood that proprietary rights other than copyright (including patent rights) are reserved.
3. If the author is a U.S. Government employee and this work was done in that capacity the assignment applies only to the extent allowable by U.S. law. If at least one co-author is *not* a government employee, said author should sign the agreement.
4. If the author is an employee of the British Government then HMSO will grant a non-exclusive licence to publish this paper in the Journal in any form or media provided British crown copyright and user rights (including patent rights) are reserved.
5. The author warrants that the manuscript is the author's original work, and has not been published before. (If excerpts from copyrighted works are included, the author will obtain written permission from the copyright owners and show credit to the sources in the manuscript.) The author also warrants that the article contains no libellous or unlawful statements, and does not infringe on the rights of others.
6. If the work was prepared jointly the author agrees to inform co-authors of the terms of the agreement, and to sign on their behalf.

With the qualifications listed above I assign to John Wiley & Sons Limited, the copyright of my paper entitled ______________________________

____

for publication in ______________________________

______________________ Signed

______________________ Date

If the paper is rejected this assignment is null and void.

JOURNAL OF PATHOLOGY, VOL. **143**: 223–239 (1984)

AIDS: HISTOPATHOLOGICAL ASPECTS

PETER R. MILLARD
Department of Histopathology, John Radcliffe Hospital, Oxford, U.K.

Received 6 December 1983
Accepted 2 February 1984

KEY WORDS—AIDS, acquired immune deficiency syndrome.

INTRODUCTION

Few doctors within any specialty can be unaware of the acquired immune deficiency syndrome (AIDS) as a new and lethal disorder. Since it appeared in the U.S.A. in 1979 the syndrome has been carefully monitored by the Centers for Disease Control, Atlanta from which statistics and reviews have been regularly issued. These reviews[1,2] and others[3,4] provide basic reference sources. The early pattern and progression of the disease has been observed and risk groups identified. Within the U.S.A. 71 per cent of the sufferers are male homosexuals (overall sex incidence male:female, 14:1);[5] another 17 per cent are intravenous drug abusers of either sex whilst the minority are haemophiliacs (1 per cent) and Haitians.[6,7] Similar risk groups have been described in at least 20 other countries and amongst all sufferers the mortality reaches 80 per cent within a 2-year period, 90 per cent of whom are aged between 20 and 49 years.[5] In the United States 48 per cent of cases occur in New York and 20 per cent in California, suggesting an infectious agent as the basis for the disease. Corroborative evidence is provided by person-to-person spread usually involving sexual transmission but also from the use of pooled factor VIII concentrates and blood. The epidemic nature of the disease, 70 new cases occurring each month, as well as the repetition of the risk groups of affected patients in separate geographical areas add further to the belief for an infectious cause. If such an agent does exist, however, casual contact with sufferers is not sufficient to result in transmission since there have been no cases amongst exposed medical or laboratory staff who lack the risk factors associated with AIDS. The causative agent(s) remains unrecognized but because of similarities between the epidemiology of AIDS and hepatitis B, viruses, such as hepatitis B (HBV), cytomegalovirus (CMV) and human T-cell leukaemia/lymphoma (HTLV) virus are the main areas of investigation. The emergence of an apparently similar disease in two strains of monkey also supports an infectious hypothesis and provides a model for studying the disease and tracing its origins.[8–10] Attention has been drawn to similarities between the practices and age groupings of the affected Rhesus monkeys and the homosexual patients with AIDS[11] but, unfortunately, hopes of rapidly identifying a transmissable agent may not be fulfilled because of the six months to two years incubation period for the disorder.

The common feature of all AIDS patients in every group is a profound and apparently irreversible depression of cell mediated immune responses. There is a quantitative reduction in a helper lymphocyte subset which is reflected by a reversal of the T-helper/T suppressor ratio. This is manifest by lymphopenia, skin-test anergy and depressed *in vitro* responses to mitogens. Diminished natural killer cell activity and the appearance of autoantibodies in particular to platelets[12] and cell nuclei[13] are other consequences. These findings have also been identified amongst the 'at risk' patients without the fully developed syndrome and are thus regarded as laboratory indices of the disorder and its prodromal stages. Complement responses and humoral immunity remain intact although hypergammaglobulinaemia may be evident particularly in the early phases. In patients with Kaposi's sarcoma without AIDS there is an increased incidence of HLA-DR5.[14] A similar increase in

0022–3417/84/080223–17 $01.70

HLA-DR5 has been found amongst homosexuals with AIDS and Kaposi's sarcoma but its relationship to the tumour or to the cellular immunodepression is of uncertain significance.

The clinical consequences of the immune depression are multiple severe infections and uncommon tumours. The organism first associated with the syndrome and now regarded as a marker is *Pneumocystis carinii.* Other intracellular organisms embracing the entire range of micro-organisms have been encountered with multiple infections being the rule. The characteristic tumour is the Kaposi sarcoma with 95 per cent of the examples being found in homosexuals with AIDS.[5] This is regarded as a marker for the syndrome but B-cell lymphomas of the Burkitt's type may also develop. These lesions are generally associated with severe wasting and lymphadenopathy which have been seen in some patients prior to the fully developed syndrome. A minority of patients have had autoimmune thrombocytopenic purpura.[12]

Amongst the plethora of reports on AIDS scattered references are made to histopathological findings and only a few direct studies relating to specific facets have been published. With the wide awareness of the syndrome and its gradual dissemination from the United States individual pathologists are soon likely to encounter examples of AIDS and the purpose of this article is to assemble the diverse histopathologic features reported to date. Many of them mark AIDS apart from other causes of immunodepression and the opportunity is, therefore, taken to compare the findings in AIDS patients with those in organ transplant patients who are a well-defined and well-monitored group with similar immunosupression.

PNEUMOCYSTIS CARINII PNEUMONIA

Pneumonia associated with *Pneumocystis carinii* was described in 1938[15] and has been a cause of infection in a variety of immunocompromised individuals including premature and malnourished infants.[16] The protozoon occurs as cysts enclosing trophozoite forms which, in mice (in the presence of a specific opsinizing antibody), are engulfed and destroyed by macrophages.[17] The organism has rarely been seen outside the lung and spread is by inhalation from infected persons. Reactivation can then occur but since focal epidemics develop in susceptible populations, it is possible that healthy hospital staff can act as carriers. The appearance in the lungs is the major method of recognition since *in vitro* cell culture has only recently been achieved.[18] Diagnosis at present relies upon light and/or electron microscopic examination of lung (transbronchial biopsies) or aspirates from the bronchial tree.

Pneumonia is the presenting diagnosis in 51 per cent of patients with AIDS and when associated with Kaposi's sarcoma occurs in 58 per cent.[1] In the first examples of AIDS some patients had recurrent episodes of pneumonia and in some the pneumonia was fatal.[19,20] The pneumonia was commonly associated with other microbial infections including *Candida* species and *Herpes* viruses, particularly CMV. This pattern of infection has been maintained and occurs in all the AIDS groups of patients. The features of the pneumonia are similar to those in other affected patients with filling of individual air sacs with granular foamy eosinophilic material amongst which cysts are occasionally encountered. The cysts and their enclosed trophozoites are more readily appreciated by electron microscopy.

CYTOMEGALOVIRUS (CMV)

The observation that 93·5 per cent[21] and 86·9 per cent[22] of homosexuals have raised titres to the cytomegalovirus and the knowledge that the virus may be transmitted via blood, saliva, urine and semen has led to serious consideration of this virus as the putative agent for AIDS. Additional circumstantial evidence is that immunodepression comparable to that in AIDS can be produced by this virus[23,24] and that there is a close association between CMV and Kaposi's sarcoma. The virus has been cultured from cells of Kaposi's sarcoma in non-AIDS patients and CMV-related antigens and CMV-DNA and RNA have been recognized in the tumour cells.[25] Additionally, these patients had raised anti-CMV titres.

There are several difficulties in accepting all of these statements. CMV is a widely dispersed virus capable of persistency and of latency with reactivation. Titres are, therefore, common amongst the general population and the raised titres reported amongst homosexuals may reflect the upset of the helper and suppressor T cell function and release of antibody producing B cells rather than active or widespread infection. While CMV can induce immunodepression there is no evidence to date that this is a long lasting or irreversible phenomenon as is found in AIDS. AIDS patients are exposed to a very wide range of foreign proteins including microbes and drugs, all of which could produce similar suppressive effects, and many of them are present in association with CMV infection. The immune deficit of AIDS thus must not, on present evidence, be regarded as solely arising from CMV infection. Finally, since the studies relating CMV-DNA and RNA with Kaposi's tumour there have been considerable advances in nuclear biology techniques. It is now appreciated that there are homologies between the genomes of CMV and human DNA and that therefore the finding of CMV-DNA within human tumour cells using whole genome probes is of questionable significance.[26] To overcome this difficulty viral DNA fragments from a number of restrictive enzyme digests must be subcloned and absence of hybridization with cellular DNA demonstrated by hybridization on Southern blots.[27] Preliminary studies incorporating some of these techniques have failed to show any virus-specific DNA sequences in Kaposi tumours[28] but obviously further studies are needed.

What, however, is undisputed is the widespread nature of CMV inclusions within AIDS patients and the presence of these inclusions within otherwise normal and abnormal tissues (Figs 1, 2). Epithelial cells are predominantly affected and inclusions within endothelial cells are not as common. The sero-conversion amongst homosexuals leading to the appearance of anti-CMV titres, and also the presence of IgM antibodies further indicates that infection is active.[22] In some of these patients this is very probably due to reactivation. The impact of CMV in AIDS and potential AIDS patients is therefore undeniable but the importance of the virus as cause or effect remains open. The recent finding of AIDS and CMV infection in Rhesus monkeys following inoculation with tissue homogenates from monkeys with AIDS[10] illustrates this as well as the need for further clarification.

KAPOSI'S SARCOMA

Moritz Kaposi, a Hungarian dermatologist, first recognized this tumour in the skin in 1872 but by the end of his Directorship of the Department of Dermatology in Vienna he had also collected examples with systemic spread.[29] This division of the tumour into two broad groups with different geographical, population, and behavioural patterns and prognosis (Table I) persists and has been added to by a mixed pattern developing in transplant recipients.[30] Tumours in these patients incoporate features of both forms and so do the tumours in the AIDS patients who have systemic and cutaneous lesions, often with an aggressive mode of spread.[14, 30–32] Even so, it is difficult to assess the tumour's role as a cause of death. Systemic involvement has rarely been extensive and over twice as many AIDS patients are reported as dying from infections (46 per cent) as from Kaposi's sarcoma (22 per cent).[5, 33] The histopathological features of the tumour are well described[34] and these features are shared by the tumours in AIDS patients[31] (Fig. 3). Early small lesions can cause difficulty in recognition and may be confused with inflammatory lesions. The altered subsets of lymphocytes found in the circulation have been observed in the cells infiltrating the tumour deposits both within skin and lymph nodes.[35, 36] The possible relationship between CMV and the tumour is outlined above.

Preliminary ultrastructural studies have demonstrated occasional individual necrotic endothelial cells in the vessels of Kaposi's sarcoma associated with AIDS but not in similar tumours from non-AIDS patients.[37] The feature that remains undetermined is the cell of origin of the tumour.

Kaposi sarcoma is clearly not a lymphoma. Studies relying upon electron microscopy and histochemical findings have suggested a wide range of cells (Table II) but for none has the evidence for a cell of origin been conclusive. The most popular hypothesis is that the tumour arises from endothelial cells and some immunocytochemical studies with polyclonal antibodies to Factor VIII-related antigen support this.[38] These studies on paraffin embedded material revealed positive staining both in the tumour spindle cells and within vascular endothelial cells and Modlin *et al.*[39] had similar results using frozen sections of Kaposi tumours from AIDS patients. However, in other comparable studies of non-AIDS tumours using paraffin sections Factor VIII-related antigen was confined to vessels and was not seen in the spindle cells.[40] Using both polyclonal and monoclonal antibodies for Factor VIII-related antigen and paraffin sections of a disseminated Kaposi's sarcoma from a homosexual with AIDS we have found the same results as these latter workers even when

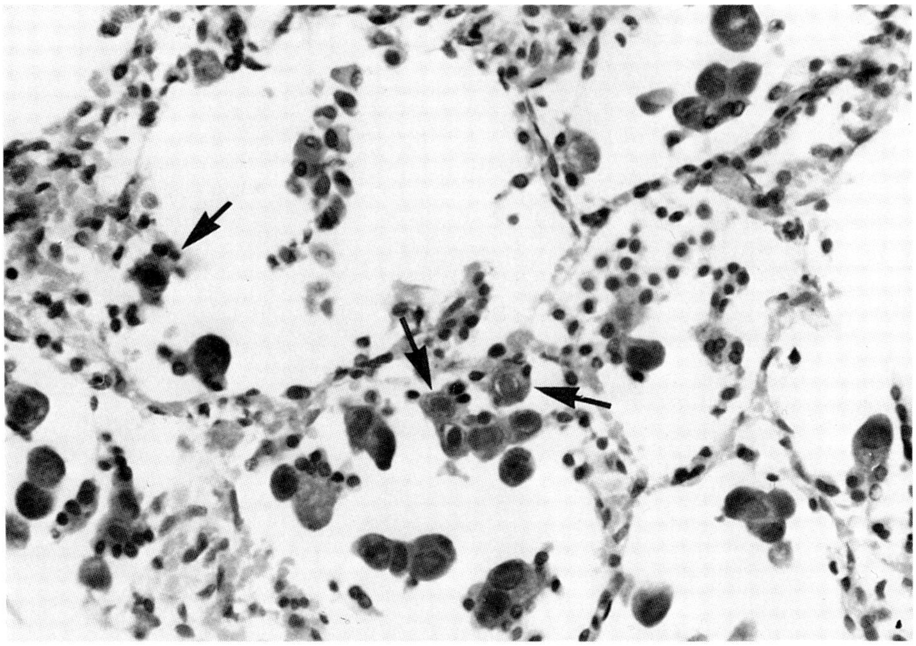

Fig. 1—Lung from a 39-year-old male with AIDS. Many alveolar cells include cytomegalovirus inclusion bodies. Organizing pneumonia and oedema were other features. The patient had presented with *Pneumocystis carinii* infection but none was seen at autopsy. Haematoxylin and eosin, ×500

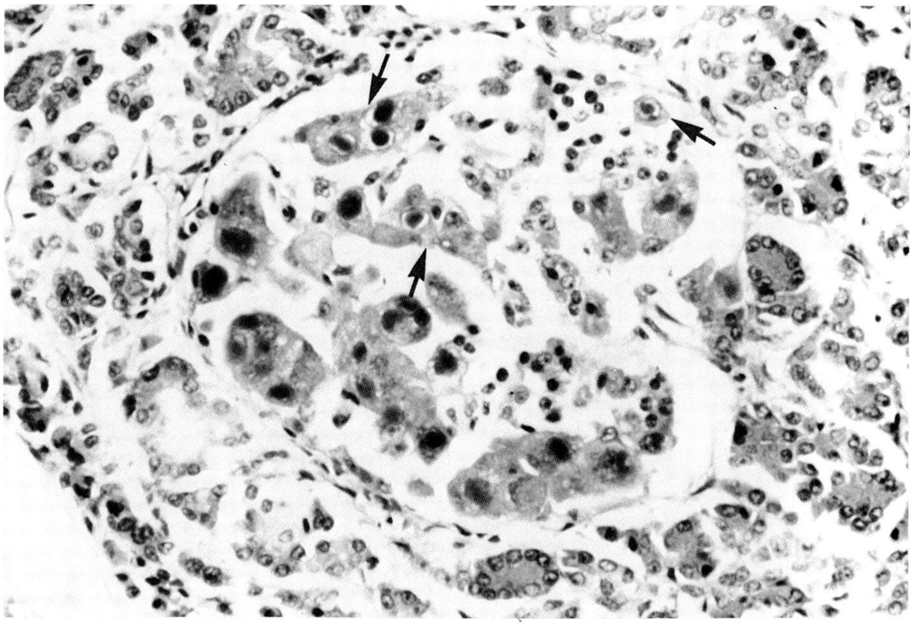

Fig. 2—Pancreatic islet from a 39 year old male with AIDS. Many of the cells include typical owl's eye inclusion bodies characteristic of the cytomegalovirus. No other abnormal features were found in the pancreas. Haematoxylin and eosin, ×140

Table I—Kaposi's sarcoma

	Europe/U.S.A.	Africa	Transplant patients
Incidence	0·6%	9%	4·9%
Age (years)	70 (>50)	40 (>50) Children	43
M:F	9:1; 15:1	4·7:1; 33·3:1	2·3:1
Population	Mediterranean, Central European and Jewish	Blacks	Mixed
Main pattern	Cutaneous	Systemic	Mixed
Course	Over decades with regression in some	Rapid, progressive and fulminant	Mixed
Second tumour	30%	Rare	Occurs

(Taylor *et al.*;[101] D'Oliveira and Torres;[102] Penn;[30] Safari *et al.*;[45] Templeton[34].)

prior trypsin and protease incubation was incorporated (Fig. 4). The distribution of Factor VIII-related antigen is not confined to endothelial cells but also occurs in megakaryocytes, platelets,[41] mast cells[42] and the glomerular mesangium.[43] Kaposi's sarcomas are in part characterized by diffuse haemorrhage and the cutaneous lesions particularly contain mast cells (Table II) both of which may contribute to Factor VIII-related antigen staining. Frozen section specimens in such circumstances may also permit diffusion of the antigen from cells harbouring Factor VIII-related antigen to adjacent cells. Although in paraffin sections modification of the antigen might be anticipated this is probably not occurring since in these tumours Factor VIII-related antigen is demonstrable within the vascular endothelium (Fig. 4).[40] Until there are uniform results with this antigen there must be reservations about accepting endothelium as the cell of origin and the tumour is probably best considered as arising from a multipotential primitive mesenchymal cell.[34, 44]

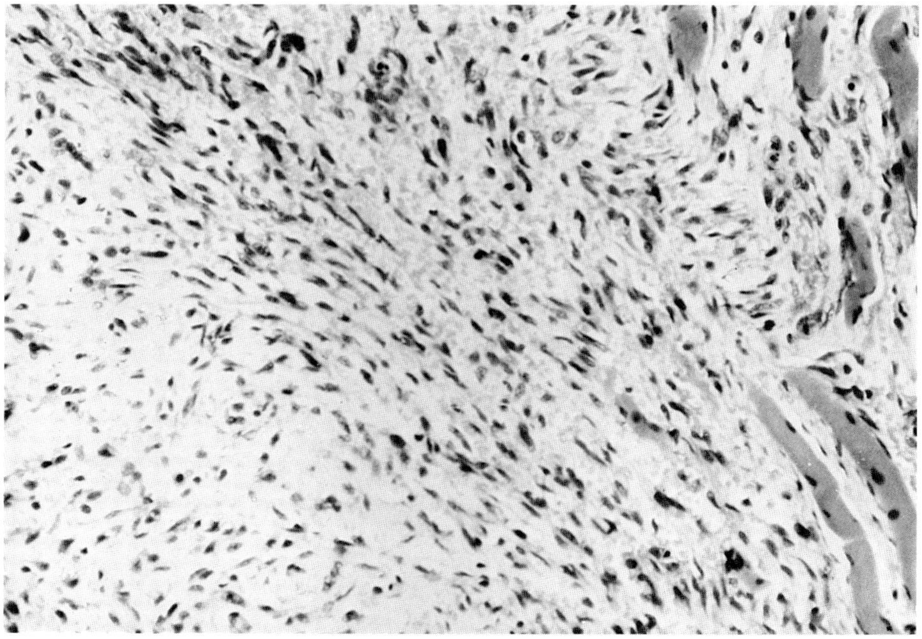

Fig. 3—Tongue from a male with AIDS. The spindle cells are uniform with no mitotic forms and arranged in bundles replacing the skeletal muscle. Spaces filled with red cells separate the bundles. Abundant iron pigment was present. The primary lesion was in the lower leg and other deposits were found in the lungs, oesophagus, rectum and lymph nodes. Haematoxylin and eosin, ×180

Table II—Cells identified by electron microscopy in examples of Kaposi's sarcoma

Endothelial cells
Perithelial cells
Fibroblasts
Undifferentiated mesenchymal cells
Smooth muscle cells
Myofibroblasts
Schwann cells
Mast cells
Histiocytes

(Harrison and Kahn;[44] Templeton [34].)

LYMPHOMAS

Any patient with a neoplastic condition has a greater chance of developing a further malignancy than age-sex-matched controls; incidences vary between 5 and 10 per cent of cancer patients.[45] Patients with Kaposi's sarcoma demonstrate this phenomenon (Table I) but the incidence is higher than in controls with other malignancies as is the occurrence of malignancy in the lymphoreticular system which has an increase of more than 20-fold.[45] These non-Hodgkins lymphomas are often associated with the Epstein–Barr virus (EBV) and are predominantly diffuse B-cell tumours (follicle centre, B-cell immunoblastic) with Burkitt's lymphoma as one of the commoner histological patterns.[45] A similar relationship between Kaposi's sarcoma and B-cell lymphomas exists in transplant recipients[46] and the pattern is repeated in AIDS patients.[47] As with transplant patients, lymphomas often develop in the brain, an otherwise uncommon site for lymphomas.[46,48] The lymphomas in AIDS are also EBV associated.[47]

LYMPHADENOPATHY

Both Kaposi's sarcoma and lymphoma can underlie the lymphadenopathy found in AIDS patients (Fig. 5).[49,50] The lymphadenopathy is also regarded as a prodromal or early phase of the full AIDS syndrome when many but not all patients will have immunological deficits.

The commonest cause is an explosive reactive hyperplasia centring upon the follicles, some of which may coalesce.[49–51] The germinal centres show evidence of destruction and regeneration with cellular debris and many mitoses. Within the

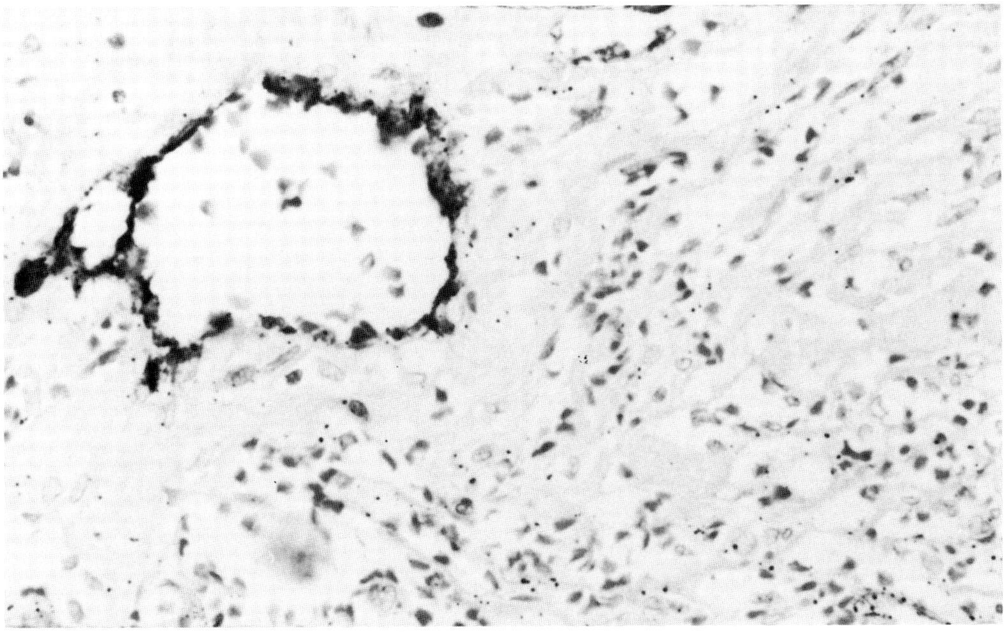

Fig. 4—Kaposi sarcoma as in Fig. 3. Paraffin section exposed to a monoclonal antibody to Factor VIII-related antigen following protease digestion. The endothelial cells of the vessel are stained but not the surrounding tumour cells. Diaminobenzidine, ×500

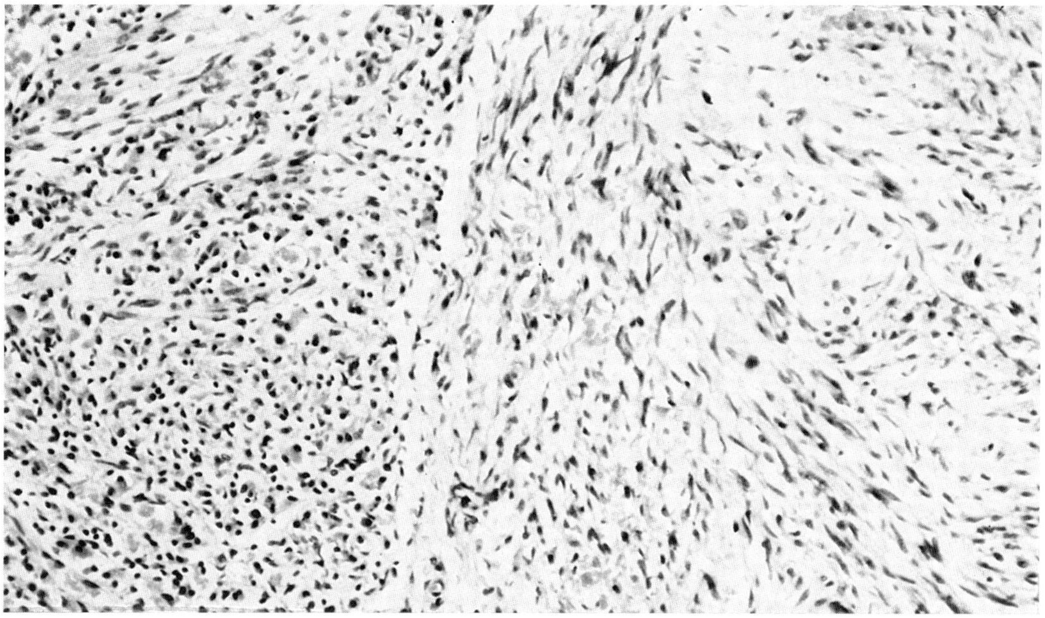

Fig. 5—Mesenteric lymph node from a 39-year-old male with AIDS. Lymphoid tissue is replaced by foamy macrophages (left) harbouring acid fast bacilli (Fig. 9). Kaposi's sarcoma is present on the right. Haematoxylin and eosin, ×180

paracortex there are aggregates of immunoblasts, lymphocytes, histiocytes and varying numbers of plasma cells. Blood vessels are invariably hyperplastic. Other features are filling of the sinusoids with mononuclear histiocytic cells and neutrophil polymorphs. This change has accounted for 82 per cent of the changes in the lymph nodes.[49,50] Paracortical hyperplasia and total lymphocyte depletion with or without hyalinization of the follicles are rarer findings in biopsy studies but have been seen at autopsy.[52–54] Associated with lymph node changes of this type there has been lymphoid atrophy within the thymus and spleen (Fig. 6).[52,53,55] Most of the changes are reactive and to an inapparent cause but as far as the homosexuals affected are concerned, must in part, represent a consequence of their lifestyle in which there is exposure to a wide range of infections. A consistent organism, however, has not been identified although rare cases have been associated with CMV infection[56] and with atypical mycobacteria.[54] The classical changes associated with *Toxoplasma* infection have not been recorded even in AIDS sufferers infected with this organism.

Vesicular rosettes have been found in lymph node cells from 17 of 18 AIDS patients by electron microscopy[57] and may infer that viruses play a particularly important aetiological role in the lymphadenopathy. The rosettes were formed of clusters of vesicles around a dense core with no supporting membrane and were randomly dispersed within the cytoplasm of lymphoid cells and particularly plasma cells. These rosettes are comparable with tubuloreticular structures recognized as hallmarks of some virus infections and have been reported in 80–90 per cent of specimens from various tissues including lymph nodes from 64 patients with AIDS.[58] Even so, the structures illustrated in both these reports are not exactly comparable to tubuloreticular bodies. This in part may be due to inadequate preservation of tumour material previously embedded in paraffin blocks and subsequently used for ultrastructural studies. Alternatively, it may be because the vesicular rosettes are entirely unrelated to tubuloreticular bodies. A recent ultrastructural study of freshly fixed biopsies discounts some of these criticisms since well illustrated tubuloreticular bodies were found in endothelial cells, histiocytes and lymphocytes from 10 AIDS patients.[59] Even if such bodies are present this obviously does not prove active infection but is consistent with latent or previous viral infections which, in view of the clinical background of these patients is, even the most cautious have to accept, a strong possibility.

Within reactive lymph nodes from patients with AIDS, changes in T- and B-cells similar to those in

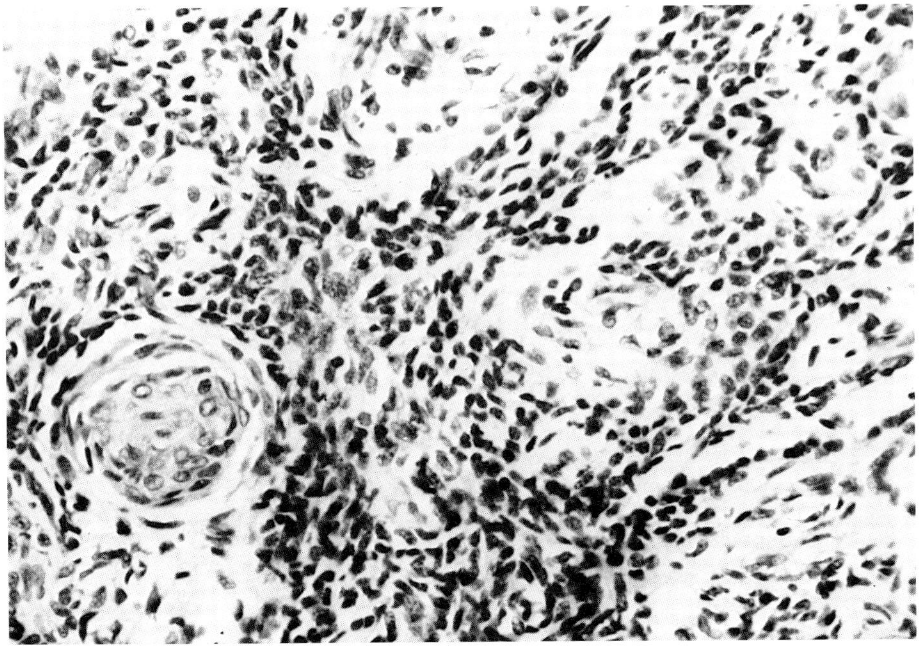

Fig. 6—Thymus from a 39-year-old male with AIDS. Lymphoid tissue is reduced and the Hassall's corpuscle is atrophic. Very few corpuscles were present within the thymus. Haematoxylin and eosin, ×500

the circulation have been demonstrated.[36, 60] B-cells were in large numbers not only in the follicular centres but also in the interfollicular and surrounding mantle zones. The T-cells in the interfollicular regions showed the same inverted ratio of helper to suppressor cells seen in the circulating cells and T-suppressor cells were also seen in large numbers in the mantle zones and follicle centres. All of these findings were in marked contrast to the patterns in control hyperplastic lymph nodes in which T-helper cells predominated and in which few of these or T-suppressor cells occurred in the B-cell rich follicular centres. From these observations it has been argued that the B-cell hyperplasia is the cause of the systemic immune deficit; infection stimulating the B-cell response, encouraging B-cell lymphoma and the migration of suppressor T-cells into the follicular centres. B-cell proliferation is, thereby, reduced and microbial proliferation released.[36] To sustain this point of view it will be necessary to perform similar studies on lymph nodes of individuals in the incubation and early stages of AIDS. It would also be necessary to confirm the result in established cases in whom lymph nodes do not harbour Kaposi's sarcoma unlike seven of the ten lymph nodes previously reported.[36]

TOXOPLASMA GONDII

This protozoon rarely causes progressive disease in individuals with normal immune responses.[15] Prior to the recognition of AIDS, infection was known as a cause of abortion and neonatal death with microencephalopathy and mental retardation, and as a complication in immunocompromised patients including transplant recipients, particularly those with cardiac grafts.[61, 62] Depressed cellular responses and diminished macrophage activation seem necessary for clinical infection to occur and the greater immunosuppression received by heart recipients as opposed to other organ recipients is in keeping with this observation. Humans act as the intermediate host while domestic animals (in particular cats) serve as a reservoir with cat faeces, human blood and tissues (including transplanted organs) acting as transmission sources.[15]

In AIDS patients the organisms have had major effects upon the central nervous system, a site of predilection in any infected person.[15,63] Myocarditis and pneumonitis, the other main manifestations, have been less common[64] and the typical lymphadenopathy has not been reported. In the brain there is a necrotizing encephalitis centring on the basal ganglia, which can be symmetrically involved, and the lining of the ventricles which leads to thickening and irregularity (Fig. 7). Microscopically large and small granulomas with diffuse inflammation and necrosis are evident. The diagnosis of necrotizing encephalitis is significantly helped by recognition of the cysts in uninvolved and less commonly in necrotic and granulomatous brain. These oval cysts are readily evident in haematoxylin and eosin stained slides where they contain multiple granular basophilic organisms (Fig. 8). Since it is only the non-encysted tachyzoite form that is associated with tissue inflammation and necrosis[15] a means of identification would be of considerable diagnostic assistance. A peroxidase–antiperoxidase method for recognizing tachyzoite forms in paraffin sections has been reported[65] and if this test can be reproduced it will provide an important part of the armamentarium for studying brain biopsies of AIDS patients. Unresolved is the dilemma of whether the brain injury is due to reactivation of a latent infection or a sequel of a newly transmitted infection.[66] It is probable that it is the latter but prospective serological studies of potential AIDS patients will be necessary to prove this.

ATYPICAL MYCOBACTERIA

AIDS has come to prominence since 1979 and within 3 years atypical mycobacteria, especially *Mycobacteria avium-intracellulare* complex (MAC), have had devastating effects on the sufferers.[67–69] Other atypical mycobacteria that have been recognized include *M. gordonae* and *M. scrofulaceum* and in some patients more than one example has been identified.[54,70] The infection occurs late in the course of the syndrome and if diagnosed, is very difficult to treat. All too often it is recognized only at autopsy. Previously, the MAC organisms rarely infected humans and only 14 examples were reported prior to 1982. These occurred in patients with widespread malignancy[67] but not amongst transplant recipients in whom there were infections by other atypical mycobacteria.[71] Almost all tissues of the body have been infected including the blood[68] and a remarkable finding is the poverty of the body's

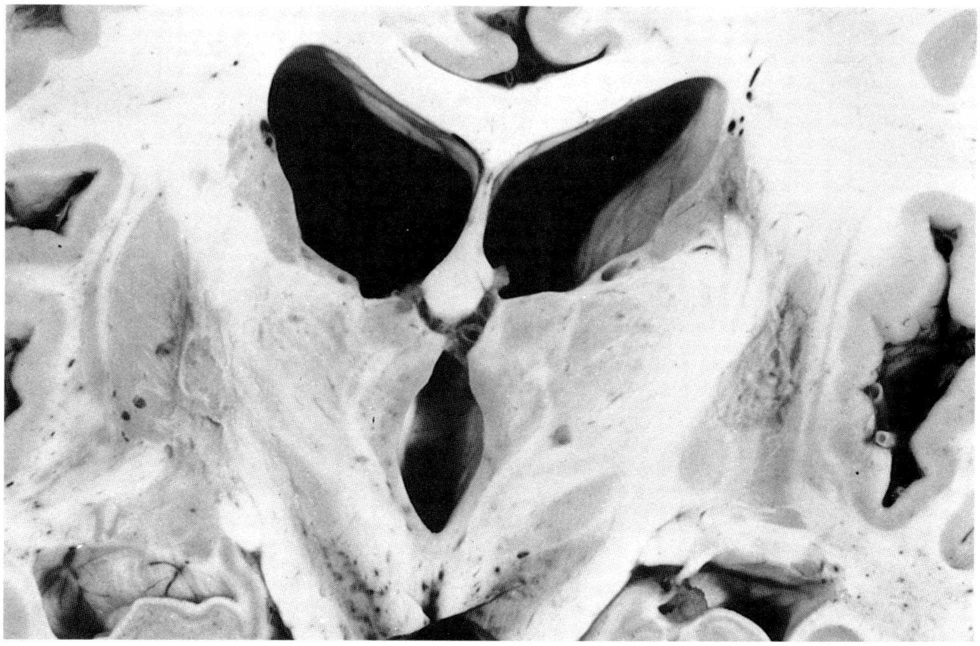

Fig. 7—Basal ganglia softening and necrosis which encroaches upon the lateral ventricle. A brain biopsy 6 months prior to death revealed *Toxoplasma gondii*. Temporary symptomatic improvement occurred with sulphadiazine, pyrimethamine, folinic acid and steroids. No *Toxoplasma* cysts were found at autopsy

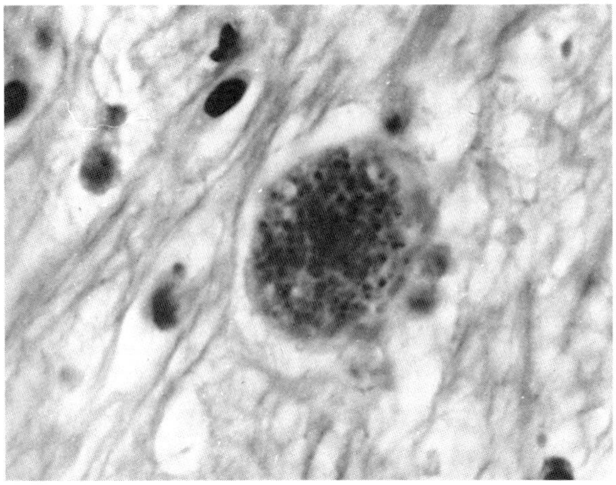

Fig. 8—*Toxoplasma* cyst in brain of a black Zambian girl of 27 years with AIDS and dying from cerebral toxoplasmosis. Haematoxylin and eosin, ×720

reaction.[54, 67] The typical tissue changes associated with mycobacterial infections, such as caseating granulomas, cavitation and necrosis are not conspicuous and may be entirely absent (Figs 5, 9). It is, therefore, recommended that any tissue from AIDS patients should be stained by the Ziehl–Neelsen technique and adoption of such a policy has revealed abundant acid-fast bacilli both intracellularly and free within otherwise normal tissues and normal bone marrow aspirates (Fig. 8).[72] Ziehl–Neelsen positivity is not peculiar to mycobacteria and in AIDS sufferers the protozoan cryptosporidiosis must be differentiated.[73] This parasite has caused diarrhoea, bleeding and death in immunodeficient individuals and in AIDS patients.[74–76]

DISCUSSION

The observations above do not embrace all of the histopathological features associated with AIDS. Others include fungal infections, of which the commonest are *Cryptococcus neoformans* and *Candida albicans*.[6, 19, 52, 77, 78] The sequelae of Epstein-Barr and hepatitis B virus infections[13, 79, 80] are frequently found in some AIDS risk groups. Examples of other protozoan infections, e.g. *Entamoeba histolytica,* have similarly not been discussed.[52, 81] In none of these examples, however, are there any histological features or pathogenetic mechanisms unique to

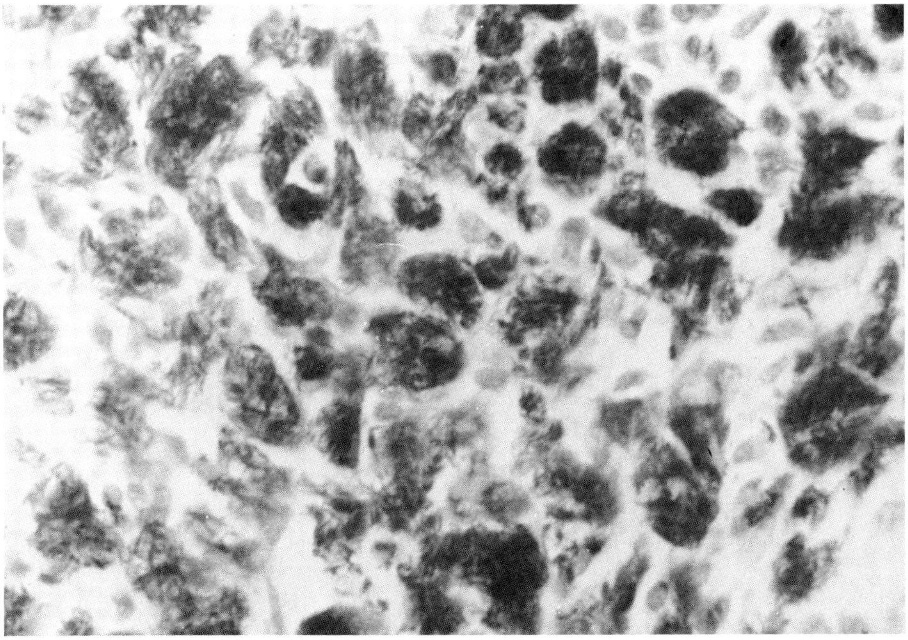

Fig. 9—Acid fast bacilli within macrophages and lying free in the mesenteric lymph node illustrated in Fig. 5. There were no caseating or non-caseating granulomas and the diagnosis was only appreciated after Ziehl–Neelson staining. Ziehl–Neelson, ×720

AIDS or related to other circumstances in which these organisms are encountered. What, nevertheless, is peculiar to AIDS is the number of infections amongst the victims as well as the number recognized in each individual sufferer. Anyone examining tissues from these patients must therefore be constantly aware of the possibility of infection by multiple micro-organisms, many associated with sexual transmission. The precautions to be observed in examining these tissues have been detailed and are basically those observed in the handling of tissues potentially contaminated with HBV.[82,83]

Immunodeficiency

Those changes which have been discussed, unequivocally reveal the ravages of infection and neoplasia but cannot be regarded as demonstrating a common cause of AIDS. Inevitably, most of the changes reported are those in homosexuals, the largest 'at risk' group, but there are already differences recognized in the other 'at risk' groups, e.g. the lower incidence of Kaposi's sarcoma and higher incidence of tuberculosis in the Haitians.[6,7,77,81] No single lesion has yet emerged as common to all sufferers. This observation is in spite of the common denominator of immunodeficiency whose morphological hallmark could be the atrophy of lymphoid tissues and Hassall's corpuscles within the thymus (Fig. 6) which although developing with age, is greater than that found in age-matched non-AIDS patients.[53,55] Even this change has not been uniform since in some patients the corpuscles persist although diminished in number and calcified[53] whilst in one patient hyperplasia of the corpuscles was apparent.[64] In most thymuses there were foci of plasma cells with similar groups of cells in the spleens and lymph nodes. At autopsy, particularly, lymphocyte depletion within the spleen and lymph nodes has been found[52,53] and, whilst this may be interpreted as a reflection of immunodepression, these features are also present in any patient with severe systemic illness and/or infection of the type found in AIDS. As an alternative cause for all of these lymphoid changes a graft versus host reaction has been suggested, the foreign lymphocytes entering the host following rectal trauma.[13] Such a reaction could account for the extreme wasting found in AIDS patients but more definitive evidence is needed to sustain such an interpretation.

Role of infection

The high incidence of infections is probably correctly regarded as a sequel to immunodeficiency, but an alternative viewpoint is that the constant antigenic stimulus associated with these infections induces the basic immunodeficiency.[2,4,84] This hypothesis is obviously difficult to prove since, by the time of presentation, there have been and invariably are multiple infections. However, since analogies can be made between HBV infection and AIDS as well as because of the high index of viral infections particularly by *Herpes* viruses, CMV, HBV and EBV in AIDS patients at any stage in the development of this disorder,[2,13,21,22,79,80,85,86] consideration has been given to the possibility that these organisms may provide the basis of AIDS. Similar infections with these viruses can occur in other groups of patients but do not have such devastating effects and amongst AIDS patients no single virus has emerged as a common denominator. The possibility of an unrecognized organism, comparable to the emergence of *Legionella* as a cause of pneumonia, does nevertheless remain and the close epidemiological similarities with HBV[2,80] make viruses particular targets for investigation. Nevertheless, other forms of persistent antigenic stimulation cannot be discounted since any stimulus of this type can be associated with immunodepression and the lifestyles of the majority of those with AIDS gives ample opportunity for exposure to a wide range of antigens. Drugs and spermatozoa have been incriminated[13,84] but no definite evidence for a causative role has emerged. The greatest difficulty in accepting any of these agents as the inducing factor, however, is that the immunodepression produced by them is reversible while that of AIDS is persistent and irreversible.

Contrasts with organ transplantation

Organ transplantation and other iatrogenic and disease-associated immunosuppressive conditions have resulted in a similar spectrum of infectious complications to those in AIDS. In organ transplant recipients a similar range of neoplasms also occurs.[46] The infective changes are attributed to depressed cellular immunity and the neoplasms in the transplant recipients to a combination of the altered cellular immunity and persistent antigenic stimulation arising from the foreign graft, possibly also influenced by immunostimulation from infective organisms. Of the immunosupressed patients, those with organ transplants have been the most closely monitored and it is, therefore, of interest to compare the findings amongst them with those made in AIDS patients.

Microbial infections—Microbial infections of all types occur in transplant recipients and involve a similar spectrum to those in AIDS.[87,88] However, not all organ recipients have recurrent and/or multiple infections and the number of organisms infecting an individual transplant recipient, even in the early phases of this therapy, seem fewer than those that an AIDS patient can anticipate. Furthermore, in AIDS patients protozoal and atypical mycobacterial infections are commoner and fungus infections less so than in the transplant recipients; organisms associated with sexual transmission are obviously an especial hazard for AIDS sufferers. The greatest difference, however, between the two groups is in the tumours they manifest.

Tumours—Tumours of all types are encountered by transplant recipients in greater numbers than in the general population and the greatest number of these are EBV related B-cell lymphomas.[46] These occur at a rate 350 times greater than in the general population and show the peculiarity that in 87 per cent of affected patients they are confined to the brain. While AIDS patients develop similar lymphomas, these are not as frequent or the most commonly found tumours (Table III). It has been suggested that, in the AIDS patients, death occurs before lymphomas have had time to appear.[89] This may be incorrect since the average time span for lymphomas to develop in transplant patients is 25 months[46] and, obviously, in some the tumours will be present before this interval. AIDS patients usually survive for two years from diagnosis but some for longer if account is taken of the incubation period of six months to two years. During this period immunodepression is present and if relevant to the development of B-lymphomas should induce them.

Table III—Tumours associated with AIDS and organ transplantation

	Kaposi sarcoma	B-lymphomas
General population*	0·6%	4%
Transplant receipts*	4·9%	33%
AIDS patients†	>35%	>8%

* Penn.[30,46]

† Curran;[1] Brynes *et al.*;[103] Fernandez *et al.*;[49] Guarda *et al.*;[50] Ioachim *et al.*;[51] Ziegler *et al.*[60] Both of these figures are minimum estimates. That for Kaposi sarcoma is from the mode of presentation and does not take account of patients developing the tumour after their first presentation. That for lymphomas is from the references which include a total of 120 lymph node examinations and does not include patients with extra-nodal presentations.

Transplant patients, in contrast to those with AIDS, have a lower incidence of Kaposi's sarcoma[30] although in both groups the incidence is greater than that found in the general population (Tables I and III). The reason for the reversed incidence of lymphomas and Kaposi's sarcoma between these two groups of patients is unclear. Both harbour the viruses (EBV and CMV) presently associated with each tumour[87,88] and both have a similar pattern of immunodepression affecting loss of T-helper cells and natural K-cells (tumour surveillance cells).[88] The transplant patients differ in having the graft's antigenic stimulus potentially promoting excessive B-cell proliferation and, thereby, the emergence of these B-cell lymphomas[91] but similar attributes could be given to the effect of multiple infections in AIDS patients. The decrease in K-cells, while consistent with the overall increase of tumours in both groups, does not explain why this increase is restricted to mainly one tumour and why the tumour is different in each group of patients. Hypotheses invoking the release of angiogenesis factors as the stimulus for the development of Kaposi's sarcoma, particularly by CMV which exhibits tropism for endothelial cells,[84] must be regarded with scepticism until an endothelial origin of this tumour is established and the relationship between it and CMV is clarified. Since CMV inclusions do not predominantly occur in endothelial cells, the tropism of the virus for endothelial cells may be neither strong nor exclusive, providing further doubt for the role of CMV and/or endothelial cells in Kaposi's sarcoma. Even should this suggestion be correct, similar circumstances exist within both transplant and AIDS patients (including the prevalence of CMV infections) and yet Kaposi's sarcoma remains rare in transplant recipients (Table III).

Recently it has been suggested that the HTLV virus (human T-cell leukaemia/lymphoma virus) promotes tumours in AIDS patients because of the occurrence of lymphomas and the finding of raised titres to this virus in 25 per cent of a group of AIDS patients.[76,92] This hypothesis has been justly criticized[93] since the lymphomas in AIDS are B-cell and HTLV is associated with T-cell lymphomas. In addition, HTLV is not cytopathic and is not associated with T-cell destruction and depletion. HTLV is probably yet another example of infection in AIDS and the antibody levels may reflect the diminished T-suppressor response and release of B-cells and their products. Similar studies in transplant patients may result in similar conclusions.

Carcinomas—The carcinomas of the tongue, penis and anus found in AIDS[94–96] are exclusive to the homosexual group amongst whom they were recognized as a hazard prior to AIDS; the epidemic nature of the syndrome makes it unlikely that any of these patients were in fact unrecognized examples of AIDS.[97] Dramatic increases in these tumours and other carcinomas have not otherwise occurred in AIDS. This contrasts with the high number of epithelial cancers, especially of the skin and cervix, that develop in transplant patients which may be partly related to papilloma viruses as well as environmental factors.[46,98]

These variations in patterns of infection and neoplasia between AIDS patients and patients with organ transplants imply that the immunodepression not only differs but, because of the infections encountered, that the immune depression of AIDS is more severe than that associated with transplantation. The irreversible nature of the immunodepression of AIDS also favours this conclusion and similar differences between AIDS and other immunodeficient states may be anticipated.

Macrophage defect

A further aspect of the unique nature of immunodepression in AIDS is the macrophage defect. Many of the protozoal infections that occur, as well as the mycobacterial infections, are all indicative of a defect in macrophage killing although phagocytosis is clearly not impaired. A single example of Whipple's disease amongst these patients[99] is yet further evidence of this defect since, in Whipple's disease, a decreased index of macrophage phagocytosis and of intracellular killing of fungi have been demonstrated.[100] The disorder of macrophage function in AIDS can be explained by the deficit in T-helper cells and the resultant impaired recruitment of macrophages but it could also be a primary effect of the AIDS inducing agent.

The urgent need to identify the cause of AIDS is self-evident and on present experience there seems little reason to abandon the infectious hypothesis. The possibilities include an undiscovered organism or the identification of a new virulent strain of a recognized organism. There is equally the possibility that one agent may be responsible for the infections and another for the neoplastic complications but until such conundrums are resolved the relentless progression of this disease can be anticipated.

ACKNOWLEDGEMENTS

Much of this material was prepared for a lecture to IMLS South Region Immunology Discussion Group. Advice has been given by Drs Helen Chapel, G. Pasvol, I. Burns and R. Eglin, and by A. J. Chaplin, S. Patel and G. Richardson. Mrs R. Hunt kindly prepared the typescript.

REFERENCES

1. Curran JW. AIDS—two years later. *New Eng J Med* 1983; **309:** 609–610.
2. Francis DP, Curran JW, Essex M. Epidemic acquired immune deficiency syndrome: epidemiologic evidence for a transmissible agent. *J Nat Cancer Institute* 1983; **71:** 1–4.
3. Lancet. Acquired immunodeficiency syndrome. *Lancet* 1983; **i:** 162–164.
4. Waterson AP. Acquired immune deficiency syndrome. *Brit Med J* 1983; **286:** 743–746.
5. MMW Report. Acquired immunodeficiency syndrome (AIDS) update—United States. *Morbid Mortal Weekly Report* 1983; **32:** 389–391.
6. Pape JW, Liautaud B, Thomas F, Mathurin J-R, St. Amand M-MA, Boncy M, Pean V, Pamphile M, Laroche AC, Johnson W. Characteristics of the acquired immunodeficiency syndrome (AIDS) in Haiti. *New Eng J Med* 1983; **309:** 945–950.
7. Pitchenik AE, Fischl MA, Dickinson GM, Becker DM, Fournier AM, O'Connell MT, Colton RM, Spira TJ. Opportunistic infections and Kaposi's sarcoma among Haitians: evidence of a new acquired immunodeficiency state. *Ann Int Med* 1983; **98:** 277–284.

8. Henrickson RV, Osborn KG, Madden DL, Anderson JH, Maul DH, Sever JL, Ellingsworth LR, Lowenstine LJ, Gardner MB. Epidemic of acquired immunodeficiency in Rhesus monkeys. *Lancet* 1983; **i:** 388–390.
9. Letvin NL, King NW, Daniel MD, Aldrich WR, Blake BJ, Hunt RD. Experimental transmission of Macaque AIDS by means of inoculation of Macaque lymphoma tissue. *Lancet* 1983; **ii:** 599–602.
10. London WT, Madden DL, Gravell M, Dalakas MC, Houff IA, Sever JL, Henrickson RV, Maul DH, Osborn KG, Gardner MB. Experimental transmission of simian acquired immunodeficiency syndrome (SAIDS) and Kaposi-like skin lesions. *Lancet* 1983; **ii:** 869–873.
11. Hapke MR. AIDS in monkeys and men. *Lancet* 1983; **i:** 1097–1098.
12. Morris L, Distenfeld A, Amorosi E, Karpatkin S. Autoimmune thrombocytopenic purpura in homosexual men. *Ann Int Med* 1982; **96:** 714–717.
13. Sonnabend J, Witkin SS, Purtilo DT. Acquired immunodeficiency syndrome, opportunistic infections and malignancies in male homosexuals: a hypothesis of etiologic factors in pathogenesis. *JAMA* 1983; **249:** 2370–2374.
14. Friedman-Kien AE, Laubenstein LJ, Rubinstein P, Buimovici-Klein E, Marmor M, Stahl R, Spigland I, Kim KS, Zolia-Pazner S. Disseminated Kaposi's sarcoma in homosexual men. *Ann Int Med* 1982; **96:** 693–700.
15. Ryning FW, Mills J. *Pneumocystis carinii, Toxoplasma gondii,* cytomegalovirus and the compromised host. *West J Med* 1979; **130:** 18–34.
16. Burke BA, Good RA. *Pneumocystis carinii* infection. *Medicine* 1973; **52:** 23–51.
17. Masur H, Jones TC. The interaction *in vitro* of *Pneumocystis carinii* with macrophages and L-cells. *J Exp Med* 1978; **147:** 157–169.
18. Pifer LL, Woods D, Hughes WT. Propagation of *Pneumocystis carinii in vitro* cell culture. *Infect Immunol* 1978; **20:** 66–68.
19. Gottlieb MS, Schroff R, Schanker HM, Weisman JD, Fan PT, Wolk RA, Saxon A. *Pneumocystis carinii* pneumonia and mucosal candidiasis in previously healthy homosexual men. Evidence of a new acquired cellular immunodeficiency. *New Eng J Med* 1981; **305:** 1425–1431.
20. Masur H, Michelis MA, Greene JB, Onorato I, Stouwe RAV, Holzman RS, Wormser G, Bretiman L, Lange M, Murray HW, Cunningham-Rundles S. An outbreak of community-acquired *Pneumocystis carinii* pneumonia. Initial manifestation of cellular immune dysfunction. *New Eng J Med* 1981; **305:** 1431–1438.
21. Drew WL, Mintz L, Miner RC, Sands M, Ketterer B. Prevalence of cytomegalovirus infection in homosexual men. *J Infect Dis* 1981; **143:** 188–192.
22. Mintz L, Drew WL, Miner RC, Braff EH. Cytomegalovirus infections in homosexual men: an epidemiological study. *Ann Int Med* 1983; **99:** 326–329.
23. Carney WP, Rubin RH, Hoffman RA, Hansen WP, Healey K, Hirsch MS. Analysis of T lymphocyte subsets in cytomegalovirus mononucleosis. *J Immunol* 1981; **126:** 2114–2116.
24. Kornfield H, Stouwe RAV, Lange M, Reddy MM, Grieco MH. T-lymphocyte subpopulations in homosexual men. *New Eng J Med* 1982; **307:** 729–731.
25. Giraldo G, Beth E, Huang ES. Kaposi's sarcoma and its relationship to cytomegalovirus. III. CMV DNA and CMV early antigens in Kaposi's sarcoma. *Int J Cancer* 1980; **26:** 23–29.
26. Peden K, Mounts P, Hayward GS. Homology between mammalian cell DNA sequences and human herpesvirus genomes detected by a hybridization procedure with high-complexity probe. *Cell* 1982; **31:** 71–80.
27. Southern EM. Detection of specific sequences among DNA fragments separated by gel electrophoresis. *J Mol Biol* 1975; **98:** 503–517.
28. Ruger R, Bornkamm GW, Fleckenstein B. The genome of human cytomegalovirus strain AD 169 contains five different regions with homologies to cellular DNA. *The 8th International Herpesvirus Workshop* 1983; 221.
29. Bluefarb SM. Kaposi's Sarcoma. Charles C. Thomas and Blackwell Scientific Publications: Oxford 1957.
30. Penn I. Kaposi's sarcoma in organ transplant recipients: report of 20 cases. *Transplantation* 1979; **27:** 8–11.
31. Hyme KB, Greene JB, Marcus A, William DC, Cheung T, Prose NS, Ballard H, Laubenstein LJ. Kaposi's sarcoma in homosexual men—a report of eight cases. *Lancet* 1981; **ii:** 598–600.
32. Gottlieb GJ, Ackerman AB. Kaposi's sarcoma: an extensively disseminated form in young homosexual men. *Human Pathology* 1982; **13:** 882–892.
33. MMW Report. Acquired immunodeficiency syndrome (AIDS) update—United States. *Morbid Mortal Weekly Report* 1983; **32:** 309–311.
34. Templeton AC. In: Sommers SC, Rosen PP, eds. Pathology Annual Part 2. 1981: 315–336.
35. Cochran AJ, Nestor MS, Groopman JE, Ahmed AR. Tumour infiltrates in acquired immunodeficiency syndrome patients with Kaposi's sarcoma. *Lancet* 1983; **i:** 416.
36. Modlin RL, Meyer PR, Ammann AJ, Rea TH, Hofman FM, Vaccaro SA, Conant MA, Taylor CR. Altered distribution of B and T lymphocytes in lymph-nodes from homosexual men with Kaposi's sarcoma. *Lancet* 1983; **ii:** 768–771.
37. McNutt NS, Fletcher V, Conant MA. Kaposi's sarcoma: ultrastructural comparison to other

vascular growths in skin. *Lab Invest* 1983; **48:** 56A.
38. Nadji M, Morales AR, Ziegles-Weissman J, Penneys NS. Kaposi's sarcoma: immunohistologic evidence for an endothelial origin. *Arch Pathol Lab Med* 1981; **105:** 274–275.
39. Modlin RL, Hofman FM, Kempe RA, Taylor CR, Conant MA, Rea TH. Kaposi's sarcoma in homosexual men: an immunohistochemical study. *J Amer Acad Dermatol* 1983; **8:** 620–627.
40. Burgdorf WHC, Mukai K, Rosai J. Immunohistochemical identification of Factor VIII-related antigen in endothelial cells of cutaneous lesions of alleged vascular nature. *Amer J Clin Path* 1981; **75:** 167–171.
41. Piovella F, Nalli G, Malamani GD, Majdino I, Frassoni F, Sitar GM, Ruggerl A, Dellorbo C, Asceri E. The ultrastructural localisation of Factor VIII antigen in human platelets, megakaryocytes and endothelial cells utilising a ferritin-labelled antibody. *Brit J Haem* 1978; **39:** 209–213.
42. Kindblom L. Factor VIII related antigen and mast cells. *Acta Path Microbiol Immunol Scand* 1982; **90A:** 437–441.
43. Sinclair RA, Bourne CAJ. Factor VIII detected within glomerular mesangium. *Lancet* 1983; **i:** 1448–1449.
44. Harrison AC, Kahn LB. Myogenic cells in Kaposi's sarcoma: an ultrastructural study. *J Path* 1978; **124:** 157–160.
45. Safai B, Mike V, Giraldo G, Beth E, Good RA. Association of Kaposi's sarcoma with second primary malignancies: possible etiopathogenic implications. *Cancer* 1980; **45:** 1472–1479.
46. Penn I. Tumors arising in organ transplant recipients. *Adv Cancer Res* 1978; **28:** 31–61.
47. Ziegler JL, Miner RC, Rosenbaum ER, Lennette E, Shillitoe E, Casavant C, Drew WL, Mintz L, Gershow J, Greenspan J, Beckstead J, Yamamoto K. Outbreak of Burkitt's-like lymphoma in homosexual men. *Lancet* 1982; **ii:** 631–633.
48. Gapen P. Neurological complications now characterising many AIDS victims. *JAMA* 1982; **248:** 2941–2942.
49. Fernandez R, Mouradian JA, Metroka C. The histopathology of lymphadenopathy in homosexual males with acquired immunodeficiency syndrome. *Lab Invest* 1983; **48:** 25A.
50. Guarda LA, Butler JJ, Mansell P, Hersh EM, Reuben J, Newell GR. Lymphadenopathy in homosexual men: morbid anatomy with clinical and immunologic correlations. *Amer J Clin Pathol* 1983; **79:** 559–568.
51. Ioachim HL, Lerner CW, Tapper ML. Lymphadenopathies and lymphoma in immunocompromised homosexual men. *Lab Invest* 1983; **48:** 39A.
52. Reichert CM, O'Leary TJ, Levens DL, Simrell CR, Macher AM. Autopsy pathology in the acquired immunodeficiency syndrome. *Amer J Path* 1983; **112:** 357–382.
53. Fligiel S, Naeim F. Immunopathologic findings in male homosexual patients with acquired immunodeficiency syndrome. *Lab Invest* 1983; **48:** 25A.
54. Freeman ML, Talbot GH. Non-granulomatous mycobacterial lymphadenitis in homosexual patients. *Lab Invest* 1983; **48:** 27A.
55. Elie R, Laroche AC, Arnoux E, Guerin J-M, Pierre G, Malebranche SR, Seemayer TA, Dupuy J-M, Russo P, Lapp WS. Thymic dysplasia in acquired immunodeficiency syndrome. *New Eng J Med* 1983; **308:** 841.
56. Spiers ASD, Robbins CL. Cytomegalovirus infection simulating lymphoma in a homosexual man. *Lancet* 1982; **i:** 1248–1249.
57. Ewing EP, Spira TJ, Chandler FW, Callaway CS, Brynes RK, Chan WC. Unusual cytoplasmic body in lymphoid cells of homosexual men with unexplained lymphadenopathy. *New Eng J Med* 1983; **308:** 819–822.
58. Sidhu GS, Stahl RE, El-Sadr W, Zolla-Pazner SB. Ultrastructural markers of AIDS. *Lancet* 1983; **i:** 990–991.
59. Kostianovsky M, Kang YH, Grimley PM. Disseminated tubuloreticular inclusions in acquired immunodeficiency syndrome (AIDS). *Ultra Path* 1983; **4:** 331–336.
60. Ziegler T, Tubbs R, Alanis A, Calabrese Petras R, Weinstein A, Ahmad M, Bergfeld W. Lymph node immunohistology in homosexual males with acquired immunodeficiency. *Lab Invest* 1983; **48:** 97A.
61. Luft BJ, Yehudith N, Araujo FG, Stinson EB, Remington JS. Primary and reactivated toxoplasma infection in patients with cardiac transplants: clinical spectrum and problems in diagnosis in a defined population. *Ann Int Med* 1983; **99:** 27–31.
62. Nagington J, Martin AL. Toxoplasmosis and heart transplantation. *Lancet* 1983; **ii:** 679.
63. Luft BJ, Conley F, Remington JS. Outbreak of central nervous system toxoplasmosis in Western Europe and North America. *Lancet* 1983; **i:** 781–783.
64. Al'Khafaji K, Rotterdam H, Lerner CW, Tapper ML. Autopsy findings in six patients with acquired immunodeficiency syndrome. *Lab Invest* 1983; **48:** 2A.
65. Conley FK, Jenkins KA, Remington JS. *Toxoplasma gondii* infection of the central nervous system: use of the peroxidase–antiperoxidase method to demonstrate *Toxoplasma* in formalin fixed, paraffin embedded tissue sections. *Human Path* 1981; **12:** 690–698.
66. Feldman HA. Epidemiology of toxoplasma infections. *Epidemiol Rev* 1982; **4:** 204–213.
67. Greene JB, Sidhu GS, Lewin S, Levine JF, Masur

H, Simberkoff MS, Nicholas P, Good RC, Zolla-Pazner SB, Pollock AA, Tapper ML, Holzman RS. *Mycobacterium avium-intra cellulare:* a cause of disseminated life threatening infection in homosexuals and drug abusers. *Ann Int Med* 1982; **97:** 539–546.
68. Zakowski P, Fligiel S, Berlin GW, Johnson BL. Disseminated *Mycobacterium avium intracellulare* infection in homosexual men dying of acquired immunodeficiency. *JAMA* 1982; **248:** 2980–2982.
69. Elliott JL, Hoppes WL, Platt MS, Thomas JG, Patel IP, Gansar A. The acquired immunodeficiency syndrome and *Mycobacterium avium intracellulare* bacteremia in a patient with hemophilia. *Ann Int Med* 1983; **98:** 290–293.
70. Croxson TS, Ebanks D, Mildvan D. Atypical mycobacteria and Kaposi's sarcoma in the same biopsy specimens. *New Eng J Med* 1983; **308:** 1476.
71. Lloveras J, Peterson PK, Simmons RL, Najarian JS. Mycobacterial infections in renal transplant recipients. *Arch Int Med* 1982; **142:** 888–892.
72. Cohen RJ, Samoszuk MK, Busch D, Lagios M. Occult infections with *M. intracellulare* in bone marrow biopsy specimens from patients with AIDS. *New Eng J Med* 1983; **308:** 1475–1476.
73. Angus KW. Cryptosporidiosis in man, domestic animals and birds: a review. *J Roy Soc Med* 1983; **76:** 62–70.
74. Honig C, Soave R. Cryptosporidium in acquired immunodeficiency syndrome. *Lab Invest* 1983; **48:** 36A.
75. Koch KL, Shankey V, Weinstein GS, Dye RE, Abt AB, Current WL, Eyster ME. Cryptosporidiosis in a patient with hemophilia, common variable hypogammaglobulinemia, and the acquired immunodeficiency syndrome. *Ann Int Med* 1983; **99:** 337–340.
76. Andreani T, Le Charpentier Y, Brouet J-C, Lachance J-R, Modigliani R, Galian A, Liance M, Messing B, Vernisse B. Acquired immunodeficiency with intestinal cryptosporidiosis: possible transmission by Haitian whole blood. *Lancet* 1983; **i:** 1187–1191.
77. Mildvan D, Mathur U, Enlow RW, Romain PL, Winchester RJ, Colp C, Singman H, Adelsberg BR, Spigland I. Opportunistic infections and immune deficiency in homosexual men. *Ann Int Med* 1982; **96:** 700–704.
78. Malerbranche R, Guerin JM, Laroche AC, Elie R, Spira T, Drotman P, Arnoux E, Pierre GD, Pean-Guichard C, Morisset PH, Mandeville R, Seemayer T, Dupuy JM. Acquired immunodeficiency syndrome with severe gastrointestinal manifestations in Haiti. *Lancet* 1983; **ii:** 873–878.
79. Schreeder MT, Thompson SE, Hadler SC, Berquist KR, Zaidi A, Maynard JE, Ostrow D, Judson FN, Braff EH, Nylund T, Moore JN, Gardner P, Doto IL, Reynolds G. Hepatitis B in homosexual men: prevalence of infection and factors related to transmission. *J Infect Dis* 1982; **146:** 7–15.
80. Ravenholt RT. Role of Hepatitis B virus in acquired immunodeficiency syndrome. *Lancet* 1983; **ii:** 885–886.
81. Baker RW, Peppercorn MA. Gastrointestinal ailments of homosexual men. *Medicine* 1982; **61:** 390–405.
82. Conte JE, Hadley WK, Sande M. Infection-control guidelines for patients with the acquired immunodeficiency syndrome (AIDS). *New Eng J Med* 1983; **309:** 740–744.
83. Quinn TC. Precautions for patients hospitalised with acquired immunodeficiency syndrome. *Infect Control* 1983; **4:** 79–80.
84. Levy JA, Ziegler JL. Acquired immunodeficiency syndrome is an opportunistic infection and Kaposi's sarcoma results from secondary immune stimulation. *Lancet* 1983; **ii:** 78–80.
85. Siegal FP, Lopez C, Hammer GS, Brown AE, Kornfeld SJ, Gold J, Hassett J, Hirschman SZ, Rundles CC, Adelsberg BR, Parham DM, Siegal M, Rundles SC, Armstrong D. Severe acquired immunodeficiency in male homosexuals manifested by chronic perianal ulcerative *Herpes simplex* lesions. *New Eng J Med* 1981; **305:** 1439–1444.
86. Rogers MF, Morens DM, Stewart JA, Kaminski RM, Spira TJ, Feorino PM, Larsen SA, Francis DP, Wilson M, Kaufman L. The Task Force on Acquired Immune Deficiency Syndrome. National case-control study of Kaposi's sarcoma and *Pneumocystis carinii* pneumonia in homosexual men: part 2, laboratory results. *Ann Int Med* 1983; **99:** 151–158.
87. Ahern MJ, Comite H, Andriole VT. Infectious complications associated with renal transplantation: an analysis of risk factors. *Yale J Biol Med* 1978; **51:** 513–525.
88. Peterson PK, Ferguson R, Fryd DS, Balfour HH, Rynasiewicz J, Simmons RL. Infectious diseases in hospitalised renal transplant recipients: a prospective study of a complex and evolving problem. *Medicine* 1982; **61:** 360–372.
89. Ciobanu N, Andreeff M, Safai B, Koziner B, Mertelsmann R. Lymphoblastic neoplasia in a homosexual patient with Kaposi's sarcoma. *Ann Int Med* 1983; **98:** 151–155.
90. Stiller CR, Keown PA. Immunologic monitoring: current perspectives and clinical implications. *Transpl Proc* 1981; **13:** 1699–1711.
91. Frizzera G, Hanto DW, Gajl-Peczalska KJ, Rosai J, McKenna RW, Sibley RK, Holahan KP, Lindquist LL. Polymorphic diffuse B-cell hyperplasia and lymphomas in renal transplant recipients. *Cancer Res* 1981; **41:** 4262–4279.
92. Essex M, McLane MF, Lee TH, Falk L, Howe

CWS, Mullins JI, Cabradilla C, Francis DP. Antibodies to cell membrane antigens associated with Human T-cell leukaemia virus in patients with AIDS. *Science* 1983; **220:** 859–862.
93. Black PH, Levy EM. The human T-cell leukemia virus and AIDS. *New Eng J Med* 1983; **309:** 856.
94. Cooper HS, Patchefsky AJ, Marks G. Cloacogenic carcinoma of the anorectum in homosexual men: an observation of four cases. *Dis Colon Rect* 1979; **22:** 557–558.
95. Conant MA, Volberding P, Fletcher V, Lozada FI, Silverman S. Squamous cell carcinoma in sexual partner of Kaposi sarcoma patient. *Lancet* 1982; **i:** 286.
96. Lozada F, Silverman S, Conant M. New outbreak of oral tumors, malignancies and infectious diseases strikes young male homosexuals. *Calif Dent J* 1982; **10:** 39–42.
97. Frederick P Li, Osborn D, Cronin CM. Anorectal squamous carcinoma in two homosexual men. *Lancet* 1982; **ii:** 391.
98. Lutzner M, Orth G, Dutronquay V. Detection of human papillomavirus type 5 DNA in skin cancers of an immunosuppressed renal allograft recipient. *Lancet* 1983; **ii:** 422–424.
99. Autran B, Gorin I, Leibowitch M, Laroche L, Escande JP, Hewitt J, Marche CL. AIDS in a Haitian woman with cardiac Kaposi's sarcoma and Whipple's disease. *Lancet* 1983; **i:** 767–768.
100. Lukacs G, Dobi S, Szabo M. A case of Whipple's disease with repeated operations for ileus and complete cure. *Acta Hepato-Gastroenterol* 1978; **25:** 238–242.
101. Taylor JF, Templeton AC, Vogel CL, Ziegler JL, Kyalwazi SK. Kaposi's sarcoma in Uganda: a clinico-pathological study. *Int J Cancer* 1971; **8:** 122–135.
102. D'Oliveira JJG, Torres FO. Kaposi's sarcoma in the Bantu of Mozambique. *Cancer* 1972; **30:** 553–561.
103. Brynes RK, Chan WC, Spira TJ, Ewing EP, Chandler FW. Morphological features of the unexplained lymphadenopathy of homosexual men. *Lab Invest* 1983; **48:** 11A.

JOURNAL OF PATHOLOGY, VOL. **143:** 241–247 (1984)

THE IMMUNOCYTOCHEMICAL DETECTION OF *HERPES SIMPLEX* VIRUS IN CERVICAL SMEARS—A VALUABLE TECHNIQUE FOR ROUTINE USE*

RICHARD L. ADAMS, DAVID R. SPRINGALL† AND MAX M. LEVENE

Regional Cell Pathology and Cytogenetic Service, Wandle Valley Hospital, Mitcham Junction, Surrey CR4 4XL, U.K.

AND

TIMOTHY E. C. BUSHELL

Royal West Sussex Hospital, Chichester, West Sussex, U.K.

Received 30 November 1983
Accepted 23 December 1983

SUMMARY

Herpes simplex virus type 2 is demonstrated in routine cervical smears by immunocytochemistry. Optimum antibody dilution and suitable fixation were determined and immunostaining results were found to compare favourably with those obtained by screening Papanicolaou-stained smears or by virus culture methods (virus isolation). Results obtained for immunostaining of smears from 158 patients agreed with those of virus isolation in 47 of 50 cases where virus isolation was performed. It is suggested that this immunocytochemical technique is valuable in detection of *Herpes simplex* virus in cervical smears, offering an inexpensive and rapid laboratory diagnosis with advantage to both patient and clinician.

KEY WORDS—Cell culture, cervical smears, cytology, *Herpes simplex* virus, immunocytochemistry, virus isolation.

INTRODUCTION

Herpes simplex virus type 2 (HSV2) is among viruses suspected of promoting carcinogenesis in the uterine cervix.[1] In the U.K. over the last 5 years there has been a steady increase of about 12 per cent per annum in the number of reported cases of genital herpetic infection.[2] Clearly, there is a need for sensitive and accurate laboratory techniques for HSV detection. Current detection methods include identification of characteristic multinucleated giant cells in Papanicolaou-stained cervical smears, observation of the cytopathic effects of the virus on cultured cells (virus isolation) and electron microscopy. These techniques have limitations. Cytology gives equivocal results. Virus isolation methods and electron microscopy are costly, both in time and resources.

The aim of this work was to detect HSV2 infections in routine cervical smears by an immunocytochemical technique. Suitable fixation methods, storage of specimens and optimum dilution of antibody were determined. The immunocytochemical method was evaluated by comparing results with those obtained by screening Papanicolaou-stained smears and by virus isolation.

MATERIALS AND METHODS

Cytological smears

These were collected from 158 patients attending the clinics of genito-urinary medicine at St

*This work was presented in part to the 2nd meeting of The Immunocytochemistry Club of Great Britain on 15 March 1983 at The Royal Postgraduate Medical School, Hammersmith Hospital, London.

†Addressee for correspondence: Dr D. R. Springall, Regional Cell Pathology and Cytogenetic Service, Wandle Valley Hospital, Mitcham Junction, Surrey CR4 4XL, U.K.

0022–3417/84/080241–07$01.00

Helier Hospital, Carshalton, The Fletcher Laboratory, Chichester, and The South London Hospital for Women, London. At least two cervical smears were taken from each of 84 patients suspected clinically of having an herpetic infection of the genitalia, and from 74 patients with no clinical signs or previously detected herpetic infection. One smear was processed for Papanicolaou staining and screened for cellular changes characteristic of HSV infection. Remaining smears were processed for immunocytochemical staining. All smears received were adequate.

Virus isolation

Specimens from 50 of the patients attending the clinics were routinely sent for virus isolation tests at the Department of Virology, West Park Hospital, Epsom, Surrey, or the Department of Microbiology, St Richard's Hospital, Chichester, Sussex.

Histological specimens

Cervical biopsy specimens were taken from three patients attending for laser treatment of cervical lesions at St Helier Hospital, Carshalton. Patients either had previous history of genital Herpes, though with no current symptoms, or were clinically negative and with no record of such infection (controls). Biopsy material was embedded in O.C.T. compound (R. A. Lamb) and snap-frozen in melting Arcton (ICI Ltd) previously frozen in liquid nitrogen.

Cryostat sections (5 μm thick) were collected on poly-L-lysine-coated slides[3] to ensure adherence of sections throughout staining. Sections were fixed as for cytological material and immunostained for HSV2.

Cell cultures

This material was used as positive controls of immunostaining and to check cross-reactivity of antibodies. Cultures of HEL (human embryo lung) cells, grown at 37°C in Eagle's Minimum Essential Medium (Gibco) plus 10 per cent fetal calf serum (T.C. Services) and 5 per cent human serum, were inoculated with suspensions of HSV1 or HSV2 (1 ml per flask) obtained from the Department of Virology, West Park Hospital, Epsom, Surrey.

After 48 h, cells were removed by adding EDTA solution (140 mM NaCl, 1·5 mM KH_2PO_4, 2·7 mM KCl, 8·1 mM Na_2HPO_4, 0·54 mM EDTA disodium salt) to the vessel, and shaking gently. Following centrifugation, the cells were pipetted onto poly-L-lysine-coated slides, gently smeared, fixed (see below) before they were air dried, and stained immunocytochemically.

Fixation for immunocytochemistry

Optimum fixation for both cytological and histological specimens was determined by fixing slides of HSV-positive material (prepared from HSV-infected cell cultures) by a variety of methods for times from 5 to 30 min. Fixatives were acetone, methanol, 10 per cent formol saline, Bouin's fluid, 'Sprayfix' (Histolab Ltd), 1 per cent carbowax in 50 per cent aqueous alcohol, 1 per cent carbowax in methylated spirit or 1 per cent carbowax in acetone.

In this study, the most suitable fixatives were judged as those giving adequate preservation of cell and tissue structure without grossly altering the antigenicity of HSV proteins.

Titration of antibody

Rabbit antisera (Dakopatts) to HSV1 and HSV2 were obtained from Mercia Brocades. Optimum dilution was determined by performing the selected immunocytochemical technique on smears known to contain HSV2-positive material. Primary antibody dilutions were 1:50, 1:100, 1:250 and 1:500 in Tris-buffered saline (TBS: 0·9 per cent NaCl in 5 mM Tris–HCl buffer, pH 7·6) containing 2 per cent normal swine serum (NSS).

Specificity of antibody

Duplicate smears prepared from HSV1-infected cell cultures were immunostained one with anti-HSV1, the other with anti-HSV2. The results were compared to see whether the anti-HSV2 was detecting HSV1 antigen.

Immunostaining

The technique used was the unlabelled antibody enzyme method of Sternberger.[4] All incubations were carried out at room temperature in a damp chamber. Endogenous peroxidase was blocked with 0·5 per cent (w/v) hydrogen peroxide in

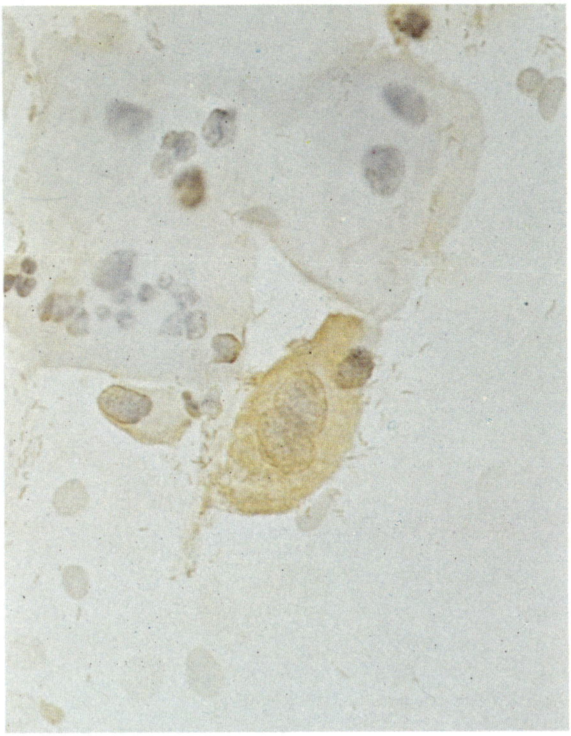

Plate 1—(a) Cervical smear fixed in methanol and immunostained for HSV2, showing strong immunoreaction in a binucleate intermediate squamous cell. Peroxidase–antiperoxidase method PAP, ×375

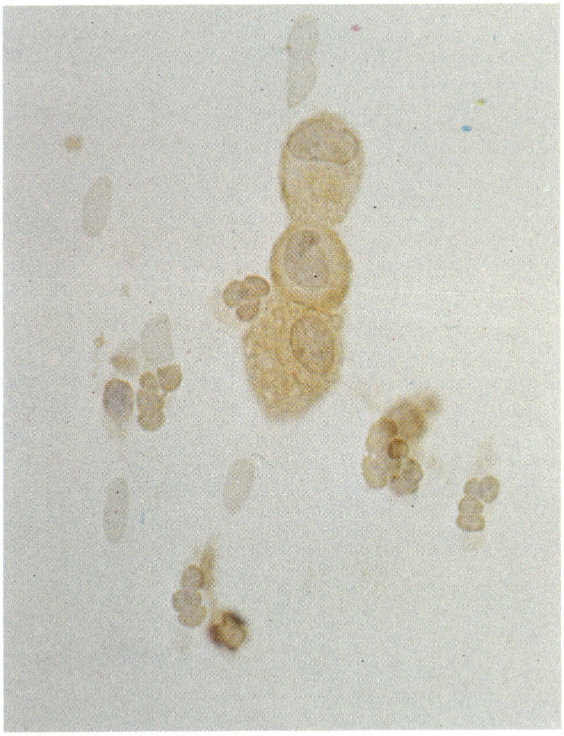

Plate 1—(b) Cells in a methanol-fixed cervical smear showing strong cytoplasmic immunoreactivity for HSV2. Though strong staining is visible in the cytoplasm, there is also some immunoreactivity in the nucleus. PAP, ×375

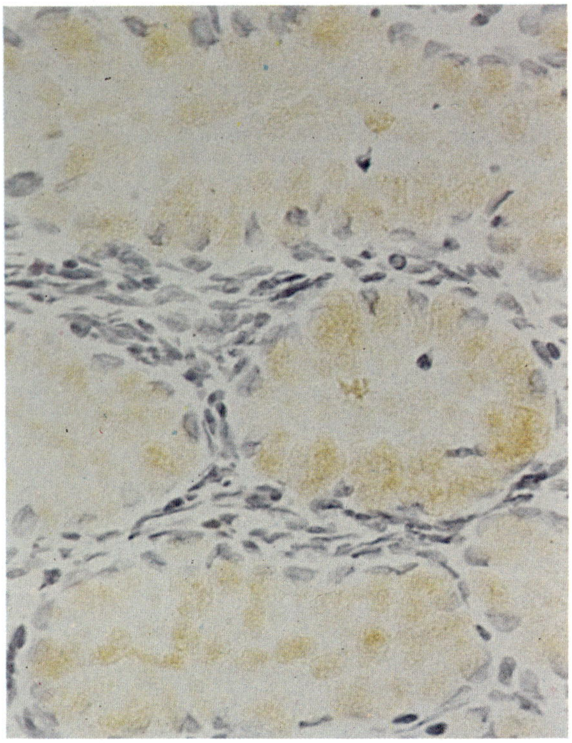

Plate 1—(c) Cryostat section of cervical biopsy specimen, post-fixed in methanol and immunostained with anti-HSV2. Strong immunoreactivity is seen in the cells of the sub-epithelial glands. PAP, ×245

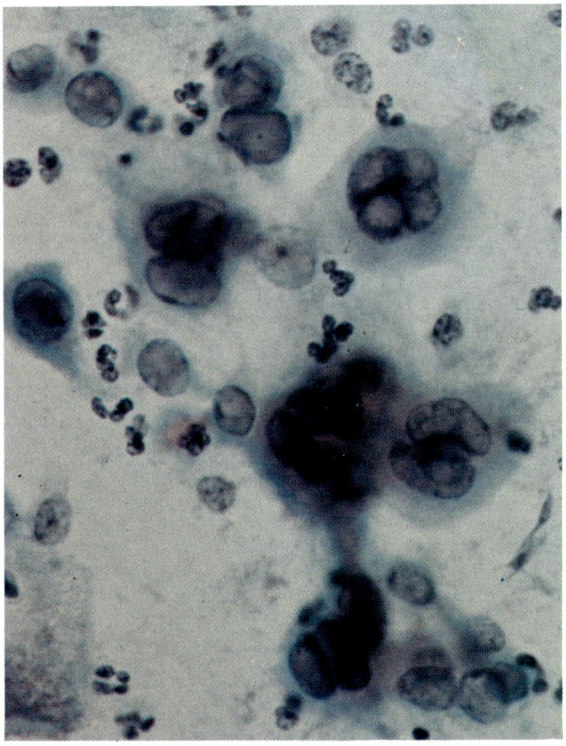

Plate 1—(d) Cervical smear from a patient with genital *Herpes simplex*. The giant multinucleate cells are characteristic of this infection. Papanicolaou, ×360

methanol for 30 min. Slides were then washed for 15 min in three changes of TBS containing 0·2 per cent Triton X-100 (BDH Ltd). Inclusion of Triton X-100 in the first wash aids subsequent spreading of antibody over the slide and enhances immunostaining. Incubation with NSS diluted 1:20 with TBS for 10 min was followed by drainage of excess serum from slides and application of appropriately diluted primary antibody for 60 min. Smears and sections were then washed as before in TBS, and swine anti-rabbit immunoglobulins (Dakopatts) diluted 1:100 in 2 per cent NSS was applied for 30 min. After washing in TBS, slides were treated with rabbit PAP (peroxidase-anti-peroxidase complex, from Dakopatts) diluted 1:200 in TBS, for 30 min. Slides were then washed again in TBS. Peroxidase activity was revealed with a freshly prepared solution of 5 mg of 3,3′-diaminobenzidine tetrahydrochloride (DAB, from BDH Ltd) in 10 ml of TBS containing 5 μl of 100 vol. hydrogen peroxide. Finally, slides were washed for 15 min in running tap water, counterstained lightly with Harris' haematoxylin, dehydrated in alcohol, cleared in xylene and mounted in Styrolite (R. A. Lamb). The procedure is complete in just over 4 h.

Positive and negative control material was included with each batch of slides immunostained. Positive controls were cultured cells inoculated with HSV2. Negative controls of immunostaining were of three types: omission of the primary antiserum, the use of primary antiserum absorbed with HSV2, and replacement of anti-HSV2 with an inappropriate antibody.

RESULTS

Formol saline destroyed HSV2 immunoreactivity in all cases. Other fixatives gave varying degrees of immunostaining and cellular preservation. Acetone or methanol fixation for 10 min gave the best results. This is in accord with the findings of Pearson and co-workers.[5] Although adequate immunostaining was seen after storing the smears dry at 4°C for up to 1 month after fixation, better results were obtained if the slides were stored wet in TBS. Such storage was found to enhance immunoreactivity of both smears and sections compared with those stored dry.

Optimal dilution of the anti-HSV2 was 1:100. This gave strong specific staining and a minimum of background staining.

Antiserum to HSV2 gave only very faint immunostaining in smears of HSV1-infected cells, whereas strong reactivity was obtained with these when using anti-HSV1. The antibody to HSV1 gave only a very weak immunostaining reaction with HSV2-infected cells.

Cytological material

None of the Papanicolaou-stained smears from the 158 cases examined showed obvious cellular changes suggestive of HSV infection.

Results of immunostaining of those patients with clinical signs or past history of genital HSV infection are given in Table I, those with no such clinical signs are given in Table II. Of the 158 smears tested by immunocytochemistry for HSV2, positive results were obtained in 26. Of these, 20 had either a history or clinical signs of HSV infection or a positive VI test; 6 were from cases with no clinical signs of HSV and a VI test was not performed.

Three of the nine immunocytochemistry and virus isolation positive cases showed no clinical signs of an herpetic infection.

Smears were obtained from 108 patients who were not tested by virus isolation. Fifteen of these cases were immunocytochemically positive for HSV2, of which nine had clinical signs suggestive of HSV.

In HSV2-positive smears, strong immunostaining was seen in 5–10 per cent of cells throughout

Table I—Immunostaining in smears of patients clinically suspected of having genital HSV infection

Immunostaining	VI positive	VI negative	VI not done
Positive	6	2	9
Negative	1	22*	44

*Two of these cases were HSV-positive by VI for vulval lesions, but negative for cervix.

Table II—Immunostaining in smears of patients with no history or signs of HSV infection

Immunostaining	VI positive	VI negative	VI not done
Positive	3	0	6
Negative	0	16	49

Table III—Immunostaining for HSV2 in cervical biopsy specimens

Biopsy No.	History	Immuno-staining
1	Clinically negative for HSV2 but with previous history of infection	+
2	Clinically negative for HSV but with genital warts	−
3	No clinical symptoms of viral disease	−

the smears. Positively stained cells were mainly of intermediate squamous type (Plate 1a, b).

No positive staining was found in slides immunostained with antiserum absorbed with HSV, nor where the primary antiserum was either omitted or replaced with an inappropriate antibody. In all cases the positive control material (HSV2-infected cultured cells) had strong immunoreactivity.

Histological material

The results of immunostaining of three biopsy specimens are given in Table III. In the biopsy that showed reaction with anti-HSV2, the immunostaining was confined to glandular tissue (Plate 1c). Sections from control cases and controls of immunostaining were all negative.

DISCUSSION

Initial results suggest that the immunocytochemical technique is as effective as the methods in current use for the detection of cervical infection by *Herpes simplex,* such as the screening of Papanicolaou-stained smears, virus isolation and electron microscopy.

The efficiency of each detection method may be governed by the stage of infection. For example, diagnosis of HSV in Papanicolaou-stained smears depends on particular changes being present in the smear. As multinucleate giant cells characteristic of herpetic infection[6] (see also Plate 1d) are not immediately obvious after infection by the virus, early detection of HSV in such smears may be impossible. Conversely, once the infection has reached the latent phase and virus has migrated to dorsal root ganglia,[7] the characteristic changes in cells are no longer apparent and diagnosis may again be impeded.

Virus isolation methods give positive results over a wider range of virus-induced changes, permitting earlier detection of HSV2 in cervical tissues than is possible by conventional cytology. The virus isolation technique currently offers the most accurate means of detecting genital herpetic infection. Unfortunately, it is both costly and time-consuming, often taking a week to complete.[8] Important determinants in virus isolation are the clinical stage of the lesion and whether the attack is an initial or recurrent infection.[9] Other factors may be important. For example, higher titres of virus are present in vesicular rather than ulcerative herpetic lesions[10] and the mean duration of virus excretion in an initial attack is longer than in the recurrent genital disease.[11,12]

In the present study, comparison of virus isolation results with the immunocytochemical technique showed a 92 per cent correlation in cases positive for HSV (corresponding Papanicolaou-stained smears were all negative) and 97 per cent in HSV-negative cases. Our results show that the anti-HSV2 used in this study is unlikely to have given any false positive results due to cross reaction with HSV1. However, the infecting HSV type may not influence the subsequent pathological changes. It is not possible to distinguish between HSV1 and HSV2 infections by the virus isolation technique. Perhaps then, the case which was positive by virus isolation but negative by immunocytochemistry was an HSV1 infection. Within the last decade, it has become increasingly clear that not all cervical herpetic lesions are due to HSV2, but that HSV1 is frequently involved. A recent study in Sheffield[13] using DNA fragmentation techniques showed no significant difference in the frequency of HSV1 and HSV2 in cervical infections. This result is corroborated by a report from Japan[14] that 50 per cent of genital strains isolated from women and detected by serological and virological methods are HSV1. However, it is possible that type 2 may recur more readily. If HSV is involved in cervical carcinogenesis, perhaps both types 1 and 2 are involved.

Three of the nine immunocytochemistry and virus-isolation-positive cases were clinically negative for HSV infection, suggesting that detection of the virus immunocytochemically and virologically may be possible in the latent phase of infection. The quiescent state of HSV2 is not fully understood. Latent virus is thought to reside in neurons of local sensory ganglia[7] and most evidence suggests that it is non-replicating during this period. Demonstration of HSV2 by immunocytochemistry in the glandular tissue of cervical biopsy material suggests that some virus particles—or viral DNA that is still being at least partially transcribed to produce viral protein that is immunostainable, but without replication to produce more virus particles—may remain locally in underlying cervical glands.

The immunocytochemical technique for detection of HSV2 in cervical smears is a useful addition to the methods of detection currently in use, showing excellent correlation with virus isolation techniques. Specimens do not require any special transport scheme, may be taken at the same time as a routine cervical smear, and the technique offers the advantages of speed and low cost.

ACKNOWLEDGEMENTS

The authors wish to thank the staff of the Department of Virology, West Park Hospital, Dr F. Davidson, Department of Genito-urinary Medicine, St Helier Hospital, and Dr B. Nunneley and Dr Elizabeth Hicks of The South London Hospital for Women, for their help and for supplying some of the material used in this study. We also wish to acknowledge the invaluable assistance of Mrs A. M. Burt in cell culture work and Mr C. Perry for supplying biopsy material.

REFERENCES

1. Nahmias AJ, Josey WE, Naib ZM, Luce CF, Guest BA. Antibodies to *Herpesvirus hominis* types 1 and 2 in humans. II Women with cervical cancer. *Am J Epidemiol* 1970; **91:** 547–552.
2. Office of Population Censuses and Surveys, Communicable Disease Surveillance Centre of The Public Health Laboratory Service. *Communicable Disease Statistics 1982*. London: H.M.S.O., 1983 (series MB2 no. 9).
3. Huang WM, Gibson SJ, Facer P, Gu J, Polak JM. Improved section adhesion for immunocytochemistry using high molecular weight polymers of L-lysine as a slide coating. *Histochem* 1983; **77:** 275–279.
4. Sternberger LA. The unlabelled antibody peroxidase-antiperoxidase (PAP) method. In: Immunocytochemistry, 2nd edn. New York: Wiley, 1979: 104–169.
5. Pearson NS, Fleagle G, Docherty JJ. Detection of *Herpes simplex* virus infection of female genitalia by the peroxidase–antiperoxidase method alone or in conjunction with the Papanicolaou stain. *J Clin Microbiol* 1979; **10:** 737–746.
6. Stern E, Longo LD. Identification of HSV in a case showing cytological features of viral vaginitis. *Acta Cytol* 1963; **7:** 295–299.
7. Cook ML, Bastone VB, Stevens JG. Evidence that neurones harbour latent *Herpes simplex* virus. *Infect Immunity* 1974; **9:** 946–957.
8. Jarrat M. *Herpes simplex* infection. *Arch Dermatol* 1983; **119:** 99–103.
9. Moseley RC, Corey L, Benjamin D, Winter C, Remington ML. Comparison of viral isolation, direct immunofluorescence, and indirect immunoperoxidase techniques for detection of genital *Herpes simplex* virus infection. *J Clin Microbiol* 1981; **13:** 913–918.
10. Spruance SL, Overall JC Jr, Kern ER, Krueger GG, Pliam V, Miller W. The natural history of recurrent *Herpes simplex labialis*. *New Engl J Med* 1977; **297:** 69–75.
11. Adams HG, Benson EA, Alexander ER, Vontver LA, Remington MA, Holmes KK. Genital herpetic infection in men and women: clinical course and effect of topical application of adenine arabinoside. *J Infect Dis* 1976; **133** (suppl.): A151–A159.
12. Corey L, Reeves WC, Chiang WT, Vontver LA, Remington M, Winter C, Holmes KK. Ineffectiveness of topical ether for the treatment of genital *Herpes simplex* virus infection. *New Engl J Med* 1978; **299:** 986–991.
13. Barton IG, Kinghorn GR, Walker MJ, Al-Omer LS, Potter CW, Turner EB. Association of HSV1 with cervical infection, *Lancet* 1981; **ii:** 1108.
14. Kawana T, Kawaguchi T, Sakamoto S. Clinical and virological studies on genital herpes. *Lancet* 1976; **ii:** 964.

JOURNAL OF PATHOLOGY, VOL. **143**: 249–258 (1984)

YORKSHIRE REGIONAL LYMPHOMA HISTOPATHOLOGY PANEL: ANALYSIS OF FIVE YEARS' EXPERIENCE

C. C BIRD, I. LAUDER, H. S. KELLETT, I. CHORLTON, N. BARNES, C. DARWIN, R. A. CARTWRIGHT AND R. BOYKO

Department of Pathology, University of Leeds, Leeds LS2 9JT, U.K., Department of Histopathology, Castle Hill Hospital, Cottingham, U.K. and Yorkshire Regional Cancer Organisation, Cookridge Hospital, Leeds, U.K.

Received 22 March 1984
Accepted 23 March 1984

SUMMARY

Five years' experience of operating a Regional Lymphoma Histopathology Panel is described. During this period, approximately 1400 cases were registered of which nearly 1200 were confirmed as malignant lymphoma. Complete concordance of diagnosis was achieved between submitting pathologists and the Panel in two-thirds of cases of Hodgkin's disease and just over half of non-Hodgkin's lymphoma. Most discrepancies in diagnosis were found to be of clinical importance in terms of prognosis and/or therapeutic management of patients. In approximately two-thirds of such instances disagreement arose because of wrong assignment of tumour grade within the main lymphoma class but in one-third of cases the main class of lymphoma was wrongly designated. Panel members experienced similar diagnostic problems as submitting pathologists although to a lesser extent. The existence of the panel has not reduced the proportion of cases causing diagnostic difficulty for submitting pathologists or panel members during the 5 year study period. The principal cause of death was ascertained from death certificates and autopsy findings in nearly half the cases dying during the study period. In approximately half of these infection (largely pulmonary) played a major role while most of the remainder died of various cardiovascular, pulmonary or renal disorders. There was no specific pattern relating to the main lymphoma class. It is concluded that whilst the panel fulfils a useful function in resolving diagnostic difficulties and standardizing lymphoma diagnosis its role is restricted somewhat by the limitations imposed by conventional morphological assessments.

KEY WORDS—Malignant lymphomas, Hodgkin's disease, non-Hodgkin's lymphomas.

INTRODUCTION

The difficulties associated with the histopathologic diagnosis of lymphomas are well recognized. Eventually these may be resolved by the identification of specific tumour markers capable of demonstration by routine immunohistological analysis.[1] However, the logistical and technical problems associated with such analyses currently preclude their widespread application except in centres where special facilities and expertise in lymphoma diagnosis exist.

Employing more traditional morphological techniques it has been suggested that the accuracy of diagnosis and consistency in classification can be better achieved by a panel of pathologists with a special interest in lymphoma diagnosis.[2,3] Such a panel has been established in Yorkshire since 1977 and we report here on our experience during the first 5 years of its existence. In addition to providing a referral diagnostic service for the region, the panel sought to determine the extent and categories of diagnostic difficulty and to establish the true incidence of lymphomas arising in a large unselected population of 3·5 million persons. Efforts were made also to determine the cause of death in patients suffering from these malignancies.

0022–3417/84/080249–10$01.00

MATERIALS AND METHODS

Case registrations

All suspected cases of lymphoma occurring in the Yorkshire Health Region (approximate population 3·5 million) during the period November 1977–November 1982, were eligible for registration with the Panel. Cases were drawn from 18 hospitals and 46 pathologists contributed material to the study. To register a case, representative sections stained by haematoxylin and eosin together with a special registration form were sent by post to the Central Coordinating Office at Cookridge Hospital in Leeds. The registration form contained essential patient details together with the submitting pathologist's diagnosis. On receipt, case and specimen details were recorded in a special file, and copies of the form, together with the sections despatched to the reviewing Panel.

Review procedure

The Reviewing Panel comprised four pathologists with a special interest in the histopathologic diagnosis of lymphomas. The sections and registration form were circulated as rapidly as possible by post and each panel member established the diagnosis independently. Each in turn acted for several months as first reviewer to provide the submitting pathologist with a rapid opinion on each case (generally within 48 h of registration). Where there was unanimity of diagnosis, this was recorded as the Final Panel Diagnosis. To resolve problematical cases, regular review meetings were held (2–3 month intervals) to reconcile differences and the Final Diagnosis was achieved by consensus. Occasionally, further material (blocks and/or slides) was requested to assist in the review procedure. The results of surface marker studies were available for only a small proportion of cases but were used wherever possible for confirmation of diagnosis.

Classification employed

Standard morphological criteria as formulated in the Rye classification[4] for Hodgkin's disease and the British National Lymphoma Investigation (BNLI) classification[5] for non-Hodgkin's lymphomas were used. The BNLI classification was employed as many of the registered cases were entered in BNLI therapeutic trials. The classifications were summarized on the registration form in a format suitable for computer coding and analysis. The submitting pathologist and panel members independently marked the appropriate diagnostic code.

Analysis of results

Patient and diagnostic information has been analysed as shown in the various tables. Differences in diagnosis between the submitting pathologist and panel and amongst panel members were assessed to determine their clinical importance. Discrepancies in diagnosis were considered to be clincally important where they might result in an alteration in prognosis (favourable $\rightleftharpoons$ unfavourable) or therapeutic management. Such discrepancies generally arise when the grade within a main lymphoma category or when a main category of lymphoma is wrongly assigned (see Tables V and VI). Statistical analyses were determined by tests of trend involving chi-squared statistics or chi-squared test for association on $2 \times k$ tables.

Table I—Cases submitted to Yorkshire Regional Lymphoma Histopathology Panel: 1977–1982

Final panel diagnosis	1977–1978	1978–1979	1979–1980	1980–1981	1981–1982	Total (%)
Hodgkin's disease	82	91	71	56	91	391 (28·3)
Non-Hodgkin's lymphoma	145	144	167	158	175	789 (57·1)
Mycosis fungoides	1	3	2	1	1	8 (0·6)
Malignant histiocytosis	1	0	4	2	2	9 (0·7)
Angioimmunoblastic lymphadenopathy	0	1	4	6	2	13 (0·9)
Myeloma	4	1	6	5	6	22 (1·6)
Metastatic carcinoma	3	9	10	4	12	38 (2·7)
Reactive hyperplasia	23	19	17	16	11	86 (6·2)
Inadequate biopsy	8	3	4	5	6	26 (1·9)
Total	267	271	285	253	306	1382 (100)

Table II—Crude incidence of lymphomas in Yorkshire Region compared with England and Wales

Lymphoma type	Incidence/100 000 population year			
	Yorkshire Region*		England and Wales†	
	Male	Female	Male	Female
All lymphomas	9·7	7·2	10·4	7·5
Hodgkin's disease	3·8	2·0	3·6	2·1
Non-Hodgkin's lymphoma	5·49	5·2	6·8	5·4

* Population Yorkshire Region = 3·5 million; Data for the period 1975–1979.
† Data derived from Registrar General's figures for 1977.

RESULTS

Cases registered

During the 5 year period, 1382 cases suspected as lymphoma were submitted to the panel (Table I). Of these, 1180 (85 per cent) were confirmed as lymphomas. Comparison with data gathered from a variety of sources for a regional epidemiological study revealed that virtually 100 per cent of lymphomas occurring within the Yorkshire Region were registered with the panel. Six per cent of the initially registered cases were considered to show reactive hyperplasia and 3 per cent comprised metastatic carcinomas. In only 2 per cent of instances was the material submitted considered inadequate for diagnostic purposes. The incidence rates of the main types of lymphoma in the Yorkshire Region calculated from verified diagnoses are shown in Table II. In general, the rates are comparable to those for England and Wales as a whole.

Lymphoma subtypes

As shown in Table I approximately one-third of all lymphomas comprised Hodgkin's disease (HD) and two-thirds non-Hodgkin's lymphoma (NHL). Nodular sclerosis was the commonest subtype (53 per cent) of HD (Table III) with the lymphocyte depletion form the least common (12 per cent). Thirty-one per cent of NHL were of follicular type with the remainder manifesting a diffuse growth pattern (Table IV). In this series, if the tumour contained any follicular component, it was classified as follicular in type. Taken individually, the commonest subtype of non-Hodgkin's lymphoma was diffuse large undifferentiated cell (24 per cent). No attempt has been made to subdivide this subtype further since the results of surface marker studies were available for only a small proportion of cases. The least common subtypes of NHL were diffuse intermediate lymphocytic (8 per cent) and follicular large follicle cell (2 per cent).

Table III—Relative incidence of Hodgkin's disease subtypes in adults and children (< 15years)

Subtype	No. cases (%)				
	Adults		Children		Total
	Male	Female	Male	Female	
Lymphocyte predominance	43 (18)	11 (9)	4 (24)	0 (0)	58 (15)
Nodular sclerosis	117 (48)	79 (62)	6 (35)	4 (67)	206 (53)
Mixed cellularity	53 (22)	17 (13)	7 (41)	2 (33)	79 (20)
Lymphocyte depletion	28 (12)	20 (16)	0 (0)	0 (0)	48 (12)
Total	241 (100)	127 (100)	17 (100)	6 (100)	391 (100)

Sex difference analysis:

	χ^2	*d.f.*	
Overall	39·96	1	$p<0{\cdot}01$
Adults	35·31	1	$p<0{\cdot}01$
Children	5·26	1	$p=0{\cdot}02$
Disease subtypes	14·21	3	$p<0{\cdot}01$

Table IV—Relative incidence of non-Hodgkin's lymphoma subtypes in adults and children (<15 years)

Subtype		Adults Male	Adults Female	Children Male	Children Female	Total
		No. cases (%)				
Follicular	Small follicle cell	61(15)	57 (16)	2 (15)	0 (0)	120 (15)
	Mixed small & large follicle cell	57 (14)	50 (14)	0 (0)	0 (0)	107 (14)
	Large follicle cell	8 (2)	10 (3)	0 (0)	0 (0)	18 (2)
Diffuse	Small lymphocytic	52 (12)	39 (11)	0 (0)	0 (0)	91 (12)
	Intermediate lymphocytic	38 (9)	24 (7)	1 (8)	0 (0)	63 (8)
	Poorly differentiated lymphocytic	43 (10)	33 (9)	7 (54)	8 (100)	91 (11)
	Mixed small and large lymphocytic	61 (15)	49 (14)	0 (0)	0 (0)	110 (14)
	Large undifferentiated cell	98 (23)	88 (25)	3 (23)	0 (0)	189 (24)
	Total	418 (100)	350 (100)	13 (100)	8 (100)	789 (100)

Sex differences:	χ^2	*d.f.*	
Overall	6·75	1	$p<0{\cdot}01$
Adults	6·02	1	$p=0{\cdot}01$
Children	1·19	1	$p=0{\cdot}28$
Follicular versus diffuse	2·71	1	$p=0{\cdot}09$
Disease subtypes	2·77	7	$p=0{\cdot}9$

Relative incidence in adults and children (<15 years)

Overall, both HD (Table III) and NHL (Table IV) are significantly more common in males than females (M:F ratio 2:1 for HD; 1·2:1 for NHL; $p<0{\cdot}01$). Both types of lymphoma were rare in children (6 per cent of cases of HD and 3 per cent cases of NHL). In both adults and children the nodular sclerosis form of HD was significantly more common in females than males ($p<0{\cdot}01$) whereas lymphocyte predominance and mixed cellularity forms of HD were less common ($p<0{\cdot}01$). In NHL, no significant sex differences were found in relation to the pattern of disease (follicular versus diffuse) or the specific histological subtypes of disease. In children, the follicular form of NHL was rare (2/21 cases) whilst by far the commonest variety was the diffuse poorly differentiated lymphocytic (lymphoblastic) subtype (15/21 cases).

Site of presentation

In HD 366/391 cases (94 per cent) presented as nodal enlargements whilst only 25/391 cases (6 per cent) were extranodal in origin. By contrast, in NHL 537/789 cases (68 per cent) presented with lymphadenopathy and 252/789 cases (32 per cent) had an extranodal origin. The commonest extranodal sites of origin were gastrointestinal tract and skin.

Concordance of diagnosis between submitting pathologist and panel in Hodgkin's disease

Overall, greater concordance of diagnosis was achieved with HD than with NHL ($p<0{\cdot}01$). In HD concordance of diagnosis between the submitting pathologist and the panel was achieved in 242/358 (68 per cent) of evaluable cases (Table V). This was greatest with nodular sclerosis (71 per cent) and mixed cellularity (74 per cent) subtypes and least with lymphocyte depletion (48 per cent) subtype. Where differences in diagnosis occurred attempts were made to assess their importance in terms of prognosis and/or treatment. In 96/116 (83 per cent) of such instances clinically important discrepancies in diagnosis were considered to have occurred (Table V). In approximately two-thirds of these cases, another form of HD with a differing prognosis was preferred. With lymphocyte predominance and nodular sclerosis forms of disease, the commonest alternative was mixed cellularity whereas with mixed cellularity and lymphocyte depletion, the commonest alternative was nodular sclerosis. However, in one-third of cases, a diagnosis of NHL was proposed: with the lymphocyte depletion form, most commonly the diffuse large undifferentiated cell subtype of NHL was suggested, whilst for nearly half the cases of lymphocyte predominance a follicular form of NHL was proposed.

Concordance of diagnosis between submitting pathologist and panel in non-Hodgkin's lymphoma

Less concordance was achieved between submitting pathologists and the panel for NHL (Table VI) than for HD (55 per cent versus 68 per cent). No statistically significant differences were detected between the recognition of the follicular (52 per cent) or diffuse (56 per cent) growth pattern nor the different subtypes ($p>0.3$). Greatest concordance was achieved with the diffuse small lymphocytic subtype (65 per cent) and least with the intermediate lymphocytic form (45 per cent). Assessment of the clinical importance of diagnostic differences in terms of prognosis or therapy revealed these to be significantly less common than for HD (158/332 versus 96/116 cases; $p<0.01$). In just over two-thirds (71 per cent) of these discrepancies another grade of NHL was proposed. This occurred with approximately equal frequency with follicular and diffuse forms of disease. With follicular lymphoma the most common discrepancy resulted from a failure to recognize a minor component with a follicular growth pattern. In diffuse lymphomas discrepancies arose most commonly because of incorrect assignment of morphological subtype. This occurred with greatest frequency with the poorly differentiated lymphocytic (lymphoblastic) subtype which was most commonly misdiagnosed as intermediate or small lymphocytic subtype. In nearly one-third of cases the discrepancy arose from designating NHL as HD.

Concordance of diagnosis between submitting pathologist and panel by year of case entry

Using the results in Table VII, no significant trend was shown to emerge in the concordance of

Table V—Hodgkin's disease: concordance between diagnosis of submitting pathologist and panel

Final panel diagnosis	No. cases (%)	No. cases complete concordance (%)	No. cases difference important (%)†	Alternative diagnosis proposed‡
Lymphocyte predominance	54 (100)	26 (48)	22 (41)	9 HD II; 13 NHL
Nodular sclerosis	193 (100)	137 (71)	49 (25)	35 HD II; 14 NHL
Mixed cellularity	70 (100)	52 (74)	16 (23)	14 HD I; 2 NHL
Lymphocyte depletion	41 (100)	27 (66)	9 (22)	3 HD I; 6 NHL
Total	358 (100)*	242 (68)	96 (27)	

* Thirty-three cases excluded where submitting pathologist failed to provide initial subtype classification.
† Difference considered clinically important when prognosis and/or treatment could have been altered.
‡ HDI = lymphocyte predominance or nodular sclerosis subtypes (favourable prognosis).
HDII = mixed cellularity or lymphocyte depletion subtypes (unfavourable prognosis).
NHL = non-Hodgkins' lymphoma NOS.

Concordance:

	χ^2	*d.f.*	
Overall: HD versus NHL	15·94	1	$p<0.01$
Disease subtypes	11·82	3	$p=0.01$
Nos. of clinically important differences HD versus NHL	43·38	1	$p<0.01$
Alternative diagnosis subtypes	13·69	3	$p<0.01$

Table VI—Non-Hodgkin's lymphoma: concordance between diagnosis submitting pathologist and panel

Final panel diagnosis		No. cases (%)	No. cases complete concordance (%)	No. cases difference important (%)†	Alternative diagnosis proposed‡
Follicular	Small follicle cell	110 (100)	57 (52)	19 (17)	12 NHL II; 7 HD
	Mixed small and large follicle cell	100 (100)	52 (52)	22 (22)	11 NHL II; 11 HD
	Large follicle cell	18 (100)	10 (56)	7 (39)	5 NHL II; 2 HD
Diffuse	Small lymphocytic	82 (100)	53 (65)	10 (12)	10 NHL II
	Intermediate lymphocytic	58 (100)	26 (45)	15 (26)	14 NHL II; 1 HD
	Poorly differentiated lymphocytic	90 (100)	48 (53)	28 (31)	24 NHL I; 4 HD
	Mixed small and large lymphocytic	100 (100)	54 (54)	22 (22)	16 NHL I; 6 HD
	Large undifferentiated cell	179 (100)	105 (59)	35 (20)	21 NHL I; 14 HD
	Total	737 (100)*	405 (55)	158 (21)	

* Fifty-two cases excluded where submitting pathologist failed to provide initial subtype classification.
† Difference considered clinically important when prognosis and/or treatment could have been altered.
‡ NHL I = all follicular and diffuse small and intermediate lymphocytic subtypes (favourable prognosis).
NHL II = diffuse poorly differentiated, mixed small and large lymphocytic and large undifferentiated cell subtypes (unfavourable prognosis).
HD = Hodgkin's disease NOS.

Concordance:

	χ^2	*d.f.*	
Follicular versus diffuse	1·02	1	$p=0{\cdot}31$
Subtypes	7·42	7	$p=0{\cdot}39$
Alternative diagnosis	χ^2	*d.f.*	
Diffuse versus follicular	5·88	1	$p=0{\cdot}02$
Subtypes	18·21	7	$p=0{\cdot}01$

Table VII—Concordance between diagnosis of submitting pathologist and panel by year of case entry

Year	Hodgkin's disease			Non-Hodgkin's lymphoma		
	No. cases entered (%)	No. cases complete concordance (%)	No. cases difference important (%)†	No. cases entered (%)	No. cases complete concordance (%)	No. cases. difference important (%)†
1977–1978	73 (100)	46 (63)	20 (27)	130 (100)	74 (57)	24 (19)
1978–1979	84 (100)	52 (62)	28 (33)	135 (100)	74 (55)	28 (21)
1979–1980	65 (100)	48 (74)	15 (23)	155 (100)	84 (54)	34 (22)
1980–1981	53 (100)	35 (66)	16 (30)	149 (100)	83 (56)	37 (25)
1981–1982	83 (100)	61 (74)	17 (21)	168 (100)	90 (54)	35 (21)
Total	358 (100)*	242 (68)	96 (27)	737 (100)‡	405 (55)	158 (21)

* Thirty-three cases excluded where submitting pathologist failed to provide initial subtype classification.
† Difference considered important when prognosis and/or treatment would have altered.
‡ Fifty-two cases excluded where submitting pathologist failed to provide initial subtype classification.

Chi-squared test for trend:

	χ^2	*d.f.*	
HD	2·51	1	$p=0{\cdot}11$
NHL	0·20	1	$p=0{\cdot}6$

diagnosis between the submitting pathologist and the panel during the 5 years of the panel's existence (HD $p=0{\cdot}11$; NHL $p=0{\cdot}6$). In particular, the concordance rate did not increase during this period and no change was observed in the proportion of important diagnostic discrepancies occurring.

Concordance of initial diagnosis amongst panel members

It was of interest to determine whether the panel members experienced similar diagnostic difficulties as submitting pathologists. As shown in Table VIII for HD, panel members achieved greater initial concordance of diagnosis amongst themselves (74 per cent) than submitting pathologists (68 per cent) did with the panel, although this barely achieved statistical significance ($p=0{\cdot}05$). Greatest concordance was achieved with the nodular sclerosis subtype (83 per cent) and least with lymphocyte predominance subtype (59 per cent). In general, the differences of opinion were also of lesser importance from the prognostic and therapeutic point of view (17 per cent versus 27 per cent). These differences however, were not statistically significant ($p=0{\cdot}07$).

Similar findings were obtained for NHL (Table VIII). The overall rate of initial diagnostic concordance was significantly better (66 per cent compared with 55 per cent for submitting pathologists and panel; $p<0{\cdot}01$) and important diagnostic discrepancies were considered to have occurred in 16 per cent of cases (compared with 21 per cent for submitting pathologists and panel). This again did not achieve a level of statistical significance ($p=0{\cdot}14$). Least diagnostic concordance (48 per cent) was achieved with the diffuse intermediate lymphocytic form of disease.

Concordance of intial diagnosis amongst panel members by year of case entry

As shown in Table IX both for HD and NHL, the initial concordance of diagnosis and the import-

Table VIII—Concordance initial diagnosis amongst panel members

Final panel diagnosis		No. cases (%)	No. cases complete concordance (%)	No. cases* difference important (%)
			Hodgkin's disease	
Lymphocyte predominance		58 (100)	34 (59)	15 (26)
Nodular sclerosis		206 (100)	171 (83)	20 (10)
Mixed cellularity		79 (100)	50 (64)	23 (29)
Lymphocytic depletion		48 (100)	34 (71)	9 (19)
Total		391 (100)	289 (74)	67 (17)
			Non-Hodgkin's lymphoma	
Follicular	Small follicle cell	120 (100)	86 (72)	12 (10)
	Mixed small and large follicle cell	107 (100)	72 (67)	8 (7)
	Large follicle cell	18 (100)	12 (67)	3 (17)
Diffuse	Small lymphocytic	84 (100)	59 (70)	12 (13)
	Intermediate lymphocytic	63 (100)	30 (48)	26 (41)
	Poorly differentiated lymphocytic	98 (100)	63 (64)	16 (16)
	Mixed small and large lymphocytic	110 (100)	60 (55)	29 (26)
	Large undifferentiated cell	189 (100)	136 (72)	17 (9)
Total		789 (100)	518 (66)	123 (16)

* Difference considered clinically important when prognosis and/or treatment could have been altered.

Concordance rates: pathologist/panel versus panel

	χ^2	*d.f.*	
HD	3·62	1	$p=0{\cdot}05$
NHL	18·32	1	$p<0{\cdot}01$

Clinically important differences: pathologist/panel versus panel

	χ^2	*d.f.*	
HD	3·09	1	$p=0{\cdot}07$
NHL	2·21	1	$p=0{\cdot}14$

Table IX—Concordance initial diagnosis amongst panel members by year of case entry

Year	Hodgkin's disease		Non-Hodgkin's lymphoma	
	No. cases entered (%)	No. complete concordance (%)	No. cases entered (%)	No. complete concordance (%)
1977–1978	82 (100)	59 (72)	145 (100)	97 (67)
1978–1979	91 (100)	62 (68)	144 (100)	91 (63)
1979–1980	71 (100)	52 (73)	167 (100)	106 (64)
1980–1981	56 (100)	39 (70)	158 (100)	107 (68)
1981–1982	91 (100)	77 (85)	175 (100)	117 (67)
Total	391 (100)	289 (74)	789 (100)	518 (66)

Chi-squared test for trend:

	χ^2	*d.f.*	
HD	2·51	1	$p=0{\cdot}11$
NHL	0·20	1	$p=0{\cdot}6$

ance of diagnostic discrepancies amongst panel members did not alter significantly during the 5 year study period (HD $p=0{\cdot}11$; NHL $p=0{\cdot}6$).

An attempt was made to assess the extent of disagreement amongst panel members where unanimity of diagnosis was not achieved. In approximately two-thirds of such cases, disagreement resulted from one dissenting opinion. This did not relate to any specific panel member or lymphoma subtype. Only rarely (<2 per cent of cases) did major differences of opinion occur when more than two members held differing opinions. There were no differences between HD and NHL in the extent of disagreement observed.

Cause of death in lymphoma patients

Autopsy was performed in only a small proportion of cases dying during the study period. However, death certificates were available for examination in 444 instances. In 225 of these cases the cause of death was expressed only in terms of the original malignancy. In the remaining 219 cases, the primary cause of death was ascribed to factors other than the malignancy *per se*. In 56 cases autopsy findings were available for checking the accuracy of death certification information. In seven instances major discrepancies were found between the primary cause of death recorded in the death certificate and the autopsy report although in five of these cases, the type of malignancy was correctly assigned. In the other two instances, the malignancy was incorrectly designated as being epithelial in origin. The primary cause of death recorded in the death certificates of the 219 evaluable cases, are summarized in Table X. In nearly half the cases infection, largely pulmonary, was considered to be the major factor contributing to death. Details were not given of the causative organisms involved. Cardiovascular disorders, principally myocardial ischaemia and cardiac failure, were the main cause of death in approximately a quarter of cases. The remainder comprised a heterogeneous group of conditions largely involving the lungs, liver and kidneys. Bone marrow failure was considered a relatively rare cause of death.

DISCUSSION

The feasibility of operating a Regional Histopathology Panel for diagnosis of lymphomas has been established by this study. It requires a central reference point (Co-ordinating Office) for registration and collection of material and co-ordination of panel activities. This can be managed with the minimum of clerical assistance. The panel has been found to subserve a number of useful functions. Firstly, it offers a review mechanism for standardization of tumour diagnosis and classification on which clinical management may be based. Secondly, it provides reliable diagnoses for evaluation and comparison of therapeutic procedures. Thirdly, it provides a reliable data base for epidemiological studies of malignancies that appear to be rising in incidence (HMSO, Cancer Statistics 1974–1979). Lastly, it provides a rapid referral service for contributing pathologists who may have

Table X—Primary cause of death in 219 cases of Hodgkin's disease and non-Hodgkin's lymphoma as recorded in death certificates

Primary cause of death	No. cases (%) Hodgkin's disease		Non-Hodgkin's lymphoma	
Infection: pulmonary	22	27 (46)	60	78 (49)
other	5		10	
Cardiovascular disorder:				
myocardial ischaemia				
cardiac failure	7		31	
haemorrhage	2	10 (17)	6	45 (28)
thrombosis	1		8	
Pulmonary disorder:				
oedema	0		4	
fibrosis	3	7 (12)	2	20 (13)
embolism	1		8	
failure NOS	3		6	
Liver disorder:				
acute necrosis	4		1	
cirrhosis	2	7 (12)	1	3 (2)
hepatorenal failure	1		1	
Renal failure		3 (5)		9 (6)
Bone marrow asplasia		0		2 (1)
Cachexia NOS		0		1 (1)
Shock NOS		2 (3)		1 (1)
Injury NOS		2 (3)		1 (1)
Chronic pancreatitis		2 (2)		0
Total		59 (100)		160 (100)

limited experience of diagnosis of these malignancies. The latter function has proved particularly useful for pathologists participating in the study.

The study has also confirmed that many difficulties still persist in achieving accuracy and consistency of lymphoma diagnosis by pathologists without special expertise in these malignancies. This proved most marked with NHL where concordance of diagnosis between the submitting pathologist and panel was obtained in just over half the cases. Although greater concordance was achieved for HD a substantial proportion of cases (approximately one-third) remained where diagnostic differences of clinical importance occurred. With both forms of lymphoma most differences resulted from assigning the wrong grade to the tumour but in nearly one-third of cases the main class of lymphoma was wrongly designated. However, it is notable that panel members experienced similar problems although to a lesser extent. In most instances this resulted from a dissenting opinion being expressed by one (but not always the same) panel member. Consensus in diagnosis was ultimately achieved by reconciling such differences at regular review meetings. When the results were analysed by year of entry, it was apparent that repeated exposure to such diagnostic problems did not lead to any significant reduction in the difficulties experienced either by the contributing pathologists or the panel members. This suggests that the difficulties inherent in conventional morphological assessments of lymphomas are unlikely to diminish without recourse to more objective methods of analysis. It is to be hoped these will emerge from current immunohistological studies directed towards identification of specific tumour markers.

The unselected nature of this series and the virtual 100 per cent registration rate, permit accurate assessments of the relative incidence of the different forms of lymphoma within a large population containing mixed ethnic groups. It was found that about one-third of cases comprised HD and two-thirds NHL. Both forms of malignancy were comparatively rare in children (6 per cent cases of HD and 2 per cent cases of NHL). Nodular sclerosis greatly exceeded other forms of HD in frequency and was significantly more common in females than males at all ages. Approximately one-third of NHL were of follicular type whilst the remainder had a diffuse growth pattern. Numerically, the large undifferentiated cell subtype (24 per cent) comprised the most common variety of NHL, although in children the most frequent form was the poorly differentiated lymphocytic (lymphoblastic) subtype (approximately 75 per cent cases). The great majority of cases of HD (94 per cent) presented as nodal enlargements whereas nearly one-third of NHL were extranodal in origin with the gastrointestinal tract and skin being most commonly involved.

Attempts were made also to assess the primary cause of death in patients with lymphoma by examination of death certificates since only a small proportion of cases dying were autopsied. In approximately half the cases, the cause of death was expressed in terms of malignancy only. In approximately a quarter of the remainder it was possible to check the accuracy of death certification against autopsy findings. In general, agreement between the two sources of information was satisfactory although in a few cases, major discrepancies were observed in the primary cause of death (but not the type of malignancy) recorded. Using death certificate data for over 200 evaluable cases, it was found that death was attributable to infection (largely pulmonary) in nearly half the cases. Various cardiovascular, pulmonary and renal disorders contributed to death of most of the remainder but there was no specific pattern relating to the main classes of lymphoma. Bone marrow failure by itself, was considered a rare cause of death although haemopoietic and immunological deficiencies seem certain to have contributed to a significant extent in deaths arising from infection or haemorrhage.

It must be concluded from this study that some improvement in the accuracy of lymphoma diagnosis can be achieved by referral of conventionally prepared histological sections to a Review Panel with a special interest in the diagnosis of these malignancies. However, diagnostic problems still persist especially for NHL and emphasize the need for development of more objective and readily applicable methods for lymphoma diagnosis.

ACKNOWLEDGEMENTS

We are grateful to all pathologists in the Yorkshire Region for their participation in this study. The contribution of the late Dr G. Storey who was a member of the Panel from 1977–1981 is gratefully acknowledged. We wish to thank also Mrs Gladys Betty and Mr I. Grigor for their assistance. This study was supported by the Yorkshire Regional Cancer Organisation and the Yorkshire Cancer Research Campaign.

REFERENCES

1. Lauder I, Bird CC, Child JA, Grigor I. Surface membrane phenotypic expression in malignant lymphomas with an assessment of initial treatment responses. 1984; submitted for publication.
2. Kim H, Zelman RJ, Fox MA *et al.* Pathology Panel for lymphoma clinical studies: a comprehensive analysis of cases accumulated since its inception. *J Natn Cancer Inst* 1982; **68:** 43.
3. Veleg Garcia E, Durant J, Gamus R, Bartolucci A. Results of a uniform histopathologic review system of lymphoma cases. *Cancer* 1983; **52:** 675.
4. Lukes RJ, Butler JL. The pathology and nomenclature of Hodgkin's disease. *Cancer Res* 1966; **26:** 1063.
5. Bennett MH, Farrer-Brown J, Henry K, Jeliffe AM. Classification of non-Hodgkin's lymphoma. *Lancet* 1974; **ii:** 405.

JOURNAL OF PATHOLOGY, VOL. **143**: 259–265 (1984)

IMMUNOSTAINING OF NEURON-SPECIFIC ENOLASE IS A VALUABLE AID TO THE CYTOLOGICAL DIAGNOSIS OF NEUROENDOCRINE TUMOURS OF THE LUNG

DAVID R. SPRINGALL*†, PETER LACKIE*, MAX M. LEVENE†, PAUL J. MARANGOS‡ AND JULIA M. POLAK*

**Department of Histochemistry, Royal Postgraduate Medical School, Hammersmith Hospital, London, U.K., †Regional Cell Pathology and Cytogenetics Services, Wandle Valley Hospital, Mitcham Junction, Surrey, U.K. and ‡National Institute of Mental Health, Bethesda, Maryland, U.S.A.*

Received 30 November 1983
Accepted 13 December 1983

SUMMARY

The neuroendocrine marker neuron-specific enolase (NSE) has been reported to be detectable by immunohistochemistry in paraffin sections of neuroendocrine neoplasms of the lung. There is no study of immunodetection of NSE in cytological smear preparations from these tumours. We have examined 10 cases of small cell carcinoma of the lung, using cells obtained from serous fluids or bronchial biopsies, and found all but one had NSE-like immunoreactivity. No such immunoreactivity was found in 26 serous fluids and 19 biopsies from non-small-cell carcinomas. It is suggested, therefore, that immunostaining for NSE is a valuable aid to the cytological diagnosis of small cell carcinoma of the lung.

KEY WORDS—Cytology, immunocytochemistry, lung tumours, neuroendocrine tumours, neuron-specific enolase, small cell carcinoma, tumour markers.

INTRODUCTION

Small cell carcinoma of the lung (SCCL) comprises about 20 per cent of bronchial carcinomas[1] and has the poorest prognosis with a 5 year survival of 2 per cent.[2] However, treatment by combined chemotherapy and radiotherapy has been found to prolong survival in patients with small cell carcinoma of the lung; other lung tumours respond better to surgery.[3] It is, therefore, of great importance to distinguish such small cell carcinomas from other lung tumours correctly. Since cytopathology is often in the forefront in diagnosing lung tumours, especially with the advent of fibre-optic bronchoscopy (brush smears as well as biopsies) and the increasing use of fine-needle aspiration, a rapid and reliable diagnostic test would be very advantageous.

There is considerable evidence that small cell carcinoma of the lung and carcinoid tumour cells are related to neuroendocrine cells of the respiratory tract. The neuroendocrine nature of carcinoid tumours is suggested by the presence of many neurosecretory granules similar to those found in normal neuroendocrine cells.[4,5] However, in small cell carconoma of the lung the granules in the tumour cells are sometimes very sparse, requiring extensive tissue sampling to establish their presence.[5–7]

Neuron-specific enolase (NSE), or γ-γ enolase, is an isomer of the glycolytic enzyme enolase which

Addressee for correspondence: Dr Julia M. Polak, Department of Histochemistry, Royal Postgraduate Medical School, Hammersmith Hospital, Du Cane Road, London W12 0HS, U.K.

This work was presented in part to the 147th meeting of the Pathological Society of Great Britain and Ireland, Edinburgh, July 1983.

0022–3417/84/080259–07 $01.00

is found in neuroendocrine cells and nerves throughout the body. Using immunohistochemical techniques, with antibodies to NSE, it is now possible to detect neuroendocrine cells[8–10] and tumours derived from them[11] at the light microscopical level. High levels of NSE have been detected by radioimmunoassay in sera of patients with small cell carcinoma of the lung[12] and in cell cultures of these tumours.[13] Sheppard and co-workers[14] have shown that in a good proportion of cases of small cell carcinoma of the lung, sections of routine formalin-fixed, wax-embedded tumour had NSE immunoreactivity.

The aim of this study was to see if immunostaining for NSE in cytological preparations would help in the diagnosis of neuroendocrine neoplasms of the lung.

MATERIALS AND METHODS

Serous fluids

Pleural fluids were obtained from cases of small cell carcinoma of the lung, and pleural and ascitic fluids from patients with various tumours (see Table I). The fluids were centrifuged at 1000× *g* for 5 min and the supernatants discarded. Sedimented cells were smeared onto poly-L-lysine-coated slides[15] and either fixed immediately or allowed to dry before fixation. Fixatives used were Bouin's fluid, 10 per cent formol saline, methanol, acetone or 70 per cent aqueous alcohol containing 5 per cent acetic acid. Smears were fixed for 20 min at room temperature.

If sufficient cell material remained after making smears, cell buttons were prepared. Cells were aliquoted and each aliquot was suspended in one of the above fixatives for 20 min, resedimented by centrifuging and then embedded in 3 per cent agar. After processing to wax, 5 μm sections were cut for morphology and immunostaining.

Biopsies

Bronchial biopsies were obtained from the Endoscopy Clinic at St Helier Hospital, Carshalton, Surrey, and Mayday Hospital, Thornton Heath, Surrey. Imprints were made by gently touching the biopsy onto 2 slides coated with poly-L-lysine which were then fixed immediately, one in formol saline, the other in methanol, for 20 min.

The biopsies were fixed in 10 per cent formol saline and routinely processed to wax. Sections 5 μm thick were cut for histopathological diagnosis and immunostaining.

Electron microscopy

Cells from serous fluids, or small pieces (1 mm cube) cut from biopsies were fixed in 3 per cent glutaraldehyde (electron microscopy grade) in 0·1 M cacodylate buffer pH 7·2 for 90 min, washed twice in the same buffer (centrifuging to sediment the cell specimens) and postfixed in 1 per cent osmium tetroxide. After dehydrating and embedding in Araldite, thin sections were cut, stained in uranyl acetate and lead citrate, and examined in an electron microscope for the presence of neurosecretory granules.

Antibodies

Antiserum to purified rat brain NSE[16] was raised in New Zealand White rabbits and characterized as described previously.[17]

Immunostaining

The unlabelled antibody enzyme (peroxidase anti-peroxidase [PAP]) technique of Sternberger[18] was used. Sections were dewaxed in xylene, and endogenous peroxidase in sections and smears was blocked using a 0·15 per cent solution of hydrogen peroxide in methanol or distilled water. After washing in phosphate-buffered saline (PBS–0·15 M NaCl in 0·01 M phosphate buffer, pH 7·3) and incubating for 10 min in 3 per cent normal goat serum in PBS, sections and smears were incubated overnight with anti-NSE (1:4000 in PBS containing 0·1 per cent bovine serum albumin) at 4°C. This was followed by 30 min incubation at room temperature in goat anti-rabbit Ig (Miles Labor-

Table I—NSE immunoreactivity in cells from serous fluids and bronchial biopsies

	Total	NSE positive
Small cell carcinoma of lung	10	9
Squamous carcinoma	20	0
Adenocarcinoma	9	0
Undifferentiated carcinoma	8	0
Others	8	0

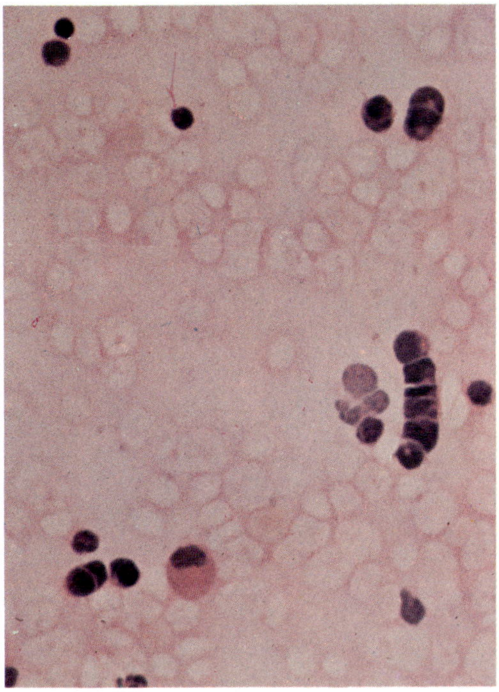

Plate 1—(a) Cell deposit of pleural fluid aspirated from patient with small cell carcinoma of the lung. Tumour cells show the characteristic small cell type morphology, with pronounced nuclear moulding. Methanol-fixed smear. Haematoxylin and eosin, ×307

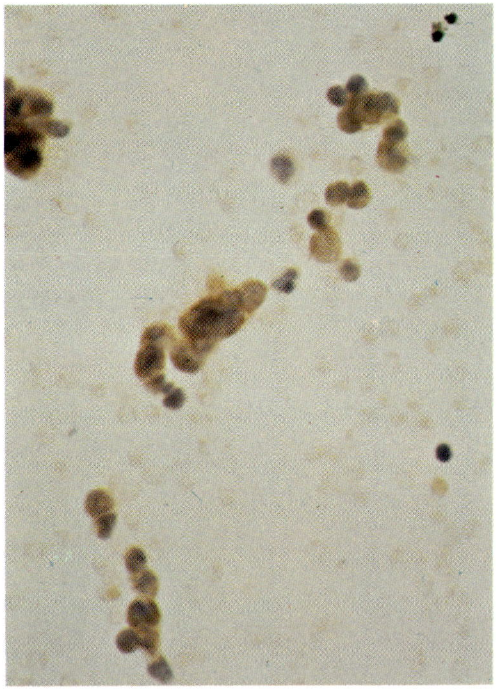

Plate 1—(b) Smear from the same fluid as in Plate 1(a), fixed in methanol and immunostained with antibody to NSE. Strong immunoreactivity is obtained with the tumour cells, as revealed by the brown staining. Peroxidase–antiperoxidase (PAP) method with diaminobenzidine (DAB) as chromogen, light haematoxylin counterstain, ×307

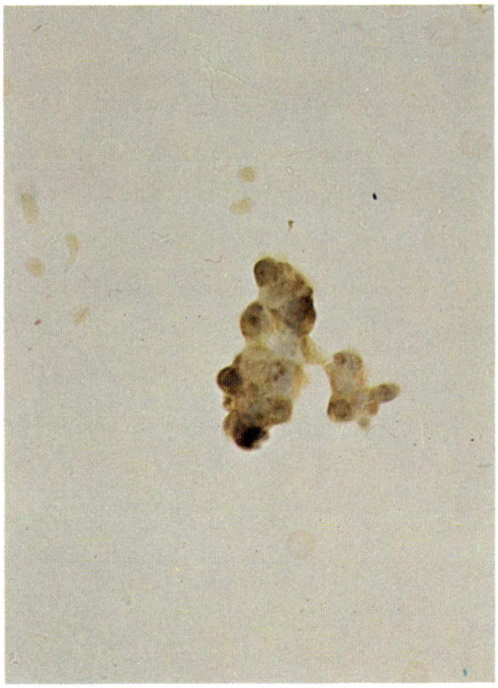

Plate 1—(c) Smear of cells from pleural fluid aspirated from another patient with small cell lung carcinoma fixed and immunoreacted as in Plate 1(b). Again intense brown immunostaining is seen in tumour cells. PAP method, DAB chromogen, haematoxylin counterstain, ×307

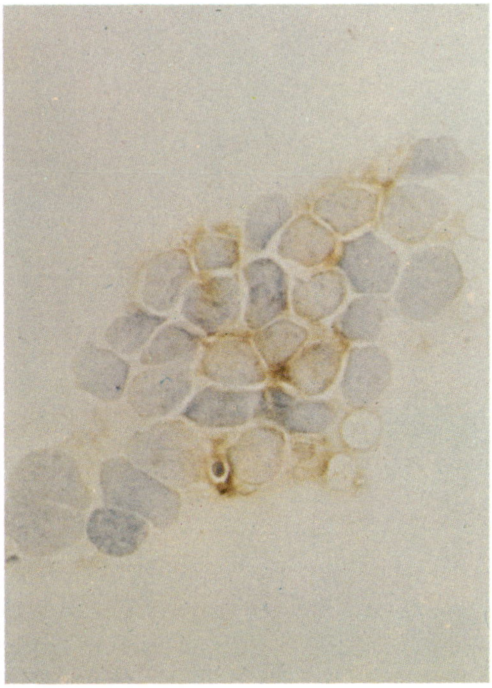

Plate 1—(d) Tumour cells in a methanol-fixed imprint made from an endoscopic bronchial biopsy and immunostained for NSE. Strong NSE immunoreactivity is seen in most of the cells, but less at the periphery of the cluster where cells have dried before fixation. PAP method, DAB chromogen, haematoxylin counterstain, ×638

atories), diluted 1:200 and then rabbit PAP complex (UCB Bioproducts), diluted 1:300, with 3×5-min washes in PBS between steps. Peroxidase activity was revealed using 3,3′-diaminobenzidine.[19] Sections and smears were counterstained with haematoxylin.

The controls of immunostaining used were absorption of anti-NSE with purified NSE (1·0 nmol/ml of diluted antiserum) and substitution of normal rabbit serum or PBS for anti-NSE.

RESULTS

Immunoreactivity was abolished by absorption of anti-NSE with purified NSE (1·0 nmol/ml diluted antibody) or by omission or substitution of anti-NSE with normal rabbit serum.

Smears

Results of immunostaining of cells from serous fluids and biopsy imprints are given in Table I. Tumour cells from all small cell carcinoma of the lung cases had intense immunoreactivity for NSE (Plate 1). No such reactivity was seen in any of the smears from the other cases.

Of the biopsy imprints, reaction with anti-NSE was seen only in the small cell carcinoma of the lung cases. Of eight such cases, seven were immunoreactive for NSE. Immunostaining was moderate ($n=4$) to strong ($n=3$) and the intensity did not correlate with the sub-type of small cell carcinoma of the lung (five intermediate and two oat cell). The case which had no reaction with anti-NSE was of intermediate type.

Of the fixatives used, formol saline and methanol were best for immunostaining, the others gave poor results. Air-drying before fixation of smears abolished all immunoreactivity, and superior results were obtained if the fixed smears were rinsed and kept in PBS rather than allowed to dry before immunostaining.

Sections

In all cases immunoreactivity in sections, whether from cell buttons or biopsies, was weaker

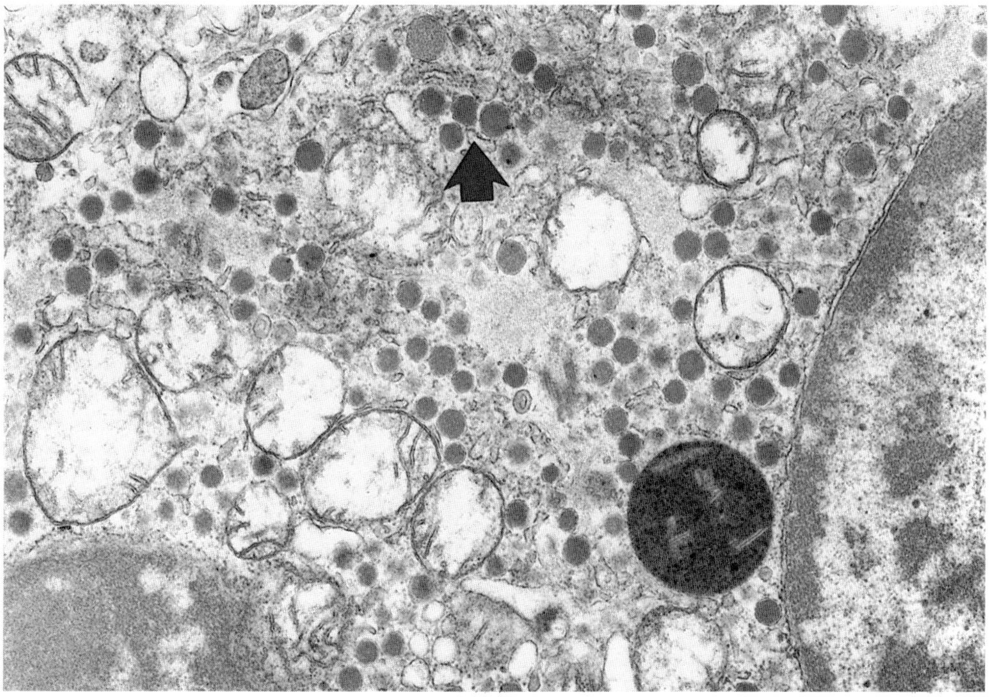

Fig. 1—Electron micrograph of ultrathin section of endoscopic bronchial biopsy from a case of small cell lung carcinoma, showing electron-dense, membrane-bound neurosecretory granules (arrow) in a tumour cell. Glutaraldehyde and osmium tetroxide fixation, resin section, lead citrate and uranyl acetate stain, ×25 000

than that in the corresponding smear or imprint, regardless of fixative used.

Electron microscopy

Material from six small cell carcinoma of the lung cases (two serous fluids, four biopsies) was examined electron microscopically. Of these, four cases had neurosecretory granules in the cytoplasm of tumour cells (Fig. 1). Two cases, both biopsies, had no granules in the sections examined, one of these being the case which was not immunoreactive for NSE.

DISCUSSION

We have shown that NSE immunostaining is a useful tool for detection of small cell carcinoma of the lung in cytological preparations. This has been previously demonstrated in histological preparations,[14] but not before in cytological material. Our results demonstrate that in all cases, stronger immunostaining was obtained in smears of cells from serous fluids or biopsy imprints than in sections of corresponding cell buttons or whole biopsies prepared by conventional wax histology techniques. This is not wholly surprising since single cells or small groups of cells are more rapidly and reproducibly fixed than are pieces of tissue and, furthermore, are not subjected to processing in dehydrating reagents and hot wax. This must help to preserve the antigenicity of NSE, avoiding its destruction or possible diffusion due to over- or under-fixation and processing.

Although our number of cases is considerably smaller than that of Sheppard and co-workers,[14] in this series we have found NSE immunoreactivity to be present in a higher proportion of cases by cytology than they found in histological material. It is, therefore, possible that tumour material processed cytologically may be more suitable for immunostaining than that processed histologically. Furthermore, immunostaining results are obtained quickly with cytological preparations since no embedding or sectioning is required.

When material was obtained from serous fluids and in four of the eight small cell carcinoma of the lung biopsies, confirmation of the diagnosis of small cell carcinoma was attempted by electron microscopic examination of the tumour cells. Of these six cases, two had no obvious neurosecretory granules in the section examined. One of the cases was typical oat cell carcinoma histologically, the other was of intermediate type and did not react with anti-NSE. Despite the probable neuroendocrine origin of small cell carcinoma of the lung, in many cases some or even all of the tumour cells have been reported to be devoid of neurosecretory granules.[4,5,7,20] Therefore, although the first case probably was a true small cell carcinoma, since it had NSE-like immunoreactivity and an 'oat cell' appearance, it is not possible to say with certainty that the other was genuinely small cell carcinoma of the lung.

Since cytology or fibre-optic bronchoscopy are often the techniques used to diagnose lung tumours, it is suggested that immunostaining of cytological preparations and of biopsy imprints with antibodies to NSE is of great value in the detection of small cell lung carcinoma. Antibody to NSE has not been commercially available until recently but is now obtainable from Dakopatts a/s (Mercia Brocades Ltd, Weybridge, Surrey) and Polysciences; the former is currently recommended. Immunostaining for NSE in cytological preparations may permit a correct classification of a tumour as small cell carcinoma of the lung without recourse to more invasive surgery, which is pointless in a tumour which responds better to radio- or chemotherapy.[3] Furthermore, NSE immunostaining may prove especially valuable for detecting small cell carcinoma of the lung metastases in other sites, such as lymph node, where fine-needle aspiration biopsy is used and the material obtained is processed cytologically rather than histologically.

REFERENCES

1. Weiss W. Small cell carcinoma of the lung: epidemiology and etiology. In: Greco A, Oldham RK, Bunn PA, eds. Small Cell Lung Cancer. New York, 1981: 1.
2. Huhti E, Sutinen S, Saloheimo M. Survival among patients with lung cancer: an epidimiologic study. *Am Rev Resp Dis* 1981; **124:** 13.
3. Weiss RB. Small cell carcinoma of the lung: therapeutic management. *Ann Int Med* 1978; **88:** 522.
4. Bensch KG, Gordon GB, Miller LR. Electron microscopic and biochemical studies on bronchial carcinoid tumor. *Cancer* 1964; **18:** 592.
5. Fisher ER, Palekar A, Paulson JD. Comparative histopathologic, histochemical, electron microscopic and tissue culture studies of bronchial

carcinoids and oat cell carcinomas of lung. *Am J Clin Pathol* 1978; **64:** 165.
6. Bensch KG, Corrin B, Pariente R, Spencer H. Oat cell carcinoma of the lung: its origin and relationship to bronchial carcinoid. *Cancer* 1968; **22:** 1163.
7. McDowell EM, Barrett LA, Trump BF. Observations on small granules in the human bronchial epithelium and in carcinoid and oat cell tumors. *Lab Invest* 1976; **34:** 202.
8. Schmechel DE, Marangos PJ, Brightman MW. Neuron specific enolase is a marker for peripheral and central neuroendocrine cells. *Nature* 1979; **276:** 834.
9. Wharton J, Polak JM, Cole GA, Marangos PJ, Pearse AGE. Neuron specific enolase as an immunocytochemical marker for the diffuse neuroendocrine system in human fetal lung. *J Histochem Cytochem* 1981; **29:** 1359.
10. Bishop AE, Polak JM, Facer P, Ferri GL, Marangos PJ, Pearse AGE. Neuron specific enolase: a common marker for the endocrine cells and innervation of the gut and pancreas. *Gastroenterol* 1982; **83:** 902.
11. Tapia FJ, Polak JM, Barbosa AJA, Bloom SR, Marangos PJ, Dermody C, Pearse AGE. Neuron specific enolase is produced by neuroendocrine tumours. *Lancet* 1981; **i:** 808.
12. Carney DN, Marangos PJ, Ihde DC, Cohen MH, Bunn PA, Minna JD. Serum neuron specific enolase: a marker for disease extent and response to therapy of small cell lung cancer, *Lancet* **i:** 1982; March, 583.
13. Marangos PJ, Gazdar AF, Carney DN. Neuron specific enolase in human small cell carcinoma cultures. *Cancer Letters* 1982; **15:** 67.
14. Sheppard MN, Corrin B, Bennett MH, Marangos PJ, Bloom SR, Polak JM. Immunohistochemical localisation of neuron specific enolase (NSE) in small cell carcinomas and carcinoid tumours of the lung. *Histopathology* 1984; **8:** 171.
15. Huang Wei-Min, Gibson SJ, Facer P, Gu J, Polak JM. Improved section adhesion for immunocytochemistry using high molecular weight polymers of L-lysine as a slide coating. *Histochemistry* 1983; **77:** 275.
16. Marangos PJ, Zis AP, Clark RL, Goodwin FK. Neuronal, non-neuronal and hybrid forms of enolase in brain: structural, immunological and functional comparisons. *Brain Res* 1978; **150:** 117.
17. Marangos PJ, Zomzely-Neurath C, Luk DCM, York C. Isolation and characterisation of the nervous system specific protein 14-3-2 from rat brain. *J Biol Chem* 1975; **250:** 1884.
18. Sternberger LA. In; Immunocytochemistry, 2nd edn, New York, 1979: 104–169.
19. Graham RC, Karnovsky MJ. The early stages of absorption of injected horseradish peroxidase in the proximal tubules of mouse kidney. Ultrastructural cytochemistry by a new technique. *J Histochem Cytochem* 1966; **14:** 291.
20. Li Wei-i, Hammar SP, Jolly PC, Hill LD, Anderson RP. Unpredictable course of small cell undifferentiated lung carcinoma. *J Thorac Cardiovasc Surg* 1981; **81:** 34.

JOURNAL OF PATHOLOGY, VOL. **143**: 267–274 (1984)

GASTRIC EPITHELIAL CELL PROLIFERATION IN MONKEYS FED 3,4,3′,4′-TETRACHLOROBIPHENYL

GREGORY M. BECKER* AND WILBUR P. MCNULTY

Oregon Regional Primate Research Center, 505 NW 185th Avenue, Beaverton, Oregon 97006, U.S.A.

Received 4 February 1983
Accepted 15 June 1983

SUMMARY

Rhesus monkeys *(Macaca mulatta)* fed diets containing 1 or 3 mg/kg of 3,4,3′,4′-tetrachlorobiphenyl (3,4-TCB), became moribund after 7–14 weeks. In the body of the stomach the mucosa was thick and cystic gastric glands penetrated the muscularis mucosae. The zymogenic and parietal cells were replaced by or converted into mucus-secreting cells. Autoradiographs of animals labelled with [^{3}H]thymidine showed that in control monkeys gastric epithelial cell proliferation was limited to the isthmus and neck regions of the glands throughout the stomach. In the 3,4-TCB-fed animals most DNA synthesis also occurred in these regions, but [^{3}H]thymidine labelled cells were also seen in the bases of the glands. The labelling indices were not elevated, and therefore the submucosal glands and cysts in this lesion may develop by a failure of the newly formed, downward migrating cells to differentiate and lose their proliferative capacity.

KEY WORDS—Gastric mucosa, gastric epithelium, polychlorinated biphenyls.

INTRODUCTION

Mixtures of chlorobiphenyls, called polychlorinated biphenyls (PCBs),[1] are highly toxic to animals, including man.[2,3] We have demonstrated[4] that the non-*ortho* substituted 3,4,3′,4′-tetrachlorobiphenyl (3,4-TCB) is more toxic in monkeys than commercial mixtures of PCBs and produces the identical lesions as higher levels of commercial mixtures of PCBs.[5,6]

Different species show widely different responses to PCBs.[3] Rhesus monkeys are particularly sensitive to PCBs and develop acneiform lesions in the skin at dietary levels of only 2·5 ppm within 1–2 months.[5] Rhesus monkeys also develop alopecia, periorbital oedema and erythema, anaemia, hypoproteinemia, bone marrow atrophy,[5] thymic involution,[4] hyperplasia of the biliary ducts (McNulty, unpublished data) and the lesion under study here, a mucous hyperplasia of the gastric epithelium with submucosal cyst formation.[6,7] Somewhat similar lesions occur in swine[8] and rats,[9] but have not been reported in any of the human victims of accidental poisoning in Japan. In a previous study[6] of this PCB-induced gastric lesion we described an apparent arrest of differentiation of the proliferative cells of the isthmus and neck zones into parietal and zymogenic cells. Only mucus-secreting cells were being formed.

The hyperplasia seen in this lesion suggests an alteration in the normal dynamic equilibrium of proliferation, maturation and cell loss, which maintains the steady-state number and distribution of cell types in the normal gastric mucosa. We looked for a disturbance of proliferation by analysing the spatial distribution and relative numbers of DNA-synthesizing cells by autoradiography.

* Present address: Department of Veterinary Microbiology and Pathology, Washington State University, Pullman, WA 99164, U.S.A.

0022–3417/84/080267–08$01.00

MATERIALS AND METHODS

3,4,3',4'-Tetrachlorobiphenyl

Pure 3,4-TCB (Analabs, Inc., CT), determined to be free of tetra- and pentachlorodibenzodioxins and dibenzofurans at detection limits of 1 and 5 ppm, respectively,[4] was used without further purification.

Animals

Six immature individually caged male rhesus monkeys *(Macaca mulatta),* 2–4 years of age and weighing 2·5–4·5 kg were fed 120 g of diet cakes twice daily and weighed once weekly. Daily observations were made to determine the status of each animal's health. Three of the animals were fed control diets and three were fed toxic 3,4-TCB diet cakes until they showed loss of appetite, skin lesions, weight loss and behaviour changes.

Diets

The diets consisted of moist cakes, each weighing about 40 g, containing 50 per cent by weight ground Purina Monkey Chow, 37 per cent water, 11 per cent bananas, 0·7 per cent vitamin mixture and a 0·4 per cent corn oil solution containing 3,4-TCB. The final 3,4-TCB content of the diet was 3 mg/kg, or 3 parts per million (ppm) for the first animal, and 1 ppm for the second and third animals. The control diets contained corn oil without 3,4-TCB.

Labelling of cells in the S-phase with [^{3}H]thymidine

After overnight fasting, each animal received intravenously 0·5 mCi of [^{3}H]thymidine (New England Nuclear) per kg of body weight at 09:00 hours. One hour later, the stomach and adjoining oesophagus and duodenum were removed from the living, anaesthetized animal and immediately placed in fixative containing 4 per cent formaldehyde and 1 per cent glutaraldehyde in a pH 7·4 buffer containing 150 mM Na^+ and 84 mM PO_4^{3-}.[10]

Autoradiography

Full-thickness sections of gastric wall, 0·3 × 1·5 cm were cut from along the entire length of the greater curvature, including adjacent portions of the oesophagus and duodenum. The tissue specimens were embedded in glycol methacrylate,[11] and sectioned at 2 μm. Unstained slides were washed, dried, and dipped into Kodak NTB2 liquid emulsion (Eastman Kodak Co.) diluted to 1 : 1 and warmed to 45°C. The slides were dried, stored for 4 weeks at −20°C, developed in undiluted Kodak D-19 at 15°C for 6 min, and stained with methylene blue and basic fuchsin. The background grain count was low: 1·5 grains per 1000 μm^2. Gastric epithelial cells were considered labelled if three or more silver grains were seen over the nuclei, but usually many more silver grains were present.

Morphometry

Measurements were made with a light microscope equipped with a drawing tube attachment, whose field of view encompassed the active area of the digitizing tablet of a Zeiss MOP-3 digital measuring instrument interfaced to a Tektronics 4051 microcomputer. The cursor of the measuring instrument was equipped with a light which appeared superimposed over the magnified image seen through the microscope. The distances between about 300 [^{3}H]thymidine labelled cells and the muscularis mucosae were measured from each section. Frequency distribution histograms were constructed of these distances for each tissue block for each animal. Similarly, mucosal thickness was measured along each section.

The relative frequency of [^{3}H]thymidine labelled cells in S-phase was determined by superimposing a rectangular grid over the microscope field with its 200 μm wide side placed along the muscularis mucosae; all the labelled cells within the confines of the rectangle were counted. The grid was then shifted to another position along the muscularis mucosae in a random manner. Ten such measurements were made from each section from each stomach and the results were expressed as the mean number of labelled cells per 200 μm long length of muscularis mucosae in each section.

The labelling indices were also determined in a conventional manner. The labelled epithelial cells were counted in a particular gastric gland, and all the nonlabelled cells between the uppermost and lowermost labelled cells were also counted. As parietal cells were never seen labelled, they were not considered to be potentially proliferative cells and, therefore, were not counted with the nonlabelled cells. Measurements were made on 15 glands from each section.

RESULTS

Clinical observations

All the monkeys appeared healthy and were gaining weight at an average rate of 75 ± 10 g (S.E.M.) per month while they were maintained on control diet cakes. Once placed on experimental diets containing 3,4-TCB, the animals immediately began to lose weight, even though they eagerly ate the toxic diet. The one animal on the 3 ppm 3,4-TCB diet lost weight at the rapid rate of 480 g per month. He became moribund and was killed after only 53 days of toxic feeding. To slow the development of toxic signs, the other two animals, which were fed at a later date, were fed 3,4-TCB at a dietary level of only 1 ppm. At this lower level of toxicity the animals lost weight at a rate of 110 and 350 g per month and were killed when they became moribund after 97 and 55 days, respectively, of toxic feeding.

Other signs of toxicity were observed: hair loss, hyperkeratosis of the nail beds, chloracne and swelling of the eyelids with loss of the eyelashes. These changes, which were first noted after 3 weeks of toxic feeding, have been described.[6] Upon dissection, the toxic-fed animals had thickened gastric rugae with focal areas of haemorrhage. No abnormalities were noted in the three control animals.

Light microscopic findings

Hyperplasia of the gastric mucosa was very obvious in two out of three of the 3,4-TCB fed animals and was identical to that seen in monkeys fed commercial mixtures of PCBs.[6,7] The total thickness of the gastric mucosa, including submucosal cysts, was greatest in the body region, 2–4 mm, but other less striking alterations occurred in all stomach sections of all the toxic fed animals. In the cardia the gastric glands were dilated and nearly all epithelial cell types were converted to mucus-secreting cells. In the body, hyperplastic, irregular glands frequently penetrated the muscularis mucosae. Parietal cells, numerous in the control animals, were only rarely seen in the 3,4-TCB-fed animals. The gastric glands were also irregular and dilated in the antra of 3,4-TCB-fed animals and in the duodenum of one of the toxic fed animals the Brunner's glands appeared dysplastic.

Autoradiography of cells in S-phase

Control animals and animals with signs of severe chronic 3,4-TCB toxicity were injected with [^{3}H]thymidine, killed 1 h later, and autoradiographs were prepared of the gastric mucosae (Figs 1, 2). In the autoradiographs of control animals, labelled epithelial cells occurred exclusively in the lower foveolae and the neck regions of the gastric glands throughout the stomach, from the cardia to the pylorus (Fig. 1). The labelled cells were mucous neck cells in the neck region and immature surface epithelial cells in the bases of the foveolae. Parietal and zymogenic cells were not labelled. In the 3,4-TCB-fed animals (Fig. 2) labelled epithelial cells were seen throughout the gastric glands from below the muscularis mucosae in submucosal cysts, to relatively high in the foveolae, although no surface epithelial cells on the surface lining the lumen of the stomach were labelled. Some of these labelled cells were tall, cylindrical and contained large numbers of secretory granules and others were short and cuboidal with few mucus granules. In both the control and 3,4-TCB-fed animals, the labelled cells were morphologically indistinguishable from their unlabelled neighbours and were seen either in clusters or randomly dispersed among neighbouring cells.

The distance from each labelled cell to the muscularis mucosae was measured in each section taken from the cardia to the pylorus of the stomachs. Labelled cells beneath the muscularis mucosae were not counted. Frequency distribution histograms were prepared for each section which showed the distance of the labelled cells above the muscularis mucosae. In the control animals, the distances appeared normally distributed. Few labelled cells were between 50 and 100 μm above the muscularis mucosae; none were less than 50 μm above it. In contrast, in the 3,4-TCB-fed animals, many of the frequency distributions were skewed toward the base of the glands, or were very broad (platykurtic) or narrow (leptokurtic). Labelled cells were found less than 100 μm above the muscularis mucosae in significantly more sections in the 3,4-TCB-fed animals than in the controls (*t*-test, $p < 0{\cdot}01$). The median distance values appeared to be shifted downward in the 3,4-TCB-fed animals compared to the controls, but the difference was not statistically significant. The median distances were divided by the mucosal heights (Fig. 3) in order to compensate for the variation of mucosal heights, both

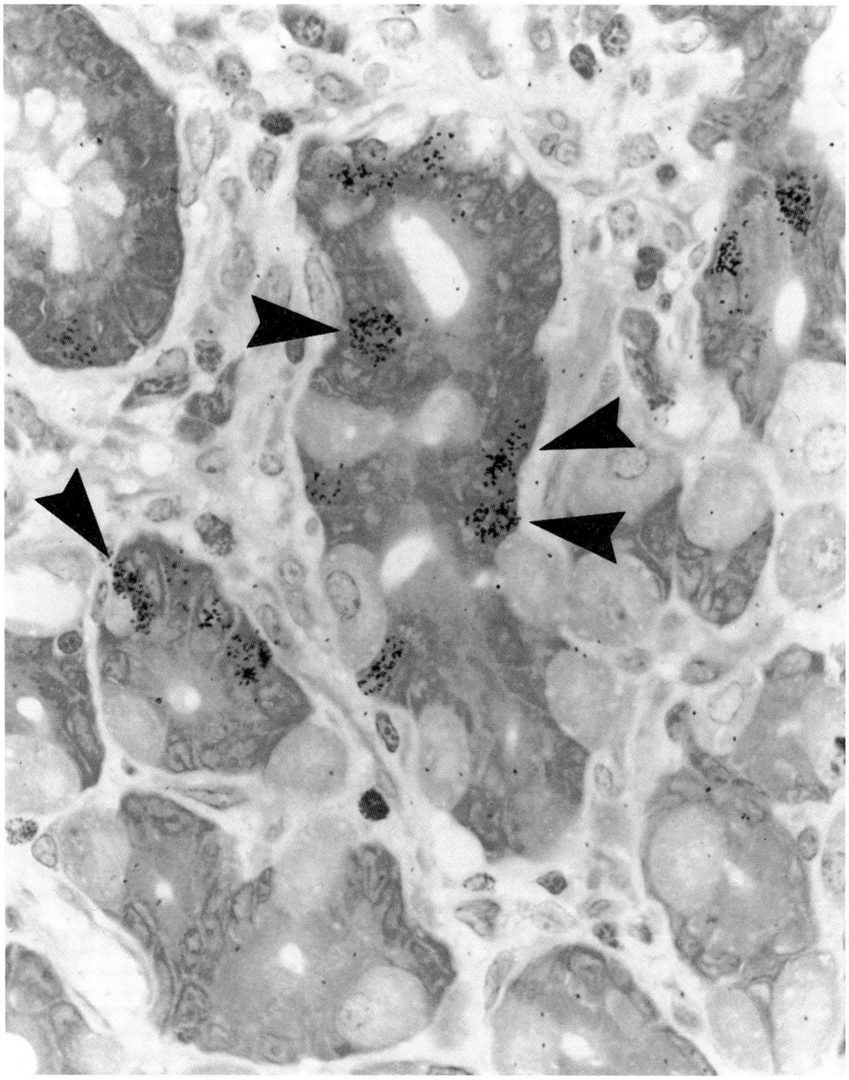

Fig. 1—Autoradiograph of the mucous neck region of gastric glands in a control animal. The animal was injected with [^{3}H]thymidine 1 h before sacrifice. Silver grains can be seen over numerous mucous neck cells. The large pale ovoid cells are parietal cells, which were not labelled. Glycol methacrylate section, 2 μm; coated with liquid photographic emulsion and exposed for 1 month before development. Stained with methylene blue and basic fuchsin. ×1000

among the controls and among the 3,4-TCB treated animals. In the controls the ratio was between 0·4 and 0·6 in most of the sections, but was significantly lower (*t*-test, $p<0.01$), only 0·15 to 0·3 in the body region of the 3,4-TCB-fed animals. This indicates that, even though the mucosal height increased in the body of the stomachs in the 3,4-TCB-fed animals, the height of the zone of proliferation did not also increase to maintain the same relative position within the glands.

The number of labelled epithelial cells per 200 μm of muscularis mucosal length for sections taken along the greater curvature is shown in Fig. 4. No increase in labelled cells was seen in the 3,4-TCB-fed animals; their numbers were even significantly less (just distal to the cardia) compared to the controls (*t*-test, $p<0.05$). In two of

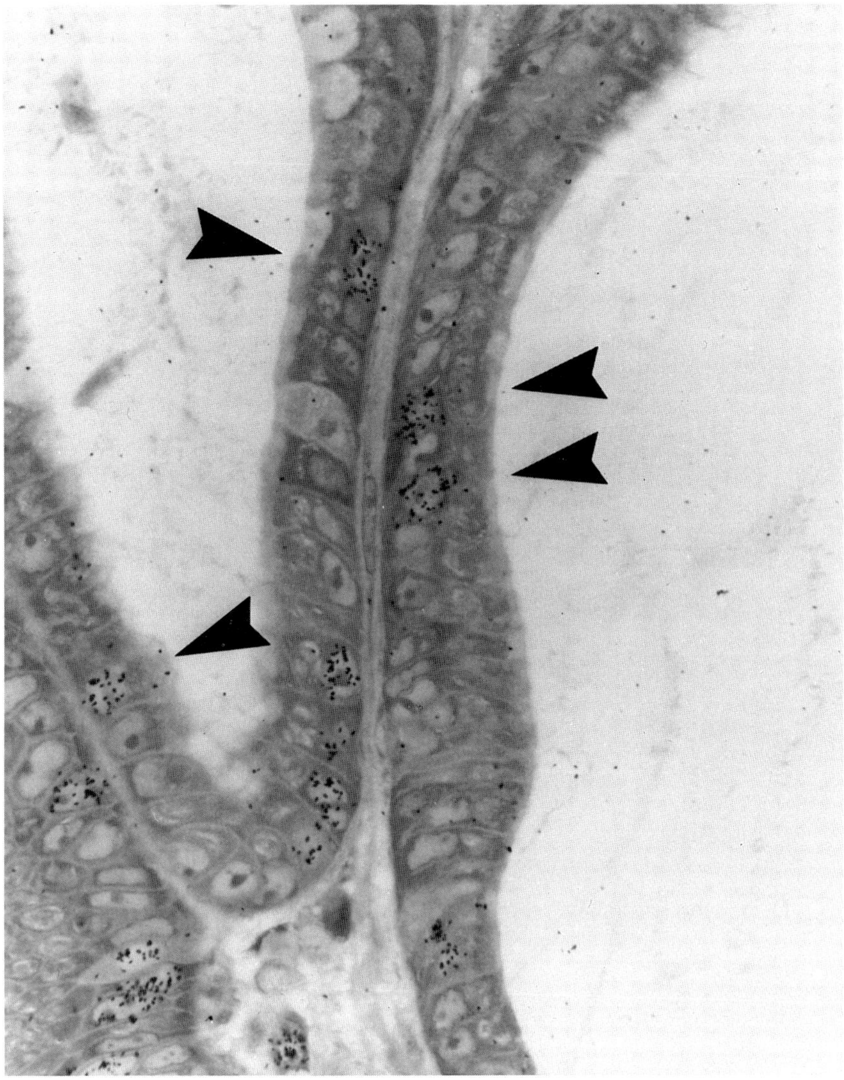

Fig. 2—Autoradiograph of the middle region of gastric glands from a monkey fed 1 ppm of 3,4-TCB for 55 days. Labelled mucus-secreting cells line the cystic, dilated glands. As in Fig. 1, the animal was injected with [^{3}H]thymidine 1 h before sacrifice. Glycol methacrylate section, 2 μm; coated with liquid photographic emulsion and exposed for 1 month before development. Stained with methylene blue and basic fuchsin. $\times$1000

three of the controls, and in two of three of the 3,4-TCB-fed animals, the relative number of labelled cells was 3- to 10-fold greater in the distal body and antral regions than in the cardiac and fundic regions. The number of labelled cells expressed per unit area in sections of mucosae showed similar relative changes, as did the labelling indices (LIs) determined conventionally.

The mean of the LIs in the ectopic cystic glands in the submucosa in the body region of the 3,4-TCB-fed animals was only 7·9 per cent $\pm$1·2 (S.E.M), significantly less (*t*-test, $p<0{\cdot}01$), than the mean of the LIs in the primary proliferative zone above the muscularis mucosae in the same animals; there the mean was 18·1 per cent $\pm$3·6 (S.E.M). It was also significantly less than the corresponding sections from the controls, for whom the mean of the LIs was 16·1 per cent $\pm$1·4 (S.E.M).

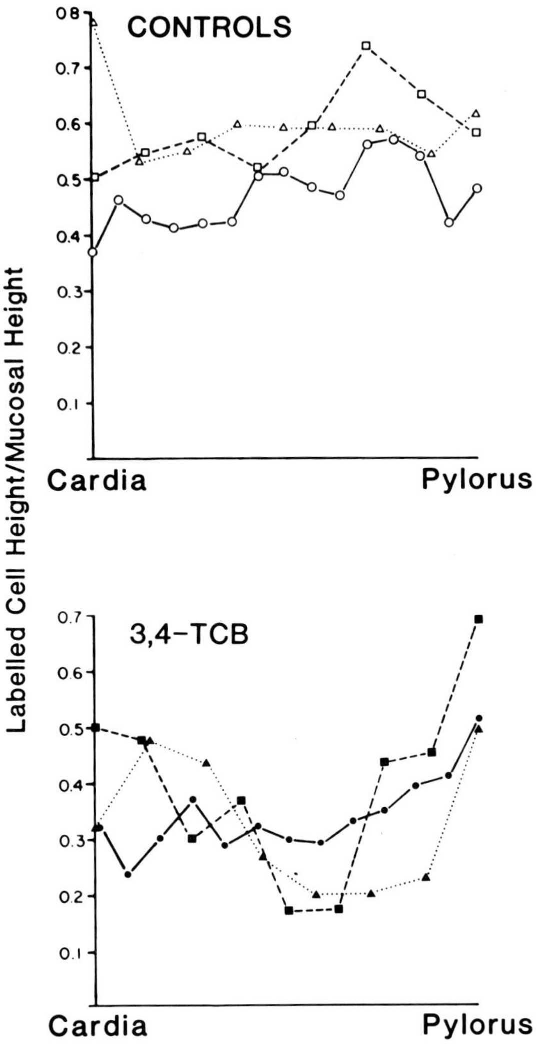

Fig. 3—Ratio of the median height of [³H]thymidine labelled gastric epithelial cells to the median gastric mucosal height (ordinate) as a function of the relative position along the greater curvature (abscissa). In the control monkeys (top graph), most of the values are between 0·4 and 0·6, but in the 3,4-TCB-fed animals (bottom graph), the ratios were significantly lower (t-test, $p<0{\cdot}01$), 0·15–0·3 in the body region of the stomachs. This indicates that, even though the mucosal height increased in the body of the stomachs in the 3,4-TCB-fed animals, the zone of proliferation did not also increase to maintain the same relative position within the glands.

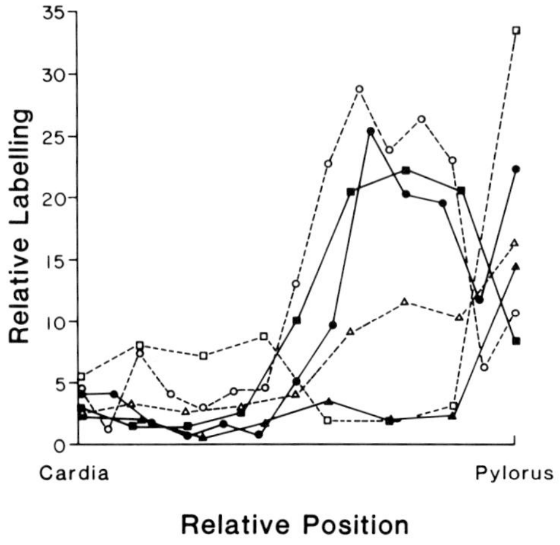

Fig. 4—Relative frequency of [³H]thymidine labelled cells, expressed as the number of labelled cells per 200 μm length of muscularis mucosae (ordinate) as a function of the relative position of the section along the greater curvature (abscissa). Each point is the mean of 10 determinations. Control animals are shown with dotted lines and open symbols, while 3,4-TCB-fed animals are shown with solid lines and symbols. The mean of the relative labelling values just distal to the cardia of the 3,4-TCB-fed animals was significantly lower (t-test, $p<0{\cdot}05$) than the mean for the corresponding region in the control animals. Notice that the relative labelling increased 3- to 10-fold progressing distally from the cardia to the pylorus in all the animals. In two of three of the controls and two of three of the toxic fed animals, the relative labelling increased sharply in the body region.

DISCUSSION

Previous studies by us[6] and others[5,7] clearly established that mixtures of PCBs and also pure 3,4-TCB,[4] when fed to monkeys at low dietary levels, induced the formation of hyperplastic, cystic gastric glands that extended beneath the muscularis mucosae to form submucosal cysts. The PCBs caused an apparent failure of cells to differentiate to zymogenic and parietal cells: only a few were seen in the bases of the gastric glands, where normally the oldest epithelial cells are found. We found that in control animals, the spatial distribution of [³H]thymidine-labelled proliferative cells approximated a normal distribution in nearly all sections of the stomach and the median position was about midway from the muscularis mucosae to the surface of the gastric mucosae. No labelled cells were seen at the base of the glands. In contrast, in 3,4-TCB-fed animals, labelled cells were frequently seen at the bases of the glands and the spatial distribution of labelled cells varied from very narrow with most of the labelled cells at or near the bases, to very broad, with labelled cells extending from the bases to the foveolae. In addition, the median position was shifted downward relative to the height of the gastric mucosae in the body of the stomach.

The development of thickened mucosae and submucosal cysts must be due to either a decrease in the rate of cell loss or an increase in the rate of cell formation, or both. Although labelled cells were found deeper in the glands in this lesion, their relative numbers as measured by labelling indices were not increased compared to the controls, and in the submucosal cysts, the labelling indices were only half the values found in the proliferative regions in the controls. One possible explanation is that the entire cell cycle of proliferating cells was shortened, including the DNA-synthesizing S-phase. If so, the rate of cell formation would be increased without an increase in the number of cells in S-phase at any given time. Alternatively, cell loss may be decreased. Non-proliferative zymogenic and parietal cells were not being formed and were replaced with mucus-secreting cells, many of which were labelled. This suggests that many or all of these mucus-secreting cells may remain in the proliferative cycle, although their rate of proliferation appears slow. Thus, normal cell ageing and loss, as occurs with the specialized zymogenic and parietal cells, may not have occurred at normal rates. Another possibility is that the rates of cell formation were indeed elevated during the development of the lesion, but declined as the animals became moribund. We cannot distinguish between these possibilities from our results. Nevertheless, labelled cells were observed in the bases of the glands in the 3,4-TCB-fed animals, but not in the controls. Therefore, it may be that cell formation was greater than cell loss in the base regions and the excess cells might have been forced through weak points in the muscularis mucosae. Submucosal glands and cysts would result from the continued proliferation of mucus-secreting cells lining these structures. Upward migration of these excess cells may be hindered, possibly by the downward migration of newly formed cells from higher in the glands. One study in hamsters[12] demonstrated that the proliferative zone of the gastric glands is firmly anchored by a stromal sheath of fibrocytes and collagen fibrils which are in contact with the basement membrane of the proliferative cells. Although we saw no clear evidence for such structures in rhesus monkeys, if present they could inhibit upward migration of cells through the mucous neck region.

Even the most irregular appearing cells were occasionally labelled with [^{3}H]thymidine, an indication that proliferation continued, even in these cells. We examined these cells by transmission electron microscopy and found the same morphologic changes we reported[6] in monkeys fed a commercial mixture of polychlorinated biphenyls, Aroclor 1242. These changes included dilated endoplasmic reticulum, irregular apices and numerous autophagic vesicles. While these changes were suggestive of cell injury and death, we never saw any evidence of an inflammatory reaction, or other signs indicative of cellular necrosis. We also did not see any evidence that the epithelial cells in this lesion penetrated the basement membrane, as reported previously,[7] rather we found that all the epithelial cells, including those in the submucosal cysts, were arranged in a single layer of columnar or cuboidal epithelium bounded by a basement membrane.

The 3,4-TCB-induced gastric lesion bears some resemblance to other gastric diseases, such as Menetrier's disease (hypertrophic gastritis) and atrophic gastritis, as we have already reported[6] in monkeys fed a commercial mixture of PCBs. The downward shift in proliferation in the 3,4-TCB-induced gastric lesion reported here is similar to the downward shift seen in *N*-methyl-*N*′-nitro-*N*-nitrosoguanidine (MNNG) induced gastric carcinoma in dogs and rodents.[13] Unlike 3,4-TCB, however, MNNG increases the labelling indices in atypical pyloric glands up to five times those of normal appearing glands.[13] while 3,4-TCB was not found to increase the labelling indices anywhere in the stomach. In addition, the MNNG-induced carcinoma has been shown to metastasize,[14,15] unlike the 3,4-TCB-induced lesion. A further difference is that the MNNG-induced changes were frequently focal, i.e. atypical glands occurred next to normal appearing glands,[13] whereas in the 3,4-TCB-induced lesion, all glands were altered.

The altered proliferation seen in the 3,4-TCB-induced gastropathy appears to be unique to this disease. This gastropathy appears to be a disturbance in the orderly process of differentiation of the several gastric cell types, encompassing either an acceleration of the proliferating cell cycle times or a lengthening of cell lifetimes or both. Since little is known about biochemical processes which govern normal differentiation in gastric mucosa, toxic chlorobiphenyls may provide a useful probe into the action, production and metabolism of such putative agents as peptide hormones, retinoids and prostaglandins.

ACKNOWLEDGEMENTS

Publication No. 1265 of the Oregon Regional Primate Research Center. Supported by grants ES-01522, RR-00163, RR-05694 and GM-07853 of the National Institutes of Health.

REFERENCES

1. Hutzinger O, Safe S, Zitko V. The Chemistry of the PCB's. Cleveland: CRC Press, 1974: 1.
2. Cordle F, Corneliussen P, Jelinek C, Hackley B, Lehman R, McLaughlin J, Rhoden R, Shapiro R. Human exposure to polychlorinated biphenyls and polybrominated biphenyls. *Environ Health Perpsect* 1978; **24:** 157.
3. Kimbrough R, Buckley J, Fishbein L, Flamm G, Kasza L, Marcus W, Shibko S, Teske R. Animal toxicology. *Environ Health Perspect* 1978; **24:** 173.
4. McNulty WP, Becker GM, Cory Helen T. Chronic toxicity of 3,4,3′,4′- and 2,5,2′,5′-tetrachlorobiphenyls in rhesus macaques. *Toxicol Appl Pharmacol* 1980; **56:** 182.
5. Allen JR. Response of the nonhuman primate to polychlorinated biphenyl exposure. *Fed Proc* 1975; **34:** 1675.
6. Becker GM, McNulty WP, Bell Mary. Polychlorinated biphenyl-induced morphologic changes in the gastric mucosa of the rhesus monkey. *Lab Invest* 1979; **40:** 373.
7. Allen JR, Norback DH. Polychlorinated biphenyl- and triphenyl-induced gastric mucosal hyperplasia in primates. *Science* 1973; **179:** 498.
8. Hansen LG, Wilson DW, Byerly CS. Effects on growing swine and sheep of two polychlorinated biphenyls. *Am J Vet Res* 1976; **37:** 1021.
9. Morgan RW, Ward JM, Hartman PE. Aroclor 1254-induced intestinal metaplasia and adenocarcinoma in the glandular stomach of F344 rats. *Cancer Res* 1981; **41:** 5052.
10. McDowell Elizabeth M, Trump BF. Histologic fixatives suitable for diagnostic light and electron microscopy. *Arch Pathol Lab Med* 1976; **100:** 405.
11. Bennett HS, Wyrick AD, Lee SW, McNeil JH. Science and art in preparing tissues embedded in plastic for light microscopy, with special reference to glycol methacrylate, glass knives and simple stains. *Stain Technol* 1976; **51:** 71.
12. Hattori T. On cell proliferation and differentiation of the fundic mucosa of the golden hamster. Fractographic study combined with microscopy and ^{3}H-thymidine autoradiography. *Cell Tiss Res* 1974; **148:** 213.
13. Deschner Eleanor E, Tamura K, Bralow SP. Sequential histopathology and cell kinetic changes in rat pyloric mucosa during gastric carcinogenesis induced by *N*-methyl-*N*′-nitro-*N*-nitrosoguanidine. *J Natl Cancer Inst* 1979; **63:** 171.
14. Sigaran MF, Con-Wong R. Production of proliferative lesions in gastric mucosa of albino mice by oral administration of *N*-methyl-*N*′-nitro-*N*-nitrosoguanidine. *Gann* 1979; **70:** 343.
15. Sugimura T, Kawachi T. Experimental stomach cancer. *Methods Cancer Res* 1973; **7:** 245.

JOURNAL OF PATHOLOGY, VOL. **143**: 275–280 (1984)

THE MONOCYTE/MACROPHAGE POPULATION OF THE NORMAL HUMAN KIDNEY

ROBERT J. MARSHALL AND ANGUS G. MACIVER

Department of Pathology, University of Southampton, South Laboratory/Pathology Block, Southampton General Hospital, Tremona Road, Southampton S09 4XY, U.K.

Received 9 March 1984
Accepted 20 March 1984

SUMMARY

There is continuing controversy over the role of mononuclear phagocytes in glomerulonephritis. It is, therefore, important to know their distribution in normal subjects. Normal kidneys (34) were assessed using three cytoplasmic markers for macrophages employing a trypsin–immunoperoxidase (PAP) technique with antibodies to α-1-antitrypsin, muramidase (lysozyme) and a further oligoclonal antibody, serum 22, developed against highly purified preparations of blood monocytes. Serum 22 detected twice as many monocytes/macrophages as anti-muramidase and four times as many as anti-α-1-antitrypsin. Most cells that showed positive staining lay in glomerular and intertubular capillaries and were considered to be blood monocytes. There was wide variation in monocyte numbers throughout different glomeruli and up to 14 monocytes could be present in a glomerulus. Not more than 1 per cent lay within the mesangium. Macrophages were virtually never seen in the interstitium, except in areas of scarring. No macrophages were present in the tubules. Monocytes and macrophages are demonstrated in greater numbers within the kidney by antisera to muramidase than to α-1-antitrypsin.

KEY WORDS—Monocyte, glomerulus, α-1-antitrypsin, muramidase.

INTRODUCTION

Mononuclear phagocytes are thought to play an important part in the pathogenesis of renal disease, particularly glomerulonephritis, tubulo-interstitial nephritis and renal allograft rejection. However, there is very little information as to the monocyte population in the normal kidney. Various cytoplasmic markers help to define monocytes within tissues, including muramidase[1] and α-1-antitrypsin.[2] Others have used an antibody to purified preparations of blood monocytes, serum 22.[3] We have investigated the distribution of monocytes/macrophages within the glomeruli, tubules and blood vessels of normal kidneys and compared their detection with the three different antisera in an immunoperoxidase technique following trypsin digestion of fixed kidney sections.

0022–3417/84/080275–06$01.00

MATERIAL AND METHODS

Blocks of normal kidney were taken from 15 autopsies and 19 nephrectomies performed for renal adenocarcinoma or nephroblastoma (Table I). Autopsy specimens came from patients aged 6–83 years, who had either died from trauma or from non-renal diseases; all had normal blood urea concentration, normal blood pressure, no evidence of proteinuria or urinary infection and had kidneys that were macroscopically and microscopically normal for age. Normal areas were sampled in four kidneys with nephroblastoma from patients aged 18 months to 8 years and in 15 kidneys with adenocarcinomas from patients aged 30–86 years. One block from each specimen was fixed in neutral buffered formalin, processed to paraffin wax and 3 μm sections examined with a trypsin–

Table I—Age and sex of patients whose kidneys were studied

	Sex	Mean age in years (range)
A. Surgical nephrectomy specimens		
(1) Nephroblastoma	2 M, 3 F	5 (1·5–8·5)
(2) Adenocarcinoma	8 M, 6 F	63 (30–86)
B. Post-mortem kidneys	1 M, 2 F	9·7 (6–14)
	2 M, 1 F	27·7 (21–36)
	4 M, 5 F	75·5 (65–83)

immunoperoxidase (PAP) technique.[4] Endogenous peroxidase was blocked by placing specimens in 0·5 per cent hydrogen peroxide in methanol for 10 min.

The following rabbit antisera were used at their respective dilutions: anti-human α-1-antitrypsin (1–500), anti-human muramidase (1–1000) and a further oligoclonal antibody (serum 22) raised against highly purified preparations of human blood monocytes,[3] used at a dilution of 1–500. A light PAS counterstain was applied to allow precise localization. Control sections omitting the first stage antibody produced no staining. Sections of lymph node and tonsil provided positive controls. In addition, a further section was examined following staining for naphthol-AS-D-chloroacetate esterase, which distinguishes neutrophil polymorphonuclear leucocytes and monocytes.

Glomeruli (30) were examined in each specimen and the number of cells counted which had been stained with each antiserum or with naphthol-AS-D-chloroacetate esterase. In each specimen, positive cells were identified as polymorphs or monocytes by their nuclear morphology, although a small proportion, 5–10 per cent, were not identified with certainty and could not be included. Peripheral total and differential white cell counts were only available for a few patients and details can, therefore, not be included. One kidney was

Table II—Mean number of monocytes detected in glomeruli and interstitium of nephrectomy and post-mortem kidneys using three different cell markers

Glomeruli

	Nephrectomy		Post-mortem kidneys	
	Mean count per glomerulus	Range	Mean count per glomerulus	Range
Alpha 1AT	1·3	0–2·5	0·4	0–1·3
Muramidase	2·6	0·2–4·8	1·6	0·1–3·3
Serum 22	4·7	0·7–6·1	3·7	1·1–8·1

Interstitium (all specimens)

	Medulla		Cortex	
	Mean count per mm^2	Range	Mean count per mm^2	Range
Alpha 1AT	2·1	0–4·3	1·2	0–2·7
Muramidase	4·6	0·4–10·4	3·3	0·4–8·0
Serum 22	8·3	0·9–16·6	6·3	1·8–13·4

perfused with normal saline until the perfusate was clear and then processed as the other specimens.

RESULTS

Glomerular cell counts

More monocytes were present in nephrectomy than post-mortem kidney specimens and the mean count per glomerulus in nephrectomy specimens was 1·3 cells with anti-α-1-antitrypsin, 2·6 cells with anti-muramidase and 4·7 cells with serum 22 (Table II and Fig. 1). In two cases, cells were counted in both left and right kidneys and their numbers were the same. α-1-Antitrypsin was even less evident in monocytes in post-mortem kidneys.

There was considerable variation between cases, as illustrated by the range shown in Table II, and the counts between glomeruli of a single case also varied greatly (Fig. 2): 0–4 with anti-α-1-antitrypsin, 0–9 with anti-muramidase, 2–23 with serum 22. There was no significant difference in monocyte numbers between males and females, nor was there significant alteration with age. No differences in glomerular macrophage counts were detected in different regions of the renal cortex.

Naphthol-AS-D-chloroacetate esterase and anti-muramidase clearly demonstrated neutrophil polymorphs within sections and up to 10 granulocytes could be counted in a single, normal glomerulus. The highest mean count was 5·3 granulocytes per glomerulus. There was a positive correlation between the numbers of neutrophil polymorphs and macrophages but slightly more polymorphs were usually present.

It was often difficult to identify accurately the exact position of a monocyte within the capillary loop or mesangium. At least 90 per cent stained cells were clearly within the lumen of the capillary but some cells lay partly in the mesangium with protrusion into the adjacent capillary. Mesangial mononuclear phagocytes were defined as cells in which a clear rim of PAS positive mesangial matrix could be identified around the whole of their periphery. Such cells were rarely detected and accounted for approximately 1 per cent glomerular mononuclear phagocytes.

Study of the perfused kidney revealed identifiable residual monocytes in glomeruli and intertubular capillaries although their number was probably reduced, being at the lower limit of the normal range. None of the antisera stained

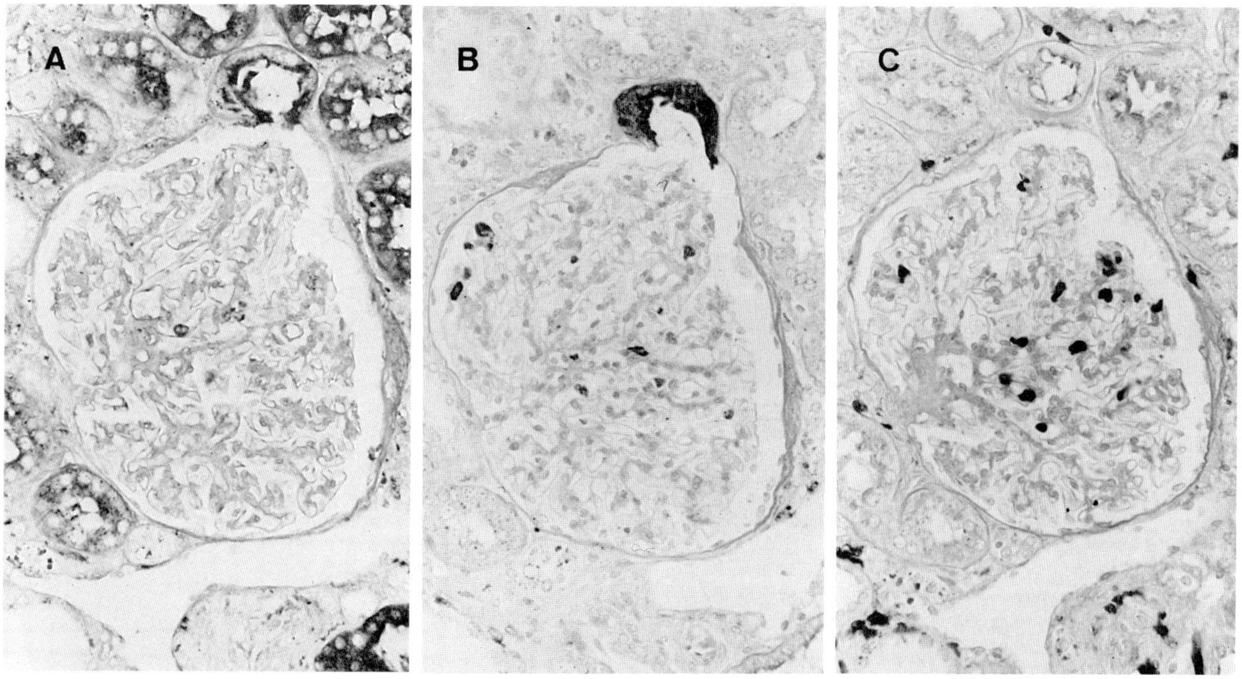

Fig. 1—Serial sections of the same glomerulus stained with (A) anti-α-1-antitrypsin, (B) anti-muramidase and (C) serum 22. Normal proximal tubules contain both α-1-antitrypsin and muramidase, acting as positive controls for the antisera. (Peroxidase–anti-peroxidase with periodic acid Schiff counterstain)

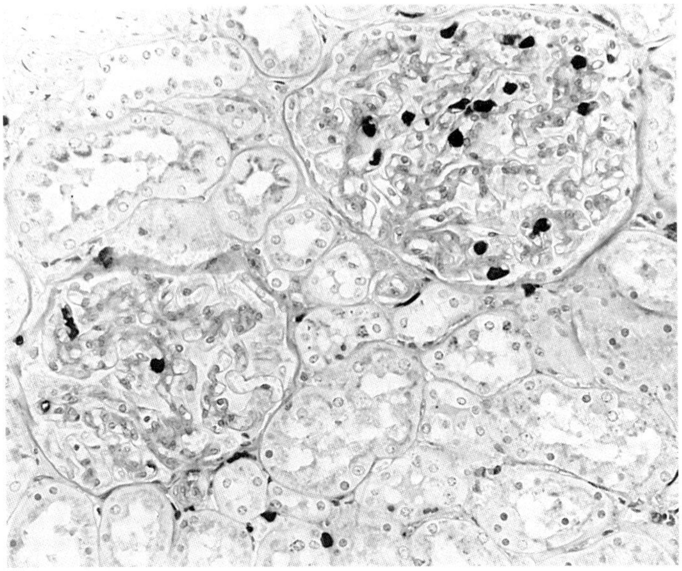

Fig. 2—Two adjacent glomeruli, one containing three, the other-15, positively staining cells. (Serum 22, peroxidase–anti-peroxidase with periodic acid Schiff counterstain)

juxtaglomerular arterioles, endothelium or visceral and parietal epithelial cells in the normal glomerulus.

Tubular and interstitial cell counts

No mononuclear phagocytes lay within the lumen of tubules nor within tubular epithelium. Anti-muramidase and serum 22 identified numerous single cells within the peritubular capillaries, particularly when they were dilated. In contrast, very few macrophages were identified within arteries, arterioles or veins. Macrophages occasionally lay in clusters but only in areas of interstitial scarring. A small number of cells lay singly in the interstitium, demonstrable by anti-muramidase and serum 22, more being present in the subcapsular area. The mean number of intracapillary and interstitial macrophages in the medulla per mm^2 was 2·1 with anti-α-1-antitrypsin, 4·6 with anti-muramidase and 8·3 with serum 22. Fewer were present in the interstitium and intracapillary position of the cortex (Table II). Nearly all (>90 per cent) cells lay within capillaries.

DISCUSSION

One of the earliest reports of monocyte involvement in glomerulonephritis was the study by Jones in 1951.[5] Subsequently, their role has been examined in more detail both in experimental[6] and human[7] glomerulonephritis and in the glomeruli of rejecting allografts.[8] Several investigators have since looked for monocytes in glomerulonephritis, using electron microscopic techniques,[6, 9–12] non-specific esterase staining of frozen sections[8, 9, 11, 13, 14] and immunoperoxidase techniques with antibodies to α-1-antitrypsin[10] or muramidase.[15]

Monocytes have also been identified in tissue cultures of normal[16, 17] and diseased[7] glomeruli and by ^{3}H-thymidine labelling of bone marrow precursors.[18] Control specimens in these studies are either not specified, not mentioned, or from biopsies with other renal abnormalities.

The mononuclear phagocyte population of the normal human kidney has never been established. Clearly such a study is required as the presence of monocytes in the normal glomerulus has been regarded as exceptional[9–11] or even denied,[8] reflecting the sensitivity of the different techniques employed.

Electron microscopy, although revealing cell structure in considerable detail, is unable to detect identifiable functional markers in non-stimulated macrophages and it is, therefore, impossible to discriminate clearly between infiltrating mononuclear cells and the native glomerular population.[9,10,19] Non-specific esterase is a recognized marker of monocytes and macrophages[20] while it is absent in normal mesangial and endothelial cells. However, it has the disadvantage of requiring frozen tissue, in which sections are thick, resolution is poor and detail obscured:[13] positive cells are said to be absent[8] or rare[9,11] in normal glomeruli. In two studies using non-specific esterase as a monocyte marker, mean counts of two or three positive cells per glomerulus were regarded as excessive.[9,11]

One study[10] has used α-1-antitrypsin as a marker for glomerular mononuclear phagocytes and a mean of 0·04 cells was reported in glomeruli. A further study,[15] using muramidase as a marker of monocyte infiltration, reported no positive cells in their control cases—two post-mortem and two-biopsy specimens with no evidence of glomerulopathy.

In our study, the mean count was 1·3 cells for surgical biopsies and 0·4 for post-mortem kidneys using anti-α-1-antitrypsin and 2·6 cells for surgical biopsies and 1·6 for post-mortem kidneys using anti-muramidase. Positive cells were always detected, even after adequate perfusion, provided at least 10 glomeruli were counted. In the examination of formalin-fixed tissue by immunoperoxidase methods, it is important that tissue sections receive adequate pre-digestion with trypsin so that cell markers can be identified.[21] Some studies of diseased kidneys have regarded the numbers of monocytes which we found in the normal kidney as being increased.[10,15] One of these studies used no trypsin pre-digestion[15] whilst the other [10] incubated the sections for only 5 min, probably an insufficient period to enhance the sensitivity of an immunoperoxidase technique. Our results show that the various markers detect different numbers of mononuclear phagocytes in the kidney and the marked increase in the detection by serum 22 suggests that different populations of mononuclear phagocytes may be present.

Most cells certainly lay within capillary lumina or were adherent to the endothelium but the exact site could not always be determined. Only about 1 per cent lay completely within the mesangium, approximately one cell in each whole normal glomerulus, 200 μm diameter. In the past, a population of mesangial macrophages has been proposed on the basis of studies of isolated, perfused rat glomeruli, from which phagocytic cells could be cultured which possessed surface Ia positive determinants as well as receptors for C3b and Fcγ.[17] Such cells were estimated to represent 1–2 per cent of the total glomerular population (5–20 cells in each whole glomerulus). The higher number in these reports may reflect a difference between species or may be the result of the very different methods used.

Since α-1-antitrypsin was first described as a marker of macrophages,[2] its use for this purpose has been enthusiastic but indiscriminate. For the identification of malignant histiocytic tumours it appears to be a most effective marker,[22] perhaps recognizing a less differentiated cell function. For normal, reactive cells, however, its effectiveness, compared with muramidase, is poor and renal tissues are much better examined using anti-muramidase or serum 22 for the detection of monocyte infiltrates. Muramidase is also a good marker of polymorph leucocytes, detecting as many as naphthol-AS-D-chloroacetate esterase. There are plentiful monocytes lying within normal renal capillaries and they are found in larger numbers than would be expected from counts of the peripheral blood. Furthermore, they remain after the intact kidney has been perfused until the perfusate is clear, suggesting that monocytes are sequestered within normal renal capillaries.

ACKNOWLEDGEMENTS

We wish to thank Dr David Jones for the supply of serum 22, the staff of the Southampton University histology laboratory and Miss Julie Foster for typing the manuscript.

REFERENCES

1. Mason DY, Taylor CR. The distribution of muramidase (lysozyme) in normal tissues. *J Clin Pathol* 1975; **28:** 124–132.
2. Isaacson P, Jones DB, Millward-Sadler GH, Judd MA, Payne S. Alpha-1-antitrypsin in human macrophages. *J Clin Pathol* 1981; **34:** 982–990.
3. Isaacson P, Jones DB. Immunohistochemical differentiation between histiocytic and lymphoid neoplasms. *Histochem J* 1983; **15:** 621–635.
4. MacIver AG, Mepham BL. Immunoperoxidase techniques in human renal biopsies. *Histopathology* 1982; **6:** 249–267.
5. Jones DB. Inflammation and repair of the glomerulus. *Amer J Path* 1951; **27:** 991–1001.
6. Kondo Y, Shigematsu H. Cellular aspects of rabbit Masugi nephritis. 1. Cell kinetics in recoverable

glomerulonephritis. *Virchows Arch (Cell Pathol)* 1972; **10:** 40–50.

7. Atkins RC, Holdsworth SR, Glasgow EF, Matthews FE. The macrophage in human rapidly progressive glomerulonephritis. *Lancet* 1976; **i:** 830–832.
8. Harry T, Bryant D, Coles GA, Davies M, Fortt W. The detection of monocytes in human renal biopsies: a prospective study. *Clin Nephrol* 1982; **18:** 29–33.
9. Hunsicker LG, Shearer TP, Plattner SB, Weisenburger D. The role of monocytes in serum sickness nephritis. *J Exp Med* 1979; **150:** 413–425.
10. Laohapand T, Cattell V, Gabriel JRT. Monocyte infiltration in human glomerulonephritis: Alpha-1-antitrypsin as a marker for mononuclear phagocytes in renal biopsies. *Clin Nephrol* 1983; **19:** 309–316.
11. Monga G, Mazzucco G, Barbiano di Belgiojoso G, Busnach G. Monocyte infiltration and glomerular hypercellularity in human acute and persistent glomerulonephritis: light and electron microscopic, immunofluorescence and histochemical investigation on 28 cases. *Lab Invest* 1981; **44:** 381–387.
12. Shigematsu H, Shishido H, Kuhara K, *et al.* Participation of monocytes in transient glomerular hypercellularity in poststreptococcal glomerulonephritis. *Virchows Arch (Cell Pathol)* 1973; **12:** 367–370.
13. Magil AB, Wadsworth LD, Loewen M. Monocytes and human renal glomerular disease. A quantitative evaluation. *Lab Invest* 1981; **44:** 27–33.
14. Monga G, Mazzucco G, Barbiano di Belgiojoso G, Busnach G. The presence and possible role of monocyte infiltration in human chronic proliferative glomerulonephritis. Light microscopic, immunofluorescence and histochemical correlations. *Am J Pathol* 1979; **94:** 271–284.
15. Jothy S, Sawka RJ. Presence of monocytes in systemic lupus erythematosus-associated glomerulonephritis. *Arch Pathol Lab Med* 1981; **105:** 590–593.
16. Camazine SM, Ryan GB, Unanue ER, Karnovsky MJ. Isolation of phagocytic cells from the rat renal glomerulus. *Lab Invest* 1976; **35:** 315–326.
17. Schreiner GF, Kiely JM, Cotran RS, Unanue ER. Characterisation of resident glomerular cells in the rat expressing Ia determinants and manifesting genetically restricted interactions with lymphocytes. *J Clin Invest* 1981; **68:** 920–931.
18. Schreiner GF, Cotran RS, Pardo V, Unanue ER. A mononuclear cell component in experimental immunological glomerulonephritis. *J Exp Med* 1978; **147:** 369–384.
19. Bradfield JWB, Cattell V. The mesangial cell in glomerulonephritis. 1. Mechanisms of hypercellularity in experimental immune complex glomerulonephritis. *Lab Invest* 1977; **36:** 481–486.
20. Yam LT, Li C-Y, Crosby WH. Cytochemical identification of monocytes and granulocytes. *Am J Clin Pathol* 1971; **55:** 283–290.
21. Mepham BL, Frater W, Mitchell BS. The use of proteolytic enzymes to improve immunoglobulin staining by the PAP technique. *Histochem J* 1979; **11:** 345–358.
22. Isaacson P, Wright DH, Jones DB. Malignant lymphoma of true histiocytic (monocyte/macrophage) origin. *Cancer* 1983; **51:** 80–91.

BOOK REVIEWS

The Reticuloendothelial System: a Comprehensive Treatise: Number 5. Cancer. Edited by R. A. HEBERMAN and H. FRIEDMAN. Plenum Press, New York and London, No. of pages: 356, illustrated. Price: U.S. $45.

Histopathologists, who spend much of their time looking at sections of malignant tumours, cannot fail to be impressed by the number of cells of the mononuclear phagocyte system which are present. On occasion, if tumours are specifically stained for macrophages, either by immunological or histochemical methods, the number of these cells appear to out-number the tumour cells. This book, which is a compilation of recent research on the interrelationships of mononuclear phagocytes and tumours, asks all the relevant questions. Not surprisingly, there are very few answers. The effect of macrophages on tumours remains unclear. They appear to affect different tumours in different animals in different ways and, in turn, to be themselves affected differently. When one adds to this the concept of macrophage heterogeneity the lack of definite answers is easily understood. The book covers almost every aspect of the relationship between macrophages and tumours including tumours of the macrophages themselves. Chapters of varying length (the longest is almost 100 pages and a book in itself) describe a multitude of experiments relating to the interaction of macrophages and tumour cells. For anyone wishing to take up the formidable challenge of this line of research this book will be indispensable, and there is also a wealth of information relating to macrophage function. It is not a book for the idly curious pathologist.

P. G. ISAACSON
University College Hospital
London

A Colour Atlas of Demonstrations in Surgical Pathology. Volume 1: The Alimentary System. ROYAL COLLEGE OF SURGEONS OF EDINBURGH. Wolfe Medical Publications, London, 1983. No. of pages: 551. Hardback. Price: £65. ISBN: 0 7234 0789 4.

For many years it was fashionable, particularly for some clinicians, to question the value of pathology museums, with their 'pots' of preserved and often pallid tissue specimens. Indeed, many American medical schools abolished their museums and tried to rely on other 'teaching materials', notably colour photographs. However, many museums have survived in this country and they remain popular not just with pathologists but with many clinicians too, especially surgeons. One of the most notable of these museums is that at the Royal College of Surgeons of Edinburgh, and this book is the first volume of a series to be produced by the College which will be based on the specimens in the College's Museum and the series of demonstration boards which have been on permanent display there for some years. With this origin, and with an editorial board consisting of 11 surgeons and one pathologst, the series will inevitably be volumes of surgical pathology. This volume is the work of a pathologist, a physiologist, a radiologist and three surgeons. The demonstrations consist not only of tissue specimens but also histological, radiological and clinical illustrations and diagrams; and the contents and format of this volume, which deals with the alimentary system, reflect this; the text is didactic, with short descriptions of the specimens (and sometimes also a short clinical history); well drawn diagrams, which make their points clearly; and x-rays, ultrasound 'scans' and endoscopy photographs. Most of the illustrations are of high quality and many still retain the Museum catalogue number. Specimens of fixed tissues predominate and, although some are outstanding, the pale brown colour of many is a serious deficiency, when compared with the vivid colours of the clinical photographs.

The numerous photomicrographs are also generally good, well reproduced and of adequate size; and it is surprising, therefore, that in a minority there is either a strong colour cast or a heavy shadow at one end of the print, as if the condenser were badly off-centre. The text also includes some terms which are now out-of-date with pathologists, and the index is too brief. Although the average size of the illustrations is relatively large, there is a lot of glossy blank white paper between them, and the result is a large heavy book, measuring 12·5 × 10·25 × 1.25 in. and weighing 6.5 lb. Still, it makes you feel that you have got something substantial in exchange for your £65. As for potential buyers, it will appeal to those lacking access to a museum and would-be surgeons (especially those studying for the Edinburgh Fellowship), but it seems unlikely to appeal to many pathologists. However, if one happens to be available, I have no doubt that pathologists in training (and their seniors) will enjoy browsing through it.

R. C. CURRAN
Medical School
Birmingham

Risk Factors in Pregnancy and Diseases of the Fetus and Newborn. RICHARD L. NAEYE and NEBIAT TAFARI. Williams and Williams, Baltimore and London, 1983. No. of pages: 361. Hardback. Price: £34. ISBN: 0 6830 6174 7.

The information presented in this book is mainly based on data acquired from the Collaborative Perinatal Project (CPP) carried out in the U.S.A. from 1959 to 1966, and from two small studies in Addis Ababa and South Africa. More than 53,000 pregnancies were prospectively documented in the CPP alone, and medical environmental and social factors have been recorded in great detail. From these and the African pregnancies a total of 2454 autopsies (post mortem rate 71 per cent) were carried out on foetuses and infants dying during an extended perinatal period. Analysis of this vast amount of data was done to identify risk factors in pregnancy which were associated with poor foetal outcome.

The information in this book is intrinsically fascinating, the authors are imaginative and confident in their approach, and the comparison of the causes of perinatal death and disease in their two very different cultures is enlightening. Unfortunately, the sheer volume of information overwhelms the readablity of the text, and there is compression at the expense of lucidity. However, due to informative chapter and section headings and a really comprehensive index, specific information and areas of interest are quickly located.

I think the information in this book is of such general academic interest to the medical and allied professions that it should be on the shelves of all medical libraries. I expect most obstetric and neonatal units will want their own copies. However, pathologists interested in the field of perinatal disease would find more practical help in the recent I.A.P. Monograph *Perinatal Diseases* of which Richard Naeye is an editor, and which is from the same publisher at a similar price.

ELIZABETH S. GRAY
University of Aberdeen

The Year Book of Pathology and Clinical Pathology. Edited by KENNETH M. BRINKHOUS. Year Book Medical Publishers, Chicago and London, 1983. No. of pages: 456. Price: £37. ISBN: 0 8151 1238 6.

This book follows the formula of 'Pathology's Greatest Hits', being a review of some 100 pathological journals. The compilers of this Year Book, the 36th in the series, are an editorial board of 27 based on the University of North Carolina. About two-thirds of the book is devoted to summaries of papers on the pathology of the various organ systems and would be of most interest to histopathologists. The remaining one-third is divided into sections on haematology, chemical pathology, microbiology and immunology with further presentations on computer applications and quality control. The aim is to cater for the entire spectrum of pathological interest.

It is clearly impossible to include in a book of this size all the significant developments in pathology during the past year. It is thus reduced to a compilation which is at best incomplete and at worst arbitrary. As a histopathologist, it was interesting to have a glimpse of recent developments in specialties such as virology or toxicology, but many of the histopathological papers selected were uninspiring, leaving one admittedly better informed but little wiser. The editors are to be praised for their efforts and the undoubted stamina required to compile such a book, surely a Herculean task. However, I believe this formula is bound to fail. A far better method is to tackle a few subjects expertly and in depth, alone the lines of the Recent Advances series. As regards investing £37, perhaps the 1982 claret . . .

A. M. ANSCOMBE
Southampton General Hospital

Histopathology of the Female Genital Tract. C. Y. GENTON. Springer-Verlag, Berlin, New York, 1983. No. of pages: 115. Soft cover. Price: U.S. $10.

This is not to be confused with *Pathology of the Female Genital Tract* from the same publishers, from which it differs in both size and content. This book is in paperback form consisting of 115 pages. For each area of the female genital tract, including placenta, there are 7 × 10 cm black and white photographs of the majority of pathological conditions that occur, with a brief description of the illustrated features. For each area 4–6 references are given and the WHO and FIGO classifications and stagings are included.

The photographs are generally clear and representative, but the nature of the paper on which they are printed has resulted in background greyness. Many of the references are out-dated and the British literature has been ignored. There is no mention of the CIN system of classification. Some areas are underrepresented, such as vulval dystrophies and endometrial hyperplasia, whilst there is undue emphasis on certain ovarian tumours.

This book may be of value to those undertaking training in gynaecology or commencing postgraduate histopathology, but a practising histopathologist would soon appreciate its limitations and turn to a more descriptive and better referenced tome, such as that mentioned above.

R. A. WALKER
University of Leicester

Malignant Lymphomas. A Pathology Annual Monograph. Edited by C. S. SUMMERS and P. P. ROSEN., 1983, No. of pages: 256. Price: $38. ISBN 0686 4747 24.

The malignant lymphomas continue to present a fascinating challenge, and it is not inappropriate that the first monograph in the Pathology Annual series should be devoted to this topic. The principal aim of this publication is not so much to provide a comprehensive review, rather to direct attention to areas of controversy and particular interest. To this end it has assembled a group of distinguished experts who present differing views and enter into lively discussion. Of particular interest is the appraisal of the National Cancer Institute Formulation which may become widely used by oncologists in future. While one can admire the spirited defence of this system, evolving knowledge regarding T-cell neoplasia is already necessitating reassessment of the classification problem. The sections dealing with histiocytic neoplasia are stimulating and should help to clarify the issues involved. Most pathologists will also welcome the excellent review of the neoplastic processes deriving from the terminal phases of B-cell differentiation. In general, this monograph is much more likely to be appreciated by experienced pathologists and lymphoma specialists rather than trainees, who might well desire a more gentle introduction to the topic. Even so, it contains a wealth of information and many excellent photomicrographs and diagrams; and it is a welcome addition to the bibliography of the subject.

F. D. LEE
Glasgow Royal Infirmary

Atlas of Colorectal Tumors. P. HERMANEK and K. KARRER, English edition by L. H. SOBIN. Butterworth Scientific, London, 1983. No. of pages: 148 (including 137 figures). Price: £35. ISBN: 4070 0340 1.

This attractive, colourful atlas covers normal bowel structure, endoscopic features, radiology, CT scanning, occult blood tests, CEA screening, surgery, epidemiology, morbid anatomy, histopathology, electron microscopy, early detection and screening methods for colorectal cancer. About half of the book is devoted to the presentation of statistical data. This is done by means of histograms, pie charts, graphs and line drawings, unfortunately often of such complexity that their impact is lost. However, there is much of interest here and I was intrigued to note that Greenland is an average risk area for colorectal carcinoma.

The illustrations of normal and morbid anatomy are very good but the photomicrographs are less satisfactory. There is a lot of space devoted to semi-micro colour and line drawings of polyps to bridge the gap between gross and histological appearances. The significance of submucosal invasion and the polyp–cancer sequence are given due weight but the presentation and discussion of epithelial dysplasia are not adequate.

The text betrays both its German origins and its American editor, but is generally accurate. Use of the terms 'scirrhous' to describe diffuse thickening of the bowel wall by carcinoma and 'circular' to mean annular are the only serious linguistic anomalies.

Both surgeons and pathologists will find the atlas of value as a ready source of up-to-date information on these important tumours and the quality of paper and of the colour plates (not, unfortunately, matched by the flimsy binding of my copy) will tempt many to purchase it for themselves.

I. C. TALBOT
Leicester Royal Infirmary

Clinical Pediatric Oncology (Third Edition). WATARU W. SUTOW, DONALD J. FERNBACH and TERESA J. VIETTI. Mosby, St. Louis and Toronto, 1984. Hardback. Price: £52. ISBN: 08016 483 43.

This book comprises 35 chapters contributed by 57 authors, all but one from North America, covering most aspects of paediatric oncology. Seventeen chapters provide a general background to the subject and cover epidemiological and aetiological aspects of childhood neoplasia, the theoretical basis of chemotherapy, uses and limitations of different investigative techniques and the role of surgery, radiotherapy and chemotherapy in the treatment of malignant disease. A chapter devoted to bone marrow transplantation includes a brief history of its development, a detailed account of graft versus host disease, the problem of infection and the current limitations of the technique. There are chapters on nursing and general care of the child with cancer both at the time of diagnosis and in the long-term, with emphasis on the team approach to total care and the needs of the whole family. A short chapter on pathology discusses differences between childhood and adult tumours and stresses the role for detailed histopathological assessment of some tumours to form a basis for rational therapy. The last general chapter is a welcome critical assessment of the long-term sequelae of cancer therapy.

The rest of the book is devoted to the presentation and management of individual tumours. Reference to tumour histopathology is made in most chapters, but in some it is very brief, in others useful textual accounts contrast with poor quality histopathology illustrations. The book does not set out to be a treatise on the histopathology of paediatric tumours but, nevertheless, contains much useful information for the pathologist who sees only occasional tumours from children. It highlights particular points for attention and is a useful source of material for case presentations and lectures, although the extensive bibliography sometimes contains few recent references. It presents a better overall view of the subject for a pathology trainee than a book on tumour pathology is likely to do.

At £52 I find it difficult to justify its place on the laboratory bookshelf of any but a very specialized unit. However, it certainly deserves a place in the library of any hospital which admits children.

J. W. Keeling
John Radcliffe Hospital
Oxford

Methods and Achievements in Experimental Pathology, Volume 11: Microanalysis and Quantification. Volume Editors: G. Jasmin and L. Proschek. S. Karger, Basel, 1984. No. of pages: vi + 109 (including 75 figures and 11 tables). Price: U.S. $98.25. ISBN: 3 8055 3717 4.

Interest in both methods and results of measurement in tissue pathology is increasing. In part this is due to demands for collaborative correlative studies with physiologists but it is also due to the advent of sophisticated electronic techniques for automating tedious counting procedures. This volume is a collection of papers on widely differing aspects of the subject. As with many multi-author volumes, both style and content are somewhat uneven. The first chapter by G. Brugal is a general essay on image analysis of microscopic preparations and provides a brave attempt at background theory for quantitative cytology. It contains introductions to concepts of measurement of shape, cell texture and colour analysis but here, as elsewhere in the book, there is a tendency to be both superficial and obscure. The last chapter on x-ray microanalysis in cytochemistry is also of a general nature. It deals in a comprehensive manner with identification and quantification of elements in cells by electron probe microanalysis. Sandwiched between these two lengthy accounts are five shorter sections dealing with practical applications of techniques which are readily available for analysis of pathological material. Computed image analysis of skeletal muscle and area estimation by manual and semi-automatic methods with special reference to myocardial infarction and breast cancer will have some immediate appeal to a practising pathologist. Of more moment perhaps are attempts in the remaining sections of the book to provide objective methods for assessing quantitative differences between normal and dysplastic tissues and cells. Of these the chapter by Herman and his colleagues describing flow cytometry points the way to more sensitive methods of diagnosing malignancy, though they do not as yet provide a definitive answer to the problem.

As U.S. $98.25 this volume of 190 pages represents a considerable outlay for the individual pathologist and, frankly, is not worth it. The natural home for this book is in the library of a well endowed university.

M. S. Dunnill
John Radcliffe Hospital
Oxford

Contemporary Issues in Surgical Pathology. Volume 3: Muscle Pathology. Edited by R. J. Heffner. Churchill Livingstone, New York, 1984. No. of pages: 235. Price: £33. ISBN: 0 443 08201 4.

This book is the third to be published in the series 'Contemporary Issues in Surgical Pathology'. Recently, there have been several large textbooks devoted to the clinical aspects of muscle disease but the objective of this book is to produce a concise account of muscle disease emphasizing the pathological approach. The book is based on the main pathological changes and the techniques that are used to evaluate them rather than a systemic classification of disease. There are 14 contributors, all from North America. The content consists of 235 pages which are arranged into 12 chapters. The opening chapter presents a clinical approach to neuromuscular disease. This is followed by a concise account of the collection and preparation of muscle biopsy specimens, a very important and often neglected step in practice. Chapter 3 presents a comprehensive account of the general reactions of muscle to injury. The following three chapters are devoted to technique; histochemistry, morphometry and fluorescence microscopy. The next section, which makes up half the book, is concerned with descriptions of the major pathological changes, namely core-genic neuromyopathies, mitochondrial myopathies, glycogen and lipid storage myopathies, systemic inflammatory myopathies and focal inflammatory diseases of muscle. The final chapter is a concise account of tumours of skeletal muscle. The book is freely illustrated and the light and electron micrographs are all of uniform high quality. The text is concise and readable. The book is aimed at the practising diagnostic pathologist and readily achieves its aim. The larger books will, no doubt, meet the specialist needs of the 'muscle men', however, the non-specialist is now being increasingly called on to interpret muscle biopsy specimens and this valuable bench book provides much useful information.

E. L. Jones
University of Birmingham

Atlas of Orthopaedic Pathology with Clinical and Radiologic Correlations, P. G. Bullough and V. J. Vigorita. Gower Medical Publishing, New York, London, 1984. No. of pages: viii + 300. Price: £49.50. ISBN: 4070 031 26.

An appropriate sub-title for this book would be Illustrated Lectures for Medical Students and Orthopaedic Surgeons. There are 14 sections dealing with normal structure, developmental anomalies and acquired disorders of formation and maintenance, injury and repair, the effects of metabolic abnormalities, haematological diseases as they affect the skeleton, the arthritides, bone and joint infections and hamartomata and neoplasms, the last chapter having a mixed bag of diseases which the authors could not include in any of the preceding categories.

The text is brief and the content is generally adequate as a basis for a lecture series, the least satisfactory section being that on injury and repair. Short bibliographies have the advantage of not overwhelming the student but suceed only if the references are well chosen. In this case there is a distinct bias to North American authors and an imbalance in the selection of the 'General Readings' which lists six books on the pathology of bone tumours but none on the arthritides. Up-to-date references are useful as a lead into the literature, but two of the 'Suggested Readings' were 'in press' at the time of printing.

Illustrations and text have been kept together. The radiographs are both well chosen and reproduced. Some of the gross specimen photographs and micrographs could be improved, the former by the elimination of highlights from the specimen surface, the latter by using the correct colour temperature. When sections have been stained by techniques other than haematoxylin and eosin, the technique has not always been stated in the caption. Some of the photomicrographs are of too low a magnification for the features described to be clearly seen.

This is not a bench book for the reporting room. It would be a very useful book for pathologist preparing lectures for medical students or orthopaedic surgeons. I would also recommend that junior histopathologists read it as an introduction to orthopaedic pathology.

C. G. Woods
Nuffield Orthopaedic Centre
Oxford

Development of the Vascular System. Ciba Foundation Symposium 100. J. Nugent and M. O'Connor (Eds). Pitman, London, 1983. No. of pages: x + 254, including 54 figures and 15 tables. Price: £25. ISBN: 0 27279732 4.

This book is composed of a series of symposium papers and the accompanying discussion. Although it covers many aspects of development of the vascular system, little emphasis is placed upon cell differentiation or pattern formation in the early stages of development; most of the symposium is devoted to morphogenesis.

The first section, which deals with development of the normal vascular system, starts with a paper on the control of embryonic heart morphogenesis. It is proposed that the extracellular matrix, synthesized by the myocardium, generates biomechanical forces which are important for cardiac morphogenesis. This is followed by an account of the growth pattern of blood vessels in the cerebral cortex and a morphological account of elastin in foetal vessels. An interesting section on structural adaptations of blood vessels to pressure is accompanied by a discussion which, at one point, centres on the problems of circulatory adaptation faced by foetal giraffes at birth and the difficulties encountered by the sea snake when held in a vertical position. The papers on vascularization of tumours discuss physical factors which influence angiogenesis and the part played by mast cells. A chapter on the role of basement membrane degradation in neovascularization is followed by a useful discussion on the whole subject of tumour angiogenesis factors. The symposium report ends with two papers, one on neovascularization of coronary intima and the other on the broad spectrum of angiogenesis defects in man.

The book is a collection of well written contributions, and the discussions following each paper and section are useful and sometimes amusing. As such, it will certainly be widely read by those specifically interested in the development of the vascular system, but it will also be of general interest to a wider audience in biological sciences and pathology.

R. O. Weller
Southampton General Hospital

Exotica: A Further Miscellany of Clinical and Pathological Experiences. William St Clair Symmers. Oxford University Press, Oxford, 1984. No. of pages: 226. Price £8·75 (clothbound). ISBN: 0 19 261225 5.

This book describes a collection of fascinating and exotic cases and might be regarded as the ultimate in histopathological one-upmanship, if the cases were not presented with such elegance and gentle humour.

I greatly enjoyed reading it. It vividly recalled to me the days of my youth when Professor Symmers and I worked in the same department. How I marvelled at his apparent effortless ability to attract the sort of cases he describes in this small volume. I still clearly remember seeing the material from his cases of thread worm granuloma, *Linguatula serrata* infestation, and *Cryptococcus neoformans* infection.

Since that time I have often wondered why I see no such cases now. Despite my occasional bursts of enthusiasm for sectioning fibrous nodules in the liver capsule not a single case of *Linguatula serrata* infestation have I found. I suspect that my failure to recognize these exotic cases is because, like most people, my daily work is diagnostic histopathology is unconsciously governed by that uninspiring old adage 'common things commonly occur'. After reading this book with its beautifully precise and elegant accounts of Professor Symmers' fascinating cases, I hope attitudes will be changed to 'uncommon things uncommonly occur, but today, if I am lucky and alert, I may encounter one'.

We cannot all hope to have a pearl pop out of the specimen and disappear down the laboratory sink (see 'He who would search for pearls must dive below', pp. 195–201) but with increased awareness of what we might be missing, at least, we might hope to increase our recognition rate of fungal infections.

I accept that orthodox documentation would have inhibited the narrative flow but we would be eternally in his debt if Professor Symmers would sometime let us into the secret of how he does it.

GERALDINE HOLMES
University of Leicester

Interpretation of Liver Biopsies, R. J. STENGER. Raven Press, New York, 1984. No. of pages: xii + 164. Price: $42.50. ISBN 0 89004 554 2.

This monograph presents a brief account of liver histopathology intended to facilitate the interpretation of human liver biopsies. Emphasis is given to clinico-pathological correlations but electron microscopy is excluded. There are 13 chapters, each concerned with one broad aspect of liver disease, such as viral hepatitis, cholestatic disorders and tumours, being preceded by three chapters which deal with the collection and processing of biopsy material and with its interpretation in general. The last of these provides a useful introduction to the subject by defining and illustrating some of the common appearances of liver damage. The book is copiously illustrated with 150 photomicrographs, 12 in colour, and all are of a very high standard. Each chapter has an adequate and up-to-date reference list.

There are now several books on liver biopsy interpretation on the market and one may wonder whether there is a need for yet one more. The main points in favour of Dr. Stenger's book are the inclusion of modern views on all important aspects of the subject, the stress on clinico-pathological correlation and the excellence of the illustrations. On the other hand, many may find it rather too concise; for example there are little more than one page of text and seven illustrations to cover the important topic of drug-induced liver injury; many uncommon, but nonetheless important, conditions are not illustrated, such as hepatoblastoma, cytomegalic inclusion disease and graft versus host disease. There are no sub-headings of disease entities and the index is rather brief. Nevertheless, the book has much to commend it as an introduction to this difficult branch of diagnostic histopathology.

R. S. PATRICK
University of Glasgow

ANNOUNCEMENTS

BENJAMIN CASTLEMAN AWARD

The Benjamin Castleman Award is sponsored jointly by the Massachusetts General Hospital and the United States–Canadian Division of the International Academy of Pathology and is financed by contributions to a fund established by former students and trainees of Dr Castleman. This award is presented at the annual meeting of the United States–Canadian Division of the International Academy of Pathology, which in 1985 will be in Toronto, 11–15 March.

This award is granted for an outstanding paper in the field of human pathology *published* in English during the calendar year 1984. The subject may represent any topic in pathology but *must* be based on human material with emphasis on morphological or anatomical approaches. On papers with multiple authorship, only one author is eligible. The Awardee must be a pathologist or pathologist-in-training who has not yet reached his 40th birthday in 1984. Papers by pathology residents, trainees and fellows are encouraged. The prize will consist of a cheque for $1000 and a certificate (travel will not be paid).

Nominations should consist of twelve (12) reprints (or preprints) of the manuscript and a letter attesting to the nominee's age, dates and places of residency training, and role in the investigation if other than the first author.

Nominations should be submitted to: United States–Canadian Division, International Academy of Pathology, 1003 Chafee Avenue, Augusta, GA 30904, U.S.A.

Deadline for receipt of nominations for the Award is 15 January 1985.

INDEX TO *JOURNAL OF PATHOLOGY* VOLUME 141

This issue of the *Journal of Pathology* contains the index material for Vol. 141 (1983) as a loose insert.

JOURNAL OF PATHOLOGY, VOL. **143**: 289 (1984)

SOCIETY SYMPOSIUM REPORT
REGULATORY PEPTIDES

At a recent symposium of the Pathological Society of Great Britain held in London at the Royal Postgraduate Medical School (R.P.M.S.) eight papers were presented on recent advances in our knowledge of regulatory peptides. Dr J. M. Polak (R.P.M.S.) set the scene by explaining that these biologically active substances are widely distributed throughout the body in typical endocrine cells and in central and peripheral nerves. They can act as classical hormones released into the circulation, as local regulators of blood flow, smooth muscle tone, glandular secretion and growth, or as neurotransmitters or neuroregulators.

In addition to the well recognized endocrine effects of excessive secretion of these substances—peptic ulceration in gastrinoma, watery diarrhoea and hypokalaemic acidosis due to tumours secreting vasoactive intestinal polypeptide (V.I.P.), etc.—S. R. Bloom (R.P.M.S.) discussed some disorders associated with deficiencies of these substances in autonomic nerves. These include two diseases with a marked deficiency of the VIPergic system: diabetic impotence and unstable bladder. VIP is known to produce vasodilation and to relax smooth muscle. A consistent reduction in nerve fibres containing somatostatin has been encountered in schizophrenic brains. These abnormalities point to chemical disorders at cellular level in all these conditions though we do not yet know how important they are in pathogenesis.

F. Cuttitta and colleagues (National Cancer Institute, Bethesda) showed that small cell lung cancers (oat cell carcinoma) not only produce bombesin-like neuropeptides but also have high affinity cell surface receptors for this substance and respond to it *in vitro* by marked enhancement of growth. G. Sorenson (Hanover, U.S.A.) showed that these cells also inappropriately express a variety of other surface receptors and transcribe the genes coding for several other regulatory polypeptides.

N. A. Wright (R.P.M.S.) used to proliferate response of the small intestine following partial resection of that organ as a model of the regulation of cell growth by peptide hormones, notably enteroglucagon and epidermal growth factor (urgogastrone), both of which appear to have trophic effects. L. D. Bell and others at Searle Laboratories described the laboratory synthesis of the human epidermal growth factor gene and the production of milligram amounts of the polypeptide by coliform bacteria with plasmids incorporating the synthetic gene. The techniques employed will almost certainly be applicable to other polypeptide hormones and their production in significant amounts will undoubtedly lead to further advances.

J. F. Jackson of Imperial College, London showed that a number of behavioural changes associated with egg laying in the marine mollusc *Aplysia* can be attributed to a set of peptides, including the egg laying hormone itself, produced in a special cell type by cleavage of a precursor polyprotein. Diverse products of a gene family in man were described by I. MacIntyre (R.P.M.S.). Thyroid C cells make two precursor proteins, the first yielding calcitonin and katacalcin while, in the second, calcitonin is replaced by C.G.R.P. (calcitonin gene related peptide). Interestingly, the latter is mainly found in central and peripheral nerves.

Thus, by combining forces, clinical practice, peptide biochemistry, molecular and cellular biology, and immunocytochemistry on normal and diseased tissues are providing and impressive picture of the profound importance of the regulatory peptides in a wide variety of physiological and pathological processes.

R. B. GOUDIE
Glasgow Royal Infirmary

Pathological Society of Great Britain and Ireland

Dutch Pathological Society

Norwegian Pathological Society

Joint Meeting, 24–25 May 1984

at

University of Bergen, Haukeland Hospital, Bergen, Norway

SYNOPSES OF PAPERS

Papers and posters presented at the meeting have not been refereed or reviewed by the *Journal of Pathology*.

These additional synopses are from the same meeting as those published in the *Journal of Pathology*, Vol. 143, No. 1, pp. A1–A6.

MORPHOMETRIC MODEL FOR ANALYSIS OF HUMAN GASTRIC BIOPSIES: FIRST RESULTS OF GRADING DYSPLASIA

B. Fringes, W. Oehlert, M. Oberholzer and A. Reith

Institute of Pathology, University of Freiburg, West Germany; Institute of Pathology, University of Basel, Switzerland; and Laboratory of Electron Microscopy and Morphometry, The Norwegian Radium Hospital, Oslo, Norway

Gastric biopsies (n=57) from 52 patients (21, 9 and 6 cases of mild, moderate and severe dysplasia, respectively, and as controls, nine cases of acute antral surface gastritis and seven patients with normal antral mucosa) were fixed in 10 per cent buffered formaldehyde, embedded in paraffin and cut perpendicular to the surface. Per HE-stained biopsy, 3–7 micrographs were taken of representative areas graded by three pathologists according to the WHO classification. In controls, isthmical and foveolar areas of the glands were micrographed. Compared to controls, the average gland area increased 2, 4 and 7 times in mild, moderate and severe dysplasia, respectively. The density of the epithelium per gland increased about 2, 3 and 6 times respectively, whereas the mean number of gland profiles decreased by 65, 69 and 82 per cent. The epithelium to interstitium ratio, being approximately 1:1 in controls, changed to 3:2 in severe dysplasia. Morphometry enables a quantitative estimate to be made of the epithelial proliferation in the different grades of dysplasia, which is considered to be a precancerous lesion.

DETERMINATION OF TOTAL NUMBER OF NUCLEI IN MOUSE UROTHELIUM

J. B. Reitan and A. Reith

Laboratory for Electron Microscopy and Morphometry, Norsk Hydro's Institute for Cancer Research, The Norwegian Radium Hospital, Oslo 3, Norway

A proper analysis of cell type distributions in cell suspensions for evaluating kinetic perturbations in tissue requires an analysis of the yield of the disaggregation method. Estimations of the number of cells in the urothelium of the mouse bladder have been in the order of 1–2 x 10^5. A morphometric model for the estimation of the number of nuclei is presented. Four inflation-fixed bladders were emptied and weighed. By systematic sampling five blocks per bladder were analysed. Micrographs of tuluidine blue stained sections were projected on a digitizing tablet. The urothelial weight was determined by assessing the percentage of urothelial area in the tissue. The number of nuclei per area, N_a, was determined and their mean caliper diameter, $\bar{D}$, was assessed by subjecting the maximal profile diameters to a Saltykov correction. By using the DeHoff and Rhines formula, $N_V = \dfrac{N_A}{\bar{D} + t}$ the number of nuclei per unit volume was determined. A total number of about 10^6 nuclei per bladder was found. This number is considerably higher than the literature values even if binuclearity is taken into account.

Pathological Society of Great Britain and Ireland

149th Meeting, 4–6 July 1984

at

The University of Leeds

SYNOPSES OF PAPERS

Papers and posters presented at the meeting have not been refereed or reviewed by the *Journal of Pathology*.

Symposium:

New Developments in Colorectal Cancer

EPIDEMIOLOGY OF COLORECTAL CANCER

R. A. Cartwright

Yorkshire Regional Cancer Organisation, Cookridge Hospital, Leeds LS16 6QB

An increasing amount is being learnt about the epidemiology of GI tract lymphomas, but this presentation will be limited to adenocarcinoma of the colorectal region. Epidemiological studies have indicated links between a wide variety of aetiological agents and increased risk of colorectal carcinoma. These range from consumption of beer to low fibre and high fat contents in the diet. However, aspects of diet cannot account for the entirety of the disease whilst there are other scattered observations which might assist in a more complete understanding of the aetiological-pathogenesis of colorectal cancer. These include, for example, aspects of inheritance, occupational studies and animal/laboratory work. In order to achieve a more complete understanding of the disease, new factors and newer epidemiological concepts are required which take into account multistage models. Analysis of the epidemiology in terms of susceptibility, initiation and promotion is discussed to highlight missing information, the limits of the epidemiological approach and the place some observations may have in the pathogenesis of the disease.

BACTERIA AND LARGE BOWEL CANCER

M. J. Hill

PHLS Centre for Applied Microbiology and Research, Salisbury, Wiltshire

Large bowel cancer has a complex etiology including genetic, hormonal and environmental (particularly dietary) factors. It has been postulated that the role of the diet in colorectal carcinogenesis is to provide substrates for the bacterial production of tumour initiators or promoters. There is a lot of evidence implicating bile acid metabolites as tumour promoters; these metabolites are produced by bacterial 7-dehydroxylase and 4-5 dehydrogenase. Recent results suggest that the bile acid metabolites are not implicated in the causation of adenomas, but cause small adenomas (with a small risk of malignancy) to grow to a large size (and with a correspondingly high malignant potential). They may also cause an increase in the severity of epithelial dysplasia in adenomatous tissues – an essential step in the dysplasia-carcinoma sequence.

EXPERIMENTAL MODELS OF COLORECTAL CANCER

M. Wells

Department of Pathology, University of Leeds, Leeds LS2 9JT

Cycasin derivates (especially dimethylhydrazine and azoxymethane) have been in use as potent inducers of intestinal tumours in rats and mice for more than twenty years. Utilising thymidine labelling experiments the rodent model of colonic cancer has made a substantial contribution to our knowledge of the relationship between cell proliferation within the crypt and the development of malignancy. Histological comparisons between animal and human tumours, however, have suffered from basic pathological misconceptions leading to the surprising failure by some workers to recognise an experimental adenoma-carcinoma sequence. Nevertheless, a proportion of animal tumours undoubtedly do arise "de novo" and such lesions are probably relevant to the pathogenesis of human cancer complicating ulcerative colitis. Information has been gained on the role of intrinsic and extrinsic factors as initiating and/or promoting factors; particularly important here are gut flora, dietary fat and their relationship to bile acids. The possible ameliorating effects of Vitamin A, bran and calcium have also been explored. Small bowel resection and jejunoileal bypass promote experimental colo-rectal carcinogenesis. This is clearly related to the adaptive hyperplasia which subsequently occurs in large bowel mucosa. In contrast, increased tumour yields following partial colectomy are confined to the anastomosis. Molecular biologists are now also focusing their attention on experimental tumours; hybridisation and sequence analysis techniques having recently demonstrated retroviral genomes in a mouse colonic neoplasm.

PROGNOSIS OF PATIENTS WITH COLORECTAL ADENOMAS

B. C. Morson

The Pathology Department of St. Mark's Hospital, City Road, London EC1V 2PS

There is now general acceptance that the colorectal adenoma is the principle precursor lesion for large bowel cancer. It occurs as a single tumour, as multiple synchronous tumours (rarely more than ten to twenty) or in the form of adenomatosis (Polyposis coli) in which the whole large bowel mucosa is covered by virtually uncountable numbers of adenomas. It is obviously desirable to obtain data about the time it takes for the adenoma-carcinoma sequence to evolve. This information has been obtained from two sources. First, a retrospective study of a large series of patients with adenomas in which it was possible to calculate the cumulative risk of developing further adenomas or cancer and second from observations on untreated patients with familial polyposis (adenomatosis). Adenoma patients are at high risk of developing further adenomas (1 in 7 at 5 yr, 1 in 3 at 10 yr and half of all patients at 15 yr). The cumulative risk of cancer is negligible at 5 yr of follow-up, about 1 in 20 at 10 yr and nearly 10% at 15 yr. The risk of cancer is greatest in patients with multiple adenomas (1 in 20 at 5 yr, 1 in 10 at 10 yr and 1 in 7 at 15 yr) and in those with "large" tumours. The magnitutde of risk reaches 100% over 35 yr in patients with untreated adenomatosis. It would appear that the evolution of the adenoma-carcinoma sequence is mostly slow being seldom less than 5 yr and on average about 10 yr but may take as much as 25 yr.

MUCIN HISTOCHEMISTRY IN PREMALIGNANT COLORECTAL EPITHELIUM

M. Isabel Filipe

Department of Pathology, Guy's Hospital Medical School, London SE1 9RT

Morphologically, epithelial dysplasia is the earliest evidence of premalignant change, and yet its interpretation has difficulties as high-lighted by the recent use of an "indefinite" category in the evaluation of epithelial dysplasia in inflammatory bowel disease. Differences in glycoprotein composition, and the demonstration of antigens or its absence in the colonic mucosa may sharpen the diagnosis of dysplasia, and help to define the "indefinite" group lesions and its natural history. Abnormal mucin patterns are observed in association with colorectal cancer. A predominance of sialomucins and decreased sulphate material, a high proportion of sialidase-labile sialic acids and decreased O-acylated derivatives characterise increasing degrees of dysplasia and malignancy. In adenomas loss of O-acylation seems to be a sensitive indicator of early malignant change. In ulcerative colitis, a significant correlation is noted between inflamed mucosa, development of cancer, presence of sialomucins and dysplasia. The co-existence of normal mucin profiles and dysplasia is uncommon. In the general population, the finding of altered mucin patterns in an otherwise normal rectal mucosa should alert the pathologist to seek an underlying pathology. Similar mucin changes are seen, albeit less common, in non-malignant conditions, by conventional histochemical methods. Lectins may increase the specificity. Lectins have shown heterogeneity of mucin carbohydrate side-chains which appear to reflect the state of cell differentiation. Peanut lectin does not bind to normal colonic epithelium, but binds avidly to mucin in carcinomas, adenomas and "transitional" mucosa, suggesting the presence of incomplete glycoproteins. Monoclonal antibodies to intestinal mucin may lead to a better understanding of colonic cell differentiation and neoplastic transformation. At present mucin profiles can provide additional criteria of malignant change in colonic biopsies and may offer a simple screening method for use on routinely processed tissues, despite its limitations.

IMMUNOHISTOLOGY OF COLORECTAL TUMOURS

Lynda G. Bobrow, Carol A. Makin and P. G. Isaacson

Department of Histopathology, University College London and The Middlesex Hospital Medical School, University Street, London WC1E 6JJ

The antigenic characteristics of tumours have been extensively studied over the past couple of decades in the search for tumour-specific markers. Several markers showed great initial promise in fulfilling this criterion, e.g. CEA (carcinoembryonic antigen) and much more recently GICA (gastrointestinal carcinoma associated) antibody, but on further study it became apparent that these were not tumour-specific. CEA is now widely used as a serological marker for clinical follow-up of patients with colorectal and other tumours. Its usefulness at the tissue level, following the development of monoclonal antibodies to various epitopes of the CEA molecule, does not appear to be altered. Currently tissue antigens and differentiation products provide a more practical perspective from which to study colorectal tumours at the tissue level. The application of a monoclonal antibody CAM 5.2 (which recognises 3 cytokeratin polypeptides) to the study of colorectal tumours will be presented. The usefulness of antibodies against secretory component, colonic mucins and HLA DR, and their relevance in the study of colorectal carcinomas, will also be discussed.

FLOW CYTOMETRY OF COLORECTAL TUMOURS

P. Quirke, J. E. D. Dyson, C. A. F. Joslin, C. C. Bird and M. F. Dixon

Department of Pathology, University of Leeds LS2 9JT

Flow cytometry using fluorescent stains allows the rapid quantitation of nucleic acid content in large numbers of single tumour cells. Colorectal tumours demonstrate a high degree of aneuploidy as assessed by the presence of non-diploid clones or the number of cells outside the normal range (>4.5C). They also vary markedly in the content of non-viable cells. Evidence is now increasing that the variation of DNA content is prognostic in these tumours and also that adenomatous polyps and mucosa from patients with long standing ulcerative colitis may also show these abnormalities. Flow cytometry may be a powerful tool in the assessment of malignant and premalignant lesions of the gastrointestinal tract.

EPITHELIAL MARKERS IN THYROID CARCINOMAS AND VARIETY OF OTHER PAPILLARY ADENOCARCINOMAS

N. W. Wilson, H. Pambakian, T. C. Richardson and Eadie Heyderman

Department of Histopathology, St. Thomas's Hospital, London SE1 7EH

Ten of each papillary, follicular, anaplastic and medullary carcinomas of the thyroid, and 5 breast, 10 ovarian, and 10 colorectal papillary carcinomas were stained for thyroglobulin, calcitonin, epithelial membrane antigen (EMA) and carcinoembryonic antigen (CEA). Affinity-purified polyclonal or monoclonal antibodies, and an indirect immunoperoxidase technique were used. All the papillary and follicular thyroid tumours, 5/10 anaplastic, and 3/10 medullary carcinomas contained thyroglobulin. One of the ten ovarian papillary carcinomas, but none of the colorectal and breast carcinomas were positive for thyroglobulin. Only the ten medullary thyroid carcinomas stained for calcitonin. 3/10 thyroid papillary, 1/10 follicular, 0/10 anaplastic, 10/10 medullary, 3/10 ovarian, and all the colorectal and breast papillary carcinomas were positive for CEA. 9/10 thyroid papillary, 7/10 follicular, 2/10 anaplastic, 3/10 medullary, and 25/25 non-thyroid papillary carcinomas were positive for EMA. The presence of calcitonin and CEA is of value in the diagnosis of medullary carcinoma, and enable its distinction from anaplastic thyroid carcinoma. Thyroglobulin is a useful marker in thyroid carcinomas. The possible reasons for its presence in one ovarian carcinoma will be discussed. EMA was present in 34/35 papillary carcinomas, but it is not a reliable marker of non-papillary thyroid carcinomas.

IMMUNOHISTOCHEMICAL STUDY OF ANAPLASTIC SMALL CELL TUMOURS OF THYROID

A. D. Burt, I. L. Brown, J. Stewart and D. J. Kerr

University Departments of Pathology and Medicine, Western Infirmary, Glasgow G11

Small cell anaplastic tumours account for 15% of all thyroid malignancies. Differentiation between those of lymphoid and those of epithelial origin is often impossible on morphological grounds but may be of therapeutic and prognostic significance. In an attempt to improve diagnostic accuracy in this respect we have examined formalin fixed paraffin embedded material from 57 anaplastic thyroid tumours and 10 well differentiated follicular and papillary thyroid carcinomas for the presence of lymphoid and epithelial markers. Detailed clinical follow up was available in 42 cases of anaplastic tumour. Sections were stained using the peroxidase-anti peroxidase technique with antibodies to common leucocyte antigen, γ_1 antichymotrypsin, epithelial membrane antigen and thyroglobulin. The use of these immunohistochemical methods has been compared with routine morphological assessment. On the basis of the correlation between histogenesis, as defined by the immunohistochemical results, and the clinical response to radiotherapy it is concluded that these antibodies represent useful diagnostic tools in the investigation of anaplastic thyroid tumours.

IN VITRO STUDY OF THYROID GROWTH AND CARCINOGENESIS

D. Wynford-Thomas, B. Stringer, P. Smith and E. D. Williams

Welsh National School of Medicine, Heath Park, Cardiff CF4 4XN

Sustained elevation of TSH induced by prolonged goitrogen treatment *in vivo* leads sequentially to (1) a marked increase in mitotic activity followed by (2) a plateau phase in which little or no growth occurs and eventually to (3) the appearance of follicular cell tumours. We have shown that the limitation of the initial phase of mitotic activity is due to a specific desensitization of the follicular cell to the mitogenic activity of TSH. To elucidate the mechanisms involved we have studied the tritiated thymidine uptake by suspension culture of reconstituted thyroid follicles obtained either from normal, plateau phase, or tumour bearing glands. Normal follicles showed a dose dependent response to TSH reaching 248±5.1% of control levels at 10 mU/ml. Repeated tests on plateau follicles showed no significant response to TSH in the same dose range. 3 tumour bearing glands have been tested so far. All showed a significant response to TSH, at 10 mU/ml 129±8.4% ($p<.02$), 146±13% ($p<.05$, and 139±6.5% ($p<.05$) respectively. The tumour bearing glands contained approximately 75% non-tumourous and 25% tumourous tissue, suggesting that the responsiveness of tumour follicles was in the same range as that of normal follicles. Our data shows (1) that the desensitization of the plateau phase cells to the mitogenic action of TSH persists *in vitro* and is therefore due to a primary change within the follicular cell itself and (2) that loss of this growth desensitizing mechanism occurs in tumour follicles. We suggest that this loss is the initial step in thyroid tumourigenesis.

TSH RECEPTORS IN EXPERIMENTAL THYROID TUMOURS

B. Jasani, B. Charnley, Y. Kajita, E. D. Williams and B. Rees-Smith

Welsh National School of Medicine, Heath Park, Cardiff CF4 4XN

Experimental thyroid tumours were produced in guinea pigs using 131-I and longterm goitrogen treatment for 20 mth. 6 of the animals were then taken off goitrogen, all were killed at 21 mth. All irradiated glands contained papillary tumours, in 3 with areas of anaplastic change. The tumours were shown to be TSH responsive for aspects of both function and growth, morphometry showed that the proportional colloid volume, 21±0.8% in animals on goitrogen, rose to 49±14% off goitrogen, and the metaphase index in animals pre-treated with vincristine was 1.1±0.8 metaphases/10^3 cells/hr in animals on goitrogen, falling to 0.01 (range 0–0.1)/10^3 cells/hr off goitrogen. TSH receptor studies were carried out by Scratchard analysis using crude membrane fractions and receptor purified 125-I bovine TSH. The binding affinities were similar in normal glands ($4.6\times10^9M^{-1}$), goitrous glands ($3.0\times10^9M^{-1}$), and tumours (mean $3.6\times10^9M^{-1}$, range 2.8 to 4.6). The binding capacity for TSH expressed as pg/mg wet weight was much higher in tumours (mean 165, range 52.7 to 280) and goitrous glands (172) than normal thyroids (25.7). However, the proportion of thyroid mass occupied by follicular cells was much greater in tumours (mean 52.7, range 40 to 65) and goitrous glands (50±2.5%) than normals (11±0.5%). When TSH binding capacity was expressed as pg/mg follicular cell weight, tumours (mean 290, range 143 to 431), goitrous glands (344) and normal thyroids (234) showed broadly similar results. We have demonstrated (i) a model for the experimental production of papillary thyroid tumours, (ii) these tumours are TSH responsive, (iii) their TSH receptor status is not significantly different from normal and goitrogen treated glands provided that allowance is made for morphological changes.

IMMUNOHISTOCHEMICAL DEFINITION OF LYMPHOCYTE SUBPOPULATIONS IN AUTOIMMUNE THYROIDITIS

Claire Smith and B. Jasani

Welsh National School of Medicine, Heath Park, Cardiff CF4 4XN

The presence of interfollicular lymphocytic infiltrate and isolated reactive lymphoid follicles and aggregates has long been recognised to constitute a pathological hallmark of autoimmune thyroiditis. With the advent of lineage specific monoclonal antibodies to lymphocyte subsets and reliable immunocytochemical techniques it has recently become feasible to analyse the functional character of these lymphocytes. Using the sensitive DNP-hapten sandwich immunoperoxidase technique in conjunction with monoclonal antibodies to primitive B-cell, Leu-3a and OKT8 markers, we have analysed the distribution of B, T-helper and T-suppressor/cytotoxic cells in thyroid tissue derived from Graves' Disease patients. Preliminary data obtained on acetone-dried frozen sections of multiple-thyroid blocks taken from the first 15 patients indicate that the interfollicular scattered lymphocyte population as opposed to that associated with the lymphoid follicles and aggregates is remarkably (>80%) rich in the T-suppressor/cytotoxic cell type with a virtual absence of B cells. The details of the staining method and the cell counting technique used will be presented. In addition the significance of the frequent and intimate apposition of predominantly T-suppressor/cytotoxic cells to the thyroid follicular cells in an immunological condition with a strong humoral component will be discussed.

ELECTRONMICROSCOPY AND IMMUNOCYTOCHEMISTRY OF DUAL POLYPEPTIDE SECRETING ENDOCRINE CELLS

G. R. Newman, B. Jasani and E. D. Williams

Welsh National School of Medicine, Heath Park, Cardiff CF4 4XN

Numerous polypeptide hormone producing cells have been described, and it has been widely assumed that one cell produces one polypeptide hormone. Immunocytochemical techniques however have shown that in a number of instances more than one polypeptide hormone is produced by the same cell – for example calcitonin and somatostatin, FSH and LH. Where electron microscope immunolocalization techniques have been used, the hormones have been localized to the same endocrine granule, although sometimes to different regions of the granule, for example glucagon and glicentin. We have demonstrated two morphologically different granules in the same cell both in normal pituitary and in abnormal pancreatic tissue, and have used serial sections and double staining at EM level to show that two separate hormones may be stored in different granules in the same cell. Some of the implications for hormone storage and production will be discussed.

PEPTIDE TYROSINE (PYY) IS CO-LOCALISED WITH GLUCAGON-RELATED IMMUNOREACTANTS IN ENDOCRINE CELLS OF GUT AND PANCREAS

A. Ali-Rachedi, I. M. Varndell, D. A. Gapp, T. E. Adrian, S. Van Noorden, S. R. Bloom and Julia M. Polak

Department of Histochemistry and Department of Medicine, Royal Postgraduate Medical School, Hammersmith Hospital, Ducane Road, London, and Department of Biology, Hamilton College, Clinton, N.Y., USA

PYY is a 36 amino acid peptide, originally reported from porcine gut, which bears striking sequence homology with members of the pancreatic polypeptide (PP) family, including NPY. For some years a PP-like immunoreactivity has been known to exist in enteroglucagon cells of the mammalian colon, although remarkably little true PP could be extracted. In order to investigate this finding, a systematic and developmental immunocytochemical study of glucagon-containing endocrine cells in the gut and pancreas has been performed using antisera to PYY, glucagon, glicentin, bovine PP and FMRFamide. Furthermore, tissue extracts have been analysed by radioimmunoassay and HPLC fractionation. In adult mammalian colon, the enteroglucagon (EG) cells have been shown to co-store (entero-) glucagon and PYY. Absorption controls have revealed that bovine PP antigen (20 nmol/ml diluted PYY antiserum) did not affect PYY immunoreactivity whereas <10 nmol PYY/ml bovine PP or FMRFamide antiserum prevents all immunostaining. No PYY immunoreactivity has been visualised in adult mammalian pancreatic A cells, whereas such a co-localisation has been observed in amphibian and reptilian pancreata. Likewise, PYY immunoreactivity has been detected by immunocytochemistry in A cells of rat foetal pancreas (14 days gestation) and also in early stages of pancreatic islet differentiation in human foetus. HPLC fractionation has revealed the PYY immunoreactivity to co-elute with natural porcine PYY marker. Large amounts of PYY (up to 129 pmol/g) were measured in 20 wk foetal human pancreas, declining to low levels at the time of birth. These findings are interpreted to confirm an earlier suggestion that colonic EG cells are ontogenetically related to pancreatic A cells.

IMMUNOPEROXIDASE STAINING IN HUMAN NERVOUS AND NEUROENDOCRINOLOGICAL TISSUES BY ANTISERA RAISED AGAINST ALDOLASES A AND C

Louise Kearns, Janice A. Royds, C. C. Rider, C. B. Taylor and W. R. Timperley

Department of Biochemistry, University of Sheffield, Sheffield, Department of Biochemistry, Royal Holloway College, University of London, Surrey and Department of Neuropathology, Royal Hallamshire Hospital, Sheffield

Aldolase is a glycolytic enzyme occurring as isoenzymes. Aldolase A occurs widely in the tissues, whereas Aldolase C is thought to be predominantly confined to the nervous system. An immunological study of the distribution of these isoenzymes was carried out using the peroxidase-immunoperoxidase technique. These studies confirm that anti-Aldolase C stains Purkinje cells very strongly; astrocytes and other neurones also stained positively but to a lesser extent. Serum raised against Aldolase A stained Purkinje cells and astrocytes strongly and other neurones weakly or not at all. Pancreatic islets, pineocytes, melanocytes within benign naevi, and isolated cells within gastrointestinal epithelium stained with anti-Aldolase C, the staining being abolished by absorbing the antiserum with purified human Aldolase C but not with Aldolase A. Studies so far have failed to show staining for Aldolase C in cardiac and skeletal muscle, liver, spleen, or pancreatic acinar cells. The staining with anti-Aldolase C was not due to cross reactivity with gamma enolase since absorption of the antiserum with gamma enolase had no effect on the staining.

ALDOLASE ISOENZYMES IN BENIGN AND MALIGNANT MELANOCYTIC LESIONS

Louise Kearns, S. Beck, Janice A. Royds, C. C. Rider, W. R. Timperley and C. B. Taylor

Department of Biochemistry, University of Sheffield, Sheffield, Department of Histopathology, Royal Hallamshire Hospital, Sheffield, Department of Biochemistry, Royal Holloway College, University of London, Surrey, and Department of Neuropathology, Royal Hallamshire Hospital, Sheffield

Aldolase is a tetrameric glycolytic enzyme with three types of subunit designated A, B and C. Aldolase C is known to be localised in brain and nervous tissue. Our own studies have, in addition, revealed the presence of Aldolase C in pancreatic islets and other APUD cells. This raises the possibility that Aldolase C, like gamma enolase may be a potential marker of cells of the APUD system and its tumours. We have therefore investigated the distribution of Aldolases A and C in 28 melanocytic lesions and in 13 other APUDomas including medullary carcinoma of the thyroid, intestinal carcinoids, and oat cell carcinoma of the bronchus, using a peroxidase-antiperoxidase technique. Melanocytes in benign naevi consistently stained strongly for Aldolase C and moderately strongly for Aldolase A. There was a marked tendency to weaker staining for both isoenzymes in malignant lesions and there was greater variation in the intensity of staining. Intestinal carcinoids and medullary carcinoma of the thyroid stained strongly for Aldolase C and moderately for Aldolase A. An occasional oat cell carcinoma stained weakly for Aldolase C but all stained negatively for Aldolase A. Aldolase C merits further study as a potential marker of tumours of the APUD system.

CHROMAGRANIN A IMMUNOCYTOCHEMISTRY: POSSIBLE CORRELATION WITH GRIMELIUS' ARGYROPHILIA

I. M. Varndell, A. E. Bishop, R. V. Lloyd, B. S. Wilson, L. Grimelius, A. G. E. Pearse and Julia M. Polak

Department of Histochemistry, Royal Postgraduate Medical School, Hammersmith Hospital, Ducane Road, London, Department of Pathology, University of Michigan Medical School, Ann Arbor, Michigan 48109, USA and Department of Pathology, University of Lund, Malmö General Hospital, S-214 01 Malmö, Sweden

In his original paper and in subsequent publications Grimelius suggested that the tissue component(s) responsible for the binding of silver ions is unlikely to be the secretory (poly)peptide product. Moreover, it has been postulated, though not proven, that argyrophilia may be attributed to a structural protein contained within certain classes of secretory granules. We have obtained results which indicate a direct correlation between argyrophilia and the presence of a structural protein – chromogranin A. Chromogranin A is a large (68,000 d) protein originally purified from bovine adrenal medulla and human pheochromocytoma. Using a monoclonal antibody to chromogranin A we have been able to demonstrate its presence in argyrophil cell secretory granules throughout the human gut and pancreas at both light and electron microscopical levels. Enterochromaffin (EC) and enteroglucagon cells of the colon and rectum are particularly immunoreactive to chromogranin A antisera. One of the most striking findings has been the localisation of chromogranin A solely to the halo of pancreatic A (glucagon-containing) cells, in direct correlation with the argyrophil reaction. No other cell type in the human pancreas has been found to exhibit chromogranin A immunoreactivity. Phaeochromocytes and calcitonin-containing cells in medullary carcinoma of the thyroid are strongly immunoreactive to applied chromogranin A antisera. Many other tumour types show a chromogranin A immunostaining pattern strikingly similar to that obtained with the argyrophilia reaction. It must be stressed that there is no proof as yet to suggest that the argyrophil reaction is totally correlated with chromogranin A immunostaining, much less that the tissue-bound reactant is the same molecule, however, the evidence does point towards an explanation for argyrophil staining.

NEUROPEPTIDE Y IN NEUROHYPOPHYSIS AND MEDIAN EMINENCE: IMMUNOCYTOCHEMICAL AND BIOCHEMICAL EVIDENCE FOR ITS PRESENCE AND ORIGIN IN THESE STRUCTURES

A. Ali-Rachedi, Y. S. Allen, J. M. Allen, S. R. Bloom and J. M. Polak

Departments of Histochemistry and Medicine, Royal Postgraduate Medical School, Hammersmith Hospital, London W12 0HS, UK

A peptide chemically related to pancreatic polypeptide (PP) has long been known to occur in rat pituitary pars nervosa. Accumulating evidence indicates that the newly identified neuropeptide Y (NPY) might be the peptide demonstrated imunocytochemically by PP antisera. By raising antisera to NPY, we report here on the occurrence and distribution of NPY-immunoreactive fibres in the neurohypophysis and median eminence of rats and guinea pigs, and on an attempt to determine their origin. NPY-immunoreactive nerve fibres were localised largely to the internal layer of the median eminence and pituitary stalk of both species, although a more diffuse distribution was observed in the rat. Several fibres were apparent in the pituitary pars nervosa, particularly in regions adjacent to the pars intermedia, although this latter region was devoid of fibres. Similarly, no immunoreactivity could be seen in the adenohypophysis (Radioimmunoassay detected values in the range 19.4–22.0 pmol/g for pars nervosa, 2.0–6.0 pmol/g for anterior pituitary). The close association of NPY-immunoreactive fibres with blood vessels in the median eminence, and a partially overlapping distribution here with catecholaminergic fibres (revealed with antibodies to tyrosine hydroxylase) suggested a largely sympathetic origin. Bilateral sympathectomy, however, and destruction of the tuberal nuclei with neonatal monosodium glutamate administration, have indicated NPY may originate dually from the hypothalamus and superior cervical ganglion. It is concluded that NPY may be an important modulator of neurohypophyseal secretion.

CHANGES IN INSULINOMA GROWTH AND PANCREATIC ISLET MORPHOLOGY DUE TO IMPLANTATION SITE

C. J. Powell, P. R. Flatt, K. Tan, C. Gray, P. Grasso and S. K. Swanston-Flatt

The Robens Institute and Department of Biochemistry, University of Surrey, Guildford

Experimental insulinomas are normally implanted subcutaneously but less than 1% of human insulinomas arise ectopically. As the site of tumour growth may significantly affect the clinical outcome the consequences of transplanting the NEDH rat insulinoma into the hepatic portal vein and pancreas were compared with a conventional subcutaneous implant. Plasma insulin levels rose and glucose levels fell most rapidly in the pancreatic transplant group. Similar, less pronounced changes developed more slowly in the hepatic transplanted group, while the subcutaneous transplant group were intermediate. Mean post-transplantation survival times were: pancreatic group 25±1, subcutaneous group 37±3, hepatic group >57 days. Four of seven hepatic transplants failed to produce a tumour at 3 mth. Tumour morphology was similar in all transplantation sites, except for one hepatic transplant which showed signs of malignancy. Pancreatic islets were atrophic with decreased insulin staining of β-cells. The islet peripheries contained pyknotic, shrunken glucagon positive α_2 cells. P.P. staining was absent or reduced, but somatostatin staining was unaffected. Additionally, some exocrine pancreatic degeneration was observed and splenic haemosiderin staining was increased. These observations were most apparent in the pancreatic transplant group and least marked in the hepatic group. Transplantation site therefore significantly affects insulinoma growth, and the subcutaneous site may not be the most appropriate for studying insulinoma development. The specific destruction of α_2 cells may be the final event which leads to death of the animal.

NESIDIOBLASTOSIS AND ISLET CELL HYPERPLASIA OF THE PANCREAS – A SECONDARY PHENOMENON – NOT A DISEASE ENTITY

W. B. Goudswaard, H. J. Houthoff, J. Koudstaal, F. T. Bosman and R. P. Zwierstra

Departments of Surgery and Pathology, University Hospital, P.O. Box 30.001, 9700 RB Groningen, The Netherlands

Ductoinsular proliferation (nesidioblastosis) and islet cell hyperplasia as a cause of organic hyperinsulinism are not yet well defined (by histometric and immunohistologic methods) in relation to the normal variablity of the pancreatic islet cell population during development and in adults. In the present study morphologic, immunohistologic (presence of insulin, glucagon, somatostatin and pancreatic polypeptide) and morphometric (endocrine volume, islet size, endocrine cell ratio's) features have been evaluated in: 1) the normal pancreas of age groups from fetal to adult (n=49); 2) nesidioblastosis (n=5); and 3) the pancreas of patients with an insulinoma (n=8). The results can be summarized and interpreted as follows: 1) for all parameters, the normal variability in all age groups was great; ductoinsular proliferation, septal islands and small islet cell groups remained present with advancing age but decreased in total numbers; 2) all parameters in the cases formerly diagnosed as pathologic nesidioblastosis were within the normal range; thus, nesidioblastosis appeared to be a pathologic non-entity; 3) prompted by this data, in 3 of these 5 cases small islet cell tumours were found during a careful second look at the pancreases; 4) in the pancreas of adults with an insulinoma, a significant islet cell hyperplasia could be demonstrated, mainly due to increased A and D cell numbers. In conclusion, nesidioblastosis is a normal feature of development and not pathologic. "Hyperplasia" – if present – is a functional and reversible feature of adaptation and in cases of organic hyperinsulinism points to the presence of an islet cell tumour.

OESTROGEN RECEPTOR STATUS OF RAT LIVER IN EVOLVING CIRRHOSIS

M. A. Parsons, V. J. M. Dangerfield, P. M. Ingleton and J. C. E. Underwood

Departments of Pathology and Zoology, The University, Sheffield

It is well established that cirrhosis may be accompanied by feminization in rats and humans. These changes in oestrogenic hormone physiology may modulate the regenerative activity of the liver and participate in the evolution of cirrhosis. Groups of three experimental intact and gonadectomised (Gdx) male and female Wistar rats received twice weekly intraperitoneal injections of 0.2 ml of 33% carbon tetrachloride (CCl_4) in arachis oil; controls received arachis oil only. After 14 weeks the livers showed extensive fibrosis and occasional cirrhosis in all CCl_4 treated rats; morphometric analysis revealed significantly less fibrosis in intact female than in Gdx female livers ($p < 0.01$). The ER concentration (fmol/mg cytosol protein) of the liver was assayed by isoelectric focusing of cryostat sections with correlative histology. The ER content of livers of CCl_4 treated Gdx females (49.6±4.0) was significantly greater than that of Gdx controls (19.6±3.9; $p < 0.01$). Livers of intact CCl_4 treated females (51.2±5.3) contained more ER than controls (25.1±8.4; $0.05 > p > 0.01$). Gonadectomy increased liver ER content of male rats, whether CCl_4 treated (17.9±3.5) or controls (13.7±2.6) compared with their intact counterparts (CCl_4 treated 3.3±1.6; control 3.0±0.5; $p<0.02$). Livers of all male rats, treated and untreated, contained significantly lower ER concentrations than CCl_4 treated females (both Gdx and intact) ($p < 0.01$). Correlations between architectural changes and ER status of the livers will be discussed.

LIVER FIBROSIS AND PITUITARY CELL HYPERPLASIA IN CARBON TETRACHLORIDE TREATED RATS

P. M. Ingleton, M. A. Parsons, J. C. E. Underwood and V. J. M. Dangerfield

Departments of Zoology and Pathology, The University, Sheffield

Because oestrogens stimulate prolactin (PRL) cell activity, and feminization often accompanies cirrhosis, we examined the pituitaries of groups of three experimental intact and gonadectomised (Gdx) male and female Wistar rats given twice weekly intraperitoneal injections of 0.2 ml of 33% carbon tetrachloride (CCl_4) in arachis oil; controls received arachis oil only. Pituitary concentrations of RIA-PRL were significantly lower in Gdx, CCl_4 treated females than in controls (1.19±0.52 v. 8.77±1.83 μg/mg, $p < 0.02$), and in both intact and Gdx, CCl_4 males compared with controls (3.84±0.64 v. 7.09±0.47 μg/mg, $p < 0.02$; 2.6±0.27 v. 5.36±0.39 μg/mg, $p < 0.02$). After 14 wk continuous treatment, despite prominent hepatic fibrosis, no differences were apparent in PRL concentrations between control and CCl_4 treated rats. Extreme changes occurred in intact females treated with CCl_4 for 14 wk then kept without treatment for a further 22 wk; in these pituitary PRL concentrations rose to 25.2±5.18 μg/mg and two of the three rats developed macroscopic hyperplasia and haematomata. PRL cells of these pituitaries were active, with abundant RER and large Golgi. Around dilated capillaries PRL cells contained only few immature secretory granules, and stained weakly for PRL. In areas remote from capillaries, PRL cells released granules into intercellular spaces. Mitoses were common and some PRL cells showed adenomatous clustering. In this study, neither male nor Gdx female rats developed similar lesions, suggesting that oestrogens may promote these changes.

MÖNCKEBERG'S MEDIAL CALCIFIC SCLEROSIS IN BREAST BIOPSIES

D. L. Ranson and J. D. Davies

Department of Pathology, University of Bristol, Bristol BS8 1TD

Mönckeberg's medial calcific sclerosis is thought to be largely confined to arteries of the limbs and genital tract. It is usually an asymptomatic condition, most cases having been discovered on routine radiological examination performed, in general, for unrelated pathology. Since July 1973 all surgically excised breast biopsies received in the University Department of Pathology at the Bristol Royal Infirmary have been routinely sliced and radiographed. During the period from July 1973 to November 1982, 2,804 breast biopsies were processed in this manner together with routine histological examination. In this study the radiological and histological appearances were reviewed for evidence of Mönckeberg's sclerosis. Nine cases showed the typical "tramline" calcification in the specimen mammogram and the characteristic microscopic medial calcification. The age range of the patients was from 35 to 89 yr, and all but two were over the age of 50 yr. The past medical history of these patients showed none of the associated medical conditions noted previously by other authors. In 7 of the 9 cases malignant breast lesions were also found in the biopsy and 4 of those were invasive ductal carcinomas. The type of calcification present in the breast arteries will be discussed with reference to Mönckeberg's original description and the findings of other authors.

USE OF ULEX EUROPEUS I AGGLUTININ AS MARKER OF ENDOTHELIUM

Rosemary A. Walker

Department of Pathology, University of Leicester, Leicester

Ulex europeus I (UEA), a lectin which binds specifically to L-fucose, has been reported to be a good marker for endothelium of human tissues, but these investigations have been restricted to frozen tissue. To establish whether the lectin could be used on routinely fixed processed tissue the binding of *UEA-peroxidase* to sections of capillary and cavernous haemangiomas, angioleimyomas, angiofibromas and angiosarcomas, selected from the routine files, has been studied. Trypsinisation has been found to be a preprequisite for staining. The endothelium of normal vessels, but not lymphatics, of capillary haemangiomas and benign tumours has a consistent positive reaction, whilst that of the larger vascular channels of cavernous haemangiomas has been more variable. The reaction in angiosarcomas has likewise varied, from 5–10% positive cells in some tumours and up to 60% in others. *UEA* can therefore be of use in the identification of vascular channels, but its value as a marker of malignant endothelium is more limited.

AXONAL PROLIFERATION IN CAROTID BODY HYPERPLASIA

P. Smith, R. Fitch and D. Heath

Department of Pathology, University of Liverpool, Liverpool

Both carotid bodies from 5 subjects free from cardiopulmonary disease were compared with those from 8 subjects with carotid body hyperplasia associated with chronic hypoxaemia or systemic hypertension. Histological sections were stained with haematoxylin and eosin or Bodian's silver protargol method to demonstrate nerves. All the hyperplastic carotid bodies showed a proliferation of elongated cells surrounding reduced cores of chief cells in each cell cluster. The elongated cells were associated with a rich network of unmyelinated nerves with smaller numbers of axons running radially towards the chief cells. Because there appeared to be more nerves in the hyperplastic organs the axonal density was measured using a Mertz semi-circle grid which, by counting the number of intercepts between axons and grid lines, provided an estimate of the total length of nerve fibres per mm^2. In the control cases the average nerve density was 12.6 mm mm^{-2}, whereas in the cases with hyperplasia it was 44.3 mm mm^{-2}, a difference which was highly significant. These findings confirm that the proliferating cells in carotid body hyperplasia are sustentacular and Schwann cells, not fibroblasts, and suggest that they develop to support an increased number of nerve axons.

NEW METHOD FOR QUANTITATING INTIMAL COMPONENT OF PULMONARY ARTERIES

June M. Fernie and D. Lamb

Institute of Occupational Medicine, Roxburgh Place, Edinburgh EH8 9SU

Quantitation of the intima of pulmonary arteries is difficult because in most disease states the changes are patchy, rarely affecting the entire circumference of an artery to a uniform extent. Also variable numbers and different size groups may be affected. The new method produced measurements of intimal area and allows artery size to be defined in terms of total length of internal elastic lamina; these measurements are unaffected by vasoconstriction. They are obtained directly from histological sections using a light microscope with a "camera lucida" attachment in conjunction with a micro-computer linked to a digitising board. The measurements produced are consistently repeatable. We considered that the extent of intimal change in a pulmonary artery was most readily understood when expressed not as an area measurement but in the form of an "Intima Index" in which intimal area is calculated as a proportion of the area enclosed by the internal elastic lamina in its theoretically unwrinkled state. Values for "Intima Index" range from >0 to $\leqslant 1$ indicating minimal through to total occlusion of the artery lumen. Relating "Intima Index" to artery size readily reveals which size of artery is most affected by intimal change and to what extent.

NEW METHOD FOR QUANTITATING MEDIAL COMPONENT OF PULMONARY ARTERIES: MEASUREMENTS AND FACTORS AFFECTING THEM

June M. Fernie, A. McLean and D. Lamb

Institute of Occupational Medicine, Roxburgh Place, Edinburgh EH8 9SU

The new method produces measurements of medial area and enables artery size to be defined in terms of total length of internal elastic lamina; these are measurements which do not vary with vasoconstriction. The measurements are obtained directly from histological sections using a light microscope with a "camera lucida" attachment in conjunction with a micro-computer linked to a digitising board. Repeatability of the measurements produced is excellent. Arteries considered "digitisable" are representative of the total muscular pulmonary artery population. We investigated the effect of several factors related to tissue preparation on the relationship between medial area and artery size. Complete distension of pulmonary arteries by an injection medium caused the internal elastic lamina to stretch by a factor of approximately 1.5. The relationship between medial area and artery size was unaffected by either the pressure/method used or lung inflation fixation or the tissue embedding medium. Tissue shrinkage was considerable with paraffin embedding and negligible with glycol ethacrylate. More arteries were considered "digitisable" in glycol methcrylate embedded tissue.

HISTOPATHOLOGY OF LARYNX FOLLOWING INTUBATION IN NEONATE

S. Gould

Department of Histopathology, University College London and The Middlesex Hospital Medical School, University Street, London WC1E 6JJ

Subglottic stenosis is a well-recognised complication of endotracheal intubation in the neonate with an incidence ranging from 2–8% of intubated infants. While often considered to be a consequence of trauma associated with prolonged intubation, the pathogenesis is poorly understood and the pathology has not been described in detail. The nature of intubation-induced injury has been investigated by examining step-sections of 43 larynges removed from neonates who had been intubated for periods ranging from 10 min to 3 mth. 17 larynges from unintubated fresh stillbirths have been used as controls. A variety of intubation-induced lesions was identified ranging in severity from simple epithelial erosions to full-thickness mucosal necrosis, perichondritis and finally destruction, with subsequent fibrosis, of arytenoid and cricoid cartilages. Although the severity of injury progressed with time, the most severe destructive injuries, including their immediate precursor lesions, developed within the first week of intubation. Prolonged intubation on its own does not appear to be an important factor in the production of severe laryngeal injury nor, therefore, the subsequent complications such as subglottic stenosis.

ARE HAEMORRHAGIC SHOCK AND ENCEPHALOPATHY (HSE) AND REYES SYNDROME (RS) CAUSED BY COMMON BACTERIAL TOXINS?

J. A. Morris, Susan Stewart and T. S. Matthews

Department of Pathology, Lancaster Moor Hospital, Lancaster, Department of Pathology, Addenbrookes Hospital, Cambridge and Department of Paediatrics, Royal Lancaster Infirmary, Lancaster

HSE is a recently recognised rare disease of infancy characterised by the acute onset of encephalopathy, fever, shock, watery diarrhoea and a bleeding tendency. Two cases of this condition are presented. One child had Staph pyogenes and the other E. coli associated nasopharyngitis. One child was only 3 wk old and was hypothermic when found. Thirty three cases are reviewed. The number of cases rises from birth to a peak at 3 mth and then falls. Heatstroke, a new virus and an environmental toxin are suggested causes but it is shown that they do not explain the data. It is proposed that common toxins produced by bacteria growing in the respiratory tract following a viral infection are a possible cause of HSE. This idea is consistent with the data and closely predicts the age distribution. Reye's syndrome is another disease of childhood in which viral respiratory tract infections predispose to an illness with a toxaemic clinical picture. A case of RS with E. coli associated nasopharyngitis is presented and it is shown that the features of RS in infancy are similar to those of HSE. A review of published cases of RS shows that the age incidence rises from birth to a peak at 4 mth followed by a progressive fall. This age distribution is a direct prediction of the common bacterial toxin hypothesis and it is difficult to reconcile with other theories of pathogenesis. The common bacterial toxin hypothesis warrants thorough investigation.

PULMONARY HISTIOCYTOSIS DUE TO AMIODARONE: HUMAN AND EXPERIMENTAL STUDY

B. Corrin, F. R. Costa-Jussa and Jean M. Jacobs

Cardiothoracic Institute, Brompton Hospital, London SW3 6HP and Institute of Neurology, Queen Square, London WC1N 3BG

Amiodarone is widely used to control cardiac dysrrhythmia and although generally quite safe there have recently appeared reports of adverse reactions in several tissues. The lungs may be affected, in which case they are generally reported as showing interstitial pneumonitis and fibrosis, but in one patient prominent foam cells were described. This paper reports such lipid pneumonia in another patient, together with comparable findings which developed in the lungs of rodents dosed with amiodarone. The changes appear to be caused by the accumulation of lamellated osmiophilic inclusions within lysosomes. The light and electron-microscopical findings are very similar to those reported in the lungs of rats treated with the tricyclic antidepressant drug iprindole and the anorectic agent chlorphentamine. These drugs are all amphiphilic in nature, i.e. they possess highly hydrophobic and hydrophilic moieties in close proximity within the same molecule. Such compounds inhibit lysosomal phospholipase and sphingomyelinase, thereby impairing normal lipid degradation.

LOCALISED BRONCHOPULMONARY AMYLOIDOSIS

P. da Costa and B. Corrin

Cardiothoracic Institute, Brompton Hospital, London SW3 6HP

Eleven patients with either localised nodular pulmonary amyloidosis or tracheobronchial amyloidosis are presented. The congophilia of the amyloid was resistant to potassium permanganate in every case, compatible with it representing immunoamyloid. This, together with the associated intense lymphocytic and plasma cell infiltration suggests a local inflammatory aetiology.

COELIAC LUNG DISEASE

C. Edwards and A. Williams

Department of Pathology, East Birmingham Hospital, Bordesley Green East, Birmingham B9 5ST

During the last decade or so there have been a number of reports of pulmonary disorders co-existing with coeliac disease. In most cases an extrinsic or intrinsic fibrosing alveolitis has been diagnosed on clinical or radiological grounds, but idiopathic pulmonary haemosiderosis and sarcoidosis have also been implicated. In a recent study of 73 patients with adult coeliac disease, 19 had physiological evidence of an interstitial lung disorder, and in 13 the respiratory problem was of sufficent severity to warrant transbronchial biopsy. In two of these patients the lung parenchyma was normal, but in the other 11 there were varying degrees of perivascular and interstitial fibrosis. Perivascular, peribronchiolar and peribronchial fibrosis was found at autopsy in a further patient with coeliac disease and lung disease. It is concluded that pulmonary fibrosis may arise as a complication of coeliac disease.

CELL CULTURES OF SMALL CELL CARCINOMA OF LUNG – VALUABLE SYSTEM FOR EVALUATION OF NEUROENDOCRINE FEATURES

D. R. Springall, P. Lackie, F. Cuttita, A. Gazdar, J. D. Minna, P. J. Marangos and Julia M. Polak

Department of Histochemistry, Royal Postgraduate Medical School, London, Regional Cell Pathology and Cytogenetic Services, Wandle Valley Hospital, Mitcham, Surrey, National Cancer Institute, Navy Oncology Branch, Bethesda, Maryland 20814, USA and Biological Psychiatry Branch, NIMH, Bethesda, Maryland 20205, USA

Small cell carcinoma of the lung (SCCL) is now believed to be neuroendocrine in nature and frequently contains immunohistochemically demonstrable neuron-specific enolase (NSE). However, regulatory peptides such as GRP (gastrin-releasing peptide – the postulated mammalian counterpart of bombesin which has part of the bombesin molecule at its C-terminus) are often only weakly immunostainable in these tumours. Cell cultures from SCCL have been used to assess the suitability of various chemotherapeutic regimens, and may provide a suitable model for pharmacological manipulations to increase intracellular peptide content (to improve immunohistochemical detection) as well as examine the role of NSE and its possible relationship to malignancy. Such a study may ultimately point correlations of these factors with tumour features such as aggressiveness and responsiveness to therapy. We have examined cells from 3 SCCL tumour lines, maintained in RPMI 1640 medium containing 10% fetal bovine serum. These were freeze dried and formalin- or p-benzoquinone-vapour fixed and wax embedded for light microscope immunohistochemistry, and glutaraldehyde fixed, resin-embedded or sectioned by cryoultramicrotomy for electron microscopy. Heterogeneity of NSE-like immunoreactivity was found in all 3 lines, and all were immunoreactive with antibodies to bombesin (which cross-reacts with GRP). After treatment of cultures with cytochalasin, the number of neurosecretory granules and immunoreactivity for regulatory peptides were increased. It is therefore suggested that cultures of SCCL are a valuable model for the investigation of immunohistochemical neuroendocrine features and permit pharmacological manipulations to facilitate intracellular detection of products which may normally be rapidly secreted.

CALCITONIN-GENE-RELATED PEPTIDE (CGRP) – A NEW REGULATORY PEPTIDE WIDELY DISTRIBUTED IN LUNG

D. R. Springall, Julia M. Polak, M. A. Ghatei, P. Lackie and S. R. Bloom

Departments of Histochemistry and Medicine, Royal Postgraduate Medical School, London, and Regional Cell Pathology and Cytogenetic Services, Wandle Valley Hospital, Mitcham, Surrey

Calcitonin-gene-related peptide (CGRP) is a regulatory peptide coded by the same gene as calcitonin. It is widely distributed in the central and peripheral nervous system of many species. Using immunohistochemical techniques on sections of benzoquinone solution – or Bouin's fluid-fixed tissue, we have examined the respiratory tract of rat (5 each of fetal days 15, 18, and 21, and 1, 7, 14, 21, 42, 63 and 84 days postnatal) for the presence of CGRP. Antibodies were raised in rabbits to whole CGRP and characterized by absorption with pure CGRP, which abolished immunoreactivity, and calcitonin, which had no effect on immunostaining. CGRP immunoreactivity was found in mucosal endocrine cells in all airways, but especially bronchioles, and in nerves surrounding trachea, bronchi, bronchioles and blood vessels. CGRP-immunoreactive nerves appeared on fetal day 21, and consistent numbers were found during development. However, CGRP-immunoreactive cells were seen earlier (fetal day 18) but their concentration decreased somewhat postnatally, in keeping with the finding of a general decrease in mucosal endocrine cells in adult respiratory tract. The nature of CGRP-containing nerves is suggested to be at least partly sensory. This is implied by their sub- and intra-epithelial localisation, the presence of CGRP in sensory neurons in nodose ganglion and the effects of surgical denervation and pharmacological manipulation (capsaicin administration) which result in depletion of pulmonary CGRP. This dual localisation of a single regulatory peptide in both endocrine cells and nerves is a novel finding for respiratory tract. CGRP is the first regulatory peptide to be found by immunohistochemistry in mucosal neuroendocrine cells of rat lung.

CALCITONIN-CONTAINING CELLS IN LUNGS OF FETAL AND NEONATAL RATS

M. C. J. Sissons, J. R. Gosney and D. Heath

Department of Pathology, University of Liverpool, Liverpool

The population of pulmonary endocrine cells containing calcitonin was studied in groups of fetal and neonatal Wistar rats ranging in age from one week of gestation to three weeks after birth. Cells containing calcitonin were identified by means of the peroxidase-antiperoxidase technique using a specific anti-calcitonin antiserum. The area of each lung section examined was measured by means of planimetry and cells immunoreactive for calcitonin were quantitatively assessed by expressing them per square centimetre of lung. Immunoreactive cells were first seen in the third week of gestation, their numbers reaching a peak 4 days prior to birth. This level was maintained at birth and for 3 weeks into the neonatal period. Cells were seen in groups (neuroepithelial bodies) and singly at all levels of the airways and alveoli. Previous studies have shown that pulmonary endocrine cells are abundant in the fetal rat and decrease dramatically in the first month of life, resulting in a view that the main function of these cells is during this early period of life. It appears that the population of cells containing calcitonin do not behave in this way.

BRONCHOPULMONARY ENDOCRINE CELLS IMMUNOREACTIVE FOR CALCITONIN IN NORMAL ADULT RAT LUNG

J. R. Gosney, M. C. J. Sissons and D. Heath

Department of Pathology, University of Liverpool, Liverpool

Bronchopulmonary endocrine cells are generally considered to be sparse in the adult rat. Most studies in this species however, have relied on silver impregnation methods as a means for their demonstration. The population of bronchopulmonary endocrine cells immunoreactive for calcitonin was studied in adult albino rats of the Wistar strain by application of the immunoperoxidase technique. A widespread distribution of strongly immunoreactive cells was revealed. These were either solitary or in corpuscular groups (neuroepithelial bodies), and were seen in both airways (particularly at points of bifurcation) and parenchyma. Whereas the majority of neuroepithelial bodies were located in bronchi and bronchioles most solitary cells were found in alveoli. Characteristically, the latter were sited on the alveolar wall immediately adjacent to an alveolar duct. Such cells immunoreactive for calcitonin almost certainly represent only a proportion of the total endocrine cell population, since the presence of other peptides such as leu-enkephalin and gastrin-releasing peptide has been demonstrated. Their function in health and role in disease is unknown.

SITE OF LYMPHOCYTE MIGRATION INTO BCG INDUCED SKIN GRANULOMATA IN RAT

A. J. Freemont

Department of Pathology, The University, Manchester M13 9PT

Lymphocyte migration from blood into mammalian lymph nodes occurs exclusively across the walls of specialised venules in the paracortex known as HEV. HEV are not restricted to lymphoid organs for identical vessels are found in sites of pathological lymphocyte accumulation in non-lymphoid tissues. Although these vessels exhibit features characteristic of HEV it is not known if lymphocytes selectively enter the tissue across their walls. This was investigated by following lymphocyte migration into cell mediated immune lesions in rats. Donor lymphocytes, obtained by thoracic duct cannulation and labelled *in vitro* with tritiated iridine were injected into syngeneic recipients intradermally inoculated with BCG vaccine 1, 2, 4 and 6 wk earlier. 15 min after injection the skin lesions and normal skin were excised and samples processed for routine microscopy, autoradiography, histochemistry and electron microscopy. Vessels identical to HEV were identified in the lesions but not normal skin. Only these vessels had radiolabelled lymphocytes in their walls and clustered about their periphery. It is concluded that vessels identical to lymph node HEV develop in areas of lymphocyte accumulation in cell mediated immune lesions in rats and are the preferred site of lymphocyte entry into the tissue.

EFFECTS OF PROSTAGLANDINS ON SECRETORY ACTIVITY IN HIGH ENDOTHELIAL CELLS OF RAT LYMPH NODES

R. W. Stoddart and A. J. Freemont

Department of Pathology, University of Manchester, Oxford Road, Manchester M13 9PT

High endothelial venules (HE venules) are the site of emigration of lymphocytes from blood to lymph nodes and are lined by secretory endothelial cells, of distinctive form. At least three secretory products are known, a sulphated glycolipid, a soluble, mucin-type glycoprotein and an insoluble glycoprotein containing N-linked saccharides. These are synthesised separately, but appear to share a common secretory pathway. *In vitro* studies using lymph node slices, radioactive sulphate sugars and quantitative autoradiography have been used to measure the effects of prostaglandins on synthesis and secretion in HE cells. 6-oxo-prostaglandin $F_1\alpha$ is a powerful and rapid inhibitor of the final stage of secretion of all products, while prostaglandins A_2, B_2, E_2, F_2 and D_2 no more than a weakly inhibitory. Synthesis of the sulphated glycolipid is slowly, but effectively, inhibited by prostaglandins E_2, F_2, and 6-oxo-$F_1\alpha$, very slowly by D_2 and is almost unaffected by A_2 and B_2. There are, therefore, two routes by which prostaglandins may affect HE cells and these have different chemical specificity. These findings suggest that the macrophages often found near HE venules might have regulatory influences.

IMMUNOHISTOCHEMICAL LOCALISATION OF FACTOR VIII-RELATED ANTIGEN IN HODGKIN'S DISEASE

J. Crocker and P. Smith

Histopathology Department, East Birmingham Hospital, Birmingham B9 5ST

The unlabelled antibody peroxidase-antiperoxidase technique for factor VIII-related antigen (FVIII RAg) has been applied to 45 lymph nodes involved by Hodgkin's disease (HD). Ten lymph nodes showing follicular hyperplasia and sinus histiocytosis were also studied. In nodular sclerosing HD, many blood vessels were present, as shown by virtue of FVIII RAg in endothelial cells. The relatively dense vasculature was present around and within HD nodules in this Rye subtype and was observed even in the cellular variant. The other 3 main subtypes of HD exhibited a paucity of blood vessels but there was striking vascularity in the hyperplastic nodes.

IMMUNOCYTOCHEMISTRY OF MONOCYTES GROWING IN HUMAN BONE MARROW CULTURE – CLUE TO ORIGIN OF LANGERHANS AND INTERDIGITATING RETICULUM CELLS

Pramila Goordyal and P. G. Isaacson

Department of Histopathology, University College London and The Middlesex Hospital Medical School, University Street, London WC1E 6JJ

Langerhans cells (LC) and interdigitating reticulum cells (IDRC) are morphologically similar cells thought to play an important role in the immune response as antigen-presenting cells. They share certain distinctive phenotypic properties, including strong HLA DR positivity and reactivity with monoclonal antibodies to the T-cell antigen T6. Animal studies suggest that these cells are derived from the bone marrow but their relationship to the mononuclear phagocyte system is controversial. Cytospin preparations of single monocyte colonies grown from normal human bone marrow were made and stained by the immunoperoxidase technique for a variety of antigens including lysozyme, alpha-1 antitrypsin, HLA DR and T6. Erythroid colonies were used as controls. Nearly all the monocytes contained lysozyme and alpha-1 antitrypsin but, significantly, a few cells in each monocyte colony stained for HLA DR and T6. Cells from erythroid colonies were uniformly negative for all antigens studied. These results provide direct evidence that LC and IDRC are derived from monocyte stem cells and therefore should be regarded as belonging to the mononuclear phagocyte system.

CHARACTERISATION OF INDUCER ACCESSORY CELLS FROM HUMAN TONSILS

B. McDowell, Andrea T. Cifelli, D. R. Katz and Julia D. Nunn

Bland-Sutton Institute of Pathology, Middlesex Hospital Medical School, London W1P 7PN

In murine systems, a distinct cell type known as the dendritic cell has been characterised by structure, phenotype and function. Those cells are probably important inducers of immune responses in lymphomedullary tissues. In human systems, a similar cell type has been identified from peripheral blood and other fluids, but a similar tissue cell has not been characterised previously *in vitro*. Using density gradient analysis, we have purified low density cell populations from human tonsil, and examined their properties using both morphologic and functional methods. These cells express HLA-D surface antigens, but lack FcR receptors and common T cell membrane markers, and show negligible proliferation in the presence of standard T cell mitogens. In functional assays, these cells can induce certain types of T cell proliferation. The features suggest that these cells are the human equivalent of the murine dendritic cell.

RETINOID EFFECTS ON MURINE PERIPHERAL LYMPHOID ORGANS

Maria Drzymala, Andrea T. Cifelli, R. Marian Hicks, D. R. Katz and J. Turton

Bland-Sutton Institute of Pathology, Middlesex Hospital Medical School, Mortimer Street, London W1P 7PN

Vitamin A acetate and Vitamin A analogues such as 13-cis-retinoic acid have been studied extensively to identify their anti-neoplastic effect. There is evidence to suggest that this effect is mediated by an immunological mechanism. A feature of mice fed diets containing these compounds is that they have enlarged lymphomedullary organs. We examined these tissues by histology at 12 wk to identify whether the enlargement was selective. There was expansion of the paracortical region, with virtually no reactive follicles recognisable. We have now examined these tissues at 4 and 7 wk to monitor the development of this selective enlargement. We have also used functional assays to show that these compounds influence accessory cell-T cell interaction. A feature of this system is that irrespective of whether the site of action is mediated via accessory cell or T cell, these compounds produce a striking increase in the number of dendritic cells which can be isolated from these organs.

STRUCTURE AND FUNCTION OF DIFFERENTIATED LEUKAEMIC CELLS

Julia D. Nunn, Andrea T. Cifelli, L. J. Fraher, G. N. Hendy, D. R. Katz and B. McDowell

Bland-Sutton Institute of Pathology and Department of Medicine, Middlesex Hospital Medical School, London W1P 7PN

The human promyelocytic cell line, HL-60, has been used as a model system for the differentiation of precursor cells into monocytes/macrophages and granulocytes. If dendritic cells and other accessory cell types are also derived from these cells, then an HL-60 differentiation pathway to generate these cells should be identifiable *in vitro*. The particular differentiation pathway we are investigating used Vitamin D_3 metabolites as inducers. This pathway is associated with decreased expression of the c-*myc* oncogene. We have shown that we can inhibit proliferation of HL-60 in a dose dependent fashion and that this is a property of D_3 metabolites hydroxylated at the C-1 site only. We are now using modulated HL-60 cells to examine whether a dendritic cell form can be identified. These questions are being monitored by (1) electron microscopy, (2) HLA-DR surface expression and (3) ability to induce alloproliferative responses.

IMMUNOHISTOCHEMICAL LOCALISATION OF LEUCOCYTE ELASTASE

J. Crocker, Rachel Jenkins and D. Burnett

Histopathology Department, East Birmingham Hospital, Birmingham B9 5ST and University Department of Immunology and The General Hospital, Birmingham

A polyclonal antiserum has been produced in sheep and is reactive against purified human leucocyte elastase. This has been applied to paraffin sections of human tissues, using the indirect immunoperoxidase method. Striking and consistent results were obtained, normal or inflammatory granulocytes being intensely positive. The reaction was "blocked" by pure elastase and activity was not observed in other cells or tissues, including histiocytic reticulum and lymphoid cells, although a weak reaction was present in gastric and ileal lining epithelium. Strong reactivity was also observed in the cells of acute and chronic myeloid leukaemia and in the granulocytes of extramedullary haemopoiesis. The technique is compared with those for the demonstration muramidase ("lysozyme"), α_1-antitrypsin and naphthol-AS-D-chloroacetate esterase.

ANALYSIS OF HUMAN LYMPHOID CELL LINE AND CHRONIC LYMPHOCYTIC LEUKAEMIA SURFACE MEMBRANE GLYCOPROTEINS

G. P. O'Connor, C. C. Bird, F. A. Lewis and P. F. Goodchild

Department of Pathology, University of Leeds, LS2 9JT

Our study of lymphoid tumour cell surface membrane glycoproteins has been extended to include a large number of human lymphoid cell lines and lymphocytes isolated from fresh blood of chronic lymphocytic leukaemia (CLL) patients. Cell surface membrane glycoproteins were labelled with I^{125}, the membranes purified and after solubilisation were electrophoresed on SDS-gradient polyacrylamide gels. After drying the gels were autoradiographed and the X-ray plates developed. Molecular weights for each band present on the autoradiographs have been calculated and compared for each cell line examined. The reproducibility of this method was confirmed by repeating the same procedure three times for each cell line tested. In a parallel study purified lymphocyte suspensions prepared from the cell lines and CLL patients were simultaneously analysed to determine their cell surface immunophenotype. Cell suspensions were incubated with appropriate dilutions of FITC labelled F $(ab')_2$ goat or burro antisera against human individual heavy or light chains or monoclonal antibodies against T-cell subset antigens. The results of attempts to correlate the glycoprotein and surface membrane phenotypes will be presented.

LECTIN HISTOCHEMISTRY OF REACTIVE TONSILLAR LYMPHOID TISSUE

J. C. Macartney and Deborah Blythe

Department of Histopathology, St. Thomas's Hospital Medical School, London

Lectins which bind selectively to saccharide residues on cell membrane and cytoplasmic glycoconjugates have been used to investigate carbohydrate expression in normal and neoplastic lymphoid tissue and as markers for subpopulations of lymphoreticular cells. Because of discrepancies in published histochemical accounts, in this study the binding of six peroxidase-labelled lectins to tissue sections of reactive human tonsillar lymphoid tissue has been examined. Binding to frozen sections has been compared with fixed embedded tissue and the effects of neuraminidase and trypsin treatment of sections investigated. Using frozen sections, with some lectins there was substantial masking of cell surface labelling by sialic acid whereas other lectins were unaffected. After neuraminidase treatment of frozen sections none of the lectins examined showed selective binding to distinct subpopulations of lymphoid cells but bound to lymphocytes and macrophages in all tonsillar compartments. After fixation, reduction or abolition of staining by all lectins was encountered. This often resulted in spurious "specific" residual staining of macrophage cytoplasm. The histochemical use of labelled lectins to identify specific lymphoreticular cell subtypes in tissue sections appears to be of doubtful validity unless frozen sections are used and the effects of neuraminidase digestion considered.

IMMUNOHISTOLOGICAL ASSESSMENT OF CUTANEOUS MANIFESTATIONS OF CHRONIC LYMPHOCYTIC LEUKAEMIA

I. Lauder, R. Greenwood, L. Parapia, M. Reid and C. C. Bird

Department of Pathology, University of Leeds; Dermatology Department, Scunthorpe General Hospital; Haematology Department, Bradford Royal Infirmary; and Pathology Department, Bradford Royal Infirmary

A series of 25 cases of immunologically proven B-cell chronic lymphocytic leukaemia were examined for evidence of cutaneous lesions. Six cases had evidence of some form of dermatosis which was usually some form of erythema. Histological assessment of fixed paraffin embedded tissue showed perivascular lymphocytic infiltrates in all cases together with more diffuse areas in most of the cases. The infiltrates were confined to the upper and mid-dermis but epidermotropism was not a prominent feature. Because of the unequivocal clinical diagnosis of chronic lymphocytic leukaemia the initial histopathological diagnosis in all cases was that the changes were considered to be suspicious of cutaneous involvement by CLL. Immunohistological studies were performed on cryostat sections from one half of the original biopsy using a range of monoclonal antibodies having both T- and B-cell specificities. In all of the cases the infiltrate was found to be exclusively of T-cell origin (UCTH1+, T11+, T6−, Ia−). The T-cells included a mixture of T_4 and T_8 cells with a ratio varying between 3 : 1 and 15 : 1. Scattered amongst the T-cells was a smaller population of Ia+, T6+ interdigitating reticulum cells. One of the six cases developed evidence of an acute leukaemia and the marker studies in a series of biopsies showed an increasing population of lysosyme positive cells indicating a myeloid or myelomonocytic origin.

DISTRIBUTION OF CYTOKERATIN-POSITIVE CELLS IN INVOLUTING HUMAN THYMUS

L. Henry and G. Anderson

Departments of Pathology, University of Sheffield Medical School and Royal Hallamshire Hospital, Beech Hill Road, Sheffield S10 2RX

The structural changes during involution of the human thymus have been established using conventional staining techniques. To supplement this information 62 thymuses have been examined with a monoclonal antibody against cytokeratin. The ages of the patients ranged from 19 wk gestation to 65 yr. The distribution of cytokeratin-positive cells will be demonstrated and related to the stage of involution.

FIBRONECTIN LOCALISATION IN NORMAL AND PATHOLOGICAL HAEMATOPOIETIC TISSUE

J. T. Reilly, J. R. G. Nash, M. J. Mackie and B. A. McVerry

Departments of Haematology and Pathology, Royal Liverpool Hospital, Prescot Street, Liverpool L7 8XP

Cryostat sections of bone marrow biopsies were stained immunoenzymatically for fibronectin using the alkaline phosphatase: anti alkaline phosphatase (APAAP) technique. In normal marrow fibronectin was present only in megakaryocytes and the walls of blood vessels. Sinusoids did not demonstrate fibronectin and there was no interstitial staining. In contrast myelofibrotic bone marrow possessed an extensive distribution of fibronectin but this did not correspond to the distribution of reticulin. Infiltrated and hypercellular marrows showed an increase in fibronectin which appeared to be related to increased marrow vacularity. Again no correlation with the reticulin pattern was evident. Myeloma and amyloid biopsies showed a background 'blush' of fibronectin which appeared to be associated with interstitial protein deposition. In contrast to platelets, other circulating blood cells, namely erythrocytes, neutorophils, eosinophils, basophils, lymphocytes, monocytes, lymphoblasts, prolymphocytes and promyelocytes had no demonstrable fibronectin. This study suggests that fibronectin does not act as a mediator of haemopoiesis *in vivo* as has been suggested by the results of experiments in non human models.

CONCOMITANT IMMUNOHISTOCHEMICAL LOCALIZATION OF FIBRONECTIN AND COLLAGEN IN SCHISTOSOMAL GRANULOMATA

M. S. Al Adnani

Department of Pathology, Faculty of Medicine, Kuwait University, P.O. Box 24923, Safat, Kuwait

Affinity purified antibodies to human collagen type 1 and III as well as antihuman fibronectin were employed immunohistochemically on formalin fixed, paraffin embedded human schistosomial granulomatous lesions. The distribution of the three connective tissue proteins was studied in 45 biopsies (30 due to Schistosomal haematobium and 15 due to Schistosomal mansoni). The granulomata were divided into early, intermediate and late according to the proportion of inflammatory cell types and the degree of fibrous tissue deposition. Only fibronectin was detected in the early granuloma where macrophages which are known to produce fibronectin, are the main cell type present. In the intermediate granuloma both fibronectin and collagen type III were localized along the fibers which also were positive by silver reticulin stain. Spindle cells (fibroblasts) and macrophages were the cell types at this stage. Collagen type I was mainly localized in the late granuloma. The hyalinized tissues were negative for the three proteins. The loose connective tissue and wall of blood vessels were constantly positive for fibronectin and collagen type III. The importance of the sequential appearance of these connective tissue proteins in the pathogenesis of various fibrotic conditions will be discussed.

DIFFERENTIAL PROTEOLYSIS AND STRUCTURAL ORGANISATION OF ELASTIC FIBRES

J. D. Davies, Faye Lovett and S. L. Mera

University Department of Pathology, Bristol Royal Infirmary, Bristol BS2 8HW

Preliminary proteolysis of tissue sections is often used to enhance immunoreactivity in routine histopathological practice. Its effects are variable, and depend upon the proteolytic enzyme used and the tissue antigen sought. We report the enzymic effects of crude and DPCC – purified trypsins, chymotrypsin, papain, bromelain, elastase, and pepsin on elastic fibres. Diminution of elastic-fibre dye staining was produced by all these proteases with the exception of DPCC-purified trypsin and chymotrypsin. The effects of preliminary proteolysis upon the immunostaining of elastic-fibre components (α-elastin, serum amyloid P component, lysozyme, and the protease inhibitors α-1 antitrypsin, α-1 antichymotrypsin and α-2 macroglobulin) were variable. The proteolytic enzymes were capable of grouping into three broad categories with differing substrate activity. The differential digestive loss and immunological exposure of the elastic-fibre components appears to be related to the structural organisation of elastic fibres in their mature and nascent forms. The study provides some evidence that within the elastin core of elastic fibrils there may also be a background matrix of glycoprotein to which are bound lysozyme and amyloid P component.

GESTATION RELATED DETECTION OF TISSUE AMYLOID P IN NORMAL HUMAN PLACENTA

A. M. Khan and F. Walker

Department of Pathology, University of Leicester, Leicester

The pentameric glycoprotein Amyloid P (AP) is normally present in human adult connective tissues but is not present in the fetus. It has been shown to be an age related glycoprotein in human skin and may be related to dermal maturation. It was decided to study AP distribution in placenta as this organ undergoes marked maturation changes and is very closely associated with the fetus. This was done by using a direct immunofluorescence technique on frozen sections of placenta from obstetric specimens of varying gestation. AP was not detected in the first trimester placenta but was invariably localised in the peri-fetal capillary zone of the chorionic villi by the third trimester. These results demonstrate that AP is age-related in the placenta and it is suggested that it may be important in the maturation of the fetal capillaries.

UNEXPECTED INORGANIC ELEMENTS IN ORAL LESIONS: RESULTS OF X-RAY ENERGY SPECTROSCOPY (XES) ON PARTICULATE MATTER IN PARAFFIN SECTIONS

D. A. Levison, P. R. Crocker, G. Lee, N. A. Shepherd and A. P. Smith

Department of Histopathology, St. Bartholomew's Hospital, London EC1A 7BE

X-ray energy spectroscopy (XES) of all particulate matter found by light microscopy in histological sections of 222 oral lesions revealed a much wider range of elements than expected from dental amalgam. Subsequent XES of a variety of endodontic materials, impression materials and toothpastes indicated possible sources for virtually all elements identified in the histopathological lesions. The range of materials identified is tabulated; histopathological lesions and probable source substances are correlated; light microscopic pointers to the elemental nature of particulate matter in sections are indicated – titanium and bismuth have characteristic appearances; possible implications of local implantation and large scale ingestion of such substances are discussed.

RESORPTIVE BEHAVIOUR IN OSTEOCLASTS IS INITIATED BY CONTACT WITH BONE MINERAL

T. J. Chambers, B. M. Thomson and Karen Fuller

Department of Histopathology, St. Bartholomew's Hospital, London EC1A 7BE

The susceptibility of several types of bony substrate to osteoclastic resorption *in vitro* was assessed. Slices of inorganic bone showed extensive tracts of uninterrupted surface excavation after incubation, while untreated bone slices tended to show discontinuous excavations of smaller total volume; demineralised bone slices were not resorbed. The endosteal surface of adult rat calvaria was also used as a substrate: the endosteum was rendered acellular and used either without further treatment or after incubation with osteoblasts or collagenase. Untreated, the endosteal surface consisted of the unmineralised fibres of the lamina limitans; incubation of calvaria with osteoblasts or collagenase resulted in loss of these fibres, to reveal the subjacent mineral front of the bone. Osteoclasts resorbed bone only from calvaria pre-treated with collagenase or osteoblasts. These experiments imply that osteoclastic contact with bone mineral is the stimulus which initiates bone resorptive behaviour in osteoclasts. One mechanism which could account for the increased osteoclastic bone resorption frequently observed in bone affected by inflammatory and neoplastic diseases is increased exposure of mineral, either through an effect on osteoblasts or through proteolytic digestion of the lamina limitans by the pathological tissue itself.

AGING OF HUMAN SKELETAL MUSCLE: EFFECT ON FIBRE SIZE, VARIABILITY, AND FIBRE TYPE CONSTITUTION

Patricia Harnden-Mayor and D. G. F. Harriman

Department of Pathology, University of Leeds, Leeds LS2 0JT

Seventy-two healthy, unaffected siblings of malignant hyperthermia-susceptible (MHS) patients were included in this study, 40 females (age range 40–74 yr) and 32 males (age range 40–65 yr) using biopsies of the same muscle (vastus medialis) in every case. The lesser diameters of fibre types 1, 2a and 2b were measured using a computer-aided image analyzer and the relative proportions of the different fibre types were calculated. The measurements for fibre types 2a and 2b were subsequently pooled by the computer to give overall results for type 2 fibres. The results for each fibre type were given as the mean fibre diameter with standard deviation and as a histogram of the distribution of fibre diameters. There was an unexpected difference in the effects of aging on males and females. The female population showed a reduction in the percentage of type 1 fibres, a decrease in fibre size and an increase in fibre size variability with advancing age, whereas in the male population there was a reduction in the percentage of type 2 fibres, with no significant decrease in fibre size or increase in fibre variability.

ALZHEIMER'S PRESENILE DEMENTIA, SENILE DEMENTIA OF ALZHEIMER TYPE AND DOWN'S SYNDROME IN MIDDLE AGE ALL FORM AN AGE RELATED CONTINUUM OF PATHOLOGICAL CHANGES

D. M. A. Mann, P. O. Yates and B. Marcyniuk

Department of Pathology, University of Manchester, Manchester M13 9PT

A loss of nerve cells from the nucleus basalis of Meynert and the locus caeruleus, averaging 70% and 60% respectively, and a reduction in nucleolar volume of 30% in surviving cells of both types, was measured in 22 patients with Alzheimer's disease (who ranged in age from 48–92 yr) when compared with 20 mentally preserved patients of similar age range. The severity of these changes was not, however, homogeneous within the Alzheimer's disease group; younger patients showed a greater cell loss and reduction in nucleolar volume as well as a greater frequency of senile plaques and neurofibrillary tangles than older patients in whom the level of change approached that in old age alone. There were only slight differences in extent of cell loss from and reduction in nucleolar volume in nucleus basalis and locus caeruleus in 6 patients over 50 yr of age with Down's syndrome (who also showed extensive plaque and tangle formation in cerebral cortex) when compared with 6 of the Alzheimer's disease patients of equivalent age. It is calculated that presenile Alzheimer's disease, senile dementia of Alzheimer type and Down's syndrome in middle age all form an age-related continuum of pathological changes.

SUBCHRONIC (90 DAYS) STUDIES USING MULTIPLE DOSE LEVELS OF TRI-ORTHO-CRESYL PHOSPHATE (TOCP): SOME NEUROPATHOLOGICAL OBSERVATIONS IN THE DOMESTIC HEN

S. K. Majeed and D. E. Prentice

Huntingdon Research Centre plc, Huntingdon, Cambridgeshire PE18 6ES

Heavy hybrid hens were dosed orally with TOCP "Tri-ortho-cresyl phosphate" for 90 days at levels of 1.0, 1.25, 2.5, 5.0, 7.5, 10.0 and 20.0 mg/kg/day. Adequate controls were present. The main purpose of the study was to compare the histological results with clinical ataxia findings. The results show that birds receiving 5.0 mg/kg/day or greater of TOCP developed clinical ataxia. Taking into account clinical and pathological findings and survival rates, 7.5 mg/kg/day was deemed to be the optimum dosage of TOCP for a positive control in 90-day neurotoxicity studies. Pathological investigations proved to be more sensitive than clinical investigations, i.e. clinically the 'no-effect' level was 2.5 mg/kg/day of TOCP, while histologically it was 1.25 mg/kg/day of TOCP.

BIOPSY SEMINAR – MUSCLE DISEASE

D. G. F. Harriman

Department of Pathology, University of Leeds, Leeds LS2 9JT

Human muscle biopsies illustrating common and rarer muscle disorders will be available for study throughout the meeting. During this session the principal features of these cases will be illustrated.

Guest Lecture

ULTRASTRUCTURAL PATHOLOGY

T. S. Beals

University of Michigan, Ann Arbor, Michigan

Applications of electron microscopy in diagnostic cytology.

ULTRASTRUCTURAL CASE SEMINAR

P. G. Toner

Department of Pathology, Royal Infirmary, Glasgow G4 0SF

A series of cases where ultrastructural analysis has contributed to the diagnosis will be presented. These will be available for study during the meeting.

IMMUNOELECTRON MICROSCOPY USING MONOCLONAL ANTIBODIES AND IMMUNOGOLD IN TISSUE SECTIONS

N. Rooney, C. A. Day and T. Gray

Department of Pathology, University of Sheffield Medical School, Sheffield S10 2RX

A method of immunostaining for electron microscopy on tissue sections is described. In general the use of monoclonal antibodies requires frozen sections of fresh tissue. Unfortunately this leads to poor cytological detail at EM. Prior fixation with glutaraldehyde preserves cytology but reduces immunostaining. Our method uses an initial fixation for 1 hr in 0.5% glutaraldehyde followed by passage through increasing concentrations of glucose before freezing. 20μ frozen sections are cut and primary and secondary immunostaining is done on glass slides. The sections are processed for electron microscopy on the slide using inverted embedding capsules. After polymerisation the capsules and sections are snapped away from the slide and the relevant area examined on the electron microscope. Using this method surface antigens can be specifically localised and interactions between identifiable cell types studied.

LIGHT, FLUORESCENCE AND ELECTRON MICROSCOPY STUDY OF POST-MORTEM CHANGES IN RAT KIDNEY TUBULES

I. E. El Shennawy, D. J. Gee and S. R. Aparicio

Department of Forensic Medicine and University Department of Pathology, St. James's Hospital, Leeds

Although post-mortem changes in the kidney are a common phenomenon in autopsy practice, their interpretation frequently creates difficulties for pathologists in making a clear distinction between changes occurring after death and pathological phenomena such as tubular necrosis. No previous systematic study of post-mortem changes of kidney left *in-situ* has been done. We studied the renal tubular alterations in rats at varying intervals after death using TEM, SEM and a newly developed fluorescent technique using aniline blue. It was found that pronounced differences exist in post-mortem behaviour between cortex, cortico-medullary junction and medulla. There are also significant differences between proximal, distal and collecting tubules. The results of this study will be described in detail. Correlation of the variations of the tubular changes in different regions of the kidney may form a basis for fairly accurate timing of death. The physiological implications of the phenomena observed may help in the understanding of the pathogenesis of tubular necrosis.

EPITHELIAL MEMBRANE ANTIGEN IN KIDNEY AND ITS TUMOURS

S. Fleming, G. B. M. Lindop and A. A. M. Gibson

University Department of Pathology, Western Infirmary, Glasgow and Pathology Department, Royal Hospital for Sick Children, Glasgow

Epithelial membrane antigen (EMA) localised by immunoperoxidase techniques is a useful marker of epithelial differentiation. Using a polyclonal anti-EMA antiserum and the PAP technique EMA distribution in the kidney during embryogenesis and in some renal tumours has been studied. We have examined 12 foetal and 10 adult kidneys and found EMA to be present on the distal tubule and collecting duct apithelium but absent from the proximal tubule and glomerular epithelium. EMA first appears during nephrogenesis at the S-shaped tubule stage where it is present on the distal tubular precursor. EMA is not seen on primitive proximal tubule or glomerular epithelium. Using the same techniques 33 primary renal carcinomas, 4 renal adenomas and 3 renal sarcomas were examined. 31/33 renal carcinomas and all of the adenomas expressed EMA while none of the sarcomas did. The renal carcinomas negative for EMA were both of the sarcomatoid variety. Renal carcinomas have previously been regarded as tumours of the proximal tubular epithelium but here we have shown that they express an antigen apparently confined, in the normal foetal and adult kidney, to distal tubular and collecting duct epithelium. The presumed histogenesis of renal carcinoma may therefore be incorrect.

RETROSPECTIVE STUDY OF HISTOLOGICAL FEATURES OF REJECTION IN RENAL HOMOGRAFTS AND COMPARISON WITH CIRCULATING T-CELL POPULATIONS

J. Wyatt, P. Guillou and S. R. Aparicio

University Departments of Pathology and Surgery, St. James's Hospital, Leeds

The early detection of rejection episodes in renal transplant patients has been claimed to be possible from the study of the changes in circulating peripheral T-cell subsets. Renal biopsy is performed to confirm rejection in patients where the clinical diagnosis is uncertain, and to assess its severity. A series of 35 patients transplanted between September 1982 and October 1983 were prospectively studied using T-cell subset data. Transplant biopsy and/or nephrectomy specimens were studied retrospectively. We graded the degree of histological rejection present using a recently described semi-quantitative method. The histological grade was compared with the circulating T-cell populations determined within 24 hr of biopsy/nephrectomy, and 4–6 days previously. No correlation was found between histology and T-cell subset data at the time of the biopsy. However, the T-cell ratio 4–6 days before biopsy/nephrectomy did vary with severity of rejection (T4/T8 ratio 1.31 ± 0.74 for mild rejection, and 2.38 ± 1.13 for severe rejection); this trend did not reach statistical significance. Follow up information was available for 6–18 mth following biopsy. The histological grading but not the T-cell assessment was found to be of prognostic value in predicting graft survival.

DEMONSTRATION OF CROSS-REACTING ANTI-DNA ANTIBODY IDIOTYPES IN RENAL BIOPSIES FROM SLE PATIENTS

C. M. Collins and D. A. Isenberg

Department of Histopathology, University College London and The Middlesex Hospital Medical School, University Street, London WC1E 6JJ

The origin of autoantibodies in SLE is unknown. Monoclonal anti-DNA antibodies from SLE patients bind to different polynucleotides of varying base composition and to other unrelated antigens. Idiotype sharing among autoantibodies from unrelated patients has been demonstrated. Cross-reacting anti-DNA antibody idiotypes were sought amongst immunoglobulins deposited in the kidneys of SLE patients. Two anti-idiotypes were used which had been previously raised in a rabbit (anti 16/6/R) and in a mouse (anti 13/15/M) by immunisation with human monoclonal antibodies from 2 SLE patients. 28 formalin-fixed, paraffin-embedded renal biopsies from 23 SLE patients and 21 control biopsies from non-lupus patients in which immune deposit had been demonstrated, were studied. The rabbit and mouse antisera were used with the trypsin-immunoperoxidase technique to visualise immune deposit in glomerular tufts. 5/23 lupus biopsies showed staining in glomerular basement membrane. 2/23 showed staining in focal proliferative lesions and 3/23 showed staining in the mesangium. In all 10/23 (43%) showed evidence of some binding. None of the 21 control biopsies showed evidence of binding. This suggests that some tissue-bound autoantibodies are derived from germ line genes which are expressed in SLE patients. The importance of these cross-reacting idiotypes in lupus nephritis remains speculative.

PERMEABILITY OF NORMAL GLOMERULAR STRUCTURES TO IgG

D. R. Davies, Thèrese Ternyck, Marie-France Belair, P. Druet and J. Bariety

Department of Histopathology, St. Thomas's Hospital, London SE1, Department of Immunochemistry, Institut Pasteur, Paris and Inserm U28, Hopital Broussais, Paris Cedex 14

In-vivo experiments, involving the injection of anti-HRP antibodies into Munich-Wistar rats with subsequent *in-situ* fixation of glomeruli and localization of antibody with horse-radish peroxidase (HRP), have shown that circulating IgG enters the mesangium and glomerular basement membrane. The sheep antibodies used in these experiments were polyclonal with a wide range of pI values (5.3–7.6). The glomerular anionic charge is believed to restrict the permeability of albumen which is also anionic at physiological pH. It is therefore possible that the charge on circulating IgG molecules will determine their penetration into normal glomeruli. Monoclonal antibodies have more restricted pI values than polyclonal antibodies. We used both a relatively anionic (pI 4.5–5.5) and a relatively cationic (pI 7–8.5) mouse monoclonal antibody to HRP to compare their penetration into glomeruli after *in-vivo* injection. The cationic antibody had a poor affinity for HRP *in-vitro* and did not give a sufficiently strong reaction *in-vivo* to be interpretable. The anionic anti HRP antibody reacted well and was shown to enter the glomerular mesangium and glomerular basement membrane, as did the polyclonal antibody. These experiments provide evidence that chemically unmodified anionic immunoglobulin can enter the glomerular extra-cellular matrix despite the glomerular anionic charge.

HETEROGENEITY OF RENAL ENDOTHELIAL CELLS FOR CLASS II ANTIGENS

A. G. MacIver, Lynne P. Trickett, P. R. Evans, J. L. Smith and M. Slapak

Southampton University Department of Pathology,
Wessex Regional Immunology Unit, Southampton and
Wessex Region Transplant Unit, Portsmouth

Both Class I and II antigens are clearly demonstrated in renal peritubular capillary endothelial cells by immunohistological techniques using monoclonal antibodies and cryostat sections. Class I antigens (HLA-ABC) are also present on the endothelium of renal arteries, glomeruli and veins. We have previously reported that HLA-DR (Class II) antigens are absent from arterial endothelium. Further studies on 16 kidneys have shown that there is variation within the Class II system. SB antigens are usually present on arterial endothelium whilst DC and other DR antigens are absent. Glomerular and renal vein endothelial cells usually contain DR and SB antigens but DC antigens are often absent (8/15 glomeruli; 6/8 renal veins). These studies emphasize the complexity of the HLA system and indicate that its role in the localisation of rejection phenomena requires further investigation.

MORPHOLOGICAL FEATURES ASSOCIATED WITH REPARATIVE AND PRENEOPLASTIC HYPERPLASIA IN RAT URINARY BLADDER

Dianne M. Creasy, H. B. Jones and W. H. Butler

BIBRA, Woodmansterne Road, Carshalton, Surrey SM5 5DS

The urothelium of the rat bladder is capable of rapid and extensive proliferation in response to injurious agents. In toxicological studies, interpretation of the significance of urothelial hyperplasia relies on the ability to distinguish a reversible reparative hyperplasia from the progressive "preneoplastic" hyperplasia which precedes overt tumour development. Using the light microscope, the transmission and scanning electron microscopes we studied the hyperplastic response induced in female F344 rat bladders by formalin and trypsin instillation, cyclophosphamide and freeze ulceration. These were compared with the urothelial changes elicited by the potent bladder carcinogen-N-butyl-4(hydroxybutyl)-nitrosamine (BBN) administered at a dose calculated to produce 100% tumour incidence. The hyperplastic response to the cytotoxic agents varied both in the cellular growth pattern and the ultrastructural features exhibited. Considerable cell and nuclear atypia were present after cyclophosphamide administration while nodular downgrowths, sub-epithelial cell nests and intra-epithelial capillary growth were observed following most of the treatments. Pleomorphic microvilli were particularly prominent after BBN treatment but were also frequently seen after formalin instillation. No qualitative differences were seen in the morphological features associated with the reparative and the "preneoplastic" hyperplasias studied.

DOSE-RESPONSE RELATIONSHIP FOR PHENOBARBITONE PROMOTION OF RAT LIVER TUMOURS INITIATED BY SINGLE DOSE DIMETHYLNITROSAMINE

H. Elizabeth Driver and A. E. M. McLean

MRC Toxicology Unit, Woddmansterne Road, Carshalton, Surrey and Laboratory of Toxicology, School of Medicine, University College London, London WC1

A single dose of 15 mg/kg dimethylnitrosamine is an effective initiator of hepatic tumour formation in rats. Subsequent promotion by Na phenobarbitone at a dose of 1,000 μg/ml in the drinking water leads to 40% or more of the rats developing hepatocellular carcinoma by 20 mth. Four days of dietary treatment designed to produce a wave of DNA synthesis at the time of initiation leads to an even greater yield of tumours and nodules after 20 mth of promotion. Lower doses of phenobarbitone (40 or 100 μg/ml), which result in a 20% or 50% increase in cytochrome P-450 and associated enzyme activity, did not promote tumour development. No carcinomas were seen in these groups, suggesting that tumour promotion and enzyme induction are not directly proportional and may be quite separate phenomena. A threshold for promotion has been demonstrated. The implications of these findings will be discussed.

COMPARATIVE STUDY OF DEVELOPMENT OF ORTHO-AMINOAZOTOLUENE INDUCED HEPATOCELLULAR CARCINOMA IN C3H AND C57/B1 MICE

Deborah J. Pritchard and W. H. Butler

British Industrial Biological Research Association, Woodmansterene Road, Carshalton, Surrey SM5 4DS

Ortho-aminoazotoluene (O-AT) was fed to adult male mice, at levels of 0.03% for up to 52 wk. A comparison was made between a high tumour incidence strain (C3H), and a low incidence strain (C57/B1), in order to study the development of the morphological events leading to hepatic neoplasms. After 52 wk of treatment, the incidence of hepatic carcinoma in the C3H mouse was 100% and in the C57/B1 was 86%. O-AT, at 0.03% in the diet was toxic to the liver as well as carcinogenic. The proliferation of bile ducts and oval cells from the periportal regions was more extensive in the C57/B1 mice, as was the degree of toxic injury, and resultant centrilobular compensatory hyperplasia. From about 24 wk of treatment small areas of basophilic cells were seen, which later appeared as more discrete foci and nodules. The distribution of foci and nodules was similar in both strains, suggesting their independence from the reactive centrilobular hyperplasia which was more extensive in the C57/B1 mice. By 52 wk of treatment large numbers of animals, of both strains, had hepatocellular carcinomas, and several discrete nodules. The development of discrete nodules and carcinoma in the later half of the feeding period appeared not to be related to the overt toxic injury produced by O-AT.

ORGAN-SPECIFIC EFFECTS ON METASTATIC GROWTH STUDIED *IN VITRO*

Elizabeth Horak, Dawn Darling and D. Tarin

Nuffield Department of Pathology, University of Oxford, John Radcliffe Hospital, Oxford OX3 9DU

Although the cells from disseminating malignant tumours rapidly arrive in all organs, they only grow in some sites, and success or failure in forming metastatic deposits is dependent upon interaction between properties of the tumour cells and the microenvironment. In the present study the influence of microenvironmental conditions of specific organs upon tumour cell survival and behaviour was investigated in tissue culture using spontaneous mouse mammary carcinomas. In co-cultures, some organs (lung, ovary) encourage the survival and the attachment of the tumour cells, while others (liver, thyroid) accelerate the process of cell destruction. The effect is due to transmittable, soluble mediators, the dose-dependency of which was established. The "stimulatory" influence is rather a preservation of the tumour cells, than a stimulation of their multiplication, as was proven with ^{125}IUdR-uptake studies. It is known that after *in vivo* inoculation, these mammary tumours develop metastases mainly in the lungs, and occasionally in the kidneys or ovaries, and the "encouraging" influences of these same organs *in vitro* are thus in good agreement with the *in vivo* observations. The findings also endorse the hypothesis that certain normal organs can suppress the formation of metastases even though cells from the same tumour have formed them elsewhere.

ASSESSMENT BY FLOW CYTOFLUOROMETRY OF RESPONSE OF TUMOURS OF UTERINE CERVIX TO RADIOTHERAPY

J. E. D. Dyson, R. I. Rothwell, P. Quirke, C. A. F. Joslin and C. C. Bird

University Department of Radiotherapy, Cookridge Hospital, Leeds 16 and Department of Pathology, University of Leeds, Leeds LS2 9JT

The technique of flow cytofluorometry enables the DNA and RNA content of individual cells, stained with nucleic acid specific fluorescent dyes, to be determined, to give DNA and RNA content profiles for tumour tissue specimens. By comparison to a diploid standard (human lymphocytes) the DNA profiles may be divided into ploidy regions and cell subpopulations of ploidy 2.5c and 4.5c and >4.5c quantitated. Non-viable degenerating cells may also be quantitated. We have applied this procedure to serial biopsies of cervical tumours, taken at approximately weekly intervals, during intracavitary radiotherapy (Cathetron). Changes in the cell sub-populations as above are plotted *versus* time elapsed since start of treatment to give a semi-quantitative indication of the response of the tumour to therapy. Rate of elimination of cell sub-populations of higher ploidy from the tumour biopsy specimens, together with increase in content of degenerating cells, used as an indication of therapeutic response, is in excellent agreement with tumour response to therapy as assessed by histopatholgical evaluation of parallel biopsy specimens. Reduction in content of these cell sub-populations, however, often precedes reduction in tumour content as determined by histopathology by 7 to 10 days, thus giving an earlier indication of therapeutic response of the tumour.

LOSS OF NUCLEAR FLUORESCENCE FROM METAPLASTIC, DYSPLASTIC AND SQUAMOUS CANCER CELLS STAINED BY FLUORESCENT PAPANICOLAOU DYES

A. de Lemos Bastos, J. M. Bastos, M. C. Moreira and Maria M. Bastos

Departamento de Patologia Experimental – Instituto Português de Oncologia de Francisco Gentil, Lisboa, Portugal

In gynaecological squamous cells normal nuclear fluorescence spectra in superficial and intermediate cells varies with the oestrogenic (yellow) and luteinic (green) phase of the ovarian cycle. The functional significance of nuclear fluorescence is supported by the fact that normal basal, parabasal and atrophic post menopausal cells show a much reduced nuclear fluorescence. The cell fluorescence of Papanicolaou (Pap) dyes is stable, can be viewed years after the staining with no apparent fading and be obtained with any excitation time. The absorption, excitation and emission spectra of Pap dyes varies with the excitation filter system, pH and solvent polarity. The Pap stain is therefore suitable to be used as a steady state multimodal emission system with each dye-cell complex identified by the absorption/excitation/emission spectra. The loss of nuclear fluorescence in metaplastic, dysplastic and cancer squamous cells is believed to be due to an alteration or loss of oxyphilic nuclear substrate. The cytochemical nature of this oxyphilic substrate could be a nuclear cytokeratin-like substance under hormonal control. The photochemical action spectra basis for this view will be discussed.

IMMUNOCYTOCHEMICAL STAINING OF BREAST CARCINOMA BY MONOCLONAL ANTIBODY NCRC 11 AND ITS PROGNOSTIC SIGNIFICANCE

I. E. Ellis, C. D. Hinton, R. A. Robins, C. W. Elston and R. W. Blamey

Department of Histopathology, Q.M.C., Nottingham, Department of Surgery, City Hospital, Nottingham, and C.R.C. Laboratories, University of Nottingham, Nottingham

The production and immunocytochemical characterization of monoclonal antibody NCRC 11 was described at a previous meeting of this Society. Staining of normal tissues shows a specific distribution virtually confined to the surface of certain epithelial cell types and similar to the distribution of antibodies raised against human milk fat globule membrane (anti E.M.A.). A series of 126 primary breast carcinomas has been studied with NCRC 11. The staining pattern seen in these tumours was quite heterogeneous. For each tumour the overall intensity of staining was assessed on a four point scale 1+, 2+, 3+, 4+. The minimum survival for each patient was 5 yr. One hundred and nineteen tumours showed positive staining. There was a highly significant relationship between staining intensity and survival (Mantel's life table analysis $X^2=63.346$; $p<0.001$). Five year survival figures are 1+ 36% (n=32): 2+ 54% (n=33): 3+ 83% (n=43): 4+ 92% (n=12). There was a weak relationship with histological grade but none with oestrogen receptor status.

β-ENOLASE AS POTENTIAL MARKER FOR RHABDOMYOSARCOMA

Janice A. Royds, S. Variend, W. R. Timperley and C. B. Taylor

Department of Biochemistry, University of Sheffield, Sheffield, Department of Pathology, The Children's Hospital, Sheffield, and Department of Neuropathology, The Royal Hallamshire Hospital, Sheffield

Twenty-one tumours diagnosed as rhabdomyosarcomas (38% embryonal,62% alveolar) by conventional light microscopy techniques were stained for α- and β-enolase using the immunoperoxidase PAP method. A control series of 3 neuroblastomas, 3 fibrosarcomas, 1 osteosarcoma and 5 Wilms sarcomas were also studied using the same technique. Enolase has 3 subunit types, α, β and γ. The α subunit is found in all tissues and is the fetal form of the enzyme; adult skeletal muscle contains the ββ isoenzyme which accounts for 3% of the soluble protein of this tissue. Positive staining for α-enolase was seen in all but one case, a small celled embryonal type. Staining for β-enolase was seen in 18 of the 21 cases of rhabdomyosarcoma (7/8 cases alveolar, 11/13 cases embryonal). None of the control tumours stained positively for β-enolase. Intensity of staining varied, the strongest being in multinucleate cells with peripheral nuclei. Cross-striations were seen in 1 of the 8 alveolar and 6 of the 13 embryonal tumours. The 3 tumours which showed no β-enolase staining contained neither rhabdomyoblasts nor cells with cross-striations but were composed of small undifferentiated cells. β-enolase appears to be a sensitive marker of muscle differentiation in rhabdomyosarcoma.

FOVEOLAR HYPERPLASIA AND GASTRIC RISK FACTORS ASSOCIATED WITH ENTEROGASTRIC REFLUX AFTER DUODENAL ULCER SURGERY

H. Thompson and F. Mosiman

Department of Histology, General Hospital, Birmingham, and Centre Hospitalier Universitaire Vaudois, Service de Chirurgie B, Lausanne, Switzerland

This study investigates the hypothesis that foveolar hyperplasia is a histological marker of entero-gastric reflux and that risk factors in gastric carcinogenesis such as intestinal metaplasia, dysplasia and chronic atrophic gastritis correlate with the pH of fasting gastric juice and the bile reflux status. Multiple endoscopic biopsies were taken from 36 asymptomatic volunteers 7–22 yr after various operations for duodenal ulcer. The patients were screened for reflux by external scanning following injection of 75 MBq of 99 mTc HIDA. The incidence and significance of risk factors including Type III sulphomucin secreting intestinal metaplasia will be assessed in relation to a pH >4.

CHANGES IN LECTIN BINDING OF LARGE INTESTINAL EPITHELIUM DURING FETAL DEVELOPMENT AND NEOPLASIA

G. T. Williams, Rosalind P. Davies and W. T. Barr

Department of Pathology, Welsh National School of Medicine, Heath Park, Cardiff CF4 4XN

Alterations in tissue carbohydrates during fetal colonic development have been studied using peroxidase-labelled lectins on formalin fixed sections, and the results related to the changes that occur in colorectal carcinomas. Fetal colon of 14, 19, 24, 30 and 36 wk development (2 of each), adult colon (26) and colorectal carcinomas (21) were studied with the following lectins (sugar specificities in parentheses): PNA (β-D-Gal(1→3)-D-GalNAc), DBA (NAc Gal), UEA (α-L-fucose), WGA (NAcGlu, sialic acid), MPA (α-D-galactose) and BSAI (α-D-galactose). Preliminary results show that the most striking changes occurred in the reactions with the apical (luminal) border of the epithelial cells, where a strong reaction in early fetuses was lost between 24 and 30 wk for PNA and between 30 and 36 wk for WGA and BSAI. The surface reaction with these 3 lectins, absent in adult colon, reappeared in colorectal carcinomas. MPA and UEA also reacted with the luminal borders of carcinoma cells, but not with fetal or adult epithelium. Changes in the lectin reactions of secreted mucin with neoplasia were not mirrored at any stage of fetal development. The results suggest that while some surface changes with neoplasia may be expressions of fetal glycosubstances, other alterations in the lectin reactions are not.

MORPHOLOGICAL ABNORMALITIES AT SITE OF HEALTHY COLONIC ANASTOMOSES FOLLOWING RESECTIONS FOR COLONIC CANCER

J. P. Sunter, M. J. Higgs and W. K. Cowan

Departments of Pathology and Surgery, Queen Elizabeth Hospital, Gateshead

The development of carcinoma at the site of anastomosis following colonic resection for carcinoma is usually assumed to represent recurrence of the original growth. But colonic cancer is multifocal, and in rodent models of intestinal cancer anastomoses are sites of enhanced tumorigenesis. It is possible therefore that some "anastomotic recurrences" in man represent metachronous second primary growths. Evaluation of the mucosa at healthy anastomoses may clarify this problem. Twenty-eight colon cancer patients, asymptomatic following resection and anastomosis, were colonoscoped as part of their follow-up, and biopsies obtained from the anastomosis and several other sites. Sections where stained by H&E, several methods for mucin and by the PAP method for CEA, randomised, and morphological changes assessed. At the anastomosis there were non-specific inflammatory changes in 11 of the 28 cases, apparent in several 2 yr after resection; focal ulceration was seen in over half these samples. Neither dysplastic nor adenomatous change was detected nor was there a consistent change in CEA pattern. In some cases mucin secretion was abnormal, resembling "transitional mucosa". It is concluded that there is morphological evidence of a continued stimulus to regenerative activity at some anastomoses, and this may represent a promoting factor enhancing further carcinogenesis.

Joint Symposium
Chromosomes and Cancer Cells

CHROMOSOME REARRANGEMENTS AND CANCER

D. G. Harnden

The Paterson Laboratories, Christie Hospital & Holt Radium Institute, Wilmslow Road, Manchester 20 9BX

Chromosome abnormalities in cancer cells are of several kinds including (1) complex abnormalities of chromosome number and morphology which appear to represent a total breakdown in control of replication of the genetic material (2) gains or losses of particular chromosomes and/or relatively simple rearrangements apparently specific for one neoplasm or subgroup of one neoplasm (3) similar abnormalities which occur regularly but not invariably in a number of different neoplasms. Some of the specific rearrangements are known to be associated with the location of cellular oncogenes. Others not yet so associated draw attention to chromosomes or regions of chromosomes which may be of interest in the initiation and progression of malignant disease. Chromosome rearrangements may not, in themselves, be sufficient for the development of cancer. Further, there may be a number of different chromosomal mechanisms involved in the carcinogenesis. Only some of these will be manifest as visible chromosome abnormalities.

CHROMOSOMES OF LEUKAEMIAS AND LYMPHOMAS

B. R. Reeves

Institute of Cancer Research, London SW3 6JJ

Leukaemias and lymphomas are the human malignancies that have been most extensively studied cytogenetically. It is now known that certain of the chromosome abnormalities found in these disorders may be regarded as common to a wide variety of cytological types; while others are more or less confined to cases with similar cytology. The cytogenetics of leukaemias and lymphomas will be discussed in the light of current concepts of the roles of chromosome changes in the initiation and progression of malignancy.

INFERENCES DRAWN FROM CYTOGENETIC STUDIES OF HYDATIDIFORM MOLES AND CHORIOCARCINOMA

Sylvia D. Lawler

Institute of Cancer Research, Royal Marsden Hospital, Fulham Road, London SW3 6JJ

On the basis of histopathology and genetics, hydatidiform moles can be defined as partial or complete. Partial moles are associated with the presence of a fetus; they are triploid, have both maternal and paternal genes, and they usually arise by dispermy. Complete moles are diploid, female, androgenetically derived and usually homozygous. About 4% of moles are diploid and heterozygous, arising by dispermy. Thus the female parent does not contribute to the nuclear DNA of complete moles. The majority of molar pregnancies subside spontaneously after evacuation, but in 10–20% of cases chemotherapy is required to treat a subsequent trophoblastic tumour, which may be invasive mole or choriocarcinoma. The opportunity to study fresh tissue from a choriocarcinoma is a rare event. Studies of the cytogenetics of choriocarcinoma after mole are usually made on cell lines and those that have been studied have been found to be heterozygous. So the question raised is whether heterozygous complete moles have more malignant potential than those that are homozygous.

CHROMOSOME ANALYSIS BY FLOW CYTOMETRY

B. D. Young and Margaret L. M. Anderson

Beatson Institute for Cancer Research, Bearsden, Glasgow

The study of chromosomal rearrangements is becoming increasingly important in the analysis of the role of oncogenes in human cancer. In our laboratory the analysis of human chromosomes by flow cytometry has been refined to the extent that the effects of particular rearrangements can be visualised. This allows quantitation of the amounts of DNA transferred in translocations and permits the isolation of sufficient quantities of translocated chromosomes to allow mapping of relevant genes. In particular we are studying the 8;22 translocation in Burkitt's lymphoma and current results will be presented. Another application of chromosome sorting is the construction of chromosome specific recombinant DNA libraries. This is of particular application for the molecular study of genetic defects which have been mapped to a certain chromosome. The current status of this field will be reviewed.

DOUBLE MINUTES AND GENE AMPLIFICATION

C. J. Bostock

MRC Mammalian Genome Unit, King's Buildings, Edinburgh EH9 3JT

Double minutes are small chromosome fragments which lack centromeres and which are visualised as paired "dots" in mitotic chromosome preparations. Although occasionally present in small numbers in spontaneous tumours, their presence in large numbers is more often associated with cells which have been selected *in vitro* for high levels of resistance to certain anti-tumour drugs. In these cases, double minutes are the cytological manifestation of the amplification of the gene that codes for the target protein of the drug. Using as an example the amplification of the dihydrofolate reductase (dhfr) gene in response to Methotrexate selection, the principal features of gene amplification will be illustrated. For example, the dhfr gene is amplified as part of a much larger unit of DNA than the gene itself, and the sequences which are built into the unit are drawn from non-contiguous parts of the genome and frequently undergo rearrangements during the early stages of amplification. Knowledge gained from these *in vitro* systems will be discussed in relation to processes that occur spontaneously in cells *in vivo* which might in some cases be partly responsible for the development of the tumour phenotype (e.g. neuroblastomas).

GENES AND CANCER

W. J. Rigby

Cancer Research Campaign, Eukaryotic Molecular Genetics Group, Imperial College, London

We can now define a number of types of gene which can contribute to the malignant phenotype. DNA tumour viruses carry oncogenes which appear to have no homologue in the cellular genome, whereas the oncogenes of strongly transforming retroviruses are transduced cellular genes. The cellular homologues of retrovirus oncogenes are normally non-oncogenic but they can become activated by a variety of mechanisms including point mutation, translocation and amplification. Such activated proto-oncogenes are thought to contribute to human disease. The protein products of oncogenes manifest a wide variety of biochemical activities. We have also identified a number of cellular targets for oncogene action. In some cases these are proteins which interact directly with oncogene-encoded proteins, in others these are genes which are activated or repressed by the transforming proteins. We are thus beginning to build up a molecular picture of the events which underlie oncogenesis.

Posters and Demonstrations

AUTOPSY VIDEOTAPES AS A TEACHING MEDIUM – LEEDS EXPERIENCE

C. Gray, C. A. R. Hay, W. A. Reid and M. Wells

Department of Pathology, University of Leeds, Leeds LS2 9JT

The autopsy has always been regarded as a valuable source of teaching material in the medical undergraduate curriculum. However, diminished clinical interest in post mortems, the reduction in hospital autopsy rates and increased student numbers have resulted in a decline in this form of teaching. In an attempt to overcome some of these problems the videotaping of autopsies has been carried out over the last three years. The necessary camera and editing expertise has been developed within the department. An expanding library of short video sequences is now available to us incorporating autopsy findings, surgical pathology, histology and illustrative clinical material including electrocardiographs and radiological investigations. From this bank tapes can then be prepared to suit varying needs, e.g. composite tapes on a particular disease process or the conventional clinicopathological format based on a single interesting case. The latter have also proved to be popular with postgraduate audiences. A further recent development has been the introduction of computer graphics whilst tapes may also be made interactive by incorporating appropriate questions. A typical example will be demonstrated and our experience presented. We hope to initiate links with other departments to exchange ideas and material.

COMPUTER ASSISTED LEARNING IN UNDERGRADUATE TEACHING

P. J. R. Harkin, M. F. Dixon, I. Lauder and W. A. Reid

Department of Pathology, University of Leeds, Leeds LS2 9JT

Computers are potentially excellent educational tools. They can be used to present tutorial information in a structured manner and to monitor student responses. Unlike human teachers, they do not make errors or become bored. Until recently, however, the cost of such computer systems has been prohibitive. We have recently developed a relatively cheap system based on the BBC microcomputer. Conventional Computer Assisted Learning (CAL) systems require a moderate degree of computer knowledge and programming skill on the part of the software author. This was not acceptable to us; so we have used an alternative approach. A system was devised whereby the computer accepts plain English text or questions, and constructs its own programs in BASIC, the standard language of the BBC microcomputer. These programs will then run independently of the creation system. Using this method, we have written a large number of tutorial programs which are currently forming part of our undergraduate teaching programme in general pathology. In addition, a specially designed interface allows the tutorial programs to use colour photographs which may rapidly be accessed via a standard Revox microfiche projector. A selection of programs will be available for demonstration during the meeting.

COMPLEMENT COMPONENT DEPOSITION IN UTEROPLACENTAL (SPIRAL) ARTERIES IN NORMAL PREGNANCY

Joanna Bennett, C. S. Holgate and M. Wells

Department of Pathology, University of Leeds, Leeds LS2 9JT

The extensive structural alterations which occur in the arterial vessels of the placental bed from early pregnancy onwards, due to their invasion by extravillous trophoblast, have been well described. However, there is a paucity of data on the immunological status of these spiral arteries both in normal and abnormal pregnancy. Complement components are normally found within healthy placentae suggesting that immunological sensitisation between mother and fetus is a physiological necessity of normal pregnancy. However, there is conflicting evidence for the deposition of complement in spiral arteries. Indirect immunoperoxidase and immunogold-silver techniques were used to investigate the distribution of C1q, C3d, C4, C6 and C9 within the spiral arteries of six formalin fixed normal pregnancy hysterectomy specimens ranging in gestational age from 4 to 40 weeks. Characteristic linear deposition was observed subjacent to the endovascular trophoblast in all cases and for all complement components, suggesting classical pathway activation. Reactivity was most intense for C3d and C9. Uterine veins showed no complement deposition. Clearly, an appreciation of this phenomenon as a feature of normal pregnancy is essential before significant immunopathology can be recognised in placental bed vessels in abnormal pregnancy.

IMMUNOHISTOCHEMICAL LOCALISATION OF CYTOCHROME P-450 IN CONTROL AND DRUG INDUCED RAT TISSUES

J. R. Foster, C. R. Elcombe, R. T. Robson, C. Hayward, A. R. Boobis, D. Sesardic, J. McQuade, D. S. Davies and E. A. Lock

Central Toxicology Laboratory, ICI; Corporate Biosciences Group, ICI; and Department of Clinical Pharmacology, Royal Postgraduate Medical School, Hammersmith Hospital, London

Cytochrome P-450 constitutes the major drug metabolising system of the liver and as such plays a key role in the detoxification and in some instances activation of absorbed chemicals. In order to study the distribution of this enzyme system, a number of mouse monoclonal antibodies (Mab's) were raised against a preparation of hepatic cytochrome P-450 isolated from β-naphthoflavone (BNF)-induced rats. The Mab's have now been used in an immunoperoxidase cytochemical assay to localise cytochrome P-450 in control, BNF treated and sodium phenobarbitone (NaPb)-treated rats. In addition to studying the distribution of the enzyme system in the liver, cytochrome P-450 was also localised in the kidney, adrenals and olfactory epithelium of the nasal cavity. Although the Mab's were raised against BNF-induced cytochrome P-450 some were also found to cross react strongly with both control and NaPb-induced cytochrome P-450. In liver from control animals cytochrome P-450 was seen to be fairly evenly distributed over the liver lobule, and although BNF-treatment increased the staining intensity, distribution remained unchanged. In contrast, treatment with NaPb produced a distinctive centrilobular enhancement of staining. Both kidney and adrenal gland showed specific staining of the cortex and this was enhanced following treatment with NaPb or BNF.

SYNOVIAL FLUID MAST CELLS IN DIAGNOSIS OF INFLAMMATORY ARTHRITIS

A. J. Freemont and J. Denton

Department of Rheumatology, University of Manchester Medical School, Manchester M13 9PT

Differentiating between primary inflammatory arthropathies is hampered by their similar clinical presentations and synovial histology. Routine cytological analysis of synovial fluid also has limited diagnostic application because there is no single cell specific to any one disease and the proportions of the cell types present are much the same in all these arthropathies. One cell type largely ignored in the analysis of synovial fluid is the mast cell. In this study synovial fluids from the knees of 97 patients with seropositive rheumatoid arthritis (RA), 37 with seronegative RA, 27 with ankylosing spondylitis (AS), 46 with Reiter's disease, 36 with psoriatic arthritis, 42 with gout, 5 with SLE and 83 with osteoarthrosis were examined for mast cells in conventional cytospin preparations stained Jenner-Giemsa. Mast cells were identified in fluids from 48% of patients with AS, 36% with Reiter's disease and 22% with psoriatic arthritis which compares with between 0 and 6% for all the other disorders. The presence of mast cells in the synovial fluid of a patient with primary inflammatory arthropathy strongly suggests the patient has ankylosing spondylitis, Reiter's disease or psoriatic arthritis.

PATHOLOGY OF MECKEL SYNDROME

B. H. Ruebner, Mary Ann Jammal, W. Ellis, and J. Bernstein

Department of Pathology, School of Medicine, University of California, Davis, CA 95616, USA

Six cases of the Meckel Syndrome were studied. This lethal, autosomal recessive disorder is classically defined as a triad of cystic renal dysplasia, encephalocele, and polydactyly. Since description of the first case in 1822, a broad spectrum of associated anomalies and variations of the classic triad have been recognized. Therefore, questions arise as to what features are minimally necessary to define Meckel Syndrome and what morphologic heterogeneity falls within the boundaries of this syndrome All of our six cases had cystic renal dysplasia of the classic pattern with huge kidneys demonstrating a paucity of glomeruli, fibrosis, and irregular cystic spaces. The other features of this syndrome were not consistently found and particular heterogeneity was noted with respect to CNS lesions. A highly vascular occipital encephalocele was found in four of our cases. Micropolygyria, cortical heterotopia, incomplete formation of cerebellum, and hydrocephalus were also findings of note. Also hepatic fibrosis and bile duct proliferation, which have not been commonly appreciated as salient features of Meckel Syndrome, were found in five of our cases. Our findings suggest that the CNS abnormalities of Meckel Syndrome are extensive and that a hepatic lesion is a significant part of this syndrome. These further classifications of the pathology in Meckel Syndrome may be useful in diagnosis of this disorder so that affected families may be counselled appropriately.

THE USE OF DOUBLE-STAINING TECHNIQUE IN LECTIN BINDING STUDIES

Sheila M. Day and Rosemary A. Walker

Department of Pathology, University of Leicester, Leicester

Double staining methods are increasingly being applied in immunohistochemistry but there has been little use of this approach in lectin histochemistry, where it could be of value when investigating the binding of lectins that have the same sugar specificity. Such a technique has been used to consider the binding of fucose-specific lectins to normal and malignant human breast tissue. *Lotus tetragonolobus (LTA)-peroxidase* and *Ulex europeus I (UEA)-alkaline phosphatase* have been applied in combination to frozen sections. The reaction product of peroxidase gives a brown colour, of alkaline phosphatase a red colour, and the combined product *orange-brown*. In normal breast the epithelial cells either reacted only with *LTA* or had a combined staining pattern. The carcinomas were varied in their reactions, having differing proportions of cells with single staining or combined reactions. Some tumours differed from normal breast in containing cells that reacted only with *UEA*. The double-staining method has been of value in giving a more accurate identification of differences in the binding to human breast of lectins with similar specificities.

RETRIEVAL OF CELLS FROM LOW CONCENTRATION SUSPENSIONS AND SUBSEQUENT IDENTIFICATION USING SURFACE MARKERS

N. M. Pettigrew and F. Baldwin

Department of Pathology, University of Manitoba, 770 Bannatyne Avenue, Winnipeg, Manitoba, R3E 0W3, Canada

Standard surface marker analysis using monoclonal antibodies on cells in suspension requires a relatively large number of cells and is unsuitable for analysis of samples where few cells may be present (e.g. CSF, fine needle aspirate biopsies, or effusions). Cells stained in suspension may be lost in an unpredictable manner during washing or when cells are subsequently deposited on a slide. Fluoroscein activated cell sorter techniques and also computer assisted cell recognition procedures similarly required a high concentration of cells. Obtaining a maximum number of viable cells on slides was made possible by modified cytocentrifugation which allowed the majority of cells (mouse peritoneal cells, human peripheral blood mononuclear cells, human cerebrospinal fluid cells) from 0.5 ml or smaller aliquots of fluid with low cellularity to be centrifuged on to a 2 mm diameter area of coated slides. The small amount of fluid required for each preparation enabled multiple slides to be made from a small sample of suspended cells and permitted quantitation of mononuclear cell subpopulations. The technique has been applied to CSF from patients with and without neurological disease as well as fine needle renal aspirates and effusions.

ORGAN-SPECIFIC EFFECTS ON METASTATIC TUMOUR GROWTH: STUDIES INVOLVING TRANSPLANTATION TECHNIQUES

Elizabeth Horak, Dawn Darling and D. Tarin

Nuffield Department of Pathology, University of Oxford, John Radcliffe Hospital, Oxford OX3 9DU

After IV or IA inoculation the disaggregated tumour cells of mouse spontaneous mammary carcinomas arrive in every organ but form metastases only in some of them. Further studies indicate that normal organs contain diffusible factors which encourage or suppress survival and adhesion of tumour cells *in vitro,* and these findings correlate with the organ distribution of mammary tumour deposits *in vivo.* This study was, therefore, undertaken to test whether a *direct* link can be demonstrated between these *in vivo* and *in vitro* phenomena. The method was to re-implant specific organ fragments already proven to have effects on tumour cells *in vitro.* By labelling tumour cells with fluorescein isothiocyanate (FITC) it was found that some tumour cells invade the tissue fragments *in vitro;* and after re-implantation of the organ fragments the cells within formed implant-derived tumours (IDT). Some IDTs formed metastases spontaneously. The higher incidence of metastasis found among tumours that can form IDTs than among undisturbed mammary tumours in general indicates that the organs "select" a population of cells with higher metastatic/invasive capability. The organs which the tumour cells most frequently invade are the same as those in which experimental metastases occur and as those which stimulate the survival/attachment of tumour cells *in vitro.*

DNA/RNA CONTENT OF TESTICULAR TUMOURS AS ASSESSED BY FLOW CYTOMETRY

P. Quirke, J. E. D. Dyson, J. Sutton, C. K. Anderson, C. C. Bird and W. G. Jones

Department of Pathology, University of Leeds, Leeds LS2 9JT and Department of Radiotherapy, Cookridge Hospital, Leeds 16

The DNA/RNA content and the number of degenerating cells have been measured prospectively on a small series of testicular tumours using flow cytometry. Whole live cells were stained using acridine orange and ethidium bromide, and excited by an argon ion laser. Seminomas appear to be composed of a single clone in nearly all the samples measured with ploidy levels of 2C, 3C and 4C. The small number of teratomas and mixed tumours were diploid except for one malignant teratoma undifferentiated at 4C.

ULTRASTRUCTURE OF SEMINOMA OF TESTIS WITH PARTICULAR REFERENCE TO INTERCELLULAR JUNCTIONS

J. R. Goepel and P. D. Norris

Department of Pathology, Sheffield University and Weston Park Hospital, Sheffield

15 cases of testicular seminoma have been examined; in one material was retrieved from paraffin wax, 2 were fixed in gluteraldehyde, the remaining 12 in formal saline. Areas of typical seminoma all showed tight or intermediate junctions; in most cases they were scanty but occasionally many were present. Two cases showed a dense accumulation of

fibrillar material either side of tight junctions within the adjacent cytoplasm. True desmosomes were present in four cases in areas otherwise typical of seminoma. As would be expected, islands of trophoblast had desmosomes between adjacent cells. The presence of desmosomes in a seminoma may represent ultrastructural differentiation of germ cells toward a teratoma. One such case of seminoma was associated with alpha-fetoprotein in occasional tumour cells.

IMAGE ANALYSIS IN HISTOLOGICAL DIAGNOSIS OF VERRUCOUS SQUAMOUS CARCINOMA OF THE LARYNX

L. Michaels, J. Cooper, C. J. Brewer, V. J. Hyams

Institute of Laryngology and Otology (University of London), 330 Gray's Inn Road, London WC1X 8EE and
Armed Forces Institute of Pathology, Washington, D.C., USA 20306

Verrucous squamous carcinoma is a highly differentiated neoplasm which is difficult to diagnose in biopsy and, in particular, to distinguish from benigh squamous papilloma. Image analysis of photographs of 10 squamous papillomas of the larynx was carried out to test the proposition that the cells of verrucous carcinoma are larger than those of squamous papilloma. Diagnosis of these neoplasms had been made by standard histological and clinical criteria. In each case the margins of epidermoid cells and their nuclei at 1200× magnification were outlined on a graphic tablet using the cursor, and mean cell area, mean nuclear area and mean nuclear cytoplasmic area ratio were calculated from the measurements so obtained. Mean cell and nuclear areas were both significantly larger ($p < 0.1$) in verrucous carcinoma than in squamous papilloma. Verrucous carcinoma cells gave a mean cell area of above 300 square micrometers and squamous papillomas below 250 square micrometers. Variations in fixation, paraffin embedding or section thickness did not significantly affect the measurements. A knowledge of the mean cell area, in particular, may be of assistance in the early histological diagnosis of verrucous carcinoma.

MORPHOLOGICAL STUDY OF PANCREATIC CARCINOMA AND ASSOCIATED LESIONS

J. Chen and S. I. Baithun

Department of Morbid Anatomy, The London Hospital, London E1 1BB

Three hundred and ninety-one cases of primary pancreatic tumours (275 autopsy and 116 surgical), excluding endocrine tumours, were studied histologically. Carcinoma of the exocrine pancreas formed the largest group (98.5%). Ductal adenocarcinoma was the commonest type (78.8%) and was divided into 4 sub-types, papillary (1%), well (5.7%), moderately (33.9%) and poorly differentiated adenocarcinoma (38.2%). Papillary carcinoma was separated from the well differentiated tumours, because of its different morphological appearances and behaviour. Other special morphological types of pancreatic carcinoma, pleomorphic (7.2%), mucinous (2.1%), adenosquamous (3.4%), acinar (1%), microadenocarcinoma (0.8%), cystadenocarcinoma (2.6%) and oncocytic carcinoma (0.3%) are also represented. In 248 cases a search was made for changes in the pancreas duct epithelium. These were compared with duct epithelium in a control group of 100 pancreases from autopsies of patients with non-pancreatic cancer. The following incidences were found for pancreatic and non-pancreatic cancers respectively: mucous cell hypertrophy, 41.0% and 17%; squamous metaplasia 4.4% and 4.0; simple hyperplasia 88.3% and 26.0%; papillary hyperplasia 49.6% and 12.0%; atypical hyperplasia 8.1% and 0%; ductular hyperplasia 8.0% and 7.0%. These results show association between hyperplasia and dysplasia of the ducts, with carcinoma.

APPLICATION OF IMMUNOHISTOCHEMISTRY AND HISTOCHEMISTRY TO THE DIFFERENTIAL DIAGNOSIS OF CHORDOMAS

J. Salisbury and P. G. Issacson

Department of Histopathology, University College London and The Middlesex Hospital Medical School, University Street, London WC1E 6JJ

The differential diagnosis of chordomas includes both chondrosarcoma and normal cartilage. We have studied ten cases of chordoma and compared these with five cases of chondrosarcoma and examples of normal cartilage and notochord. Sections of formalin-fixed, paraffin-embedded tissue were stained by the PAP technique for lysozyme and S-100 protein. Fresh tissue was available from two cases each of chordoma and chondrosarcoma respectively and imprint and cryostat sections of these were stained for alpha naphthyl esterase, as were cryostat sections of normal cartilage and notochord. Normal cartilage, chondrosarcomas and notochord from fetuses of between ten and twenty-eight weeks' gestation all stained positively for S-100 protein and lysozyme. Chordomas, however, while positive for S-100 protein did not stain for lysozyme. Alpha naphthyl acetate esterase activity was demonstrated in chordomas, notochord and chondrosarcoma but could not be demonstrated in normal cartilage. Thus, absence of lysozyme, which appears to be associated with neoplastic transformation of notochord, serves to distinguish chordomas from chondrosarcoma and normal cartilage. Demonstration of alpha naphthyl acetate esterase in chordomas appears to be an additional helpful feature in its differential diagnosis since this enzyme is not present in normal cartilage. Although the number of cases studied is small, the presence of this enzyme in chondrosarcomas as opposed to normal cartilage may be a useful diagnostic feature.

IMMUNOHISTOLOGICAL ASSESSMENT OF EPITHELIAL TUMOURS USING PANEL OF ANTIBODY MARKERS

J. J. Mikel, C. C. Bird, R. G. French, I. Lauder, A. J. Baczkowski and M. Gani

Departments of Pathology and Mathematics, University of Leeds, Leeds LS2 9JT and Unilever Research, Colworth House, Sharnbrook, MK44 1LQ

Six epithelial markers (one polyclonal and the remainder monoclonal antibodies) were used to stain a wide range of epithelial tumours (23 histogenetic tumour types, 84 tumours in total) by the indirect immunoperoxidase technique. All tissues were formalin fixed and paraffin embedded. Four of the markers (antikeratin, F1/10/F3, F3/14/E7, E29) gave sufficiently strong staining reactions to be considered diagnostically useful. With these both tumours and their normal epithelial counterparts were examined quantitively for strength and area of staining reaction and gave similar results in 33 – 48% of cases, depending on the antibodies used. Tumour stained more strongly than normal epithelium in 24 – 28% of cases and less strongly in 23 – 43% of cases. Staining results in lymph node metastases were frequently different from those in the primary tumour. Two main points of diagnostic importance revealed were: (1) the staining of dysplasia in colonic mucosa and colonic adenomas and (2) the staining of plasma cells in various sites and its particular relevance to examining bone marrow for tumour metastases.

POSSIBLE RELATIONSHIPS BETWEEN MONOCYTIC CELLS IN LYMPHOMATA

Sarah Matthews, A. J. Freemont, Carolyn J. P. Jones and R. W. Stoddart

Department of Pathology, The University, Manchester M13 9PT

Immunocytochemical markers, lectin binding characteristics and cellular morphology have been used to explore the interrelationships of cells of seemingly monocytic lineage in a range of human lymphomata. Using paraffin-embedded tissue from reactive and neoplastic lymph nodes the distribution of α_1 antitrypsin ($\alpha_1$at) and lysozyme and the patterns of lectin binding (using avidin) were examined. Three categories of cells could be identified. The first were rounded (15–20 μm diameter), stained strongly for lysozyme and $\alpha_1$at and bound Concanavalin A and wheatgerm agglutinin (WGA). The second were larger, had long, arborescent, cytoplasmic processes (apposed to nearby cells), stained weakly for lysozyme and $\alpha_1$at, and bound Concanavalin A without trypsin treatment. They also bound erythro-phytohaemagglutinin and pea lectin after exposure to trypsin. The third category had features intermediate between the others. Cells of the first type closely resembled blood monocytes and occurred near small vessels, while cells of the second type were associated with nodular areas and occasionally contained phagocytic debris. Cells of the intermediate type occurred between the others, suggesting a developmental sequence, reflected in the saccharide sequences expressed upon and within them.

MAST CELL CONTENT AND DISTRIBUTION IN LYMPHOMATA

Carolyn J. P. Jones, Sarah Matthews, A. J. Freemont and R. W. Stoddart

Department of Pathology, The University, Manchester M13 9PT

Mast cell counts per unit area of section have been analysed for a series of formalin-fixed, paraffin embedded, normal, reactive and lymphomatous human lymph nodes. Counts were made over 10 random low-power (×250) fields on each of 9 sections of each node. A fixation procedure was used which was shown to give good preservation of mast cells and they were stained either with acid toluidine blue or with an avidin-peroxidase method. Elevated mast cell counts were found in most reactive nodes, some being very marked. Greatly depleted mast cell densities were seen in immunoblastic, diffuse lymphocytic and lymphocyte-predominant Hodgkin's lymphomata. Considerable, but less marked depletion of mast cells occurred in centrocytic, centrocytic/centroblastic and most lymphocyte-depleted Hodgkin's lymphomata, while the mast cell contents of other forms of Hodgkin's disease and histocytic lymphomata were only slightly lower than normal. In all cases mast cells were generally absent from follicular and nodular areas and in some lymphomata were confined to the rims of the nodes. They were particularly associated with areas of fibrosis and were notably low in tumours with a high mitotic index.

EPIDEMIOLOGICAL ASPECTS OF LYMPHOMA IN YORKSHIRE REGION

C. J. O'Brien, N. Barnes, R. Cartwright, C. C. Bird and I. Lauder

Department of Pathology, Leeds University, Leeds LS2 9JT

Marked variation in the incidence of lymphoma, based on Cancer Registry figures, have been noted in different areas within this Region. In order first to validate this impression we have reviewed large numbers of cases from three selected areas of the Region, submitted during the period 1963–1967. These cases formed a heterogenous group variously coded by the local pathologists as malignant lymphoma, reactive lymphoid tissue, anaplastic carcinoma, etc. In this way we hoped to correct possible false positive or false negative diagnoses of lymphoma. These cases were reviewed "blind" and classified according to the BNLI system. The results have then been compared with those from the period 1978–1982 during which time lymphoma cases have been reviewed and diagnosed by a five man Lymphoma Panel. Results of our historical review have differed somewhat from the original Cancer Registry figures. Our comparative study indicates a marked overall increase in the incidence of lymphoma generally in the areas studied together with some variation in the relative incidence of various subtypes. These results will now form the basis for an epidemiological study of possible environmental influences on the incidence of lymphoma in this Region.

JOURNAL OF PATHOLOGY, VOL. **143:** vii–viii (1984)

KEY WORD INDEX

Acquired immune deficiency syndrome (AIDS), 223
Alveolar macrophages, 117
Amyloid P component, 183
Anabolic androgens, 211
α-l-Antitrypsin, 275
Appendix, 51
APUD cell, 51
Autoimmune disease, 11

Basement membrane, 193
Breast carcinoma, 39, 187
Bronchiolar clearance, 117
Breast disease, 39
Bronchiolar epithelium, 127

Cancer, 1
Carcinogenesis, 211
Carcinoid tumours, 199
Cell culture, 241
Cerebral haemorrhage, 177
Cervical smears, 241
Chagas' disease, 93
Children, 183
Cirrhosis of the liver, 81
Clara cells, 127
Collagenases, 193
Conducting tissue, 93
Cytology, 241, 259
Cytopathology, 147
Cytoskeleton, 17

Diagnosis, 147
Diagnostic histopathology, 205
Diffuse nodular hyperplasia, 81
Dysplasia, 211

Enterochromaffin cell, 51
Enzyme-histochemistry, 205

Fetus, 183

Gastric epithelium, 267
Gastric mucosa, 267
Giant cells, 17
Glomerular basement membrane, 57
Glomerulus, 57, 275
Glycosidases, 39

Hepatic injury, 31
Herpes simplex virus, 241
Histochemical stains, 199
Histochemistry, 39
Hodgkin's disease, 69, 249
Hypertension, 177

Immunocytochemistry, 241, 259
Immunohistochemistry, 205
Immunoperoxidase, 199

Juvenile xanthogranuloma, 205

Lacrymal gland, 11
Langhans giant cells, 17
Liver, 81, 211
Lung clearance, 117
Lung tumours, 259
Lymph nodes, 187
Lymphocytic infiltration, 11

Malignant lymphomas, 69, 249
Mice, 211
Microfilaments, 17
Microtubules, 17
Mesothelioma, 147
Metastatic spread, 187
Microaneurysms, 177
Monocyte, 275
Morphometry, 69
Muramidase, 275
Myocarditis, 93

Neuroendocrine cell, 51
Neuroendocrine tumours, 259
Neuron-specific enolase, 259
Non-Hodgkin's lymphoma, 69, 249

Oncogenesis, 1
Oncogenetic retroviruses, 1

Pleural biopsy, 147
Polychlorinated biphenyls, 267
Portal hypertension, 31
Prealbumin, 199
Proteinuria, 57

Pulmonary hypertension, 31
Pulmonary vasculature, 31

Scanning EM, 127
Schwann cell, 51
Sjögren's syndrome, 11
Skin, 183
Small cell carcinoma, 259

Trimethyl phosphorothioate toxicity, 127
Tumour invasion, 193
Tumour markers, 259

Urinary bladder, 103

Virus isolation, 241

X-irradiation, 103

AUTHOR INDEX

Adams, R. L., 241
Adamson, I. Y. R., 117
Andrade, S. G., 93
Andrade, Z. A., 93
Anim, J. T., 177
Antonakopoulos, G. N., 103

Barnes, N., 249
Becker, G. M., 267
Berry, R. J., 103
Bird, C. C., 249
Bliss, D. J., 57
Bowden, D. H., 117
Boyko, R., 249
Brewer, D. B., 57
Bushell, T. E. C., 241

Cartwright, R. A., 249
Chorlton, I., 249
Crocker, J., 69

Darwin, C., 249
Degreef, H., 205
Desmet, V. J., 205

Facchetti, F., 205
Fukuto, T. R., 127

Gandy, J., 127

Hartveit, F., 187
Herbert, A., 145
Hicks, R. M., 103
Horne, C. H. W., 199

Imamura, T., 127

Kasuga, T., 31
Kellett, H. S., 249
Khan, A. M., 183
Kofi, A. D., 177

Lackie, P., 259
Lesna, M., 211
Lauder, I., 249
Levene, M. M., 241, 259
Liddle, N., 199

MacIver, G., 275
McKinnell, R. G., 193
McNulty, W. P., 267
Marangos, P. J., 259
Marshall, R. J., 275
Matsubara, O., 11, 31
Millard, P. R., 223
Miller, I. D., 199
Millikin, P. D., 51
Mutum, S. S., 81

Nakamura, T., 31
Nasu, M., 11

Ogilvie, D. J., 193

Polak, J. M., 259
Papadimitriou, J. M., 17
Paul, J., 1

Reid, W. A., 199
Rigby, P. J., 17

Sadigursky, M., 93
Shields, S. E., 193
Shilkin, K. B., 147
Snowball, S., 211
Springall, D. R., 241, 259

Tarin, D., 193
Taylor, W., 211

Uehara, T., 31

Van Den Oord, J. J., 205
Vanneste, A., 205

Walker, F., 183
Walker, R. A., 39
Weinbren, K., 81
Whitaker, D., 147
Wolf-Peeters, C. De, 205

Yamamoto, H., 11

PUBLISHING AGREEMENT

1. It is our custom to request authors to vest the worldwide copyright of their papers in John Wiley & Sons Limited for the full term of copyright and we would be grateful if you would confirm your acceptance of these terms by signing and returning the agreement below. We will not withhold permission for any reasonable request from you to publish any part of this paper in connection with any other work by you, provided the usual acknowledgements are given regarding copyright notice and reference to the original publication.
2. If it is appropriate, the author's employer may sign this agreement, and in any event the employer may reserve the right to use the paper internally or for promotional purposes only, by so indicating on this agreement. It is understood that proprietary rights other than copyright (including patent rights) are reserved.
3. If the author is a U.S. Government employee and this work was done in that capacity the assignment applies only to the extent allowable by U.S. law. If at least one co-author is *not* a government employee, said author should sign the agreement.
4. If the author is an employee of the British Government then HMSO will grant a non-exclusive licence to publish this paper in the Journal in any form or media provided British crown copyright and user rights (including patent rights) are reserved.
5. The author warrants that the manuscript is the author's original work, and has not been published before. (If excerpts from copyrighted works are included, the author will obtain written permission from the copyright owners and show credit to the sources in the manuscript.) The author also warrants that the article contains no libellous or unlawful statements, and does not infringe on the rights of others.
6. If the work was prepared jointly the author agrees to inform co-authors of the terms of the agreement, and to sign on their behalf.

With the qualifications listed above I assign to John Wiley & Sons Limited, the copyright of my paper entitled ______________________________

____

for publication in ______________________________

______________________ Signed

______________________ Date

If the paper is rejected this assignment is null and void.